ANNALS OF
THE NEW YORK ACADEMY
OF SCIENCES

Volume 570

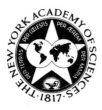

EDITORIAL STAFF

Executive Editor
BILL BOLAND

Managing Editor
JUSTINE CULLINAN

Associate Editor
STEVEN E. BOHALL

The New York Academy of Sciences
2 East 63rd Street
New York, New York 10021

VITAMIN E

BIOCHEMISTRY AND HEALTH IMPLICATIONS

ANNALS OF THE NEW YORK ACADEMY OF SCIENCES

Volume 570

VITAMIN E

BIOCHEMISTRY AND HEALTH IMPLICATIONS

Edited by Anthony T. Diplock, Lawrence J. Machlin, Lester Packer, and William A. Pryor

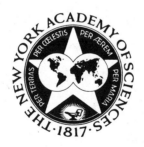

The New York Academy of Sciences
New York, New York
1989

Library of Congress Cataloging-in-Publication Data

Vitamin E : biochemistry and health implications / edited
  by Anthony T. Diplock . . . [et al.].
  p. cm. — (Annals of the New York Academy of Sciences,
ISSN 0077-8923 ; v. 570)
  Result of a conference held in New York City on Oct.
31-Nov. 2, 1988, by the New York Academy of Sciences.
  Includes bibliographical references.
  ISBN 0-89766-535-X (pbk. : alk. paper). — ISBN
0-89766-536-8 (pbk. : alk. paper)
  1. Vitamin E—Physiological effect—Congresses. 2.
Vitamin E—Health aspects—Congresses. I. Diplock,
Anthony T. II. New York Academy of Sciences. III.
Series.
  [DNLM: 1. Vitamin E—congresses. W1 AN626YL
v. 570 / QU 179 V8384 1988]
Q11.N5 vol. 570
[QP772.T6]
500 s—dc20
[612.3'99]
DNLM/DLC
for Library of Congress   89-14048
                                                                CIP

PCP
Printed in the United States of America
ISBN 0-89766-535-X(cloth)
ISBN 0-89766-536-8(paper)
ISSN 0077-8923

ANNALS OF THE NEW YORK ACADEMY OF SCIENCES

Volume 570
December 26, 1989

VITAMIN E: BIOCHEMISTRY AND HEALTH IMPLICATIONS [a]

Editors and Conference Organizers
ANTHONY T. DIPLOCK, LAWRENCE J. MACHLIN,
LESTER PACKER, AND WILLIAM A. PRYOR

CONTENTS

[a] This volume is the result of a conference entitled Vitamin E: Biochemistry and Health
Implications, held in New York City on October 31-November 2, 1988, by the New York
Academy of Sciences.

Financial assistance was received from:

- BASF CORPORATION, CHEMICALS DIVISION
- EASTMAN CHEMICAL PRODUCTS, INC.
- EISAI COMPANY, LTD.
- HENKEL CORPORATION, FINE CHEMICALS DIVISION
- HOFFMANN-LA ROCHE INC.

Preface

LAWRENCE J. MACHLIN

Hoffmann-La Roche Inc.
Nutley, New Jersey 07110-1199

Scientific interest in vitamin E in the six years since the last New York Academy of Sciences Conference has been spurred by the explosion of interest in free radical biochemistry and biology and the increasing acceptance of vitamin E as the major membrane-bound antioxidant. Moreover, the need for vitamin E in humans has now been firmly established, and an increasing number of epidemiological studies have linked vitamin E status to lowered risk of a number of chronic health problems. We know considerably more detail about the absorption, transport, and biochemical function of the vitamins, thanks to increased sophistication in methodology. Moreover, its role in maintaining the health of the nervous and cardiovascular systems and its role in a number of age-related health problems, such as cancer, cataracts, and maintenance of immunity, is becoming increasingly evident. It is the hope of the organizers that we will not only bring the state of the science up to date, but also capture some of the scientific excitement generated by research of this important vitamin.

Vitamin E: Introduction to Biochemistry and Health Benefits

LESTER PACKER AND SHARON LANDVIK

Department of Physiology-Anatomy
University of California, Berkeley
Berkeley, California 94720

BACKGROUND

The naturally occurring tocopherols and tocotrienols present in plant oils have long been known to be essential components of the diet of animals and humans. Most indications point to the critical role that vitamin E plays in membranes where it is present only in a very low ratio, sometimes one molecule for two- to three-thousand lipids.[1,2]

Biochemical Implications

Despite its low molar concentration in membranes, vitamin E effectively serves as the major lipid-soluble chain-breaking antioxidant, preventing lipid peroxidation and modulating the metabolism of the arachidonic acid cascade initiated by lipoxygenase and/or cyclooxygenase (see FIG. 1).

Vitamin E appears to be highly efficient as an antioxidant. It is further known from chemical and biochemical studies that after being oxidized and prior to its decomposition, vitamin E can be rereduced. Ascorbic acid (vitamin C) and glutathione are major water-soluble intracellular antioxidants (reductants) in the cytosol that generate reduced vitamin E. This reaction is dependent on the concentration of these substances and/or the enzymes that maintain them in their reduced form.[3,4]

VITAMIN E DEFICIENCY STATUS

Young animals are susceptible to vitamin E deficiency often due to some abnormality or disease that slows vitamin E absorption or transport. Usually in such cases, premature babies or children show symptoms of vitamin E deficiency resulting in anemia, and neuromuscular and neurological disorders. Frequently, the vitamin E deficiency effects are exacerbated by the necessity of employing 100% oxygen inhal-

1

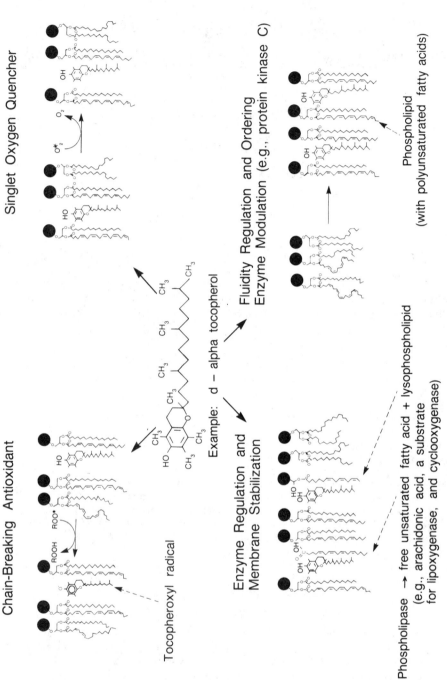

FIGURE 1. Vitamin E as a biological response modifier.

ation therapy in very low birth weight infants. Nevertheless, high doses of vitamin E or vitamin E analogues have proven useful in the management of these disorders.[1,5]

A paradox exists inasmuch as adult animals on a vitamin E-deficient diet never develop symptoms of deficiency. It is more difficult to deplete the tissues of older animals of vitamin E than it is weanling animals that are placed on vitamin E-deficient diets. Moreover, in the young animals it is difficult to totally deplete vitamin E from tissues even after prolonged exposure to dietary E deficiency; lower tissue levels of vitamin E become stabilized under such conditions. Two explanations for these findings are that redistribution of vitamin E between body tissues occurs and/or oxidized products like the free radical form of vitamin E (tocopheroxyl radical) may be regenerated. Vitamin E in its oxidized free radical (tocopheroxyl radical) form is a relatively unreactive radical, which therefore inhibits propagation of chain reactions of lipid peroxidation. Vitamin E radical (tocopheroxyl radical) reductase activity has recently been discovered in liver mitochondrial and microsomal membranes (Maguire, Wilson and Packer, unpublished results, and reference 3). Thus the tocopheroxyl radical may be regenerated to the native form of vitamin E. Different forms of tocopherol present in the diet may have differing abilities to exhibit redistribution and regeneration. D-Alpha-tocopherol is the major biological dietary component with the most prominent antioxidant activity, but other vitamin E forms may also be important as biological response modifiers.

VITAMIN E REQUIREMENT

Determination of requirements for vitamin E are complicated by variations in susceptibility of dietary and tissue fatty acids to peroxidation and the difficulty in demonstrating vitamin E inadequacies in healthy adults. Vitamin E requirements may vary fivefold, depending on dietary intake and/or tissue composition; high polyunsaturated fat intakes increase vitamin E requirements due to the increased peroxidative potential of body tissues.[6]

VITAMIN E ROLE IN PREVENTION OF FREE RADICAL DAMAGE

Using breath pentane output as a measure of lipid peroxidation, studies have demonstrated that intake of 1000 IU vitamin E for 10 days significantly decreased breath pentane excretion in healthy adults consuming a normal diet. Study results may be significant in view of research evidence showing a role for free radical-related damage in normal body processes and in certain diseases and protective effects of vitamin E in controlling peroxidation in body tissues.[7]

AGING

Research has shown that free radical damage accumulates during the aging process, and evidence is increasing that lipid peroxidation may be an important factor in making aging less than the long and healthy process it should be.[8] Animal and human studies have demonstrated protective effects of vitamin E and the other antioxidants on free radical reactions and peroxidative damage in the aging process.[9,10]

CANCER

Reactive oxygen species have been implicated in the process of cancer initiation, and promotion and research evidence suggests that vitamin E and the other antioxidants alter cancer incidence and growth by functioning as anticarcinogens, quenching free radicals or reacting with their products. Evidence from epidemiological studies and controlled animal studies suggest that vitamin E, alone or in combination with other antioxidants, decreases the incidence of certain forms of cancer.[11]

ARTHRITIS

Increased free radical production has been observed in animal and human studies on arthritis. Animal data has demonstrated that vitamin E has beneficial effects on symptoms of arthritis, and results of limited human studies in patients with osteoarthritis suggest that vitamin E therapy is significantly more effective than placebo in relieving pain and also results in greater improvement of mobility.[12,13]

CIRCULATORY CONDITIONS

Excessive platelet aggregation is a significant factor in development of atherosclerosis. Studies have shown that vitamin E supplementation significantly decreased induced platelet aggregation in healthy adults and reduced elevated platelet aggregation rates in patients with high blood lipid levels and in oral contraceptive users.[14–16] In coronary artery disease patients undergoing coronary bypass surgery, free radical concentrations did not increase significantly during or after bypass surgery in a group of patients pretreated with 2000 IU vitamin E 12 hours before surgery, whereas free radical levels progressively increased during surgery in unsupplemented patients.[17]

CATARACTS

It is commonly accepted that oxidative mechanisms have an important role in cataract development. Research to date indicates that vitamin E delays or minimizes cataract development in isolated animal lenses and in animal studies and that high plasma antioxidant concentrations may reduce cataract risk in adults.[18,19]

EXERCISE

Strenuous physical exercise is associated with an increased rate of lipid peroxidation, and animal studies have demonstrated that vitamin E is consumed by body tissues in periods of increased physical exercise.[20] In a study of mountain climbers, vitamin E supplementation (400 IU/day) prevented a reduction in physical performance and an increase in breath pentane output associated with prolonged exposure to high altitudes.[21]

AIR POLLUTION

Animal research has demonstrated that vitamin E may be an important component of the lung's defense against peroxidative damage, helping to protect against the injurious effects of smoke and smog.[22] A protective role for vitamin E against the harmful effects of pollution has also been documented in studies of smokers.[23,24]

SUMMARY

Free radical-mediated damage has been implicated in cellular changes that occur over time in the aging process and in development of degenerative diseases. Research results to date have demonstrated that vitamin E and the other antioxidants function to prevent or minimize peroxidative damage in biological systems and suggest that adequate antioxidant defense can protect the body from the high free radical concentrations that are unavoidable at the present time.

REFERENCES

1. BIERI, J. G., L. CORASH & V. S. HUBBARD. 1983. Medical uses of vitamin E. N. Eng. J. Med. **308:** 1063.
2. KRISHNAMURTHY, S. 1983. The intriguing biological role of vitamin E. J. Chem. Ed. **60:** 465.

3. PACKER, L., J. MAGUIRE, R. MEHLHORN, E. SERBINOVA & V. KAGAN. 1989. Mitochondria and microsomal membranes have a free radical reductase activity that prevents chromanoxyl radical accumulation. Biochem. Biophys. Res. Commun. **159**(1): 229.
4. WEFERS, H. & H. SIES. 1988. The protection by ascorbate and glutathione against microsomal lipid peroxidation is dependent on vitamin E. Eur. J. Biochem. **174**: 353.
5. CARPENTER, D. 1985. Vitamin E deficiency. Semin. Neurol. **5**: 283.
6. HORWITT, M. K. 1986. Interpretations of requirements for thiamin, riboflavin, niacin-tryptophan and vitamin E plus comments on balance studies and vitamin B6. Am. J. Clin. Nutr. **44**: 973.
7. LEMOYNE, M. et al. 1987. Breath pentane analysis as an index of lipid peroxidation: a functional test of vitamin E status. Am. J. Clin. Nutr. **46**: 267.
8. HARMAN, D. 1984. Free radical theory of aging: the free radical diseases. Age **7**: 111.
9. MEYDANI, M., C. P. VERDON & J. B. BLUMBERG. 1985. Effect of vitamin E, selenium and age on lipid peroxidation events in rat cerebrum. Nutr. Res. **5**: 1227.
10. WARTANOWICZ, M. et al. 1984. The effect of alpha-tocpherol and ascorbic acid on the serum lipid peroxide level in elderly people. Ann. Nutr. Metab. **28**: 186.
11. WATSON, R. R. & T. K. LEONARD. 1986. Selenium and vitamins A, E and C: nutrients with cancer prevention properties. J. Am. Diet. Assoc. **86**: 505.
12. BLANKENHORN, G. 1986. Clinical efficacy of spondyvit (vitamin E) in activated arthroses. Z. Orthop. Ihre Gvenzgeb. **124**: 340.
13. MACHTEY, I. & L. OUAKNINE. 1978. Tocopherol in osteoarthritis: a controlled pilot study. J. Am. Geriatr. Soc. **26**: 328.
14. RENAUD, S. et al. 1987. Influence of vitamin E administration on platelet functions in hormonal contraceptive users. Contraception **36**: 347.
15. STEINER, M. 1983. Effect of alpha-tocopherol administration on platelet function in man. Thromb. Haemostasis **49**: 73.
16. SZCZEKLIK, A. et al. 1985. Dietary supplementation with vitamin E in hyperlipoproteinemias: effects on plasma lipid peroxides, antioxidant activity, prostacyclin generation and platelet aggregability. Thromb. Haemostasis **54**: 425.
17. CAVAROCCHI, N. C. et al. 1986. Superoxide generation during cardiopulmonary bypass: Is there a role for vitamin E? J. Surg. Res. **40**: 519.
18. CREIGHTON, M.O. et al. 1985. Modelling cortical cataractogenesis VII. Effects of vitamin E treatment on galactose-induced cataracts. Exp. Eye Res. **40**: 213.
19. JACQUES, P. F. et al. 1988. Antioxidant status in persons with and without senile cataract. Arch. Ophthalmol. **106**: 337.
20. PACKER, L. 1984. Vitamin E, physical exercise and tissue damage in animals. Med. Biol. **62**: 105.
21. SIMON-SCHNASS, I. & H. PABST. 1988. Influence of vitamin E on physical performance. Int. J. Vit. Nutr. Res. **58**: 49.
22. SEVANIAN, A., A. D. HACKER & N. ELSAYED. 1982. Influence of vitamin E and nitrogen dioxide on lipid peroxidation in rat lung and liver microsomes. Lipids **17**: 269.
23. PACHT, E. R. et al. 1986. Deficiency of vitamin E in the alveolar fluid of cigarette smokers. J. Clin. Invest. **77**: 789.
24. SHARIFF, R. et al. 1988. Vitamin E supplementation in smokers. Am. J. Clin. Nutr. **47**: 758.

Vitamin E as an *in Vitro* and *in Vivo* Antioxidant[a]

GRAHAM W. BURTON AND KEITH U. INGOLD

Division of Chemistry
National Research Council of Canada
Ottawa, Ontario K1A 0R6, Canada

The challenge we are faced with is to relate the known antioxidant properties of vitamin E, which are now well-understood at the molecular level, to the diverse range of known symptoms associated with a deficiency of the vitamin in various types of animals.[1] For example, how are we to explain the well-known effect of a lack of vitamin E upon fertility in certain animals, often misconstrued in a jovial sense in the human context (FIG. 1), in terms of the antioxidant properties of vitamin E? In approaching this challenge, it is realized that there are, *in vivo*, other factors that also are important in determining the bioactivity of vitamin E. It is evident that antioxidant capability alone is not sufficient. Clearly, the vitamin must also have the capability of not only being delivered in sufficient quantity to all vulnerable biomembranes at a sufficient rate but also of being able to be retained and maintained at the required membrane sites. Thus, we are also concerned with understanding uptake into, transport between, retention in, and, eventually, loss of vitamin E from tissues. We refer broadly to these aspects as the *biokinetics* of vitamin E.

During the past 10 years the arsenal of tools, techniques, and knowledge available to the chemist has been focused in a concerted manner on vitamin E in an effort to better understand some of its properties.[2] This paper will describe some of the successes and insights that these endeavors have yielded.

IN VITRO STUDIES

Lipid Peroxidation

Much of the recent progress in understanding the antioxidant behavior of vitamin E has depended upon developing appropriate techniques and useful models that simulate the key aspects of the phenomenon of liquid phase autoxidation, of which lipid peroxidation is a special case.[3-5] There are three features that characterize autoxidation.[6] The first feature is called the *initiation* phase, during which very low concen-

[a] The authors wish to acknowledge the support of Eastman Chemicals, Eisai Ltd., Henkel Inc., the Natural Source Vitamin E Association, the Association for International Cancer Research, and the National Foundation for Cancer Research.

7

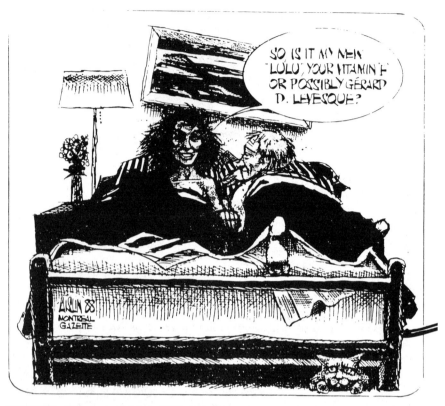

FIGURE 1. Cartoon by Aislin published in *The Gazette* (Montréal) in response to the announcement by Gérard Levesque, a minister in the Quebec government, that his government would be offering a financial incentive to Quebec residents to have more children. (Reproduced with permission.)

trations of carbon-centered free radicals are produced from a precursor molecule (reaction 1). This reaction may occur *in vivo,* for example, by a metal-ion

Initiation: Production of R· (carbon-centered radicals)   (1)

catalyzed decomposition of a lipid hydroperoxide. *In vitro,* water-soluble and lipid-soluble azo initiators (R-N=N-R) have proven to be convenient and very useful for the generation of free radicals at a known, constant, and reproducible rate. Carbon-centered radicals are produced in either the aqueous or lipid phases as the azo compound spontaneously undergoes a very slow, first-order decomposition at ambient temperature (reaction 2). A fraction of these radicals are converted

$$R\text{-}N{=}N\text{-}R \rightarrow 2R\cdot + N_2 \qquad (2)$$

to peroxyl radicals in a rapid reaction with dissolved molecular oxygen (reaction 3). This reaction, which represents the first step of the second feature of autoxidation, the *propagation* phase, involves a transformation of the chain-carrying species from a relatively unreactive carbon-centered radical to a very reactive peroxyl radical. The peroxyl radical then attacks any available peroxidizable material, either by abstraction of a hydrogen atom (reaction 4a), or possibly by addition to a double bond (reaction 4b), if one is available. The new carbon-centered radical

Propagation: $R \cdot + O_2 \rightarrow ROO \cdot$ (fast)   (3)

$ROO \cdot + RH \rightarrow ROOH + R \cdot$ (H atom abstraction)   (4a)

$ROO \cdot + RH \rightarrow ROORH \cdot$ (double bond addition)   (4b)

proceeds by way of reaction 3 to yield another peroxyl radical. Thus a chain reaction is set in motion that proceeds through the propagation reactions 3 and 4 for a potentially large number of cycles (*i.e.*, a long chain length) until the *termination* reaction between two peroxyl radicals occurs (reaction 5; the third feature of autoxidation), yielding nonradical products. The chain length of

Termination: $ROO \cdot + ROO \cdot \rightarrow$ inactive products   (5)

the propagation phase is increased by an increase in the concentration of peroxidizable substrate and by the reactivity of the peroxyl radical towards the substrate, and is decreased by an increase in the concentration of radicals and by the reactivity of the peroxyl radicals towards each other in the termination reaction.

From the practical standpoint, most types of biological membranes, often richly endowed with highly peroxidizable, polyunsaturated fat, are very susceptible to severe, oxidative damage during the propagation phase. The ideal defense against this is the complete suppression of free radical reactions. This form of *inhibition* is, in effect, the function of primary or preventive antioxidants, which act by removing precursors of free radicals or by inactivating catalysts, for example, glutathione peroxidase and metal-ion sequestering agents. When peroxyl radicals do escape through the preventive antioxidant safety screen, however, the system must then rely upon the secondary or chain-breaking antioxidant screen. Chain-breaking antioxidants inhibit peroxidation by keeping the chain length of the propagation reaction as small as possible. In contrast to preventive antioxidants, which remove catalysts or precursors such as hydroperoxides, chain-breaking antioxidants react directly with peroxyl radicals.

Simple phenols (ArOH), sterically hindered at the hydroxyl group, are excellent chain-breaking antioxidants. They react very rapidly with peroxyl radicals by the donation of a hydrogen atom from the phenolic hydroxyl group (reaction 6). Although a phenoxyl radical (ArO ·) is

Inhibition: $ArOH + ROO \cdot \rightarrow ArO \cdot + ROOH$ (6)

produced, it is unreactive in the propagative sense and is therefore unable to continue the chain reaction. The phenoxyl radical is eventually removed from the system by reaction with another radical, giving relatively stable, nonradical products. Because suitable phenols can compete very effectively with substrate for peroxyl radicals, small amounts of phenol are able to protect a large amount of peroxidizable lipid. Usually, two peroxyl radicals are removed at the expense of one molecule of phenol. The supply of antioxidant, therefore, may eventually be exhausted unless it is replenished or regenerated (see below).

How Good an Antioxidant Is Vitamin E?

In vitro studies have now established that α-tocopherol (α-TOH), the most active form of vitamin E,[1] has close to optimal properties for trapping peroxyl radicals.[7-10] In particular, the fully methylated aromatic ring and the chroman moiety ensure near-maximal stabilization of the tocopheroxyl radical formed in the rate-limiting reaction of α-tocopherol with a peroxyl radical (reaction 7). This fact means that not only does α-tocopherol react more rapidly with peroxyl

$$\alpha\text{-TOH} + \text{ROO}^{\bullet} \rightarrow \alpha\text{-TO}^{\bullet} + \text{ROOH} \qquad (7)$$

radicals, but also the greater stability of the tocopheroxyl radical ensures that it is unable to continue the chain reaction by attacking other species, including oxygen.[11] That is, it is a very effective radical "trap". The rate of peroxyl trapping by a chain-breaking antioxidant is vital for the successful protection of very reactive substrates such as polyunsaturated fat. The more rapidly an antioxidant is able to react with peroxyl radicals, the better it is able to successfully compete against the much larger amount of oxidizable substrate for the radicals. The substrate, then, is subject to less peroxidative damage. In the ideal situation, the antioxidant traps all the peroxyl radicals before they attack the oxidizable substrate.

The foregoing concept of antioxidant efficiency has been demonstrated clearly in a study of the ability of various antioxidants to inhibit the thermally initiated autoxidation of styrene.[8,10] The very high reactivity of styrene towards peroxyl radicals was used to set up a competition between styrene and each antioxidant for the peroxyl radicals generated by an azo initiator. The better the antioxidant, the smaller the amount of styrene and molecular oxygen consumed in the propagation reaction (see FIG. 2). This information can be translated directly into quantitative estimates of the rate constant for reaction 6 for each antioxidant. TABLE 1 summarizes the key findings.

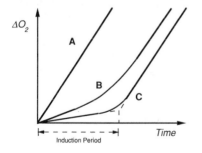

FIGURE 2. Plot of the consumption of oxygen by an oxidizable substrate (*e.g.,* styrene) in a model system with a constant production of radicals. A: no chain-breaking antioxidant; B: a poor antioxidant; C: a good antioxidant.

TABLE 1. Reactivity of Various Phenolic Chain-Breaking Antioxidants toward Peroxyl Radicals Relative to α-Tocopherol in Styrene

Structure	Compound		Relative Reactivity (α-TOH = 100)
	1a	R = phytyl (α-T-OH)	100
	1b	R = CH$_3$	119
	2		12
	3	BHT	0.4
	4a	R = H	169
	4b	R = CH$_3$	178
	4c	R = phytyl	147

Comparison of α-tocopherol with the analogue in which a methyl group has replaced the phytyl tail (1a vs 1b) confirms that reactivity is controlled by the chroman "head" group and that the tail exerts only a minor influence upon the rate of the reaction. The approximately 10-fold reduction in reactivity brought about by the more drastic structural modification present in the tetramethylmethoxyphenol, 2, indicates that the heterocyclic ring of the chroman group has a very large, enhancing effect on the rate of reaction 6. For comparison, the result obtained for the well-known commercial antioxidant, BHT (butylatedhydroxytoluene, 3) is also shown. It is approximately 250 times less reactive than α-tocopherol.

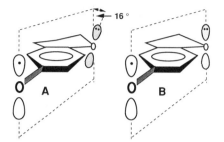

FIGURE 3. Diagram depicting the better *p*-orbital stabilizing interaction possible in the flatter dihydrobenzofuran phenoxyl radical (B) compared to the more puckered tocopheroxyl radical (A).

Are There other Phenols That Are Better Chain-Breaking Antioxidants?

On the basis of X-ray structural determinations carried out on 1b and 2, it has been concluded that the molecular architecture of the chroman heterocyclic ring confers enhanced stability on the chromanoxyl radical intermediate formed in reaction 6.[7,8] Specifically, the chroman structure facilitates additional stabilization of the phenoxyl radical through an interaction between the *p*-orbitals on the two *para*-oxygen atoms (FIG. 3A). The structure of 1b suggests that the *stereoelectronic effect* has not quite reached full expression in the chroman structure. Specifically, the *p*-orbitals on the two oxygen atoms appear to be approximately 16° out of alignment. It was anticipated that in the flatter, 5-membered ring of the analogous dihydrobenzofuran structure the two orbitals would be in near-perfect alignment (FIG. 3B). X-ray structural determinations of appropriate model compounds have indicated, on the basis of dihedral angle measurements, the deviation from perfect coplanarity in the phenoxyl would be only about 6°.[10] Indeed, significant enhancements in the range of 47-78% have been determined for the rate of reaction 6 in the model compounds 4a-4c (TABLE 1),[9,10] providing strong support for the stereoelectronic effect.

Where Is α-Tocopherol Located in the Membrane?

The full answer to this important question has remained elusive, partly because of the very low concentration of vitamin E in natural biomembranes. [13]C nuclear magnetic resonance (NMR) experiments, however, conducted on small unilamellar phospholipid vesicles containing 10 mole-percent of natural α-tocopherol (FIG. 4) labeled with ^{13}C at the 5-methyl group, have shown conclusively that the chromanol head group is very close to the surface of the membrane.[12] The flexible phytyl tail is believed to be approximately aligned, in a time-averaged sense, with the acyl chains

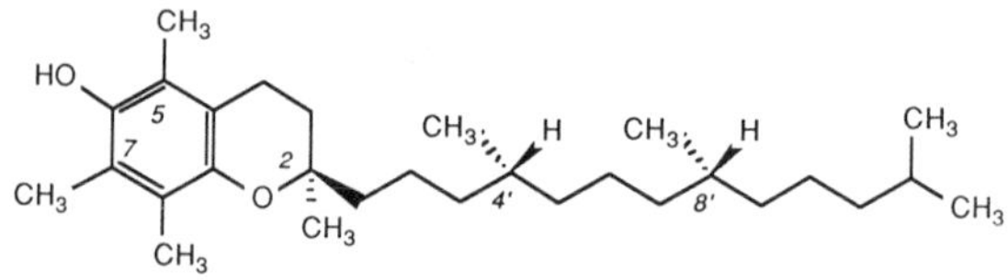

FIGURE 4. 5; 2*R*,4'*R*,8'*R*-α-Tocopherol (*RRR*-α-TOH).

in the interior of the membrane. Limited support for this has been obtained from a deuterium NMR study carried out with multilamellar egg lecithin liposomes containing specially synthesized *RRR*-α-tocopherols labeled with precise amounts of deuterium at various specific, strategic locations.[13]

The close proximity of the chromanol head group to the membrane surface is consistent with the synergistic antioxidant behavior of vitamins C and E observed in peroxidations of artificial phospholipid membranes using lipid-soluble, thermal azo initiators.[14-16] Although the two vitamins are completely sequestered and separated in their respective lipid and aqueous phases, a very significant extension of inhibition of peroxidation is obtained when both are present. Vitamin C by itself is a good antioxidant when peroxyl radicals are generated in the aqueous phase, but it is very much less effective when radicals are initially generated within a membrane.[14,15] Presumably, vitamin C cannot penetrate the membrane sufficiently to interact with a peroxyl radical present there. The most likely explanation of the synergy between vitamins C and E is that vitamin C is able to reduce the tocopheroxyl radical back to α-tocopherol. The chemical feasibility of this regeneration mechanism has been amply demonstrated in homogeneous media.[17,18]

The location of the chromanol near the membrane surface may seem paradoxical when it is realized that the unsaturation of the fatty acyl chains, and therefore the most likely site for the formation of lipid peroxyl radicals, is located well within the interior of the membrane (assuming that the NMR results for α-tocopherol in an artificial membrane are a valid reflection of the situation in a biological membrane). This hardly seems like an ideal situation for efficient antioxidant action. This paradox, however, may be understood in terms of the dynamic nature of membrane constituents. First, α-tocopherol is not fixed in its preferred location. Instead, it is expected to be very mobile, moving not only in the direction lateral to the membrane but also "oscillating" about its time-averaged position perpendicularly to the membrane surface, that is, "bobbing" up and down. Movements into the interior may be sufficiently deep to bring the chromanol group close enough to a lipid peroxyl radical. Second, it has been pointed out that when a lipid peroxyl radical is formed, the erstwhile nonpolar nature of the affected region of the tail acquires considerable polar character.[19] This process occurs in a very nonpolar region of the membrane. Therefore, it is quite possible that the portion of the acyl tail bearing the peroxyl group is "squeezed" out of the nonpolar interior toward the polar region at the membrane surface. These two effects may work in concert to bring the two molecules into much closer proximity than is at first envisaged.

The heterogeneous nature of a biological membrane, with its variable mix of proteins, cholesterol, polar head groups, and saturated and unsaturated lipid components, makes it unlikely that α-tocopherol is distributed uniformly throughout the membrane. The work by Giasuddin and Diplock[20,21] with cultured mouse fibroblasts showing the effect of α-tocopherol in enhancing the γ-linolenic (18:3), homo-γ-linolenic (20:3), and arachidonic (20:4) fatty acid composition of the phosphatidyl choline, serine, and ethanolamine components may reflect the existence of higher concentrations of α-tocopherol in membrane regions containing polyunsaturated acid residues.[1]

The Phytyl Tail Is Important for Retention of α-Tocopherol in Membranes

A physical chemical study by Maggio, Diplock, and Lucy, measuring the penetration of a series of α-tocopherols with tails of different lengths into phospholipid monolayers, has shown that the derivatives with shorter or longer tails are inferior to α-tocopherol itself.[22]

A clever experiment carried out by Niki and co-workers has shown how tightly α-tocopherol is bound in artificial phospholipid membranes.[23] Nonperoxidizable, dimyristoyl phosphatidyl choline vesicles containing an antioxidant (α-tocopherol, the tailless α-tocopherol analogue (1b), or BHT (3)) were mixed with azo-initiated, peroxidizing soybean lecithin vesicles. Only the vesicles with either BHT or the tailless analogue were able to effectively inhibit the peroxidation. The vesicles containing α-tocopherol were without effect. Clearly, BHT and 1b are able to rapidly exchange between vesicle membranes on the time scale of this experiment. The extreme insolubility in water conferred on α-tocopherol by the phytyl tail, greatly inhibits its ability to exchange between membranes in the absence of other mediating factors.

In contrast to this intermembrane exchange study, *in vitro* studies have shown that α-tocopherol readily exchanges between rat plasma and red blood cells.[24,25] The half-life for exchange is 2.2 hours at 37°C. The mechanism of this facile exchange and *in vivo* exchange, in general, still awaits elucidation.

IN VIVO STUDIES

α-Tocopherol Is the Major Lipid-Soluble, Chain-Breaking Antioxidant in Mammalian Membranes

This conclusion has been arrived at after developing a quantitative assay for lipid-soluble, chain-breaking antioxidants and using it in conjunction with a high-performance liquid chromatographic (HPLC) analysis for α-tocopherol.[26,27] The assay uses an azo initiator to produce peroxyl radicals in styrene at a constant and known rate. A known amount of lipid from a biological sample is added, and the length of time that oxidation is inhibited (the *induction period*) is measured. Knowing the rate of production of radicals and using the fact that each molecule of α-tocopherol traps two peroxyl radicals, the amount of α-tocopherol equivalent to the measured induction period can be calculated. The results of the lipid peroxyl-antioxidant titration are then compared with the amount of α-tocopherol measured directly by HPLC. In this manner it has been shown that vitamin E accounts for most, if not all, of the lipid-soluble antioxidant in human blood[26,27] as well as in various rat tissues and tumors.[28,29] Even in the case of humans with a severe deficiency in vitamin E, no evidence has been found in plasma for the existence of compensating levels of other antioxidants.[30]

β-Carotene has been shown to possess chain-breaking antioxidant properties at the low oxygen partial pressures typically found in mammalian tissues.[31] The lipid peroxyl-antioxidant titration method is run under normal atmospheric oxygen pressure. Under this condition, β-carotene behaves more like a pro-oxidant than an antioxidant. Therefore, the interpretation of results of titrations conducted under atmospheric oxygen may need to be qualified. Unless the amount of β-carotene present in the sample tissue, however, is similar to the amount of vitamin E, the contribution of β-carotene to the overall lipid-soluble chain-breaking antioxidant capacity will not be large.

Does a Better Antioxidant Show Greater Vitamin E Activity?

This question has been prompted by the enhanced reactivity toward peroxyl radicals of the dihydrobenzofuran (DHBF) series of compounds (4a-4c, TABLE 1). The synthesis of the *all-racemic* phytyl derivative (*all-rac*-phytyl-DHBF, 4c) has afforded an opportunity to answer this question.[32] Using the rat plasma pyruvate kinase (PPK) curative myopathy assay,[33] it was found in three separate assays that *all-rac*-DHBF acetate is 49-93% (mean 76%) better at decreasing the elevated level of plasma pyruvate kinase in vitamin E-deficient rats than is *all-rac*-α-tocopheryl acetate. It thus appears that the better antioxidant has more vitamin E activity.

Recently, *RRR*-phytyl-DHBF, the analogue of the natural stereoisomer of α-tocopherol (*RRR*-α-TOH; 5), has been synthesized. Surprisingly, the plasma pyruvate kinase (PPK) activities of the acetates of this compound and *RRR*-α-tocopherol are not significantly different,[34] in striking contrast to the result obtained with the corresponding *all-rac*-pair of compounds. The origin of this discrepant behavior is not presently understood. Preliminary results, however, from tissue uptake studies conducted in the study of the *RRR*-pair of compounds indicate that less of the DHBF compound is taken up in all of the eleven tissues and fluids examined. Thus, it can be inferred that an equal reduction in PPK was obtained with a smaller amount of absorbed *RRR*-phytyl-DHBF. It appears again, therefore, that the more reactive peroxyl trap has greater inherent vitamin E activity.

Stereochemistry, Absorption, Transport, Uptake, and Loss of α-Tocopherol

In addition to the requirement for optimal inherent antioxidant activity, it is obvious that for proper antioxidant function of vitamin E *in vivo,* the vitamin must be capable of being absorbed sufficiently from the gut, transported in the blood, delivered to the tissues and, ultimately, of being retained in the membranes of the cells and organelles. In order to probe these other important aspects, we have labeled α-tocopherol at specific molecular locations with precise amounts of deuterium, and we have, in a variety of studies aimed at elucidating the biokinetics of vitamin E, used gas chromatography-mass spectrometry (GC-MS) to measure changes in levels of both deuterated and nondeuterated forms in animals and humans.

The Deuterated Tocopherol / GC-MS Method

Thomas and co-workers[35] first demonstrated in 1981 the feasibility and high sensitivity of GC-MS for the measurement of concentrations of nonlabeled α-tocopherol in very small pieces of lung tissue, using deuterium-substituted α-tocopherol as an internal standard. We have synthesized multigram quantities of α-tocopherols of various stereochemistries, substituted with either 3, 6, or 9 atoms of deuterium in the aromatic methyl groups (compounds 6-11, FIG. 5) for use in biokinetic studies.[36-39] Deuterium, being a stable, heavier isotope of hydrogen, can be used in tocopherol

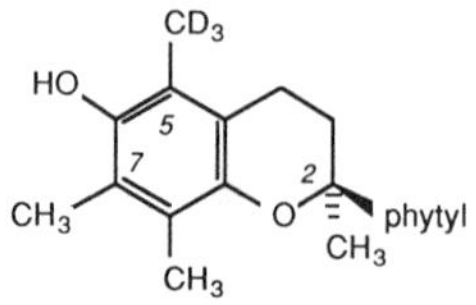

6: d_3-*RRR*-α-TOH

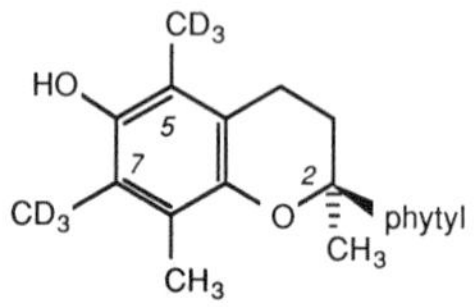

7: d_6-*RRR*-α-TOH

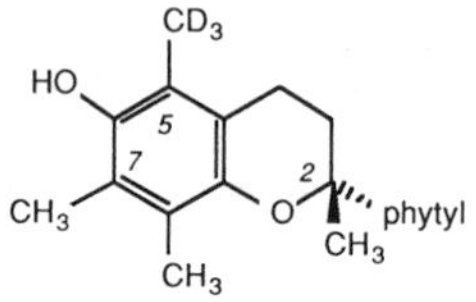

8: d_3-*SRR*-α-TOH

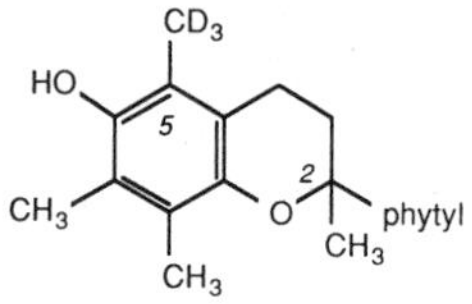

9: d_3-*all-rac*-α-TOH

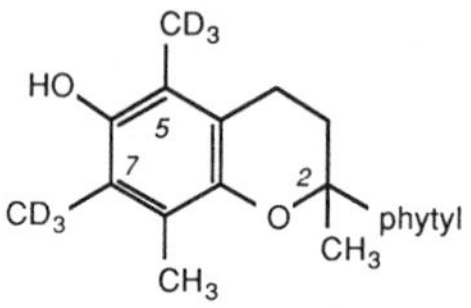

10: d_6-*all-rac*-α-TOH

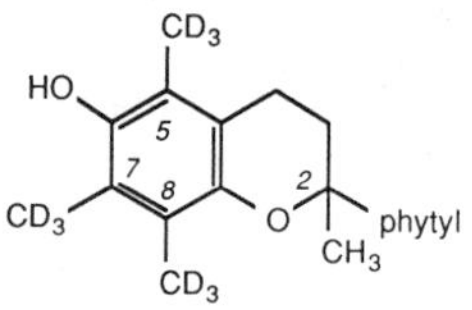

11: d_9-*all-rac*-α-TOH

FIGURE 5. Deuterated α-tocopherol stereoisomers indicating the positions and degree of substitution by deuterium.

without the hazards associated with a radioactive label. This has opened the way for long-term studies on humans and animals.

Deuterated tocopherol from an ingested dose can easily be determined in a lipid extract, along with any accompanying nonlabeled, residual α-tocopherol. As the α-tocopherol peak from an injected sample of a purified lipid extract emerges from the gas chromatograph, the mass spectrometer resolves the parent ions of the variously labeled tocopherols and determines the associated peak areas (FIG. 6). The use of d_9-α-TOH (compound 11, FIG. 5) as an internal standard (added to the weighed sample prior to extraction) has allowed the determination of the absolute concentrations of the deuterated and nondeuterated forms in the tissue.

As the following examples illustrate, deuterated tocopherols now provide us with a new experimental approach with opportunities for gaining fresh insights into some old and longstanding problems.

Turnover in Tissues

In the first application of deuterated α-tocopherol,[37] a group of weanling male rats, maintained for 4 weeks on a diet containing 36 mg/kg of the acetate of d_0-*RRR*-

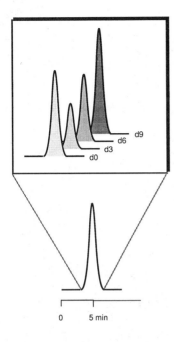

FIGURE 6. Depiction of resolution, by mass spectrometer, of α-tocopherol gas chromatography peak into component peaks corresponding to α-tocopherols containing 0, 3, 6, and 9 deuterium atoms/molecule.

α-TOH (d_0-RRR-α-T acetate) as the only source of vitamin E, were switched to a diet that was identical in all respects except that the vitamin E was replaced by the same quantity of the acetate of compound 6 (d_3-RRR-α-T acetate). The animals were sacrificed at various time intervals over the ensuing 2 months and, by analyzing lipid extracts from the excised tissues, the rate of disappearance of d_0-RRRα-TOH and the rate of appearance of d_3-RRRα-TOH, respectively, were determined. From this information, it has been found that there is a 10-fold difference in turnover rate, with lung and liver being the fastest tissues and spinal cord being the slowest tissue. More recently, we have determined rates of turnover in guinea pigs under identical conditions. Again, lung and liver are the fastest tissues. In comparing guinea pigs with rats, however, important differences are apparent. The relative ordering of some of the tissues is different, and there are also, in some cases, substantial differences in the rate of turnover when the same tissue is compared between animals. Especially noteworthy is the rate of turnover in the guinea pig brain, which is approximately three times slower than in the rat.

Stereochemistry

Although α-tocopherol has three centers of chirality at the 2, 4' and 8' carbons, it occurs naturally in only one form (RRR-α-TOH, 5). Synthetic, all-rac-α-tocopherol, on the other hand, exists as a mixture of equal amounts of all eight possible stereoisomers. The relationships between the natural, 2-ambo (the early form of synthetic vitamin E) and all-rac stereoisomers are shown in FIGURE 7.

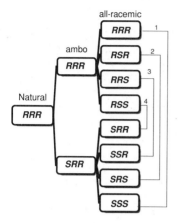

FIGURE 7. Stereochemical relationship between natural α-tocopherol (1 isomer), 2-*ambo*-α-tocopherol (2 isomers), and *all-rac*-α-tocopherol (8 isomers).

Although it is well-recognized that the *all-rac* form is less active in several bioassays,[1] most notably the rat fetal gestation-resorption assay, it is of interest, both from a practical point of view and from the need to understand better the origin of this effect, to perform bioavailability studies using appropriately deuterated forms of the stereoisomeric α-tocopherols.

The problem was approached by focusing first on the effect of changing the stereochemistry at the 2-position only. In a study identical in form to the previous turnover study, rats were switched instead to a diet containing a 36 mg/kg, 1:1 mixture of d_3-2S,4'R,8'R-α-tocopheryl acetate (d_3-SRR-α-T acetate) and d_6-RRRα-T acetate (see 8 and 7, respectively, in FIG. 5) as the sole source of vitamin E.[37] Analysis of the tissues obtained from animals sacrificed at various time intervals over a 5 month period provided a direct measure of the preference of each tissue for the RRR form over the SRR form as the animal continued to ingest equal quantities of each type of tocopherol.

Perhaps the most striking result was the discrimination shown by the brain. After 5 months, the d_6-RRR/d_3-SRR ratio had reached a value of 5-6 with no indication of an upper limiting value. By contrast, liver, the only tissue to do so, showed a substantial (initially ca. 2:1) accumulation of the SRR form over the RRR form, which decreased over a 3 week period until there was an approximately equal amount of each form. All other tissues showed RRR/SRR ratios, which eventually leveled off at values between 1 and 4.

The variable discrimination response of tissues calls into question the reliance upon animal tests for evaluating biopotencies of different tocopherol forms. It appears, based on these relative uptake results, that the assay will reflect the individual stereochemical preference of the vitamin E-depleted tissue effecting the test response. Very different responses would, for example, be expected from an assay that is based on the response of the rat brain compared to one based on the liver.

The finding concerning the brain is important because of the known neurological consequences associated with vitamin E deficiency in humans.[1] It is perhaps noteworthy that an *in vitro* study of the competitive exchange of RRR- and SRR-α-TOH between rat plasma and red cells showed that both forms transferred at the same rate into the red cells but that the SRR form was lost more rapidly from the red cell.[25] Possibly, a similar preferential loss is also occurring in the brain.

The initial accumulation of the *SRR*-isomer in the liver is a result, we suggest,[37] of the existence of the hepatic α-tocopherol-binding protein[40] facilitating the intracellular transport and eventual export into the plasma of *RRR*-α-tocopherol.

Very recently, in a direct comparison of *RRR*- and *all-rac*-α-tocopheryl acetates, a man was given eight consecutive, daily doses of a 1:1 mixture of d_3-*RRR*-α-T acetate and d_6-*all-rac*-α-T acetate (cf. 6 and 10, FIG. 5).[41] FIGURE 8 shows the initial rise and subsequent decline of the two tocopherols in the plasma. The *RRR*/*all-rac* ratio was 1.4–1.6 during the first 8 days and reached a limiting ratio of 1.9 by day 10.

Free Tocopherol versus Tocopheryl Acetate

This subject is of some interest because tocopherol occurs in food as the free (*i.e.,* nonesterified) form, whereas supplemental vitamin E is usually provided as tocopheryl acetate. Using forms of *RRR*-α-tocopherol with 3 and 6 atoms of deuterium/molecule, respectively, we have been able to determine directly the uptake in the rat and human of tocopherol derived from an oral dose of a 1:1 mixture of the free form and its acetate.[39] The results confirmed the substantially lower potency of the free tocopherol observed in previous rat bioassays. It was also found, however, that when the mixture of tocopherols was administered with laboratory diet instead of in oil, the two forms were practically equivalent. The results obtained in humans showed α-tocopherol was taken up in equal amounts from both forms.

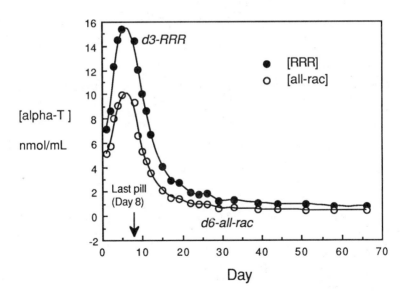

FIGURE 8. Time plot of d_3-RRR-α-TOH and d_6-*all-rac*-α-TOH in the plasma of a man during and after eight consecutive daily doses of 150 mg each of d_3-*RRR*-α-T acetate and d_6-*all-rac*-α-T acetate starting at day 0.

Absorption and Transport in Human Lipoproteins

Results obtained recently with deuterated RRR-α-tocopherol[38] confirm the concept that newly absorbed vitamin E is secreted by the intestine into chylomicrons and, subsequently, chylomicron remnants are taken up by the liver from which the vitamin E is secreted in very low density lipoproteins (VLDL). The metabolism of VLDL in the circulation results in the simultaneous delivery of the vitamin into the low density and high density lipoproteins.

SUMMARY

α-Tocopherol has near optimal activity as a chain-breaking antioxidant. Inherent antioxidant activity plays an important part in determining overall biological activity but the phytyl tail also exerts a very important influence. The new deuterated α-tocopherol/GC-MS technique is providing unprecedented insight into the importance of the stereochemistry of the phytyl tail in determining bioavailability, as well as helping to discover how rapidly and effectively absorption, transport, uptake, and loss occur. Measurements of rates of turnover in tissues indicate that differences exist between different types of animals. It is possible that these tissue differences may explain the diverse range of vitamin E deficiency symptoms observed across a wide variety of animals. It is not known what is responsible for the differences in biokinetic behavior.

REFERENCES

1. DIPLOCK, A. T. 1985. Vitamin E. *In* Fat-Soluble Vitamins. A. T. Diplock, Ed.: 154-224. Technomic Publishing Co. Lancaster, Pennsylvania.
2. BURTON, G. W. & K. U. INGOLD. 1986. Vitamin E: applications of the principles of physical organic chemistry to the exploration of its structure and function. Accts. Chem. Res. **19:** 194-201.
3. WAYNER, D. D. M. & G. W. BURTON. 1988. Measurement of individual antioxidants and radical-trapping activity. *In* Handbook of Free Radicals and Antioxidants in Biomedicine. J. Miquel, Ed. Vol 3: 223-232. CRC Press. Boca Raton, FL.
4. BURTON, G. W. & K. U. INGOLD. 1988. Mechanisms of antioxidant action: preventive and chain-breaking antioxidants. *In* Handbook of Free Radicals and Antioxidants in Biomedicine. J. Miquel, Ed. Vol 2: 29-43. CRC Press. Boca Raton, FL.
5. NIKI, E. 1987. Antioxidants in relation to lipid peroxidation. Chem. Phys. Lipids **44:** 227-253.
6. HOWARD, J. A. 1973. Homogeneous liquid phase autoxidations. *In* Free Radicals. J. K. Kochi, Ed. **2:** 3-62. John Wiley & Sons. New York.
7. BURTON, G. W., Y. LE PAGE, E. J. GABE & K. U. INGOLD. 1980. Antioxidant activity of vitamin E and related phenols. Importance of stereoelectronic factors. J. Am. Chem. Soc. **102:** 7791-7792.
8. BURTON, G. W. & K. U. INGOLD. 1981. Autoxidation of biological molecules. 1. The antioxidant activity of vitamin E and related chain-breaking phenolic antioxidants *in vitro.* J. Am. Chem. Soc. **103:** 6472-6477.

9. BURTON, G. W., L. HUGHES & K. U. INGOLD. 1983. Antioxidant activity of phenols related to vitamin E. Are there chain-breaking antioxidants better than α-tocopherol? J. Am. Chem. Soc. **105:** 5950-5951.

10. BURTON, G. W., T. DOBA, E. J. GABE, L. HUGHES, F. L. LEE, L. PRASAD & K. U. INGOLD. 1985. Autoxidation of Biological Molecules. 4. Maximizing the antioxidant activity of phenols. J. Am. Chem. Soc. **107:** 7053-7065.

11. DOBA, T., G. W. BURTON, K. U. INGOLD & M. MATSUO. 1984. α-Tocopheroxyl decay: lack of effect of oxygen. Journal of the Chemical Society, Chemical Communications 461-462.

12. PERLY, B., I. C. P. SMITH, L. HUGHES, G. W. BURTON & K. U. INGOLD. 1985. Estimation of the location of natural α-tocopherol in lipid bilayers by ^{13}C-NMR spectroscopy. Biochim. Biophys. Acta. **819:** 131-135.

13. EKIEL, I. H., L. HUGHES, G. W. BURTON, P.A. JOVALL, K. U. INGOLD & I. C. P. SMITH. 1988. Structure and dynamics of α-tocopherol in model membranes and in solution: a broad-line and high-resolution NMR study. Biochemistry **27:** 1432-1440.

14. DOBA, T., G. W. BURTON & K. U. INGOLD. 1985. Antioxidant and co-antioxidant effect of vitamin C. The effect of vitamin C, either alone or in the presence of vitamin E or a water-soluble vitamin E analog, upon the peroxidation of aqueous multilamellar phospholipid liposomes. Biochim. Biophys. Acta. **835:** 298-303.

15. NIKI, E., A. KAWAKAMI, Y. YAMAMOTO & Y. KAMIYA. 1985. Oxidation of lipids. VIII. Synergistic inhibition of oxidation of phosphatidylcholine liposome in aqueous dispersion by vitamin E and vitamin C. Bull. Chem. Soc. Jpn. **58:** 1971-1975.

16. BENDICH, A., L. J. MACHLIN, O. SCANDURRA, G. W. BURTON & D. D. M. WAYNER. 1986. The antioxidant role of vitamin C. Adv. Free Radical Biol. Med. **2:** 419-444.

17. PACKER, J. E., T. F. SLATER & R. L. WILLSON. 1979. Direct observation of a free radical interaction between vitamin E and vitamin C. Nature **278:** 737-738.

18. NIKI, E., J. TSUCHIYA, R. TANIMURA & Y. KAMIYA. 1982. The regeneration of vitamin E from alpha-chromanoxyl radical by glutathione and vitamin C. Chem. Lett. **6:** 789-792.

19. BARCLAY, L. R. C. & K. U. INGOLD. 1981. Autoxidation of biological molecules. II. The autoxidation of a model membrane. A comparison of the autoxidation of egg lecithin phosphatidylcholine in water and in chlorobenzene. J. Am. Chem. Soc. **103:** 6478-6485.

20. GIASUDDIN, A. S. M. & A. T. DIPLOCK. 1979. The influence of vitamin E and selenium on the growth and plasma membrane permeability of mouse fibroblasts in culture. Arch. Biochem. Biophys. **196:** 270-280.

21. GIASUDDIN, A. S. M. & A. T. DIPLOCK. 1981. The influence of vitamin E and membrane lipids of mouse fibroblasts in culture. Arch. Biochem. Biophys. **210:** 348-362.

22. MAGGIO, B., A. T. DIPLOCK & J. A. LUCY. 1977. Interactions of tocopherols and ubiquinones with monolayers of phospholipids. Biochem. J. **161:** 111-121.

23. NIKI, E., A. KAWAKAMI, M. SAITO, Y. YAMAMOTO, Y. TSUCHIYA & Y. KAMIYA. 1985. Effect of phytyl side chain of vitamin E on its antioxidant activity. J. Biol. Chem. **260:** 2191-2196.

24. BJORNSON, L. K., C. GNIEWKOWSKI & H. J. KAYDEN. 1975. Comparison of exchange of α-tocopherol and free cholesterol between rat plasma lipoproteins and erythrocytes. J. Lipid Res. **16:** 39-53.

25. CHENG, S. C., G. W. BURTON, K. U. INGOLD & D. O. FOSTER. 1987. Chiral discrimination in the exchange of α-tocopherol stereoisomers between plasma and red blood cells. Lipids **22:** 469-473.

26. BURTON, G. W., A. JOYCE & K. U. INGOLD. 1982. First proof that vitamin E is a major lipid-soluble, chain-breaking antioxidant in human blood plasma. Lancet **ii:** 327.

27. BURTON, G. W., A. JOYCE & K. U. INGOLD. 1983. Is vitamin E the only lipid-soluble, chain-breaking antioxidant in human blood plasma and erythrocyte membranes? Arch. Biochem. Biophys. **221:** 281-290.

28. CHEESEMAN, K. H., G. W. BURTON, K. U. INGOLD & T. F. SLATER. 1984. Lipid peroxidation and lipid antioxidants in normal and tumor cells. Toxicol. Pathol. **12:** 235-239.

29. CHEESEMAN, K. H., S. EMERY, S. P. MADDIX, T. F. SLATER, G. W. BURTON & K. U. INGOLD. 1988. Studies on lipid peroxidation in normal and tumour tissues. Biochem. J. **250:** 247-252.

30. INGOLD, K. U., A. C. WEBB, D. WITTER, G. W. BURTON, T. A. METCALFE & D. P. R. MULLER. 1987. Vitamin E remains the major lipid-soluble, chain-breaking antioxidant in human plasma even in individuals suffering severe vitamin E deficiency. Arch. Biochem. Biophys. **259:** 224-225.

31. BURTON, G. W. & K. U. INGOLD. 1984. β-Carotene: an unusual type of lipid antioxidant. Science **224:** 569-573.

32. INGOLD, K. U., G. W. BURTON, D. O. FOSTER, M. ZUKER, L. HUGHES, S. LACELLE, E. LUSZTYK & M. SLABY. 1986. A new vitamin E analogue more active than α-tocopherol in the rat curative myopathy bioassay. FEBS Lett. **205:** 117-120.

33. MACHLIN, L. J., E. GABRIEL & M. BRIN. 1982. Biopotency of α-tocopherols as determined by curative myopathy bioassay in the rat. J. Nutr. **112:** 1437-1440.

34. HUGHES, L., D. O. FOSTER, G. W. BURTON & K. U. INGOLD. Unpublished results.

35. THOMAS, D. W., R. M. PARKHURST, D. S. NEGI, K. D. LUNAN, A. C. WEN, A. E. BRANDT & R. J. STEPHENS. 1981. Improved assay for α-tocopherol in the picogram range, using gas chromatography-mass spectrometry. J. Chromatogr. **225:** 433-439.

36. INGOLD, K. U., L. HUGHES, M. SLABY & G. W. BURTON. 1986. Synthesis of 2*R*,4'*R*,8'*R*-α-tocopherols selectively labelled with deuterium. J. Lab. Comp. Radiopharm. **24:** 817-831.

37. INGOLD, K. U., G. W. BURTON, D. O. FOSTER, L. HUGHES, D. A. LINDSAY & A. WEBB. 1987. Biokinetics of and discrimination between dietary *RRR*- and *SRR*-α-tocopherols in the male rat. Lipids **22:** 163-172.

38. TRABER, M. G., K. U. INGOLD, G. W. BURTON & H. J. KAYDEN. 1988. Absorption and transport of deuterium-substituted 2*R*,4'*R*,8'*R*-α-tocopherol in human lipoproteins. Lipids **23:** 791-797.

39. BURTON, G. W., K. U. INGOLD, D. O. FOSTER, S. C. CHENG, A. WEBB, L. HUGHES & E. LUSZTYK. 1988. Comparison of free α-tocopherol and α-tocopheryl acetate as sources of vitamin E in rats and humans. Lipids **23:** 834-840.

40. CATIGNANI, G. L. & J. G. BIERI. 1977. Rat liver α-tocopherol binding protein. Biochim. Biophys. Acta. **497:** 349-357.

41. BURTON, G. W. & K. U. INGOLD. Unpublished results.

Inhibition of Oxidation of Biomembranes by Tocopherol[a]

ETSUO NIKI, YORIHIRO YAMAMOTO,
MAREYUKI TAKAHASHI, ERIKA KOMURO, AND
YUUICHIROU MIYAMA

Department of Reaction Chemistry
Faculty of Engineering
University of Tokyo
Hongo, Tokyo 113, Japan

INTRODUCTION

The rate and mechanism of inhibition of peroxidation of lipids by tocopherols in homogeneous solution are now well-elucidated,[1] whereas those in the membranes are not well-understood yet. Recently, the action of tocopherols as antioxidants in the phospholipid liposomal membranes was studied extensively.[1,2] It was found that tocopherols incorporated into liposomal membranes suppress the oxidation of phospholipids induced by free radicals generated either in the aqueous phase or within the liposomal membranes.[3-6] Tocopherols scavenge both the oxygen radicals attacking from outside the membrane and the chain-carrying lipid peroxyl radicals within the membranes to terminate the free radical chain reaction by donating the active, phenolic hydrogen atom at the 6-position to the oxygen radicals. The resulting tocopheroxyl radical, 2, may scavenge another peroxyl radical to give a stable adduct, 3, react with another tocopheroxyl radical to give a dimer, or may be reduced by, for example, ascorbic acid to regenerate the corresponding tocopherol as shown in equations I to IV, where R is the phytyl side chain and RH the reducing agent. The adduct, 3, may further react with peroxyl radicals to give an epoxide under certain conditions.[7]

[a] This study was supported by a Grant-in Aid for Scientific Research from the Ministry of Education, Science, and Culture, Japan.

23

The antioxidant activities of tocopherols in the phospholipid liposomal membranes are much smaller than those in the homogeneous solutions,[8,9] probably because of a lower chance of collision between the tocopherol and the peroxyl radical and a higher chance of chain propagation in the tightly packed structure of liposomal membranes. The lateral mobility of tocopherols within the liposomal membranes appears not to be affected significantly, however, and it has been observed that tocopheroxyl radicals interact readily with tocopherol and ascorbic acid esters incorporated within the same liposomal membranes.[2,8] On the other hand, the phytyl side chain of tocopherol reduces the mobility of tocopherol between the liposomal membranes.[10] Thus, α-tocopherol incorporated into dimyristoyl phosphatidylcholine (PC) liposomes cannot suppress the oxidation of soybean PC liposomes in the same aqueous dispersions. 2,2,5,7,8-Pentamethyl-6-chromanol, however, a model compound of vitamin E without phytyl side chain, incorporated into dimyristoyl PC liposomes, does suppress the oxidation of soybean PC liposomes in the same aqueous dispersions. It was also found that this 2,2,5,7,8-pentamethyl-6-chromanol (E_o) could penetrate the PC liposomal membranes freely.[10]

The synergistic inhibition of oxidation by a combination of vitamin E and vitamin C has received considerable attention.[1,2,11,12] It was shown clearly that ascorbic acid reduces the tocopheroxyl radical to regenerate tocopherol in the liposomal membrane system[3,4] as well as in homogeneous solution.[13,14]

On the basis of the results and knowledge obtained in these oxidations of the liposomal membrane systems, the inhibition of oxidation of erythrocyte membranes by vitamin E and related compounds has been studied. In most of the experiments, the azo compound was used in order to generate free radicals at a known and constant rate and at a specific site. The azo compound is decomposed thermally without enzyme or biotransformation to give two geminate carbon radicals and a nitrogen molecule. A small fraction of the carbon radicals recombine (equation V), but the rest of them diffuse and react with oxygen to give peroxyl radicals (equation VI), which attack lipids and proteins in the membranes. A water-soluble 2,2'-azobis(2-amidinopropane) dihydrochloride (AAPH), dissolved in water, generates aqueous free radicals, whereas lipid-soluble 2,2'-azobis (2,4-dimethylvaleronitrile) (AMVN), located within the membranes, generates free radicals in the lipid phase.

$$\underset{\text{H}_2\text{N}}{\overset{\text{HCl·HN}}{\diagdown}}\text{C}-\underset{\text{CH}_3}{\overset{\text{CH}_3}{\text{C}}}-\text{N}{=}\text{N}-\underset{\text{CH}_3}{\overset{\text{CH}_3}{\text{C}}}-\text{C}\underset{\diagdown\text{NH}_2}{\overset{\diagup\text{NH·HCl}}{}}$$

AAPH

$$\underset{\text{CH}_3}{\overset{\text{CH}_3}{\text{CH}}}-\text{CH}_2-\underset{\text{CN}}{\overset{\text{CH}_3}{\text{C}}}-\text{N}{=}\text{N}-\underset{\text{CN}}{\overset{\text{CH}_3}{\text{C}}}-\text{CH}_2-\underset{\text{CH}_3}{\overset{\text{CH}_3}{\text{CH}}}$$

AMVN

$$\text{A}-\text{N}{=}\text{N}-\text{A} \longrightarrow \text{A}\cdot + \text{N}_2 + \cdot\text{A} \begin{cases} \longrightarrow (1-e)\text{A}-\text{A} \\ \searrow 2e\text{A}\cdot \end{cases} \qquad \text{(V)}$$
$$\qquad\qquad\qquad\qquad\qquad\qquad\qquad\qquad\qquad\qquad\qquad\qquad\qquad\qquad \text{(VI)}$$

$$\text{A}\cdot + \text{O}_2 \longrightarrow \text{AO}_2\cdot \longrightarrow \text{attack membranes} \qquad \text{(VII)}$$

INHIBITION OF OXIDATION OF ERYTHROCYTE GHOST MEMBRANES

The erythrocyte membranes are susceptible to peroxidation because they are rich in polyunsaturated fatty acids; they contain hemoglobin, which may catalyze the oxidation and are continuously exposed to a high concentration of oxygen. The oxidations of erythrocytes and their ghost membranes serve as good models for the oxidative damage of biological membranes. One of the important questions was whether or not the biological membranes were oxidized by a free radical chain mechanism and, if so, how long was that chain. This is important because one molecule of initiating radical can produce many lipid hydroperoxides by chain reactions, although one molecule of nonradical species such as singlet oxygen can produce only one molecule of hydroperoxide. Thus, the chain reactions induced by a single hit of free radicals may amplify the damage of the membranes, whereas the damage from the initiation or the attack of nonradical active species might well be negligible.

The oxidations of human and rat erythrocyte ghost membranes were performed in an aqueous suspension at 37°C under air in the presence of AAPH.[15] As observed in the oxidation of phosphatidylcholine liposomal membranes, a constant rate of oxygen uptake was observed and the kinetic chain length was long, ranging from 7 to 100 depending on the experimental conditions, indicating that erythrocyte ghost membranes are oxidized by molecular oxygen by a free radical chain mechanism. Proteins as well as polyunsaturated fatty acids were oxidized. α-Tocopherol in the ghost membranes suppressed the oxidation and gave a clear induction period. α-Tocopherol decreased linearly with time during the induction period. When α-tocopherol was depleted, the induction period was over, and a fast oxidation took place.

OXIDATIVE DAMAGE OF ERYTHROCYTES AND ITS INHIBITION BY VITAMIN E

The oxidations of vitamin E-deficient and control erythrocytes were carried out in order to study the effect of vitamin E in the membranes. Vitamin E-deficient blood was obtained from Wistar strain male rats fed on a vitamin E-deficient diet for 12 weeks. The concentrations of α-tocopherol in the erythrocyte membranes from vitamin E-deficient and control rats were 25 and 308 μg/dL, respectively. The initial rate of oxygen uptake in the oxidation of erythrocytes from vitamin E-deficient rats, as 10% aqueous suspension at 37°C initiated with AAPH, was larger than those from control rats, and the vitamin E-deficient erythrocytes underwent hemolysis faster than control erythrocytes.[16] The kinetic chain length was obtained as 3.3 to 7.5, considerably larger than 1, suggesting that erythrocyte membranes are oxidized by a free radical chain mechanism. Similar results were obtained for vitamin E-deficient and control rabbits. Little hemolysis was observed even for vitamin E-deficient erythrocytes in the absence of AAPH. Interestingly, however, the extent of hemolysis was determined primarily by the amount of oxygen uptake, that is, by the extent of oxidation of the membrane independent of the presence or absence of vitamin E. This implies that vitamin E suppresses hemolysis not physically but chemically by scavenging oxygen radicals and interrupting the chain oxidation.

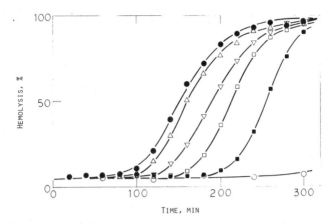

FIGURE 1. Inhibition by 3-(2,5,7,8-tetramethyl-6-chromanol)propionic acid (**4**) of oxidative hemolysis of rabbit erythrocytes (10% suspension in saline) induced by 50 mM AAPH at 37°C under air. The concentrations of **4** were 0 (●); 10.3 (△); 52.0 (▽); 103 (□); and 204 μM (■). The open circle (○) shows the results in the absence of AAPH and **4**.

Apparently, the radicals generated in the aqueous phase from AAPH attack the erythrocyte membranes, induce the chain oxidations of lipids and proteins, and eventually cause membrane damage leading to hemolysis. It has been found that AAPH induces hemolysis dose-dependently,[2] that is, the higher the AAPH concentration, the sooner the hemolysis takes place, and that the extent of hemolysis is proportional to the total amount of radicals formed.[17]

It was found that water-soluble, chain-breaking antioxidants, such as ascorbic acid and uric acid, suppressed the hemolysis of rabbit erythrocytes induced by AAPH.[2,18] FIGURE 1 shows that 3-(2,5,7,8-tetramethyl-6-chromanol)propionic acid, **4**, a water-soluble analogue of vitamin E, suppresses the hemolysis of rabbit erythrocytes induced by AAPH dose-dependently. These water-soluble antioxidants must scavenge radicals derived from AAPH in the aqueous phase before the radicals attack membranes.

Lipid-soluble antioxidants incorporated into phosphatidylcholine liposomal membranes also suppressed the hemolysis of erythrocytes induced by AAPH. FIGURE 2 shows the effects of chromanol E_n, **5**, having side chains of different length incorporated into dimyristoyl PC liposomal membranes: the shorter the side chain, the more effective in suppressing the hemolysis. FIGURE 3 shows the similar results observed for E_n', **6**, having no methyl group at the 4′, 8′, and 12′-positions at the side chain. Substantially, the same results were observed for E_n and E_n'.

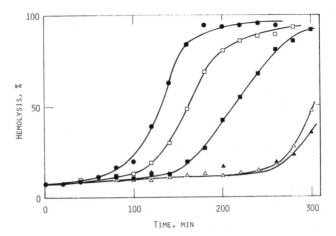

FIGURE 2. Effect of 0.30 mM chromanol E_n incorporated into 1.84 mM dimyristoyl PC liposomes on the hemolysis of rabbit erythrocytes induced by 50 mM AAPH at 37°C under air. ●:no E_n; □:E_3; ■:E_2; △:E_1; ▲:E_0.

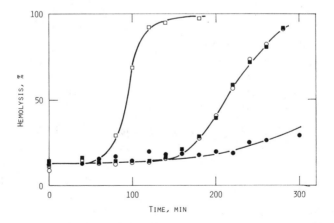

FIGURE 3. Effect of side chain of chromanols E_n and E_n' (0.30 mM) incorporated into 1.76 mM egg PC liposomes on the oxidative hemolysis of rabbit erythrocytes induced by 50 mM AAPH at 37°C under air. □:no antioxidant; ●:E_0; ○:E_3; ■:E_3'.

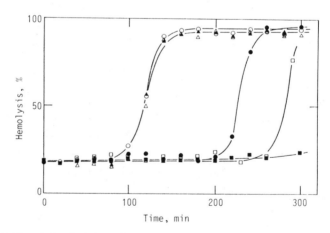

The lipid-soluble radical initiator, AMVN, incorporated into soybean PC liposomes, enhanced the hemolysis, although soybean PC alone without AMVN also induced the hemolysis. AMVN incorporated into dimyristoyl PC liposomes, however, did not induce hemolysis. FIGURE 4 shows the effects of α-tocopherol and its derivatives, incorporated into soybean PC liposomes together with AMVN, on the hemolysis of rabbit erythrocytes. α-Tocopherol suppressed the hemolysis dose-dependently, but α-tocopheryl acetate and nicotinate did not, indicating that the phenolic hydrogen is important for suppressing the oxidative damage of erythrocytes. The chromanols E_n ($n = 0,1,2,3$) incorporated into soybean PC liposomes, together with AMVN, were all effective in suppressing the hemolysis.

When 0.92 mM of dimyristoyl PC liposomes, containing 0.020 mM of either α-tocopherol or E_o, was added to the aqueous suspensions of 10% rabbit erythrocytes and 0.80 mM soybean PC liposomes, containing 0.25 mM AMVN, α-tocopherol showed little inhibitory effect, but E_o suppressed the hemolysis efficiently. This finding is consistent with the previous findings[10] that E_o incorporated into one liposomal membrane can suppress the oxidation of the other liposomes, whereas α-tocopherol cannot. Apparently, α-tocopherol with a long phytyl side chain is retained strongly within the membranes and cannot transfer from one liposome to another.

As shown in FIGURE 5, the addition of ascorbic acid delayed the hemolysis of rabbit erythrocytes induced by 1.61 mM soybean PC liposomes containing 0.25 mM

FIGURE 4. Hemolysis of rabbit erythrocytes (10% in 0.11 M NaCl aqueous suspensions, pH 7.4) in the presence of 1.16 mM soybean PC multilamellar liposomes containing 0.25 mM AMVN and α-tocopherol or its esters. $\bigcirc$:without antioxidant; $\blacktriangle$:0.1 mM α-tocopherol acetate; $\triangle$:0.1 mM α-tocopheryl nicotinate; $\bullet$:0.010 mM α-tocopherol; $\square$:0.016 mM α-tocopherol; $\blacksquare$:0.125 mM α-tocopherol.

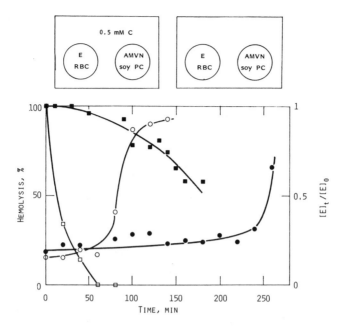

FIGURE 5. Hemolysis (circles) and consumption of vitamin E (squares) of rabbit erythrocytes (10% suspensions in saline, pH 7.4) induced by 1.61 mM soybean PC liposomes (MLV) containing 0.25 mM AMVN in the presence (solid) and absence (open) of 0.50 mM ascorbic acid at 37°C in air. Initial $[E]_0 = 0.26$ μM.

AMVN. In the absence of ascorbic acid, vitamin E in the erythrocytes decreased without any lag, but ascorbic acid reduced the rate of consumption of vitamin E. It is not clear at present whether this is due to the regeneration of vitamin E by ascorbic acid or if it is due to the direct scavenging of radicals derived from AMVN by ascorbic acid.

As shown above, vitamin E in the erythrocyte membranes, water-soluble chain-breaking antioxidants dissolved in water, and vitamin E analogues with short side chains incorporated into PC liposomal membranes suppress the oxidative hemolysis of red blood cells induced by AAPH. The results of the vitamin E-deficient and control erythrocytes show that the difference of 0.66 μM vitamin E in the erythrocyte membranes delayed the hemolysis in 30 minutes. FIGURE 1 shows that, under similar conditions, 50 μM of water-soluble vitamin E analogue is required to delay the hemolysis in 30 minutes. Furthermore, when E_0 was incorporated into dimyristoyl PC liposomes, about 100 μM was necessary to delay the hemolysis in 30 minutes. Furthermore, as shown in FIGURE 6, 1 μM of E_0 had little protective effect. These results suggest that vitamin E retained in the erythrocyte membranes protects them quite efficiently from the free radical attack and from subsequent peroxidations of lipids and proteins by the chain mechanism. The regeneration of vitamin E in the erythrocyte membranes may also contribute to the efficient protective action of vitamin E. The water-soluble antioxidants in the aqueous phase scavenge the radicals in the aqueous phase and reduce the number of radical attacks on the membranes. They cannot scavenge the lipid peroxyl radicals within the membranes and interrupt the

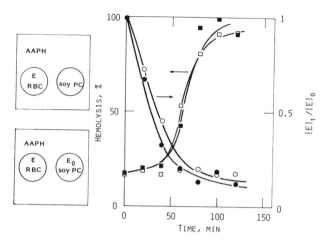

FIGURE 6. Hemolysis and consumption of vitamin E of rabbit erythrocytes (10% suspensions in saline, pH 7.4) induced by 50 mM AAPH at 37°C in air in the presence of 1.61 mM soybean PC liposomes without and with 1.01 μM 2,2,5,7,8-pentamethyl-6-chromanol (E_0). ■,●:without E_0; □, ○:with E_0.

chain reactions, however. Thus, it may be concluded that vitamin E plays a vital role in the protection of membranes from a free radical-mediated damage.

ACKNOWLEDGMENT

The authors are grateful to Professor Mino and Dr. Miki, Dr. Tamai, and Dr. Yasuda for their advice and suggestions on hemolysis experiments. The authors also acknowledge Dr. Urano and Dr. Shimasaki for generous gifts of vitamin E-deficient blood and vitamin E analogues.

REFERENCES

1. BURTON, G. W. & K. U. INGOLD. 1986. Vitamin E: Application of physical organic chemistry to the exploration of its structure and function. Acc. Chem. Res. **19:** 194-201.
2. NIKI, E. 1987. Antioxidants in relation to lipid peroxidation. Chem. Phys. Lipids **44:** 227-253.
3. NIKI, E., A. KAWAKAMI, Y. YAMAMOTO & Y. KAMIYA. 1985. Synergistic inhibition of oxidation of soybean phosphatidylcholine liposomes in aqueous dispersions by vitamin E and vitamin C. Bull. Chem. Soc. Jpn. **58:** 1971-1975.
4. DOBA, T., G. W. BURTON & K. U. INGOLD. 1985. Antioxidant and co-antioxidant activity of vitamin C. The effect of vitamin C, either alone or in the presence of vitamin E analogue, upon the peroxidation of aqueous multilamellar phospholipid liposomes. Biochim. Biophys. Acta. **835:** 298-303.

5. BARCLAY, L. R. C., A. M. H. BAILEY & D. KONG. 1985. The antioxidant activity of α-tocopherol-bovine serum albumin complex in micellar and liposome autoxidations. J. Biol. Chem. **260:** 15809-15814.

6. NIKI, E. 1987. Inhibition of oxidation of liposomal- and bio-membranes by vitamin E. *In* Clinical and Nutritional Aspects of Vitamin E. O. Hayaishi & M. Mino Ed.: 3-13. Elsevier, Amsterdam.

7. MATSUMOTO, S., M. MATSUO, Y. IITAKA & E. NIKI. 1986. Oxidation of a vitamin E model compound, 2,2,5,7,8-pentamethylchroman-6-ol, with the t-butylperoxyl radical. JCS Chem. Commun. 1076-1077.

8. NIKI, E., M. TAKAHASHI & E. KOMURO. 1986. Antioxidant activity of vitamin E in liposomal membranes. Chem. Lett. 1573-1576.

9. NIKI, E. & E. KOMURO. 1989. Inhibition of peroxidation of membranes. *In* Oxygen Radicals in Biology and Medicine. M. G. Simic, Ed.: 561-566. Plenum Press. New York.

10. NIKI, E., A. KAWAKAMI, M. SAITO, Y. YAMAMOTO, J. TSUCHIYA & Y. KAMIYA. 1985. Effect of phytyl side chain of vitamin E on its antioxidant activity. J. Biol. Chem. **260:** 2191-2196.

11. McCAY, P. B. 1985. Vitamin E: Interactions with free radicals and ascorbate. Annu. Rev. Nutr. **5:** 323-340.

12. NIKI, E. 1987. Interaction of ascorbate and α-tocopherol. Ann. N. Y. Acad. Sci. **498:** 186-199.

13. PACKER, J. E., T. F. SLATER & R. L. WILLSON. 1979. Direct observation of a free radical interaction between vitamin E and vitamin C. Nature **278:** 737-738.

14. NIKI, E., J. TSUCHIYA, R. TANIMURA & Y. KAMIYA. 1982. Regeneration of vitamin E from α-chromanoxy radical by glutathione and vitamin C. Chem. Lett. 789-792.

15. YAMAMOTO, Y., E. NIKI, J. EGUCHI, Y. KAMIYA & H. SHIMASAKI. 1985. Oxidation of biological membranes and its inhibition. Free radical chain oxidation of erythrocyte ghost membranes by oxygen. Biochim. Biophys. Acta **819:** 29-36.

16. YAMAMOTO, Y., E. NIKI, Y. KAMIYA, M. MIKI, H. TAMAI & M. MINO. 1986. Free radical chain oxidation and hemolysis of erythrocytes by molecular oxygen and their inhibition by vitamin E. J. Nutr. Sci. Vitaminol. **32:** 475-479.

17. MIKI, M., H. TAMAI, M. MINO, Y. YAMAMOTO & E. NIKI. 1987. Free-radical chain oxidation of rat red blood cells by molecular oxygen and its inhibition by α-tocopherol. Arch. Biochem. Biophys. **258:** 373-380.

18. NIKI, E., E. KOMURO, M. TAKAHASHI, S. URANO, E. ITO & K. TERAO. 1988. Oxidative hemolysis of erythrocytes and its inhibition by free radical scavengers. J. Biol. Chem. **263:** 19809-19814.

Evidence That Alpha-Tocopherol Functions Cyclically to Quench Free Radicals in Hepatic Microsomes

Requirement for Glutathione and a Heat-Labile Factor

PAUL B. McCAY, GEMMA BRUEGGEMANN,
EDWARD K. LAI, AND SAUL R. POWELL

Oklahoma Medical Research Foundation
Oklahoma City, Oklahoma 73121

INTRODUCTION

In the early part of this decade, Burk and co-workers reported that lipid peroxidation in rat liver microsomes was inhibited by the presence of glutathione.[1-4] These investigators found that the inhibition of peroxidation by glutathione was heat-labile and that this protective activity involved alpha-tocopherol.[4,5] It was concluded that the thiol may function in conjunction with a trypsin-sensitive microsomal factor[4] to protect the endoplasmic reticulum of the liver against oxidative stress that might trigger peroxidative breakdown, possibly by recycling tocopheroxyl radicals back to tocopherol, as the latter quenches free radicals formed in the initiating phase of lipid peroxidation.[5-7] The hepatic endoplasmic reticulum is the site of a number of strongly oxidizing cytochrome P-450 enzyme systems that have the capability of metabolizing some xenobiotic compounds to free radicals.[8] This report describes an investigation in which additional evidence has been obtained to support the hypothesis that a labile glutathione-dependent factor, presumably an enzyme, cycles the tocopheroxyl radical back to tocopherol, as the latter quenches free radical reactions that may be initiated by enzymic process in the hepatic endoplasmic reticulum. The latter appears to be the only organelle in animal tissues containing such a protective mechanism. The data also suggest that the recycling to the tocopheroxyl radical by ascorbic acid may not be efficient in this organelle.

32

METHODS

The rats used in these experiments were males and of the Sprague-Dawley strain supplied by Sasco, Inc., Omaha, NE.

All reagents used in this work were either of reagent grade or best grade available. The spin trapping agent, alpha-phenyl-*t*-butylnitrone (PBN) and nickel peroxide (NiO_2) were obtained from the Eastman Kodak Company, Rochester, NY. Glutathione was purchased from Boehringer Mannheim Biochemicals, Indianapolis, IN. *dl*-Alpha-tocopherol was obtained from Sigma Chemical Co., St. Louis, MO.

The tocopherol-deficient diet was prepared by ICN Nutritional Biochemical Sciences, Cleveland, OH 44128. The rats were fed this diet for 8 weeks prior to preparing microsomes from liver tissue. These microsomes still contained tocopherol, but at very low levels.

Washed liver microsomes were prepared as described previously[9] and stored at −20°. They were employed in the experiments within 48 hours, as the glutathione-dependent activity diminishes significantly beyond that time period.

The reaction systems employed to initiate lipid peroxidation were of different types (both enzymic and nonenzymic, metal-dependent and non-metal-dependent), in order to avoid the possibility that the inhibitory effect caused by glutathione was not a limited effect on a particular type of peroxidation process. System 1 produced lipid peroxidation by an enzyme-catalyzed process involved in the oxidation of NADPH by liver microsomes. System 2 promoted lipid peroxidation by a nonenzymic reaction among an ADP-Fe^{2+} complex, ascorbic acid, and heat-inactivated liver microsomes. System 3 produced lipid peroxidation initiated by the microsomal generation of trichloromethyl radicals during the cytochrome P-450-mediated metabolism of carbon tetrachloride. These enzyme-generated radicals attack membrane polyunsaturated fatty acids, which triggers the peroxidation process. This system is not dependent on the presence of low levels of iron as are systems 1 and 2. System 1 components: NADPH, 0.03 mM, 0.5 mM glucose-6-phosphate, 0.5 Kornberg units of glucose-6-phosphate dehydrogenase, 0.4 mM ADP, 0.012 mM $FeCl_3$, and 1.0 mg microsomal protein, made up to 1.0 mL final volume with 0.15 M potassium phosphate buffer, pH 7.4. System 2 components: 0.66 mM ascorbic acid, 0.4 mM ADP, 0.012 mM $FeCl_3$, 1.0 mg microsomal protein, made up to 1.0 mL with the same phosphate buffer. System 3 components: 0.3 mM NADPH, 0.5 mM glucose-6-phosphate, 0.5 M Kornberg units of glucose-6-phosphate dehydrogenase, 20 μL CCl_4, 1.0 mg microsomal protein, and the phosphate buffer, final system volume, 1.0 milliliter. Reaction time for all systems was 30 min at 37° excepting where indicated otherwise. In experiments requiring heat-denatured microsomes, the particles were warmed to 70° and then cooled to room temperature before addition to the reaction systems.

Measurement of Lipid Peroxidation

Lipid peroxidation produces a number of products derived from the oxidative chain scission of polyunsaturated fatty acids. Some of these products form derivatives with thiobarbituric acid, which have a characteristic absorption at 532 nm.[10,11] One of the end products of lipid peroxidation that has been well-characterized is malondialdehyde.[12] It has been useful to express the values for thiobarbituric acid assays as equivalents of the malondialdehyde-thiobarbituric acid derivative (which has a molar absorbancy of 1.53×10^5), and malondialdehyde equivalents have been used to express the data in this report. The procedure was as follows: each reaction system was inactivated by the addition of 0.5 mL of 35% trichloroacetic acid followed by 1.0 mL of 70% trichloroacetic acid and 2.0 mL of chloroform. The two-phased system was vortexed for 30 seconds and then centrifuged to separate the phases cleanly. One milliliter of the aqueous phase was pipetted into a cuvette (1.0 cm light path) and the optical density determined. The molar absorbancy of the malondialdehyde-thiobarbituric acid derivative is 1.53×10^5. Values obtained from the various determinations were expressed as ng/mg microsomal protein. Protein was determined by the method of Lowry et al.[13] Various control systems were included to demonstrate that lipid peroxidation did not occur unless all required components of the system were present.

Measurement of Microsomal Tocopherol Content

The method of Burton et al.[14] was employed to extract tocopherol from the microsomes in the various reaction systems. The procedure involves the following steps. Reaction systems were extracted by adding 5.0 mL of 200 mM sodium dodecyl sulfate at the end of the incubation period followed by 30 sec of mixing by vortexing. To this mixture was added 1.0 mL of absolute ethanol followed by vortexing again. After the mixing, 5.0 mL of either hexane or heptane containing 0.0625% of butylated hydroxytoluene was added, and the mixture was again subjected to vortexing for 1.0 minute. The systems were then centrifuged, and the organic top layer was recovered, the solvent removed by rotating evaporation, and the extracted material taken up into a known volume of chloroform:methanol (5:95 v/v). Analyses of the tocopherol content of the extracts were performed by high-pressure liquid chromatography according to a procedure described by Hatam and Kayden.[15] This technique used a Spherisorb ODS-II 5u column (4.6×25 cm) (a product of Custom LC, Inc., Houston, TX.) and a guard column (5.0×20.0 cm). Samples of the hexane extracts were injected into a 100 μL loop. Column elution was performed isocratically using 99:1 (v/v) methanol:water at room temperature. The flow rate was 1.0 mL/minute. Retention time and a standard curve was established using known amounts of tocopherol that were processed by the same procedure. The tocopherol content of the eluted fractions was determined by ultraviolet absorption at 294 nm and expressed as ng/mg microsomal protein.

Determination of Glutathione

The method of Sedlak and Lindsey[16] was employed to determine the glutathione content in the various systems.

Spin-Trapping Assay of Trichloromethyl Radical Generation by Rat Liver Microsomes

This spin-trapping procedure was developed in this laboratory and was the first example of the trapping of metabolically produced free radicals.[17] Liver microsomes (1.0 mg protein) were incubated with 0.3 mM NADPH, 0.1 M PBN, 0.2 mM CCl_4, and the phosphate buffer (final system volume, 1.0 mL) at 37° for 30 minutes. The microsomes generate the highly reactive trichloromethyl radicals that are trapped by PBN as relatively stable radical adducts. At the end of the reaction time, the systems were transferred into Pasteur pipettes that had had their tips sealed. The microsomal particles were centrifugally forced into the tip end portion of the pipette and assayed in an ER 200 IBM Bruker electron paramagnetic resonance (EPR) spectrometer. The rat liver microsomes used in these experiments had been kept at −20° for several days. Such microsomes remain highly active in the metabolism of trichloromethyl radicals from carbon tetrachloride, and have the added advantage that they sediment easily at low centrifugal forces, which facilitates positioning the microsomes in the sensing cavity of the EPR measurements for maximum detection of the spin-trapped radical adducts.

Production of Tocopheroxyl Radicals

The relatively stable tocopheroxyl radical was prepared by treating *dl*-alpha-tocopherol with NiO_2. Using 2.0 mL chloroform as the solvent, 125 mg of alpha-tocopherol was added along with 125 mg of solid NiO_2 and mixed by vortexing occasionally for 5.0 minutes. The reaction system was then filtered using Acrodisc CR disposable filters to remove the NiO_2. The tocopheroxyl radical persists for several hours in this hydrophobic medium and decays slowly by a second order disproportionation process. In a 2.0 mm diameter quartz sample tube, 0.2 mL of this preparation gave the characteristic signal for the tocopheroxyl radical in the EPR spectrometer.

RESULTS

Effect of Glutathione Addition on Lipid Peroxidation

TABLE 1 demonstrates that the addition of glutathione to all three reaction systems causes a marked reduction in the extent of peroxidative breakdown of microsomal membrane lipids. Even system 3 in which the metabolism of carbon tetrachloride is occurring shows a significant inhibition of oxidative lipid destruction. This system generates a flux of trichloromethyl radicals that are avidly reactive with membrane lipids, and this reaction always results in loss of most of the membrane polyunsaturated fatty acids and a significant fraction of membrane proteins within a short period.[18] The inhibition by glutathione appears to be rather specific in that neither beta-mer-

TABLE 1. Inhibition of Lipid Peroxidation by a Liver Microsomal Heat-labile Factor Requiring Glutathione[a]

System	Malondialdehyde Equivalents (OD/mg protein)
System 1: (NADPH Oxidase-dependent Peroxidation)	
Microsomes	0.027 ± 0.012
Microsomes + ADP-Fe^{3+}	0.031 ± 0.017
Microsomes + ADP-Fe^{3+} + NADPH	1.256 ± 0.186
Microsomes + ADP-Fe^{3+} + NADPH + GSH	0.291 ± 0.084
Microsomes + ADP-Fe^{3+} + NADPH + BME	0.901 ± 0.056
Microsomes + ADP-Fe^{3+} + NADPH + DTT	0.897 ± 0.083
Microsomes + ADP-Fe^{3+} + NADPH + CYS-SH	0.197 ± 0.060
System 2: (Ascorbate-Iron-Catalyzed Lipid Peroxidation)	
Microsomes	0.027 ± 0.012
Microsomes + ADP-Fe^{3+} + AA	0.654 ± 0.113
Microsomes + ADP-Fe^{3+} + AA + GSH	0.096 ± 0.031
Microsomes + ADP-Fe^{3+} + AA + BME	0.377 ± 0.233
Microsomes + ADP-Fe^{3+} + AA + CYS-SH	0.128 ± 0.038
Heated Microsomes + ADP-Fe^{3+} + AA	0.812 ± 0.129
Heated Microsomes + ADP-Fe^{3+} + AA + GSH	0.828 ± 0.141
Heated Microsomes + ADP-Fe^{3+} + AA + BME	0.794 ± 0.183
Heated Microsomes + ADP-Fe^{3+} + AA + CYS-SH	0.194 ± 0.042
System 3: (Peroxidation Associated with CCl_4 Metabolism)	
Microsomes	0.035 ± 0.0125
Microsomes + NADPH + CCl_4	0.921 ± 0.177
Microsomes + NADPH + CCl_4 + GSH	0.420 ± 0.215
Microsomes $\pm$ NADPH + CCl_4 + BME	0.805 ± 0.123
Microsomes $\pm$ NADPH + CCl_4 + DDT	0.772 ± 0.077
Microsomes $\pm$ NADPH + CCl_4 + CYS-SH	0.512 ± 0.054

[a] The data shown are averages for four experiments $\pm$ standard deviations. The experimental procedures for the thiobarbituric acid assay (expressed as equivalents of malondialdehyde), which is used as an indicator of the extent of lipid peroxidation in each system, are described in the METHODS section of the text. The concentrations of GSH, β-mercaptoethanol (BME), and cysteine (Cys-SH) in these experiments was 10 mM. The concentration of dithiothreitol (DTT) was 5.0 mM. Incubations were carried out for 30 min at $37°$. The heat lability studies on the microsomal factor were carried out using microsomes that had been heated to $80°$ for 10 minutes prior to assembling the incubation systems.

captoethanol nor dithiothreitol at a similar concentration caused any depression of the oxidative attack on the membrane. The inhibition by cysteine is a special case that will be discussed below. System 2, which promotes lipid peroxidation by a nonenzymic mechanism involving ascorbic acid and chelated iron (probably by promoting the generation of superoxide anion radicals through cyclic reduction and oxidation of the iron and subsequent Fenton-type chemistry[19]), was also inhibited, but not if the microsomes were previously heat-inactivated (TABLE 1). Glutathione was utilized during the inhibition of lipid peroxidation (FIG. 1). Glutathione was not consumed in these systems if one of the components required for lipid peroxidation was absent.

Effect of Glutathione Addition on Microsomal Tocopherol Content

The tocopherol content of the microsomes in the three types of reaction systems was determined at the beginning and the end of the incubation period (TABLE 2). After a 30 min reaction period, the tocopherol content was markedly reduced in all three systems, correlating with an extensive peroxidation of microsomal lipids. When

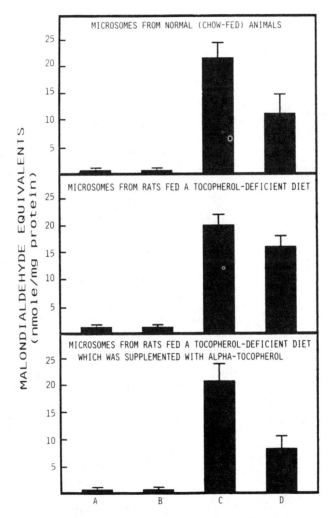

FIGURE 1. Effect of a dietary deficiency of tocopherol on the inhibition by glutathione of microsomal lipid peroxidation caused by enzymic and nonenzymic reactions. Concentration of additions and conditions of the reactions are described under METHODS. A. Microsomes alone. B. Microsomes + ADP-Fe^{3+}. C. Microsomes + ADP-Fe^{3+} + NADPH. D. Microsomes + ADP-Fe^{3+} + NADPH + glutathione.[25]

TABLE 2. Maintenance of the Tocopherol Content of Microsomes by a GSH-Dependent Factor during Peroxidative Stress[a]

System	Incubation Time (min)	Tocopherol Content (ng/mg protein)	Malondialdehyde Equivalents (OD/mg protein)
1. NADPH Oxidase-dependent Lipid Peroxidation:			
Microsomes	0	222 ± 31	0.043 ± 0.008
Microsomes	30	220 ± 45	0.046 ± 0.009
Microsomes + ADP-Fe^{3+} + NADPH	30	77 ± 32	0.713 ± 0.182
Microsomes + ADP-Fe^{3+} + NADPH + GSH (10 mM)	30	193 ± 64	0.166 ± 0.010
Microsomes + ADP-Fe^{3+} + NADPH + BME (10 mM)	30	84 ± 41	0.730 ± 0.147
2. Ascorbate-ADP-Fe^{3+}-dependent Peroxidation:			
Microsomes	0	208 ± 21	0.035 ± 0.005
Microsomes	30	192 ± 14	0.032 ± 0.008
Microsomes + ADP-Fe^{3+} + Ascorbate	30	158 ± 19	0.406 ± 0.138
Microsomes + ADP-Fe^{3+} + Ascorbate + GSH (10 mM)	30	200 ± 19	0.089 ± 0.039
Heated Microsomes	0	166 ± 24	0.044 ± 0.012
Heated Microsomes	30	144 ± 24	0.042 ± 0.004
Heated Microsomes + ADP-Fe^{3+} + Ascorbate	30	71 ± 19	0.698 ± 0.269
Heated Microsomes + ADP-Fe^{3+} + Ascorbate + GSH	30	82 ± 18	0.840 ± 0.287
3. CC1$_4$-dependent Lipid Peroxidation:			
Microsomes	0	224 ± 53	0.042 ± 0.007
Microsomes	30	217 ± 67	0.054 ± 0.007
Microsomes + CC1$_4$ + NADPH	30	37 ± 28	0.640 ± 0.133
Microsomes + CC1$_4$ + NADPH + GSH (10 mM)	30	159 ± 31	0.116 ± 0.025

[a] System compositions and incubation conditions are described in the METHODS section of the text. The values represent the averages ± the standard deviations (n = 6 for the NADPH oxidase system, n = 4 for the CC1$_4$-dependent and the ascorbate-ADP-Fe^{3+} systems). BME indicates β-mercaptoethanol. The values for microsomal tocopherol contents are given as percentages of the amount in the microsomes at the beginning of the experiment instead of absolute values because preparations of liver microsomes from different animals used in the various experiments contained different amounts of tocopherol.

glutathione was present, the loss of tocopherol was largely prevented. Addition of beta-mercaptoethanol instead of glutathione in system 1 did not sustain tocopherol levels.

Effect of Modifying the Tocopherol Content of the Microsomes

To determine if the inhibitory action of glutathione on lipid peroxidation was affected by the amount of tocopherol in the membranes, microsomes were prepared from rats fed tocopherol-deficient diets as well as rats fed the same diet but supplemented with tocopherol. The microsomes from the tocopherol-deficient rats contained low but measurable amounts of tocopherol, and FIGURE 1 shows that the inhibition of lipid peroxidation in those microsomes by glutathione was substantially less than that observed in systems with microsomes from tocopherol-supplemented diets or from rats fed a standard laboratory ration.

In order to determine whether or not the inhibition of peroxidation by glutathione required that some tocopherol must be present in the microsomal membrane, it was determined that total removal of tocopherol from microsomes could be achieved by acetone extraction of these particles, yet still leaving most of the peroxidation-promoting action of systems 1 and 2 as well as the heat-labile factor required for the inhibitory effect of glutathione active (system 3, which is cytochrome P-450-dependent, did not tolerate such extraction). Part of each batch of microsomes was extracted in the same manner, excepting that sufficient tocopherol was added to the acetone so that the extracted microsomes still contained a substantial amount of tocopherol. FIGURE 2 shows that the presence of glutathione in systems containing microsomes with no detectable tocopherol showed no inhibition of lipid peroxidation, whereas peroxidation in systems containing microsomes extracted with acetone in the same manner but still containing appreciable amounts of tocopherol was substantially inhibited. If enzymic activity in the microsomes had been heat-inactivated prior to addition to these systems, however, there was no inhibition of peroxidation in any of the reactions. This is particularly relevant in the case of peroxidation by the ascorbate-iron system in which no enzyme-link function is required except the glutathione-dependent, heat-labile factor responsible for the inhibition of lipid peroxidation.

Effect of a Dietary Deficiency in Tocopherol on the Intensity of Trichloromethyl Radical Production during Carbon Tetrachloride Metabolism

The spin-trapping procedure has been shown to be a useful method for detecting free radicals produced in microsomal systems, and can be used to make determinations of the relative number of free radicals formed in such systems during a given period of time.[20] The signal intensity or height is directly proportional to the number of radicals that are trapped. If the mechanism of inhibition of lipid peroxidation in hepatic microsomes involves quenching by tocopherol of free radicals that may be generated in that membrane followed by glutathione-dependent recycling of the resulting tocopheroxyl radical to tocopherol, the presence of glutathione in a microsomal system that is producing free radicals might be expected to result in fewer radicals

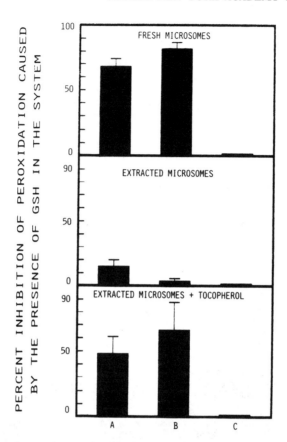

FIGURE 2. Requirement for tocopherol in the microsomal membrane to observe the inhibition of lipid peroxidation by glutathione. Microsomes were extracted with cold acetone in one of two ways: alone to remove essentially all tocopherol as described under the METHODS section, or extracted with acetone containing tocopherol so that the recovered extracted microsomes still contained at least as much tocopherol as the control microsomes. Tocopherol contents of microsomes in ng/mg protein were control microsomes, 91 ± 21; extracted microsomes, 4 ± 6; extracted + tocopherol, 170 ± 44. A. Enzymic (NADPH oxidase) system. B. Nonenzymic ascorbate-iron system. C. Same as B except that the microsomes were heat-treated before addition to the reaction system.

available for trapping by spin-trapping agents. FIGURE 3 shows that the presence of glutathione does, indeed, reduce the number of trichloromethyl radicals that are available for trapping by PBN. Addition of glutathione to such systems after the radicals have been trapped does not diminish the signal, indicating that the action of glutathione did not involve the reduction of the spin-adduct of the trichloromethyl radical.

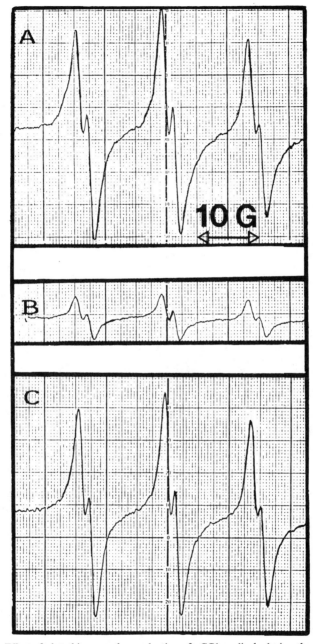

FIGURE 3. Effect of glutathione on the production of $\cdot CCl_3$ radicals during the microsomal metabolism of tocopherol. The assay for production of $\cdot CCl_3$ radicals is described under the section on spin trapping under METHODS. (A) EPR spectrum observed when microsomes were incubated with carbon tetrachloride, an NADPH-generating system, and PBN. (B) EPR spectrum of system described in A, but with 10 mM glutathione added. (C) Same as B, except the glutathione was added at the end of the incubation period.

If microsomal tocopherol has an obligatory role to play in a glutathione-dependent free radical-quenching process in the hepatic endoplasmic reticulum, lowering of the hepatic tocopherol content might be expected to decrease the efficiency of such activity. To test this possibility, rats were fed a tocopherol-deficient diet for 8 weeks while other rats were fed the same diet supplemented with tocopherol. The liver microsomes that were prepared from the deficient rats had a low tocopherol content. The microsomes from both deficient and control groups were incubated in system 3 to generate trichloromethyl radicals, and the intensity of trichloromethyl radical trapping and the effect of the presence of glutathione on that trapping process was assayed. FIGURE 4 shows that the intensity of radical trapping was markedly lower in the systems containing microsomes from tocopherol-deficient animals.

DISCUSSION

Taken as a whole, the results are consistent with tocopherol serving as an electron shuttle between a glutathione-dependent, heat-labile factor and reactive free radicals for the purpose of quenching the latter. In the absence of tocopherol, glutathione appears to have little effect on free radical processes in hepatic microsomes. In addition, if the microsomes had been warmed prior to addition to the reaction systems, glutathione also failed to inhibit lipid peroxidation even when normal levels of tocopherol were present in the microsomes. This result, together with the observation by Hill and Burk[4] that the suppression of lipid peroxidation by glutathione is eliminated by prior treatment of the microsomes with trypsin, suggests that the glutathione-dependent factor is a microsomal membrane protein.

This system appeared to compete well with the spin-trapping agent employed in this study (phenyl-t-butyl nitrone) for the reactive trichloromethyl radicals that were generated in the microsomal membrane, in that the intensity of trapping of these radicals by the spin trap was markedly decreased in microsomes containing normal levels of tocopherol. The decreased EPR signal of the trapped trichloromethyl radicals was not due to reduction of the spin adduct by glutathione, as addition of glutathione to the spin adduct after its formation demonstrates. It is possible that this system, with its efficient free radical quenching activity, may parallel the distribution of domains in the microsomal membrane that are subject to peroxidation (*i.e.*, domains containing significant amounts of polyunsaturated fatty acids). It may be significant that when glutathione is omitted from the peroxidation systems, and lipid peroxidation proceeds to its maximum extent, not all of the tocopherol in the membrane is lost (see TABLE 3). It seems possible that there are domains in the microsome in which

TABLE 3. Utilization of Glutathione during the Glutathione-dependent Inhibition of Microsomal Lipid Peroxidation[a]

System	GSH Oxidized (nmoles mL^{-1} min^{-1})
1. Microsomes + GSH	1 ± 2
2. Microsomes + GSH + NADPH (system 1)	44 ± 11
3. Microsomes + GSH + CCl$_4$	16 ± 2.5
4. Microsomes + GSH + CCl$_4$ + NADPH (system 3)	60 ± 10

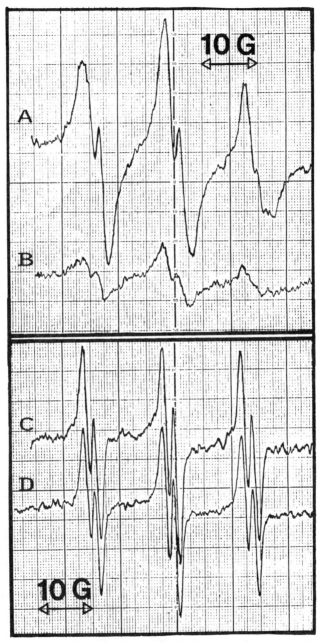

FIGURE 4. Effect of a dietary tocopherol deficiency on the capacity of glutathione to inhibit the generation of $\cdot CCl_3$ radicals during the microsomal metabolism of carbon tetrachloride. The intensity of radical production was assayed using the spin-trapping procedure and EPR spectrometry (see METHODS). The spectra shown above are typical of the trichloromethyl radical adduct of PBN. The height of the EPR signal is proportional to the number of radicals produced in the systems. A. System with microsomes from tocopherol-supplemented rats. B. Same as A, except that 10 mM was present in the reaction system. C. System with microsomes from tocopherol-deficient rats. D. Same as C, except 10 mM glutathione was present in the reaction system.

discrete pools of tocopherol exist that may not be influenced to a great extent by events taking place in other domains. The observation that lipid peroxidation proceeded well in system 2, which contained 0.66 mM ascorbic acid (55-fold greater than the Fe^{3+} content), indicates that the latter is not as effective in maintaining tocopherol in its reduced state in biological membranes as it is in single-phase solvent systems.[21,22] If the recycling of tocopheroxyl radicals to tocopherol is a major mechanism for maintenance of tissue tocopherol levels, deficiency of ascorbic acid might be expected to result in depletion of tissue tocopherol, but we are not aware of such a study having been done.

Using low-level chemiluminescence as an index of lipid peroxidation in a system similar to system 1 (NADPH + ADP-Fe^{3+}), Wefers and Sies observed that ascorbic acid produced a lag in lipid peroxidation in hepatic microsomes that were dependent on the presence of normal levels of tocopherol in the membrane.[23] By contrast, Sterrenberg et al. found no evidence that the tocopherol content of microsomes from liver and other tissues affected either the pro- or antioxidant effects of ascorbic acid on iron-mediated lipid peroxidation.[24] The possible role of ascorbic acid in maintaining tocopherol levels in animal tissues remains unclear.

The significance of the apparent limitation of the glutathione/tocopherol-dependent factor to the hepatic endoplasmic reticulum suggests that it may be a protective mechanism that evolved along with the capacity of this organelle to metabolize xenobiotics that may produce highly reactive intermediates.

REFERENCES

1. BURK, R. F., M. J. TRUMBLE & R. A. LAWRENCE. 1980. Biochim. Biophys. Acta 618: 35-41.
2. BURK, R. F. 1982. Biochem. Pharmacol. 31: 601-602.
3. BURK, R. F. 1983. Biochim. Biophys. Acta 757: 21-28.
4. HILL, K. E. & R. F. BURK. 1984. Biochem. Pharmacol. 33: 1065-1068.
5. REDDY, C. C., R. W. SCHOLZ, C. C. THOMAS & E. J. MASSARO. 1982. Life Sci. 31: 571-576.
6. HAENEN, G. R. M. M. & A. BAST. 1983. FEBS Lett. 159: 24-28.
7. HAENEN, G. R. M. M., J. N. L. T. T. TSOI, N. P. E. VERMEULEN, H. TIMMERMAN & A. BAST. 1987. Arch. Biochem. Biophys. 259: 449-456.
8. SMITH, M. T., H. THOR & S. ORRENIUS. 1984. Methods Enzymol. 105: 505-510.
9. MAY, H. E. & P. B. McCAY. 1966. J. Biol. Chem. 243: 2296-2301.
10. WARAVDEKAR, V. S. & L. D. SASLAW. 1959. J. Biol. Chem. 234: 1945-1949.
11. SAWICKI, E., T. W. STANLEY & H. JOHNSON. 1963. Anal. Chem. 35: 199-205.
12. BULL, A. W. & L. J. MARNETT. 1985. Anal. Biochem. 149: 284-290.
13. LOWRY, O. H., N. J. ROSEBROUGH, A. L. FARR & R. J. RANDALL. 1951. J. Biol. Chem. 193: 265-275.
14. BURTON, G. W., A. WEBB & K. U. INGOLD. 1985. Lipids 20(1): 29-39.
15. HATAM, L. J. & H. J. KAYDEN. 1979. J. Lipid Res. 20: 639-645.
16. SEDLAK, J. & R. H. LINDSAY. 1968. Anal. Biochem. 25: 192-205.
17. POYER, J. L., R. A. FLOYD, P. B. McCAY, E. G. JANZEN & E. R. DAVIS. 1978. Biochim. Biophys. Acta. 539: 402-409.
18. MAY, H. E. & P. B. McCAY. 1966. J. Biol. Chem. 243: 2288-2295.
19. GUTTERIDGE, J. M. 1986. FEBS. Lett. 201: 291-295.
20. McCAY, P. B., E. K. LAI, J. L. POYER, C. M. DUBOSE & E. G. JANZEN. 1984. J. Biol. Chem. 259: 2135-2143.
21. NIKI, E. 1987. Ann. N.Y. Acad. Sci. 498: 186-198.

22. NIKI, E. 1987. Br. J. Cancer [Suppl.] **8:** 153-157.
23. WEFERS, H. & H. SIES. 1988. Eur. J. Biochem. **174:** 353-357.
24. STERRENBERG, L., R. H. JULICHER, A. BAST & J. NOORDHOEK. 1985. Toxicol. Lett. **25:** 153-159.
25. McCAY, P. B. 1987. A biological antioxidant function for vitamin E: Electron shuttling for a membrane-bound "free radical reductase." *In* Fat Production and Consumption. Technologies and Nutritional Implications. Series A. C. Galli & E. Fedeli, Eds.: **131:** 149. Plenum Publishing Corp. New York.

Products of *in Vivo* Peroxidation Are Present in Tissues of Vitamin E-Deficient Rats and Dogs

EDWARD A. DRATZ,[a]
CHRISTOPHER C. FARNSWORTH,[b] ELLIS C. LOEW,[c]
ROBERT J. STEPHENS,[d] DAVID W. THOMAS,[d] AND
FREDERIK J. G. M. VAN KUIJK[a]

[a] *Department of Chemistry*
Montana State University
Bozeman, Montana 59717

[b] *Howard Hughes Medical Institute*
University of Washington Medical School
Seattle, Washington 98532

[c] *Department of Physiology*
School of Veterinary Medicine
Cornell University
Ithaca, New York 14853

[d] *Life Sciences Division*
SRI International
Menlo Park, California 94025

INTRODUCTION

Our laboratory's involvement in research on vitamin E and other antioxidants originally arose from a long-standing interest in the structure and mechanism of action of retinal rod photoreceptor membranes.[1] These membranes are very rich in the most highly polyunsaturated fatty acid known (docosahexaenoic acid, 22:6ω3). FIGURE 1 indicates the percent composition of the major fatty acids in frog retinal rod outer segment membranes and shows that they contain over 50 mole percent of 22:6ω3. Mammalian outer segments have a similar fatty acid profile, containing 45-50 mole percent 22:6ω3.[2] Photoreceptor membranes are thought to be extremely susceptible to lipid peroxidation damage because of their high concentration of polyunsaturated fatty acids and an excellent oxygen supply.[3]

In order to effectively carry out experiments on the structure and function of retinal rod membranes, we found it essential to learn how to detect and control lipid peroxidation.[3] Initially, our principal experimental material was from cattle, because cattle retinas are large and abundantly available. After considerable difficulty with unstable properties of isolated rod retinal photoreceptor membrane preparations, we noticed that the preparations were much less stable in the summer months.[3]

46

It was discovered that there was undetectable vitamin E in the cattle photoreceptors in the summertime and high levels in the winter season.[3] Low endogenous vitamin E was strongly correlated with the unstable membrane preparations.[3] This work was being done in California, where the cattle eat dry grass in the summer that is essentially devoid of vitamin E. We were surprised to see that the photoreceptor membranes apparently lost vitamin E so rapidly in the intact animal retina in the summer when the dietary intake was low. This might be explained, however, by the fact that photoreceptor membranes turn over rapidly and are completely replaced with new membranes approximately every ten days.[4]

The problems we experienced with the sensitivity of photoreceptor membrane preparations to peroxidation damage stimulated our interest in the potential relevance of vitamin E and other antioxidants in the health of animal and human retinas. Our laboratory embarked on a series of experiments where we fed rats antioxidant-deficient diets. We found retinal degeneration, photoreceptor cell death, and abnormalities in the retinal pigment epithelium adjacent to the retina in rats raised on vitamin E- and selenium-deficient diets.[5,6]

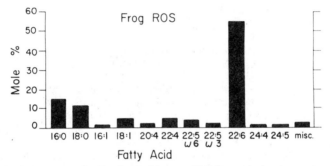

FIGURE 1. Mole percent of major fatty acids in purified frog retinal rod outer segment membranes. The membranes were highly purified with extensive precautions against loss of polyunsaturated fatty acids by oxidation.[2] The fatty acids were transesterfied with boron trifluoride in methanol and analyzed by GC on Supelco 2340.

The time that it takes for the retina to degenerate depends on the age of the animal at the time it was put on a vitamin E-deficient diet. FIGURE 2 shows the vitamin E depletion from the rat retina as a function of time for animals that were started on vitamin E-deficient diets at four different ages. The youngest animals start at somewhat lower levels of vitamin E in the retina and deplete most rapidly. Older animals build up a store of vitamin E that maintains the retinal vitamin E for longer periods of depletion. Adult rats show depletion of vitamin E in their retinas, although the depletion is much slower than we observed in the adult cattle rod outer segments. Different species apparently may show great differences in vitamin E metabolism and turnover. Retinal degeneration appears to start when the vitamin E level drops below about 20 ng/retina.[6-8] The degeneration is strongly aggravated by simultaneous deficiency of selenium,[7] another nutrient with antioxidant activity. The vitamin E distribution within microscopic regions of the retina and associated tissues has been recently studied in some detail by microdissection and gas chromatography-mass spectrometry (GC-MS) analysis of vitamin E.[8] It was found that the light-sensitive photoreceptor outer segments and the retinal pigment epithelium concentrate vitamin

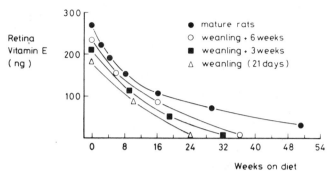

FIGURE 2. Loss of vitamin E from retinas of rats started on vitamin E-deficient diets at different ages. Weanling pigmented ACI rats were obtained from Maryland Microbiologicals and placed on vitamin E-deficient, corn oil-rich diets.[5] Animals were maintained on vitamin E-sufficient lab chow diets for the indicated time periods before switching to the deficient diets. Vitamin E was extracted with ethanol and 1% pyrogallol, followed by extraction with hexane in the presence of tocol internal standard, and analyzed by reverse phase HPLC.

E substantially relative to surrounding tissues.[8] The same regions in the eye that concentrate vitamin E also degenerate first in vitamin E and selenium deficiency[5-7] and must therefore be especially dependent on its antioxidant protection.

Interest in the role of lipid peroxidation as a causative agent in a variety of degenerative diseases has been growing rapidly in recent years.[9] Little progress, however, has been made in understanding the molecular mechanism of tissue degeneration in any of these diseases. In our opinion, the widespread reliance on the thiobarbituric acid (TBA) test for lipid peroxidation has been a major limitation to progress. The TBA test is convenient but is subject to interference and can be misleading.[10] We judged that more progress might be made if improved methods were developed to measure lipid peroxides and lipid peroxide breakdown products in tissues, and to identify their molecular structures. Erik van Kuijk began to work in the Dratz lab to develop such improved methods using GC-MS as a medical school project in 1984. The GC-MS approaches developed were found to be very powerful, and the work to be described here is largely the result of efforts by Dr. Van Kuijk with the collaboration of Dr. David Thomas at SRI International.

OVERVIEW OF METHODOLOGY

TABLE 1 summarizes the approach developed to identify and measure peroxidized lipids by GC-MS. Synthetic phospholipids, containing polyunsaturated fatty acids, were photooxidized, and the peroxidized products were characterized using a variety of methods.[11,12] Phospholipid peroxide standards are prepared in organic solvents, or mixtures of oxidized lipids are extracted from tissue samples with a modified Bligh and Dyer method.[11] The extraction method was modified to use dichloromethane instead of chloroform, which increased the recovery of the lipid peroxides, probably because $CCl_3\cdot$ radicals are generated in chloroform and not in dichlormethane.[13]

After organic solvent extraction, the peroxide functions are stabilized by reduction to alcohols with sodium borohydride. The vast majority of polyunsaturated fatty acids in biological membranes are esterified in phospholipids and triglycerides. Therefore, a gentle method was adapted to transesterify fatty acids in the complex lipids to form methyl esters[12] or pentafluorobenzyl esters.[12] The polar alcohol functions produced by reduction of the peroxides are formed into trimethylsilyl ethers and separated by capillary gas chromatography before being analyzed by mass spectrometry. (See FIG. 5 for the derivatization method used to introduce pentafluorobenzyl (PFB) esters.)

The method indicated does not form volatile esters from any free fatty acids that may be present. Therefore oxidized free fatty acids, which are largely products of enzymatic prostanoid metabolism, are not detected in the usual form of our assays. Simple modifications can be made to analyze free fatty acids and their oxidized products, if so desired.[14-16]

Four oxidized isomers are formed by photooxidation of linoleic acid ($18:2\omega$). These isomers fragment by electron ionization (EI) in the mass spectrometer, as shown in FIGURE 3. The total ion current in the mass spectrometer that results when the photooxidized phospholipid 16:0, 18:2 phosphatidylcholine is analyzed is shown in FIGURE 4a. The two oxidized fatty acid peaks are each shown to contain two nonconjugated and two conjugated derivatives. The mass spectrum of the unconjugated derivatives is shown in FIGURE 3a, and the mass spectrum of the conjugated derivatives is shown in FIGURE 3b.

Adipose tissue isolated from rats deficient in vitamin E and selenium was processed as described above and analyzed for oxidized lipids. FIGURE 4b shows that conjugated peroxidized fatty acids are detected, whereas unconjugated proxidized fatty acids are absent. The presence of these compounds is confirmed by their characteristic fragments in the mass spectrum shown in FIGURE 3c. The presence of conjugated fatty acid peroxides indicates that free radical catalyzed lipid peroxidation occurs in vivo in the antioxidant-deficient rats. Oxidized lipids could not be detected in vitamin E- and selenium-supplemented rat adipose using the methyl ester method, which has about 10 ng sensitivity.

The use of PFB esters provides about a 1000-fold increase in sensitivity (10 pg detection limit) (TABLE 1) compared to the methyl esters because the PFB esters allow effective use of the highly sensitive negative ion chemical ionization (NICI)

TABLE 1. Summary of Techniques Developed in the Course of This Study

	Methyl Ester[11,24]	PFB Ester[12]	PFB Oxime[22]
Substrate specificity		Fatty acid hydroperoxides Hydroxy fatty acids 9-oxononanoate	4-hydroxyalkenals alkanals alkenals
Detection limit	10 ng	1-10 pg	10-100 pg
MS Detection	EI[a]	NICI[b]	NICI
Main Ion	Fragments	M-H	M-PFB-HOTMS
Application	Adipose	All tissues	All tissues
GC Detection	FID[c]	ECD[d]	ECD

[a] Electron ionization
[b] NICI = Negative Ion Chemical Ionization
[c] FID = Flame Ionization Detection
[d] ECD = Electron Capture Detection

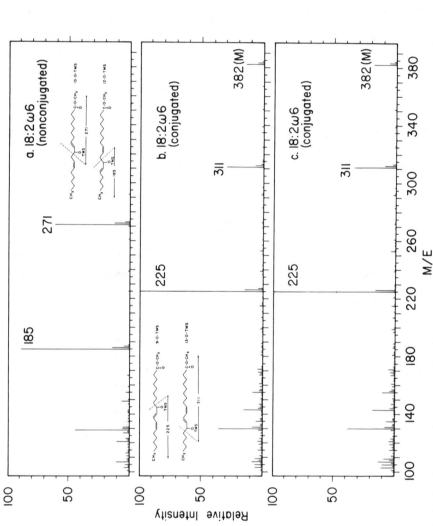

FIGURE 3. Electron ionization fragmentation patterns of the nonconjugated and conjugated oxidized linoleic acid O-TMS derivatives are shown in mass spectra a and b, respectively. These mass spectra are derived from the total ion chromatagram shown in FIGURE 4. Mass spectra were found at the maximum of peaks a and b in FIGURE 4, and mass spectrum c was obtained from peak c in lower panel, FIGURE 4.

method in the mass spectrometer. Using the PFB esters and NICI, we are able to detect traces of peroxidized fatty acids in the adipose of vitamin E-supplemented rats, but the levels are obviously much lower than in the vitamin E-deficient rats investigated.

The formation of the PFB esters is shown in FIGURE 5. The use of the PFB

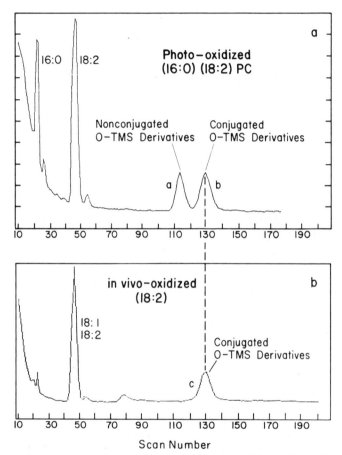

FIGURE 4. Total ion chromatograms of upper panel, photooxidized 16:0, 18:2PC standard; and lower panel, extract of vitamin E-deficient rat adipose tissue. Samples were prepared as described in the text and were separated on 5 meter DB-5 capillary columns to favor product recovery.

ester-NICI method reveals oxidized lipids in all other tissues investigated, in vitamin E-deficient, as well as in vitamin E-supplemented and lab chow-fed rats. An example of oxidized $18:2\omega3$ and oxidized $22:6\omega3$ is shown in rat retinas taken from vitamin E-deficient rats (FIGURE 6). FIGURE 6a shows an NICI GC-MS analysis using specific ion monitoring for oxidized linoleate PFB esters in a vitamin E-deficient rat retina.

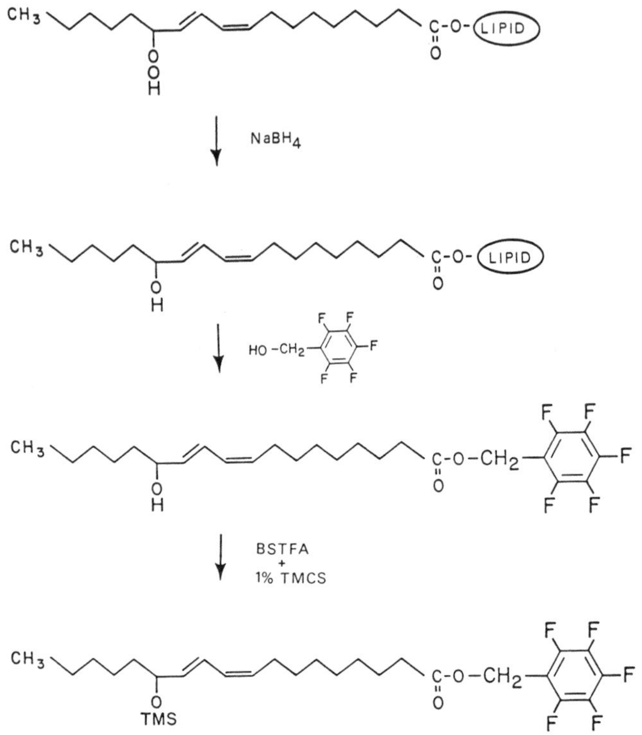

FIGURE 5. Schematic procedure for the complete derivatization and preparation of PFB esters of oxidized fatty acids for high sensitivity NICI GC-MS analysis of oxidized lipids.

The contribution of the nonconjugated products of linoleic acid is limited (peak 1 in FIGURE 6a), as discussed below.

It is surprising that the conjugated derivatives of linoleic acid (peaks 2-4) are not concentrated in one peak, but that the later eluting trans-trans stereoisomers (peaks 3 and 4), near scan numbers 174 and 180, which are weak in *in vitro* photooxidized lipids,[12] appear to be abundant in *in vivo* oxidized lipids.

FIGURE 6b shows a similar analysis for oxidized docosahexanoate-(22:6ω3). The major peak at scan number 254 (peak 5) is a mixture of conjugated and nonconjugated derivatives. The broader peaks at scan numbers 264 and 278 are a mixture of conjugated isomers. The two early eluting peaks at scan numbers 115 and 150 are impurities.

Similar chromatographic traces, as those shown in FIGURE 6, are obtained from animals from the supplemented, deficient, and chow-fed dietary groups. Lipid peroxidation products were detected in vitamin E-supplemented retinas, which indicates that lipid peroxides are formed during normal physiology, and that those normal levels can be detected with the PFB ester method. Preliminary semiquantitative analysis for lipid peroxides was attempted using endogenous arachidic acid (20:0) as reference. The 20:0 was used as an internal reference because it occurs *in vivo* at levels similar to the oxidation products. The tissue contents of 20:0 have not been well-characterized, and it is not clear whether it is endogenous to the retina or whether its presence is due to contamination with blood. This approach did not yield reproducible results, and it was abandoned.

The analysis of *in vivo* oxidized rat retinal lipids shows that there may be contributions of singlet oxygen reactions because of the occurrence of relatively low concentrations of nonconjugated lipid oxidation products. This analysis is difficult to address with certainty from these initial studies, however. A small amount of nonconjugated linoleate oxidation products was detectable in the rat retina *in vivo* (peak 1 in FIGURE 6a). Interestingly, the retina contains very little linoleic acid, and that which is present is primarily localized in the retinal pigment epithelium. Therefore, perhaps virtually all of the oxidized linoleic acid found in the retina might come from cross-contamination from the retinal pigment epithelium.

The different oxidation products from the most abundant fatty acid, docosahexaenoic acid, are not well-resolved with the low resolution chromatographic conditions employed. In addition, the resolution between conjugated and nonconjugated oxidation products of docosahexaenoic acid is limited, so the contribution of singlet oxygen-mediated oxidation to retina damage remains difficult to establish at this time. The nonconjugated and conjugated oxidation products from arachidonic acid are well-separated, but the retina has a low content of this fatty acid, as compared to the pigment epithelium. Separation of the nonconjugated and conjugated oxidation products from docosahexaenoic acid will require the use of higher resolution (longer) GC columns, despite the risk of decreased yield.[12]

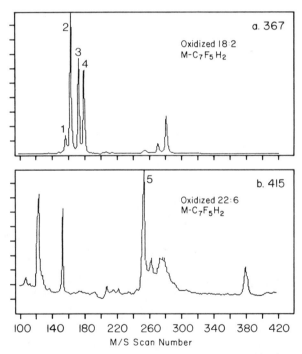

FIGURE 6. PFB ester analysis of peroxidized 22:6 fatty acid esters extracted from vitamin E-deficient rat retinas. The samples were prepared as described in the text and were analyzed by NICI GC-MS using ammonia reagent gas.

Experiments to date suggest that oxidized lipids are elevated in vitamin E deficiency, but quantitative comparison of different tissues and of the effect of vitamin E deficiency must await current developments using isotopically enriched internal standard fatty acids. The NICI method can use deuterium-labeled fatty acids, but carbon-13 or oxygen-18 labels appear to be preferable.[16–18] The use of deuterium-labeled stable isotope internal standards has been successful in our hands for analysis of the 4-hydroxyalkenals as described below.

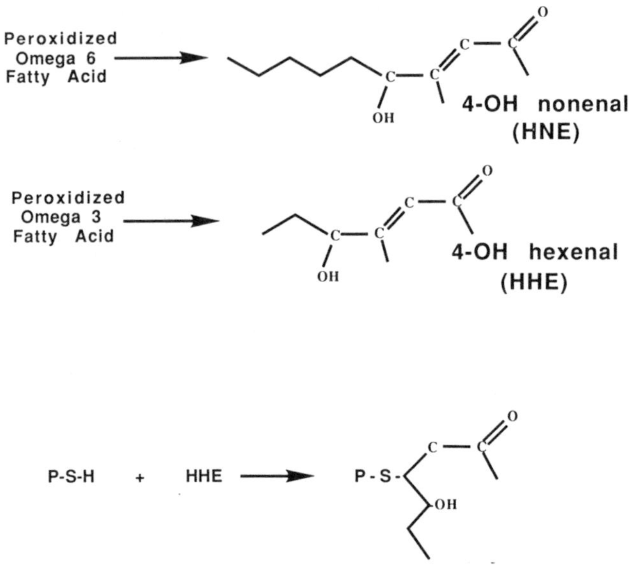

FIGURE 7. A new concept has recently been proposed that explains the mechanism of cellular damage due to lipid peroxides. The FIGURE is a schematic explanation of the formation of 4-hydroxynonenal from oxidized omega-6 fatty acids and the formation of 4-hydroxyhexenal from oxidized omega-3 fatty acids (two top reactions). These compounds irreversibly inactivate protein sulfhydryl groups at very low levels. The reaction of these compounds that inactivates protein sulfhydryl groups is also shown (bottom reaction). This reaction poisons transmembrane pumps and catabolic enzymes (such as cathepsins).

QUANTITATIVE ANALYSIS OF 4-HYDROXYALKENALS USING DEUTERATED INTERNAL STANDARDS

The 4-hydroxyalkenals are major decomposition products of oxidized polyunsaturated fatty acids, which have been reported to be specific chemical indicators of lipid peroxidation.[19,20] The 4-hydroxyalkenals have a number of powerful biological activities, such as inhibition of enzymes,[20] inhibition of calcium regulation by microsomes,[21] and reactivity with protein sulfhydryl groups.[19] FIGURE 7 shows the decomposition of oxidized omega-6 fatty acids to form 4-hydroxynonenal. The decomposition of oxidized omega-3 fatty acids is thought to form 4-hydroxyhexanal, but this has not been proven as yet. The chemical structure formed when these alkenals inactivate protein sulfhydryl groups is shown at the bottom of FIGURE 7.

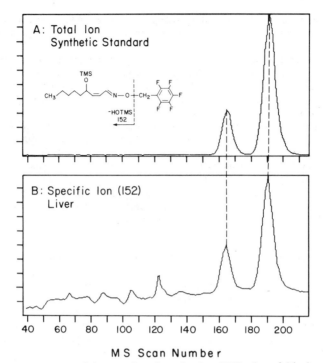

FIGURE 8. The structure of the pentafluorobenzyl oxime TMS ether of 4-hydroxynonenal is shown at the top together with NICI GC-MS traces of the strongest specific ions for an authentic standard and for an extract of rat liver.

We have developed a highly sensitive and specific GC-MS method for detection and analysis of 4-hydroxyalkenals, using NICI methods, which has about 10 pg sensitivity.[22] The method forms an O-pentafluorobenzyl oxime from the aldehyde function, as shown in FIGURE 8, followed by formation of trimethylsilyl (TMS) ethers from the alcohol functions. GC traces on nonpolar stationary phases contain two characteristic peaks for each oxime due to syn/anti isomerism around the oxime bond. This pair of peaks, in a characteristic intensity ratio favoring the syn (trans) form, is a diagnostic feature of the method that helps guard against artifactual peaks. It is theoretically possible that some other substance in the tissue overlaps with 4-hydroxyalkenal in the GC trace, and there is a distant possibly that they could also form ions with the same molecular weight. It is extremely unlikely, however, that such compounds would also have the syn/anti pair of peaks that are characteristic of the oximes analyzed.

FIGURE 9 explains how isotopic internal standards are used in GC-MS for quantitative analysis. The principal specific ions are accompanied by natural abundance

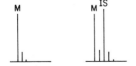

FIGURE 9. Typical spectrum obtained from a mixture of a compound (M) and its dideuterated (M + 2) internal standard (IS).

carbon-13 satellites to higher mass, as shown by the schematic mass spectrum on the left side of FIGURE 9. Known amounts of isotopically labeled internal standards are added to the extraction mixture at the beginning of the analysis. A typical mass spectrum in the presence of an M + 2 standard (*e.g.* dideuterated a di C-13 substituted) is shown on the right side of FIGURE 9. The peak height of the parent mass peak of the unknown is measured, and the M + 2 satellite height is calculated and subtracted from the M + 2 internal standard peak. Any losses in extraction, derivatization, chromatography, or changing mass spectrometer sensitivity factors are reflected in both the internal standard and the unknown. Therefore, the amount of the unknown can be determined as a simple ratio from the known amount of internal standard used in the original extraction. This assumes that the isotope labels are not scrambled in the mass spectrometer, which certainly does not occur for C-13 and is a reasonably safe assumption for aliphatic deuteriums.

Data for the analysis of 4-hydroxynonenal in the vitamin E-deficient rat retina are shown in FIGURE 10 where specific ion monitoring has been carried out for the specific 4-OH-nonenal fragment at 152 atomic mass units (amu) and for the same fragment in the dideuterated internal standard that appears at 154 amu. The 4-hydroxyalkenals are elevated in rat retinas that are degenerating due to vitamin E deficiency as shown in FIGURE 11. Similar experiments were carried out in dogs that were extremely sensitive to retinal degeneration due to vitamin E deficiency.[23] Very similar elevations of 4-hydroxynonenal were found in the vitamin E-deficient dog retina as shown in FIGURE 11. Therefore, the association of elevated 4-hydroxynonenal with retinal degeneration is not species-specific. Even larger elevations in 4-hydroxyhexenal appear to be present in the degenerating retina, which is consistent with the high levels of omega-3 fatty acids in the tissues, but truly quantitative measurements for the 4-hydroxynonenal have not been completed as yet.

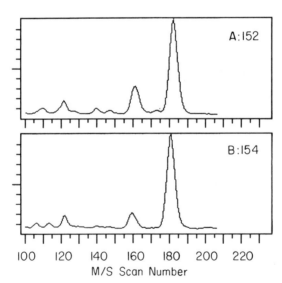

FIGURE 10. NICI GC-MS analysis of 4-hydroxynonenal in vitamin E-deficient rat retinas using double bond dideuterated 4-hydroxynonenal as an internal standard. The upper trace shows specific ion monitoring for the unknown at 152 amu, and the lower trace shows specific ion monitoring for the dideuterated internal standard at 154 amu.

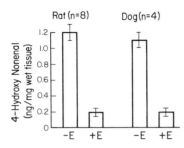

FIGURE 11. Histogram showing the amount of 4-hydroxynonenal isolated from vitamin E-deficient and vitamin E-supplemented rat and dog retinas. The dots above the bars show the standard deviations of the assays. Three retinas were analyzed in duplicate from four different animals in the case of the rats, and retinas were analyzed in duplicate from three different animals in the case of the dogs.

We initially expected to find larger elevations in 4-hydroxyalkenals in degenerating retinas than we observed in FIGURE 11. Much more may be present than we are detecting because our current extraction procedure does not appear to be recovering 4-hydroxyhexanal alkenals that are bound to protein sulfhydryl groups. The relevant 4-hydroxyalkenal chemistry is shown in FIGURE 12. The analytical procedure adds an O-substituted hydroxylamine, which extracts both free aldehydes and Schiff's-base bound aldehydes as oximes as shown on the left side of FIGURE 12. Another fraction of the 4-hydroxyalkenals is bound to protein sulfhydryl groups, as shown on the right side of FIGURE 12. These groups are not efficiently recovered by our current extraction procedures. It appears in work with tritium-labeled 4-hydroxynonenal bound to pure proteins or to cell homogenates from which we are recovering only a fraction of the total 4-hydroxynonenal present. Therefore, the nonenal recovered to date may just be the "tip of the iceberg". Work is actively in progress to modify the method to quantitatively cleave the carbon-sulfur bond to obtain quantitative or near quantitative recovery of the 4-hydroxyalkenals. We expect that this will be complete in the near future and that more detailed studies of the mechanism of involvement of the alkenals in degenerative disease can begin.

SUMMARY OF TECHNIQUES USED IN THE COURSE OF THESE STUDIES

TABLE 1 summarizes the methyl and PFB ester methods for detection of lipid peroxides in tissues. The methyl ester method is suited for analysis of lipid peroxides in adipose tissues because these appear to be depots for the lipid peroxides.[24] The PFB ester method is useful for all tissues because of its picogram sensitivity. Routine use of the PFB method for quantitative analysis will soon be possible after final development of isotopic internal standard methods are complete. The PFB-oxime method can be used for all aldehyde products of lipid peroxidation and is now being used for high sensitivity quantitative studies because we have synthesized deuterated internal standards that we have found adequate for quantitative NICI MS studies. Improvements in progress in the 4-hydroxyalkenal studies involve methods to accomplish recovery of the fraction of the compounds that are bound to protein sulfhydryl groups. It is anticipated that these new tools will allow much more penetrating investigations of antioxidant status and the role of lipid peroxidation in degenerative disease.

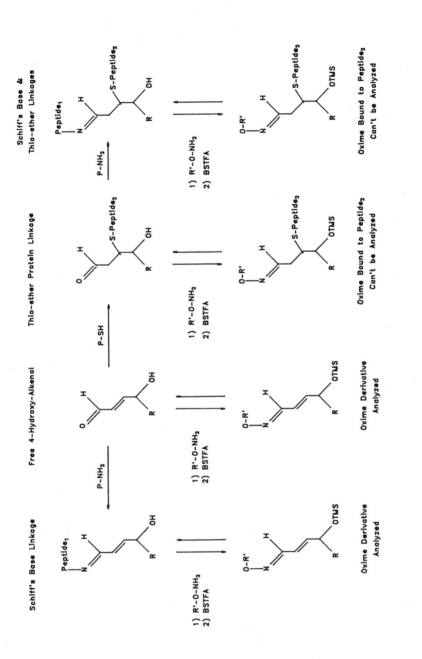

FIGURE 12. Reactions of 4-hydroxynonenal with protein amino (part A) and sulfhydryl groups (part C). Part D shows the cross-linking of proteins that can occur by sequential reaction of one molecule of 4-hydroxynonenal with amino and sulfhydryl groups.

REFERENCES

1. DRATZ, E. A., J. E. GAW, S. SCHWARTZ & W. CHING. 1972. The molecular organization of the photoreceptor membranes of rod outer segments. Nature New Biol. **237:** 99-102.
2. STONE, W. L., C. C. FARNSWORTH & E. A. DRATZ. 1979. A reinvestigation of the fatty acid content of bovine, rat and frog outer segments. Exp. Eye Res. **28:** 387-397.
3. FARNSWORTH, C. C. & E. A. DRATZ. 1976. Oxidative damage of retinal rod outer segment membranes and the role of vitamin E. Biochim. Biophys. Acta **443:** 556-570.
4. YOUNG, R. W. 1967. The renewal of rod and cone outer segments. J. Cell Biol. **33:** 61-72.
5. KATZ, M. L., W. L. STONE & E. A. DRATZ. 1978. Fluorescent pigment accumulation in retinal pigment epithelium of antioxidant-deficient rats. Invest. Opthalmol. Vis. Sci. **17:** 1049-1058.
6. KATZ, M. L., K. R. PARKER, G. J. HANDELMAN, T. L. BRAMEL & E. A. DRATZ. 1982. Effects of antioxidant nutrient deficiency on the retina and pigment epithelium of albino rats: a light and electron microscopic study. Exp. Eye Res. **34:** 339, 369.
7. KATZ, M. L., K. R. PARKER, G. J. HANDELMAN, C. C. FARNSWORTH & E. A. DRATZ. 1982. Structural and biochemical effects of antioxidant nutrient deficiency on the rat retina and retinal pigment epithelium. Ann. N.Y. Acad. Sci. **393:** 196-197.
8. STEPHENS, R. J., D. S. NEGI, S. SHORT, E. A. DRATZ & D. W. THOMAS. 1988. Vitamin E distribution in ocular tissues resulting from long-term depletion and supplementation as determined by gas chromatography-mass spectrometry. Exp. Eye Res. **47:** 237-245.
9. MARX, J. L. 1987. Oxygen free radicals linked to many diseases. Science **235:** 529-531.
10. VAN KUIJK, F. J. G. M. & H. SIES. 1988. Lipid peroxidation terminology: Thiobarbituric (TBA) or total tissue aldehyde (TTA) test. Unpublished results.
11. VAN KUIJK, F. J. G. M., D. W. THOMAS, R. J. STEPHENS & E. A. DRATZ. 1985. Gas chromatography-mass spectrometry method for determination of phospholipid peroxides I: transesterification to form methyl esters. J. Free Radic. Biol. Med. **1:** 215-225.
12. VAN KUIJK, F. J. G. M., D. W. THOMAS, R. J. STEPHENS & E. A. DRATZ. 1985. Gas chromatography-mass spectrometry method for determination of phospholipid peroxides II: transesterification to form pentafluorobenzyl esters and detection with picogram sensitivity. J. Free Radic. Biol. Med. **1:** 387-393.
13. RECKNAGEL, R. O., E. A. CLENDE & A. M. HRUSZKEWYCZ. 1977. Chemical mechanisms in carbon tetrachloride toxicity. *In* Free radicals in biology. W. A. Pryor, Ed. **3:** 97-132. Academic Press. New York.
14. STRIFE, R. J. & R. C. MURPHY. 1984. Preparation of pentafluorobenzyl esters of arachidonic acid lipoxygenase metabolites. Analysis by gas chromatography and negative-ion chemical ionization mass-spectrometry. J. Chromatogr. **305:** 3-12.
15. VAN KUIJK, F. J. G. M., D. W. THOMAS, J. P. KONOPELSKI & E. A. DRATZ. 1986. Transesterification of phospholipids or triglycerides to fatty acid benzyl esters with simultaneous methylation of free fatty acids for gas-liquid chromatographic analysis. J. Lipid Res. **27:** 452-456.
16. STRIFE, R. J. & R. C. MURPHY. 1984. Stable isotope labelled 5-lipoxygenase metabolites of arachidonic acid: Analysis by negative ion chemical ionization mass spectrometry. Prostaglandins, Leukotrienes Med. **13:** 1-8.
17. ROHWEDDER, W. K. 1985. Mass spectrometry of lipids labelled with stable isotopes. Prog. Lipid Res. **24:** 1-18.
18. FRANK, H., W. WIEGAND, M. STRECKER & D. THIEL. 1987. Monohydroperoxides of linoleic acid in endoplasmic lipids of rats exposed to tetrachloromethane. Lipids **22:** 689-697.
19. ESTERBAUER, H. 1982. Aldehydic products of lipid peroxidation. *In* Free Radicals, Lipid Peroxidation, and Cancer. D. C. H. McBrien & T. F. Slater, Eds.: 101-128. Academic Press. London.
20. SCHAUENSTEIN, E. 1967. Autooxidation of polyunsaturated esters in water: Chemical structure and biological activity of the products. J. Lipid Res. **8:** 417-428.
21. BENEDETTI, A., R. FULCERI & M. COMPORTI. 1984. Inhibition of calcium sequestration activity of liver microsomes by 4-hydroxyalkenals originating from the peroxidation of liver microsomal lipids. Biochim. Biophys. Acta **793:** 489-493.

22. VAN KUIJK, F. J. G. M., D. W. THOMAS, R. J. STEPHENS & E. A. DRATZ. 1986. Occurrence of 4-hydroxyalkenals in rat tissues determined as pentafluorobenzyl oxime derivatives by gas chromatography-mass spectrometry. Biochem. Biophys. Res. Comm. **139:** 144-149.
23. RIIS, R. C., B. E. SHEFFY, E. R. LOEW, T. J. KERN & J. S. SMITH. 1981. Vitamin E deficiency retinopathy in dogs. Am. J. Vet. Res. **42:** 74-86.
24. VAN KUIJK, F. J. G. M., D. W. THOMAS, R. J. STEPHENS & E. A. DRATZ. 1988. Lipid peroxidation products in subcutaneous adipose associated with vitamin E deficiency measured by gas chromatography-mass spectrometry. *In* Lipid peroxidation in biological systems. A. Sevanian, Ed.: 117-129. American Oil Chemist Society. Champaign, IL.

The Role of the Low Density Lipoprotein Receptor for α-Tocopherol Delivery to Tissues

W. COHN AND H. KUHN

Departments of Vitamin and Nutrition Research and Pharmaceutical Research
F. Hoffmann-La Roche and Company Ltd.
Grenzacherstrasse 124
CH-4002 Basle, Switzerland

INTRODUCTION

α-Tocopherol (vitamin E) is transported in blood within plasma lipoproteins.[1,2] In humans and in animals, α-tocopherol is distributed among all of the lipoproteins with a large portion either in the low density lipoprotein (LDL) or in the high density lipoprotein (HDL) fraction.[3-5] Recently, the high-affinity receptor for LDL has been recognized to function as a mechanism for delivery of α-tocopherol to fibroblasts in culture.[6,7] Uptake and degradation of LDL occurs, however, only in part by the specific LDL receptor first described by Goldstein and co-workers.[8] In addition, LDL can be taken up and degraded by receptor-independent processes.[9] In normal animals and normal humans, both mechanisms may be operating simultaneously. Accordingly, the LDL-specific receptor pathway is not the only mechanism for α-tocopherol transport from LDL to fibroblasts,[6,7] though the majority of the α-tocopherol enters the cells with the intact lipoprotein particle. Receptor-independent delivery of α-tocopherol to tissues may be relevant for patients homozygous for the receptor-negative form of familial hypercholesterolemia. These patients do not manifest any symptoms of vitamin E deficiency, though the LDL receptor is absent. Presently little is known about the contribution of the LDL receptor pathway in the delivery of α-tocopherol to tissues. To further understand the role of the LDL receptor pathway for the maintenance of α-tocopherol concentrations in tissues of intact animals, we have used an animal model for homozygous familial hypercholesterolemia, the Watanabe heritable hyperlipidemic (WHHL) rabbit.[10] WHHL rabbits are homozygous for a mutant allele that produces an LDL receptor that is of apparent normal molecular size but is transported to the cell surface at only one-tenth the normal rate.[11] We have compared α-tocopherol levels in plasma and in tissues of normal and WHHL rabbits. Our results demonstrate the importance of the LDL receptor pathway for vitamin E clearance in the normal rabbit, although at high LDL concentrations alternative mechanisms may become more efficient for the delivery of vitamin E to tissues.

METHODS

Animals

All experiments were performed with male, normal Burgundy (KOBU) or pure-bred WHHL rabbits. The WHHL rabbits were from a colony bred from two pairs of WHHL rabbits kindly provided by Dr. Watanabe. The animals were housed individually with free access to water and a commercial diet (normal rabbit chow: Nafag 814, Nafag Ltd., Gossau, Switzerland) containing 40 mg vitamin E (all-rac-α-tocopheryl acetate) per kilogram. At the age of 100, 200, or 450 days, animals were anesthetized with Nembutal. A catheter was implanted into the carotid artery, and blood samples were collected in EDTA tubes. The thoracic aorta was ligated directly after the arch, and a cannula was inserted in the direction of the blood flow. Blood vessels were perfused at 80 mm Hg with phosphate-buffered saline, pH 7.4, for 15 minutes, and simultaneously animals were exsanguinated through the carotid catheter. Discrete organs were then removed and weighed, and muscle and adipose tissues were sampled. Immediately after separation of the plasma, a mixture of preservatives in solution (pH 7.0) was added to obtain final concentrations of 100 μg/mL gentamycin sulfate (Sigma), 0.1 μg/mL trypsin inhibitor (Sigma), 1 mM 1,4-dithioerythrite, 0.2 mM phenylmethanesulfonylfluoride, 1 mM EDTA, and 0.05% NaN$_3$. Plasma and tissues were frozen and kept under argon at $-70°$ C for later analysis.

Preparation of Lipoproteins

For lipoprotein analysis, plasma samples from each rabbit strain were mixed, and the density (d) of the pooled plasma was increased with NaBr to d 1.21 g/mL. In order to compensate for the differing lipid contents in the plasma of normal and WHHL rabbits,[12] three samples each of 2 mL for normal and 1 mL for WHHL rabbits, respectively, were subjected simultaneously to preparative ultracentrifugation at 16° C. The lipoproteins ($d \leq 1.21$ g/mL) were isolated by flotation[13] through buffer (pH 7.5) containing 10 mM Tris, 1 mM EDTA, 1 mM 1,4-dithioerythrite, 0.2 mM phenylmethanesulfonylfluoride, 0.05% NaN$_3$, and 10 mM ε-amino-n-caproic acid (buffer A) adjusted to d 1.21 (g/mL) with NaBr. After ultracentrifugation in a Kontron TGA 65 using a Kontron TST 41.14 rotor at 38,000 rpm for 25 hours, the floating lipoproteins were recovered by tube slicing. Lipoprotein samples were adjusted to 2 mL before they were applied to density gradient ultracentrifugation. An automatic gradient maker (Mico Desaga) allowed the preparation of six identical NaBr density gradients in buffer A. Concave gradients (8 mL) from d 1.000-1.21 g/mL were produced in each tube using a two-jars gradient generator. The gradient was successively underlayered with buffer A adjusted to d 1.21 g/mL with NaBr and 2 mL of the previously isolated lipoproteins. For each rabbit strain, three lipoprotein samples were centrifuged simultaneously with a Kontron TST 41.14 rotor at 38,000 rpm for 24 hours at 16° C. Tubes were punctured with a Mico perforator; the gradient was displaced at a constant flow rate with a solution of 5.6 M NaBr, and fractions of 190 μL were collected. For each rabbit strain, analogous lipoprotein fractions were pooled before they were analyzed for α-tocopherol, cholesterol, triglycerides, phospholipids, and protein, as described below. The density of the fractions was determined in a Paar densitometer (DMA 35, Paar, Graz, Austria).

Analytical Methods

Protein in tissues and lipoprotein fractions was quantitated by the method of Markwell et al.[14] using bovine serum albumin as a reference standard. Cholesterol and triglyceride concentrations were determined enzymatically[15,16] using commercial kits (Roche Diagnostica, Switzerland). Total phospholipids were assayed as described by Cook and Daughton.[17] α-Tocopherol and retinol concentrations were determined by high-performance liquid chromatography (HPLC).[18] For the analysis of α-tocopherol, phospholipids, and protein in the lipoprotein fractions, aliquots for precipitation with trichloroacetic acid (5.8%), sodium phosphotungstate (0.3%), and $MgCl_2$ (0.154 M). After centrifugation, the sediment was washed twice with 1 N HCl at 4° C and extracted with chloroform-methanol 2 : 1 (v/v). These extracts were used for phospholipid determinations, whereas the protein residues were dried and dissolved in 0.1 N NaOH containing 1% sodium dodecyl sulfate for protein analysis. To assay α-tocopherol, precipitated lipoproteins were dissolved in 0.5 M sodium citrate, and α-tocopherol was extracted with ethanol and hexane as described.[18]

Discrete organs and tissue samples were rinsed with phosphate buffered saline, pH 7.4, before they were homogenized at 4° C with a Virtis Modell 6303 homogenizer. Homogenized tissues (300 mg wet weight) were lyophilized to apparent dryness (i.e. negligible weight loss when lyophilization was continued for another 24 hours) and extracted twice with 2 mL of hexane-isopropanol 3 : 2 (v/v) containing butylated hydroxytoluene (250 μg/mL). Extraction was promoted by sonication (5 × 30 s) at 4° C. After centrifugation, the sediment was dried under nitrogen, and tissue protein was solubilized in 0.1 N NaOH containing 1% sodium dodecyl sulfate. Aliquots of the combined hexane-isopropanol extracts were dried under nitrogen and dispersed in 10 mM Tris buffer, pH 7.4, containing 150 mM NaCl and 1 mM EDTA prior to the enzymatic determination of cholesterol and triglyceride. α-Tocopherol dissolved in hexane was determined by HPLC analysis. Unless stated otherwise, the results are expressed as means ± 1 SD. The significance of differences between mean values was calculated by the Student's t test.

RESULTS

α-Tocopherol Concentrations in Plasma and Lipoproteins

Plasma concentrations of α-tocopherol, triglycerides, and cholesterol were consistently 6 to 12 times higher in WHHL rabbits as compared to normal rabbits (FIG. 1). For both α-tocopherol and triacylglycerol, plasma levels in WHHL rabbits decreased with animal age, whereas the cholesterol status was maintained. Further studies were performed with rabbits at the age of 200 days. At this age, plasma α-tocopherol, cholesterol, triacylglycerol, and phospholipid concentrations in WHHL rabbits were elevated to ten times normal levels. By contrast, the retinol plasma status was comparable in the two strains (TABLE 1). The distribution of α-tocopherol between the plasma lipoproteins of the two rabbit strains was investigated by gradient ultracentrifugation. Fractions were monitored for α-tocopherol, cholesterol, phospholipids, triacylglycerol, and apolipoprotein (data for the latter three components not presented) in order to define lipoprotein classes. As indicated by the cholesterol profile obtained from normal rabbit plasma, peak densities for LDL and HDL were 1.022 g/mL and 1.091 g/mL (FIG. 2). In normal rabbit plasma, α-tocopherol was confined mainly to HDL; in the LDL fraction, α-tocopherol levels were markedly lower. The α-tocopherol and cholesterol contents of very low density lipoprotein (VLDL) (d < 1.008 g/mL),

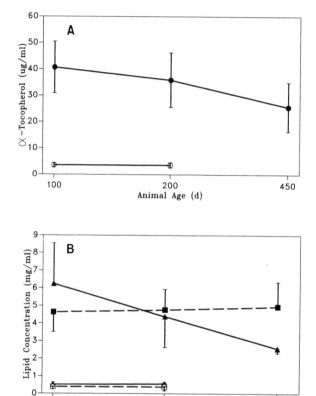

FIGURE 1. Concentrations of plasma lipids in three age groups. (**A**) α-Tocopherol levels in normal rabbits (○) and WHHL rabbits (●). (**B**) Levels of triacylglycerol in normal (△) and WHHL rabbits (▲) and cholesterol in normal (□) and WHHL rabbits (■). Values are means ± 1 SD for 5 rabbits.

intermediate density lipoprotein (IDL) (1.008–1.012 g/mL), and LDL (peak density 1.022 g/mL) in WHHL rabbits were much higher than in normal rabbits (note the different scales in FIGURES 2A and 2B for normal and WHHL rabbits). By contrast, α-tocopherol and cholesterol associated with HDL were found to be reduced.

TABLE 1. Rabbit Plasma Lipids[a]

Animals	α-Tocopherol (mg/L)	Retinol (mg/L)	Triglycerides (g/L)	Cholesterol (g/L)	Phospholipids (g/L)
Normal (N = 5)	3.57 ± 0.98	0.77 ± 0.22	0.57 ± 0.07	0.39 ± 0.22	0.43 ± 0.11
WHHL (N = 5)	35.96 ± 10.34[b]	0.68 ± 0.11	4.37 ± 1.77[b]	4.77 ± 1.16[b]	3.76 ± 0.91[b]

[a] Male rabbits of age 200 days were used; animal weights were 3.53 ± 0.16 kg for normal rabbits and 3.50 ± 0.77 kg for WHHL rabbits, respectively. N, number of animals.
[b] Significantly different from normal rabbits ($p < 0.005$).

α-Tocopherol Tissue Concentrations

Liver α-tocopherol concentrations in WHHL rabbits were not significantly different from those found in normal animals (TABLE 2), though mean concentrations were slightly higher in normal rabbits. Similar mean α-tocopherol concentrations were

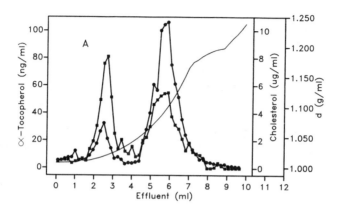

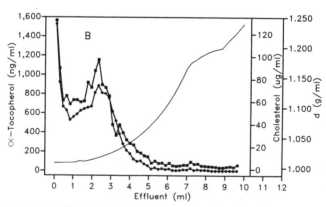

FIGURE 2. Density gradient ultracentrifugation of pooled plasma lipoproteins $d \leq 1.21$ g/mL. Lipid profiles for (**A**) normal and (**B**) WHHL rabbits. Concentrations of α-tocopherol (●) and cholesterol (■) are expressed per mL of the pooled plasma. The density gradient is represented by the continuous curve. Experimental details are described in the METHODS.

obtained when results were expressed per tissue lipid (0.51 μg/mg in normal vs 0.46 μg/mg in WHHL rabbits) or per protein (0.082 μg/mg in normal rabbits vs 0.079 μg/mg in WHHL rabbits). Inasmuch as tissue compositions in WHHL rabbits differed in several instances from those of normal animals, results (TABLE 2, FIG. 3) included lipid and protein concentrations and were expressed per milligram dry weight. In the adrenal, both α-tocopherol and cholesterol concentrations were significantly decreased

TABLE 2. Lipid and Protein Concentration of Rabbit Livers[a]

Animals	α-Tocopherol (ng/mg)	Triglycerides (μg/mg)	Cholesterol (μg/mg)	Phospholipids (μg/mg)	Protein (μg/mg)
Normal (N = 5)	46.16 ± 12.00	10.78 ± 4.86	6.62 ± 4.00	73.52 ± 14.93	561.00 ± 47.11
WHHL (N = 5)	36.96 ± 6.60	8.60 ± 3.30	12.53 ± 2.40[b]	59.66 ± 9.66	468.18 ± 67.33[b]

[a] Concentrations are expressed per mg dry weight. The values represent the means ± SD. N, number of animals.
[b] Significantly different from normal rabbits ($p < 0.05$).

in the WHHL mutant ($p < 0.05$), whereas total lipid and protein did not differ. By contrast, α-tocopherol and triacylglycerol levels in skeletal muscle and kidney of WHHL rabbits exceeded those of normal animals ($p < 0.05$). The α-tocopherol content of fat and testis was comparable in the two strains.

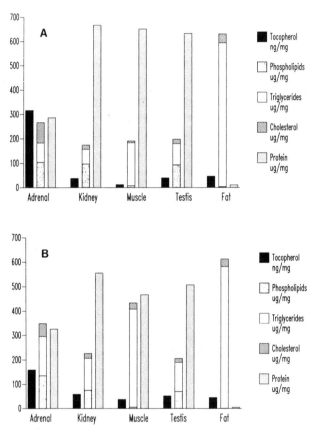

FIGURE 3. α-Tocopherol content of normal (**A**) and WHHL rabbit (**B**) tissues. Data are expressed per mg dry weight and are means for results obtained in 5 animals in each group.

DISCUSSION

In WHHL rabbits, which lack nearly all LDL receptor activity, plasma levels of α-tocopherol and major plasma lipids, that is, triglycerides, cholesterol, and phospholipids, were similarly elevated. By contrast, plasma retinol concentrations were found to be unchanged in comparison with those in normal animals (TABLE 1). Both vitamins A and E enter the circulation by way of the lymphatics within chylomicrons. In the plasma, however, retinol is transported by the retinol-binding protein,[19] whereas α-tocopherol is associated with the lipoproteins. In normal rabbits, α-tocopherol was confined mainly to HDL, the major lipoprotein fraction in rabbits,[20] and vitamin E levels in LDL were markedly lower. The α-tocopherol contents of VLDL, IDL, and LDL in WHHL rabbits were much higher than in normal rabbits. By contrast, α-tocopherol HDL levels in WHHL rabbits were found to be reduced. As for normal rabbits, α-tocopherol distribution among WHHL rabbit lipoproteins consistently paralleled the concentration profiles of the lipoproteins.

Taken together, these various observations suggest that in the WHHL rabbits, α-tocopherol plasma levels are raised as a consequence of the fact that the vitamin is transported as a component of the lipoproteins. Thus, the build-up of α-tocopherol in VLDL, IDL, and LDL fractions results from the receptor defect, which is analogous to the accumulation of a substrate behind a metabolic block.

In the WHHL rabbit, there is not only loss of LDL receptor activity, but in addition there is a 5.6-fold increase in the total metabolic production rate of LDL.[21] Moreover, these animals manifest a significant degree of hypertriglyceridemia (FIG. 1), suggesting the possibility that secretion of VLDL rather than LDL is increased. α-Tocopherol has been reported to be secreted from the liver in VLDL.[22,23] Hence, a coordinate release of α-tocopherol and VLDL might account for the finding of highly elevated α-tocopherol concentration in the VLDL fraction of the WHHL mutant (FIG. 2). In older WHHL animals, hypertriglyceridemia was somewhat diminished, and concomitantly, α-tocopherol plasma pools were lowered (FIG. 1). Because cholesterol plasma levels remained unchanged as the animals aged, the decrease in the triacylglycerol concentration is related to the portion of VLDL that is converted to LDL rather than, or as well as, to a change of hepatic VLDL secretion.

The findings in the WHHL rabbit demonstrate that an extremely high concentration of plasma α-tocopherol can be maintained in the face of a normal vitamin E diet. Under these conditions, the α-tocopherol contents of various tissues were normal or slightly elevated, except for the adrenal gland. High rates of LDL uptake occur in tissues like the liver and the endocrine glands due to the presence of significant amounts of receptor-dependent LDL transport.[24,25] In the present study, however, only the α-tocopherol content of the adrenal was found to be reduced in the WHHL mutant (FIG. 3), indicating that the comparatively high α-tocopherol steady state concentrations could not be maintained by nonreceptor means. Dietschy and co-workers[26] demonstrated that in the absence of LDL receptor activity, only the adrenal gland manifested a significantly higher rate of cholesterol synthesis, although cholesterol concentrations were still reduced in WHHL animals (FIG. 3). Thus, the adrenal gland was the only organ we could identify to actually rely on LDL uptake for supplying a portion of its α-tocopherol requirement. For normal rabbits, nearly 70% of the LDL was shown to be removed from the plasma by the liver, and 89% of this was receptor-mediated.[24] Nevertheless, the hepatic α-tocopherol content was only marginally lowered in the WHHL animals (FIG. 3), although in these animals the burden of LDL degradation is shifted away from the liver, with more than 70% of the LDL cholesterol being delivered to extrahepatic tissues.[24] In addition to uptake and degradation of LDL by the LDL receptor pathway, hepatic clearance of chylomicron remnants and HDL lipid is mediated by the apo E receptor and the HDL binding sites, respectively.[27-29] These mechanisms, combined with receptor-independent pathways, could all contribute in the delivery of α-tocopherol to liver and compensate for the lack of LDL receptor activity. For the receptor-independent LDL transport, the plasma clearance rate is constant.[24] Therefore, in WHHL rabbits, where LDL cholesterol concentrations are about 15-fold increased, the absolute clearance of LDL by receptor-independent pathways becomes much more efficient,[24] and some tissues acquire increased amounts of LDL because receptor-independent LDL uptake activity is distributed in nearly every organ in the body. In turn, this might even result in increased α-tocopherol concentrations in the WHHL rabbit and account for the elevated α-tocopherol and triacylglycerol content found in the kidney and the skeletal muscle. Despite the high concentration of plasma α-tocopherol, the tissue content in fat and testis remained unchanged.

The accumulation of α-tocopherol in the plasma as a result of LDL receptor deficiency suggests that delivery of the vitamin by the receptor pathway is important in the normal animal. Once the α-tocopherol plasma pool has built up, it can be maintained without increasing rates of intestinal absorption. Presently it is not clear how α-tocopherol steady state concentrations are adjusted in tissues. In this animal model for familial hypercholesterolemia, however, in the absence of LDL receptor activity, none of the tissues investigated was found to be vitamin E-deficient.

SUMMARY

To study the role of the LDL receptor pathway for the maintenance of α-tocopherol concentrations in tissues of intact animals, we have compared vitamin E levels in plasma and tissues of normal rabbits and WHHL rabbits. WHHL rabbits are deficient in LDL receptor activity. For WHHL rabbits, α-tocopherol plasma concentrations were elevated to 10 times normal levels. When plasma lipoprotein profiles were analyzed by density gradient centrifugation, concentrations of VLDL, IDL, and LDL were increased in WHHL rabbits, and plasma α-tocopherol was only recovered in these fractions. In normal rabbits, plasma α-tocopherol was confined mainly to the HDL fraction; levels associated with LDL were markedly lower. Despite LDL receptor deficiency, α-tocopherol concentrations in various tissues of WHHL rabbits were not found to be reduced, with the exception of the adrenal. Vitamin E levels in muscle and kidney of WHHL rabbits exceeded those of normal animals. Our results demonstrate the importance of the LDL receptor pathway for vitamin E clearance in the normal rabbit, although at high LDL concentrations, alternative mechanisms may become more efficient for the delivery of vitamin E to tissues.

ACKNOWLEDGMENTS

We gratefully acknowledge the excellent technical assistance of Francine Hoffmann. We thank Dr. Jochen Bausch (F. Hoffmann-La Roche & Co., Ltd., Basle) for analytical help with the α-tocopherol determinations.

REFERENCES

1. MACHLIN, L. J. 1984. *In* Handbook of Vitamins. L. J. Machlin, Ed.: 99-145. M. Dekker. New York.

2. GALLO-TORRES, H. E. 1980. *In* Vitamin E, a Comprehensive Treatise. L. J. Machlin, Ed.: 193-267. M. Dekker. New York.
3. BJORNSON, L. K., H. J. KAYDEN, E. MILLER & A. N. MOSHELL. 1976. J. Lipid Res. 17: 343-352.
4. PEAKE, I. R., H. G. WINDMUELLER & J. G. BIERI. 1972. Biochim. Biophys. Acta 260: 679-688.
5. BEHRENS, W. A., J. N. THOMPSON & R. MADÈRE. 1982. Am. J. Clin. Nutr. 35: 691-696.
6. TRABER, M. G. & H. J. KAYDEN. 1984. Am. J. Clin. Nutr. 40: 747-751.
7. THELLMAN, C. A. & R. B. SHIREMAN. 1985. J. Nutr. 115: 1673-1679.
8. GOLDSTEIN, J. L. & M. S. BROWN. 1977. Ann. Rev. Biochem. 46: 897-930.
9. GOLDSTEIN, J. L. & M. S. BROWN. 1977. Metabolism 16: 1257-1275.
10. WATANABE, Y. 1980. Atherosclerosis 36: 261-268.
11. SCHNEIDER, W. J., M. S. BROWN & J. L. GOLDSTEIN. 1983. Mol. Biol. Med. 1: 353-367.
12. TANZAWA, K., Y. SHIMADA, M. KURODA, Y. TSUJITA, M. ARAI & H. WATANABE. 1980. FEBS Lett. 118: 81-84.
13. HAVEL, R. J., H. A. EDER & J. H. BRAGDON. 1955. J. Clin. Invest. 34: 1345-1353.
14. MARKWELL, M. A. K., S. M. HAAS, L. L. BIEBER & N. E. TOLBERT. 1978. Anal. Biochem. 87: 206-210.
15. RICHMOND, W. 1973. Clin. Chem. 19: 1350-1356.
16. BUCOLO, G. & H. DAVID. 1973. Clin. Chem. 19: 476-482.
17. COOK, A. M. & CH. G. DAUGHTON. 1981. Methods Enzymol. 72: 292-295.
18. VUILLEUMIER, J.-P., H. E. KELLER, D. GYSEL & F. HUNZIKER. 1983. Int. J. Vit. Nutr. Res. 53: 265-272.
19. RASK, L., H. ANUNDI, J. BÖHME, U. ERIKSSON, A. FREDRIKSSON, S. F. NILSSON, H. RONNE, A. VAHLQUIST & P. A. PETERSON. 1980. Scand. J. Clin. Lab. Invest. 40 (Suppl. 154): 45-61.
20. WAKASUGI, T., H. MABUCHI, Y. SAKAI, T. SAKAI, A. YOSHIMURA, A. WATANABE, J. KOIZUMI, S. MIYAMOTO, R. TAKEDA & Y. WATANABE. 1984. J. Lipid Res. 25: 246-253.
21. BILHEIMER, D. W., Y. WATANABE & T. KITA. 1982. Proc. Natl. Acad. Sci. USA 79: 3305-3309.
22. COHN, W., F. LOECHLEITER & F. WEBER. 1988. J. Lipid Res. 29: 1359-1366.
23. BJØRNEBOE, A., G. E. BJØRNEBOE, B. F. HAGEN, J. O. NOSSEN & C. A. DREVON. 1987. Biochim. Biophys. Acta 922: 199-205.
24. SPADY, D. K., M. HUETTINGER, D. W. BILHEIMER & J. M. DIETSCHY. 1987. J. Lipid Res. 28: 32-41.
25. PITTMAN, R. C., T. E. CAREW, A. D. ATTIE, J. L. WITZTUM, Y. WATANABE & D. STEINBERG. 1982. J. Biol. Chem. 257: 7994-8000.
26. DIETSCHY, J. M., T. KITA, K. E. SUCKLING, J. L. GOLDSTEIN & M. S. BROWN. 1983. J. Lipid Res. 24: 469-480.
27. MAHLEY, R. W. & T. L. INNERARITY. 1983. Biochim. Biophys. Acta 737: 197-222.
28. GRAHAM, D. L. & J. F. ORAM. 1987. J. Biol. Chem. 262: 7439-7442.
29. PITTMAN, R. C., T. P. KNECHT, M. S. ROSENBAUM & C. A. TAYLOR, JR. 1987. J. Biol. Chem. 262: 2443-2450.

Relationship of Tocopherol Structure to Biological Activity, Tissue Uptake, and Prostaglandin Biosynthesis[a]

ANTHONY T. DIPLOCK, GUANG-LU XU,[b]
CHAI-LAI YEOW, AND MARIA OKIKIOLA[c]

Division of Biochemistry
United Medical and Dental Schools
Guy's Hospital
University of London
London, SE1 9RT, United Kingdom

INTRODUCTION

The biological activity of the tocopherols vary greatly, and this variation is only partly correlated with the antioxidant activity of the tocopherols when this is studied in a lipid medium.[1] A number of features of the tocopherol molecule evidently contribute to the biological activity, and this may be compared with the activity of either synthetic *all rac*-α-tocopherol or to the natural *RRR*-α-tocopherol. The features causing alterations in biological activity may include (1) the presence or absence of ring methyl groups in the 5, 7, and 8 positions; (2) the number of carbon atoms in the side chain; (3) the stereospecificity of the carbon atoms 2, 4', and 8'; (4) the branching of the side chain; (5) the chromanol ring as compared to a furanol ring; and (6) the point of attachment of the side chain to the ring structure. The work described in the present paper is a systematic study in which the effect of variation in the parameters listed above (1-6) was determined in a rat bioassay system and in a cultured cell system in which the uptake and effect on growth and on prostaglandin E₂ synthesis was measured on a comparative basis for a range of structurally modified compounds.

[a] The financial assistance of the Wellcome Trust, the Special Trustees of Guy's Hospital, the Nigerian Government, and the Government of the People's Republic of China is gratefully acknowledged.

[b] On leave of absence from Laboratory of Keshan Disease, Xi'an Medical University, Xi'an, People's Republic of China.

[c] Nigerian government scholar.

MATERIAL AND METHODS

Structurally Modified Tocopherols

The structures of the fifteen tocopherols employed are set out in TABLE 1. Compounds 1, 3, 7, 8, 12, and 13 were a gift from Hoffmann-La Roche, Basle, Switzerland; compound 2 was obtained from the Henkel Corporation, Chicago; compounds 4, 5, and 6 were a gift from Dr. Jack Pennock, Department of Biochemistry, University of Liverpool, England; compounds 9, 10, and 14 were a gift from Dr. K. U. Ingold, National Research Council, Ottawa, Canada; compound 11 was a gift from Dr. B. Kingsley, formerly of Cornell University, Ithaca, NY; and compound 15 was a gift from Dr. D. McHale, Cadbury-Schweppes, Slough, England.

TABLE 1. Trivial Names and Structures of the 15 Tocopherols Used in the Present Study

No.	NAME	STRUCTURE
1	All-rac-(ordl) α-tocopherol	
2	RRR-α- tocopherol	
3	2-ambo- α-tocopherol	
4	All-rac-β- tocopherol	
5	All-rac-γ- tocopherol	

TABLE 1—*Continued*

No.	NAME	STRUCTURE
6	All–rac–δ–tocopherol	8–methyl tocol
7	2 –rac–α–tocotrienol	3',7',11'–triene
8	All–rac–α–tocopherol –11,Br	
9	2–rac–α–tocopherol –11,St	
10	2–rac–α–tocopherol –13,St	

Bioassay Technique

Groups of six weanling male Wistar rats were given the vitamin E- and selenium-deficient diet,[2] based on torula yeast. The diet causes death of the rats after about 30-35 days due to massive centrilobular necrosis of the liver.[3] When the diet had been given for twenty days, the tocopherols were administered, dissolved in 0.1 mL olive oil, by stomach tube as a dose of 1 mg tocopherol per day; this dosage was continued until all the rats in the control group, which were given 0.1 mL olive oil only, had died. The day on which the rats died, and the number of survivors in each group, was recorded. Autopsies showed that the rats had died of centrilobular liver necrosis.

Tissue Culture

The techniques used followed those described previously.[4,5] Tocopherols and other lipids were added in solution in a small amount of ethanol, which has been shown to have no effect on the growth of the fibroblasts.[5] The BALB/373 A_{31} mouse cell line was used in all the experiments described here, and growth of cells was assessed by measurement of the protein content[6] of the cultures. This was shown in other experiments to be an accurate measure of growth when it was compared with measurement of cell number and DNA content.

TABLE 1—*Continued*

No.	NAME	STRUCTURE
11	2–rac–α–tocopherol –16,St	Straight–chain analogue of synthetic α–tocopherol
12	All–rac–α–tocopherol –26,Br	
13	All–rac–α–tocopherol –31,Br	
14	Dihydro–benzfuran tocopherol	
15	McHale's tocopherol (All–rac)	

NOTE: Hoffmann-La Roche supplied numbers 1, 3, 7, 8, 12, and 13; the Henkel Corporation supplied number 2; Jack Pennock supplied numbers 4-6; Keith Ingold supplied numbers 9, 10, and 14; B. Kingsley supplied number 11; and David McHale supplied number 15.

Measurement of Tocopherols

This was done by the method previously described.[7] Some small modifications to the solvent system were necessary to achieve separation of all the tocopherols studied. In the experiments in which uptake of tocopherols was measured, the membrane fraction of the fibroblast cultures was extracted with solvent prior to the analysis.

Thiobarbituric Acid-Reactive Substances (TBARS)

Aldehyde and other derivatives of lipid peroxides react with thiobarbituric acid to give a pink color that can be measured spectrophotometrically to give an approximate measurement of lipid peroxidation in liver homogenates. Rat liver homogenates were allowed to peroxidize for a standard period of time at 37° in an oxygen atmosphere in a shaking water bath in the presence or absence of the tocopherols. TBARS were measured in the homogenate by standard methods.[8]

Measurement of Prostaglandin Biosynthesis in Rat Liver Microsomal Fraction

Eleven groups of six weanling male Wistar rats were given the vitamin E- and selenium-deficient diet[2] for 24 days. During this period, one group of rats was given a daily oral dose of 1 mg all rac-α-tocopherol in 0.1 mL olive oil; a second group was given a daily oral dose of 1.5 mg butylated hydroxytoluene (BHT); four groups of rats were given drinking water containing 0.1 ppm selenium as Na_2SeO_3; and one group of rats was given the oral α-tocopherol and selenium in their drinking water. At the end of the 24-day period all rats were killed and their livers placed in ice-cold 0.9% (w/v) saline solution buffered at pH 7.4. A microsomal fraction was prepared from the livers individually. The microsomal fraction, resuspended in phosphate buffer, pH 7.4, was incubated at 37° with ^{14}C-labeled arachidonic acid (150 μg per flask); the microsomal fraction derived from the rats given no vitamin E *in vivo* was supplemented *in vitro* with either 0.01 μmolar all rac-α-tocopherol, 0.1 μmolar all rac--α-tocopherol, 1.0 μmolar all rac-α-tocopherol, or no supplement. At the end of a 45-minute incubation period, trichloracetic acid was added and the lipids extracted into 1:1 (v/v) chloroform methanol.

Prostaglandin E_2 (PGE_2) and $F_2α$ were separated by standard thin layer chromatographic methods and identified by comparison with authentic markers; in some experiments ^3H-labeled markers were added and shown to co-chromatograph with the ^{14}C-labeled prostaglandins derived from the microsomal fraction. Radioactivity was measured by liquid scintillation counting.

Measurement of Prostaglandin Biosynthesis in Cultured Mouse Fibroblasts

Mouse $BALB/3T3A_{31}$ fibroblasts were used; $8\text{-}10 \times 10^4$ cells were inoculated in petri dishes containing 4 mL Dulbecco's modified Eagle's medium (DMEM) with 10% fetal calf serum together with α-tocopherol, BHT, or sodium selenite as indicated in the individual experiments. The lipids were added in solution in a minimal amount of ethanol, which was shown in other experiments to have no effect on the parameters measured. Dishes were incubated at 37° in a 5% CO_2 atmosphere until the cells were nearly confluent. Two μg ^{3}H-labeled arachidonic acid was added, and incubation continued for a further 24 hours to allow maximum incorporation of [^{3}H]arachidonic acid into the membrane phospholipids. The medium was removed and the cells washed thrice with 3 mL warm phosphate-buffered 0.9% (w/v) saline, pH 7.4. Fresh medium with 2 μg of unlabeled arachidonic acid was added, and the incubation continued to allow release of the prostaglandins into the medium. The medium containing the prostaglandins was extracted twice with 3 mL ethyl acetate containing 0.005% (w/v) BHT, to act as an antioxidant during the extraction procedure, following acidification (0.1 m HCl) and the addition of [^{14}C]prostaglandin E_2 as an internal standard. The extracts were evaporated to dryness with N_2, dissolved in 40 μL ethanol, and chromatographed on thin layer chromatography (TLC) plates with 20:20:1 benzene: dioxene: acetic acid as developing solvent. Markers of authentic prostaglandins were also applied. The plates were dried and neutralized with NH_3 vapor; the spots were scraped off the plate following identification with I_2 vapor. ^{14}C and ^{3}H were determined by liquid scintillation counting, and the recovery of ^{3}H was corrected by reference to the added ^{14}C-labeled standard.

RESULTS AND DISCUSSION

In all the experiments described, except that given in TABLE 2, the procedures were repeated twice and the results of each experiment were consistent. The data in the TABLES are from one of these experiments only. The bioassay of tocopherols has conventionally depended upon the rat gestation-resorption test; this test is, however, costly and time-consuming and requires quite large amounts of the compounds to be tested.[9] The bioassay used in the present context was chosen because it is quick and reliable and, in particular, can be carried out with quite small amounts of the compounds concerned, which was of primary importance because in many instances only a few milligrams of compound was available. The results cannot be accorded the same certainty as the rat gestation-resorption assay, but nevertheless they give a good indication of the biological activity of the tocopherols concerned. Thus the present test is not capable, at least as used here, of distinguishing between the biological activity of *all rac*-α-tocopherol and *RRR*-α-tocopherol, the second of which is known to have a higher biopotency than the first. The results given in TABLE 2 clearly show, however, that the removal of one isopentane unit from the tocopherol side chain eliminated the biological activity of the compound. Addition of one or two isopentane units also resulted in a lessening of the biological activity, although even the 31-carbon side-chain compound had some apparent residual activity. Of particular interest is the 2-*rac*-α-tocopherol-16 St (no.11, TABLE 1), which differs from *all rac*-α-tocopherol only in the fact that it has not a branched side chain. This compound was almost

TABLE 2. Biological Activity of Tocopherols[a]

Compound and number (TABLE 1)	Rats surviving on day 39	Day of death of rats (mean and range)
None	0/6	32.3 (29-36)
All rac-α-tocopherol-11 Br (8)	0/6	32.5 (30-36)
All rac-α-tocopherol-16 Br (1)	6/6	—
RRR d-α-tocopherol (2)	6/6	—
All rac-α-tocopherol-26 Br (12)	3/6	35.7 (35-37)
All rac-α-tocopherol-31 Br (13)	1/6	30.2 (29-35)
2-rac-α-tocopherol-16 St (11)	1/6	32.2 (30-35)
McHale's tocopherol (4-side chain) (15)	0/6	32.0 (29-33)

[a] Experimental details are given in the text. One milligram of the tocopherols in 0.1 mL olive oil was administered daily to each of six rats per group from day 20 following commencement of feeding the vitamin E- and selenium-deficient diet until the end of the experiment.

devoid of biological activity, indicating clearly the vital importance of the branched side chain to the tocopherol biological activity. When the normal side chain was attached in the 4-position of the chromanol ring, there was also a complete loss of biological activity. Unfortunately, insufficient amounts of the other compounds in TABLE 1 were available to subject them to this test.

The antioxidant activity of some of the compounds studied here has been determined previously. In order to be able to compare this important parameter together in all the compounds studied, their ability to inhibit the formation of TBARS was measured in two systems: in cultured fibroblasts and in a rat liver homogenate, both alone or in the presence of ascorbic acid and Fe(II), which acts as a stressor in exacerbating the lipid peroxidation process. The results are given in TABLE 3; in general, the rate of peroxidation in the presence of ascorbic acid and Fe(II) was some five to seven times the rate observed when the stressor was not added. The data in TABLE 3 are not absolute values, but, instead, the inhibitory ability of all rac-α-tocopherol was expressed as 100%, and the inhibitory activity of all the other tocopherols was expressed relative to this. Although it is now clear that the TBARS method does not measure only the malondialdehyde degradation product derived from lipid peroxide, but includes other aldehydes such as hexanal and 4-hydroxynonenal,[10] as well as other nonlipid derivatives,[11] there is a general consensus that TBARS measurement does give a consistent and reliable approximate measure of lipid peroxidation. The data in TABLE 3 thus give a reasonable measure of the ability of the tocopherols studied to inhibit lipid peroxidation. Thus, as expected, RRR-α-tocopherol was found to be a superior antioxidant to the all rac form. The other tocopherols showed varying antioxidant ability and, in general, this was consistent with the results of other workers for those tocopherols that had been studied previously. Thus β- and γ-tocopherols exhibited 70-80% of the activity of α-tocopherol, whereas δ-tocopherol was somewhat less active, as was α-tocotrienol. The short-branched chain 11-Br compound was about 50% as active as α-tocopherol, whereas the straight chain 11-St compound was a very poor antioxidant. The 15-St compound, which differs from α-tocopherol only in the branching of the side chain, was a very poor antioxidant in the ascorbate/Fe(II) stressed systems, but showed 54-67% of the activity of the branched chain analogue in the unstressed systems. The tocopherols with side chains longer than α-tocopherol were poorer antioxidants, in particular the 31-Br compound.

TABLE 3. Inhibition by Tocopherols of Formation of Thiobarbituric Acid-Reactive Substances (TBARS) in Cultured Mouse Fibroblasts and Rat Liver Homogenates[c]

Compound and number (TABLE 1)	Percentage inhibition			
	Cultured cells		Liver homogenate	
	Alone	With Fe^{2+} ascorbate	Alone	With Fe^{2+} ascorbate
RRR-α-tocopherol (2)	110 ± 5	114 ± 8	109 ± 14[b]	108 ± 12[b]
2-ambo-α-tocopherol (3)	57 ± 6	82 ± 9[b]	—	—
All rac-β-tocopherol (4)	74 ± 3	80 ± 8[b]	72 ± 12	78 ± 10
All rac-γ-tocopherol (5)	85 ± 11	74 ± 6	72 ± 15	75 ± 12
All rac-δ-tocopherol (6)	60 ± 6	45 ± 7	59 ± 11	58 ± 16
All rac-α-tocotrienol (7)	62 ± 3	39 ± 17	50 ± 3	65 ± 15
All rac-α-tocopherol-11 Br (8)	58 ± 4	59 ± 7	54 ± 9	55 ± 6
2-rac-α-tocopherol-11 St (9)	30 ± 2	23 ± 6	18 ± 7	20 ± 14
2-rac-α-tocopherol-13 St (10)	58 ± 7	36 ± 9	64 ± 17	26 ± 11
2-rac-α-tocopherol-15 St (11)	67 ± 5	28 ± 2	54 ± 10	11 ± 2
All rac-α-tocopherol-26 Br (12)	65 ± 9	35 ± 11	57 ± 9	18 ± 3
All rac-α-tocopherol-31 Br (13)	27 ± 5	32 ± 9	44 ± 13	35 ± 7
Dihydrobenzifuran tocopherol (14)	49 ± 3	19 ± 7	44 ± 12	21 ± 6
McHale's 4-side chain tocopherol (15)	69 ± 12	67 ± 15	70 ± 10	22 ± 9

[a] Inhibitory effect of *all rac*-α-tocopherol was expressed as 100%, and the effect of the other tocopherols was expressed relative to this. Experimental details are given in the text. Values given are mean ± standard deviation.

[b] The value given was significantly different from the value for *all rac*-α-tocopherol in all cases not marked with this symbol ($p > 0.01$ or a higher level of significance).

The dihydrobenzfuran tocopherol analogue had less than 50% of the activity of α-tocopherol, and the 4-side chain compound had about 70% of the activity except in the stressed liver homogenate system. Thus alterations in any of the parameters (1-6) in the INTRODUCTION result in loss of antioxidant activity of the tocopherol analogue.

The uptake of the tocopherols in the fibroblasts and their effect on growth of the cells was studied together, and the results are given in TABLE 4. In view of the marked differences in biological activity of the various tocopherols that had been reported by others, it was thought to be important to determine what effect the alteration in the structure might have on the uptake of the tocopherol into cells and what, if any, the relationship of this to the biological activity was, judged in this instance in terms of the stimulation of growth of the cells. The media used for these experiments, like most tissue culture media, were deficient in vitamin E,[4] and addition of *all rac-α*-tocopherol usually resulted in a stimulation in the rate of growth of about 25-30% in the experiments reported here. The stimulatory effect of the other tocopherols was calculated relative to the growth stimulating effect of *all rac-α*-tocopherol, which was expressed as 100% (TABLE 4). The greater biopotency of *RRR*-α-tocopherol was partly related to its increased uptake by the cells; all other tocopherols had a lower level of uptake and a lower biopotency than *all rac-α*-tocopherol. The uptake and biopotency of β-tocopherol was not significantly different from α-tocopherol, whereas both parameters for γ- and δ-tocopherol were lower; the uptake of δ-tocopherol was only 50% of α-tocopherol, yet its biopotency was 72%, which suggests that poor membrane transport of this tocopherol may, in part at least, account for its low biological activity. A particularly striking feature of these results is that the straight side-chain tocopherols had, in general, very weak biopotency, even though, as in the case of the 13-St and 15-St analogues, their uptake was only slightly lower than that

TABLE 4. Uptake and Biopotency of Tocopherols in Cultured Mouse Fibroblasts[a]

Compound and number (TABLE 1)		Uptake (percent)	Biopotency (percent)
RRR-α-tocopherol	(2)	112 ± 6	135 ± 4
2-*ambo*-α-tocopherol	(3)	69 ± 9	49 ± 11
All rac-β-tocopherol	(4)	83 ± 11[b]	93 ± 6[b]
All rac-γ-tocopherol	(5)	62 ± 8	71 ± 9
All rac-δ-tocopherol	(6)	51 ± 14	72 ± 9
All rac-α-tocotrienol	(7)	47 ± 10	23 ± 6
All rac-α-tocopherol-11 Br	(8)	35 ± 3	59 ± 7
2-*rac*-α-tocopherol-11 St	(9)	38 ± 5	13 ± 2
2-*rac*-α-tocopherol-13 St	(10)	81 ± 7	34 ± 8
2-*rac*-α-tocopherol-15 St	(11)	85 ± 9[b]	37 ± 7
All rac-α-tocopherol-26 Br	(12)	42 ± 6	(−5)[c]
All rac-α-tocopherol-31 Br	(13)	38 ± 2	(−8)[c]
Dihydrobenzfuran tocopherol	(14)	86 ± 9[b]	76 ± 11
McHale's 4-side chain tocopherol	(15)	18 ± 3	10 ± 7

[a] Uptake into the cells and biopotency (growth stimulation) of *all rac-α*-tocopherol are expressed as 100%, and these parameters for other tocopherols were expressed relative to this. Experimental details are given in the text. Values given are mean ± SD.

[b] The value given was significantly different from the value for *all rac-α*-tocopherol in all cases not marked with this symbol ($p > 0.01$ or a higher level of significance).

[c] These tocopherols appeared to be either without activity or slightly inhibitory of growth of the cells.

TABLE 5. Prostaglandin Synthesis in Rat Liver Microsomal Fraction[a]

Rat diet and treatment *in vivo*	Radioactivity (dpm/mg protein)		Addition *in vitro*
	$F_2\alpha$	E_2	
Basal $(-E,-Se)$	129 ± 19	287 ± 27	None
	256 ± 36[b]	397 + 47[b]	0.01 μmolar E
	181 ± 41[c]	302	0.1 μmolar E
	64 ± 21	132 ± 22[b]	1.0 μmolar E
Basal + E	89 ± 19[b]	181 ± 34[b]	None
Basal + BHT	134 ± 16	286 ± 39	None
Basal + Se	128 ± 27	276 ± 33	None
	324 ± 41[b]	446 ± 47[b]	0.01 μmolar E
	298 ± 25[b]	337 ± 22[b]	0.1 μmolar E
	70 ± 16[b]	138 ± 27[b]	1.0 μmolar E
Basal + E + Se	70 ± 8[b]	170 ± 12[c]	None

[a] Experimental details are given in the text. Vitamin E (100 mg/kg *all rac*-α-tocopherol) and BHT (150 mg/kg) were added to the diets where indicated, and selenium (0.1 ppm Se as Na_2SeO_3) was added to the drinking water.
[b] Significantly different from basal with no E addition *in vitro* ($p > 0.001$).
[c] Significantly different from basal with no E addition *in vitro* ($p > 0.01$).

of α-tocopherol. The branched side chain is thus shown to be of particular significance as a requirement for high biological activity. The larger branched side-chain analogues (26 Br and 31 Br) were taken up rather poorly and had no biological activity at all; in fact they tended to inhibit cell growth. The dihydrobenzfuran analogue was taken up well by the cells and had quite a high biopotency in this system in contrast to the 4-side chain analogue, which was poorly taken up and had little biological activity.

Several authors have reported that vitamin E influences prostaglandin synthesis,[12] and this seemed to us to be an ideal system in which to test the biological activity of the tocopherol analogues under study. In particular, this system was thought to have great relevance to the question of the localization of tocopherol in biological membranes and to the structural specificity that may be involved in this. The initiation of the prostaglandin cascade depends upon the cleavage by phospholipase A_2 from attachment to a phospholipid that is intimately a part of the membrane structure. Thus, modification by tocopherol of the compactness of the membrane in the manner proposed previously might modify the activity of phospholipase A_2 and thus might modify the availability of free arachidonic acid; there is evidence that tocopherol has an effect on phospholipase A_2 activity.[13] The antioxidant activity of vitamin E might, in addition, have modulating effects on the arachidonic acid cascade. In some preliminary experiments, a rat liver microsomal system was used to study prostaglandin biosynthesis. Great difficulty was, however, experienced because in some experiments, α-tocopherol appeared to stimulate prostaglandin synthesis, whereas in others there was no effect or the added tocopherol was inhibitory. When it was established that this was not experimental variability but that a real phenomenon was involved, a series of careful experiments was carried out in which vitamin E at several different levels was added to a vitamin E-deficient diet, and also several different levels of tocopherol covering a wide range were added to the microsomal fraction *in vitro*. The result of one such experiment, in which 100 mg *all rac*-α-tocopherol was added *in vivo*, are given in TABLE 5; the possible effect of the synthetic antioxidant BHT and of selenium was also investigated. At this level of inclusion of α-tocopherol in the diet, microsomal fraction prepared from the livers of rats supplemented with vitamin E produced significantly less prostaglandins than did the microsomal fraction prepared from vitamin E-deficient or vitamin E- and selenium-deficient rats. The addition of BHT at a concentration equimolar with the vitamin E added, or of selenium, were without effect on the synthesis of prostaglandins. Addition of α-tocopherol *in vitro* at three different levels gave consistent significant results at each level of inclusion, irrespective of whether selenium had been added to the diet or not, although there was some evidence of a synergistic effect between vitamin E and selenium, which proved, however, not to be statistically significant. Addition *in vitro* of 0.01 μmolar α-tocopherol caused a consistent significant stimulation of prostaglandin synthesis; 0.1 μmolar α-tocopherol was somewhat less stimulatory and 1.0 μmolar α-tocopherol gave a consistent significant inhibitory effect. These effects, moreover, were observed irrespective of the presence, or absence of, selenium in the diet of the rats. A possible explanation of these apparently paradoxical results was that low levels of α-tocopherol stimulated prostaglandin synthesis by virtue of the antioxidant properties of the vitamin. As the level of α-tocopherol inclusion was raised by two orders of magnitude, the membrane could be expected to become more compact, which, it is supposed, caused an inhibition of phospholipase A_2 activity and a consequent decrease in prostaglandin biosynthesis.

To test the above hypothesis, experiments with the analogues of tocopherol, described in the earlier part of this paper, were carried out. The hypothesis[14] that proposes that there is stereospecificity of the tocopherol side chain in the membrane-stabilizing effect of the vitamin would predict that the tocopherols that have side chains different from α-tocopherol might be expected to show the stimulatory effect of the vitamin on prostaglandin synthesis but not the inhibitory effect, which is thought to require stereospecificity of the side chain in stabilizing the membrane structure. The rat liver microsomal system was replaced by cultured mouse fibroblasts in which it was possible to demonstrate prostaglandin synthesis. In a series of preliminary experiments (not given here), we were able to demonstrate that the addition of *all rac*-α-tocopherol to the growth medium caused stimulation of prostaglandin synthesis at low levels of inclusion (0.01 μM) and was inhibitory at higher levels (1.0 μM). This system was therefore used to test the ability of different levels of most of the tocopherols given in TABLE 1 to affect the biosynthesis of PGE$_2$; the results are given in TABLE 6.

Addition of 0.01 μM *all rac*-α-tocopherol resulted in a 3.5-fold increase in PGE$_2$; *RRR*-α-tocopherol caused a fivefold increase, and addition of 1 μM of the tocopherols caused an inhibition, respectively, of one-third to one-ninth of the control values. 2-*ambo*-α-Tocopherol showed a weak stimulatory response and no inhibition at the higher level, and β-, γ-, and δ-tocopherols all showed some biphasic response, as did all the branched chain analogues, although in some instances there was no inhibitory effect at the higher concentration. α-Tocotrienol and the 16-St analogue showed about a 2.5-fold stimulatory effect at the lowest level of inclusion, and this stimulatory effect was also seen at the high level of addition. The 4-side chain tocopherol (15) showed a fourfold stimulatory effect when 0.01 μM was added, and this same stimulatory effect was observed at the highest level of inclusion. These results were interpreted as indicating that alteration of the tocopherol side chain does indeed discriminate between two important functions for α-tocopherol, one dependent on the antioxidant ability of the vitamin and the other depending upon the stereospecificity of the side chain.

CONCLUSION

RRR-α-tocopherol had the greatest antioxidant activity, was taken up best by cells, and had the largest biological activity of all the tocopherols studied here. Alteration of the 2R configuration to the 2S form resulted in a large loss of biological activity. With regard to the ring methyl groups, alpha tocopherol > beta tocopherol > gamma tocopherol > delta tocopherol, with respect to biological activity, only partly related to cellular uptake. The insertion of three double bonds in the side chain to form α-tocotrienol resulted in loss of about half the biological activity. Replacement of a branched side chain by a straight side chain of equivalent length resulted in considerable reduction in the biological activity. Prostaglandin synthesis was stimulated by a low level of the straight-chain analogue, but there was no inhibition at the higher concentration. Replacement of the chromanoxy ring by a furanoxy ring resulted in only a small loss of biological activity. The 4-side chain tocopherol was not taken up by cells. When added to cultured cells *in vitro,* however, it stimulated prostaglandin

TABLE 6. Prostaglandin E_2 Synthesis in Cultured Mouse Fibroblasts[a]

Compound and number (TABLE 1)	Tocopherol additions to medium			
	0	0.01 μmolar	0.1 μmolar	1.0 μmolar
All rac-α-tocopherol	(1) 1.8 ± 0.3	6.7 ± 1.2[b]	2.8 ± 0.4[c]	0.6 ± 0.1[c]
RRR-α-tocopherol	(2) 1.8 ± 0.3	9.3 ± 0.8[c]	1.1 ± 0.3[b]	0.2 ± 0.0[c]
2-*ambo*-α-tocopherol	(3) 1.8 ± 0.3	3.9 ± 0.8[b]	2.7 ± 0.6[b]	2.1 ± 0.3
All rac-β-tocopherol	(4) 1.8 ± 0.3	8.6 ± 0.9[c]	2.3 ± 0.4	0.9 ± 0.2[b]
All rac-γ-tocopherol	(5) 1.8 ± 0.3	6.2 ± 1.3[c]	1.6 ± 0.2	0.9 ± 0.3[b]
All rac-δ-tocopherol	(6) 1.8 ± 0.3	3.2 ± 0.7[b]	1.7 ± 0.1	1.0 ± 0.4[b]
All rac-α-tocotrienol	(7) 1.8 ± 0.3	5.4 ± 0.6[c]	5.8 ± 0.3[c]	4.8 ± 0.3[c]
All rac-α-tocopherol-11 Br	(8) 1.8 ± 0.3	4.9 ± 0.5[c]	1.7 ± 0.4	1.8 ± 0.2
2-*rac*-α-tocopherol-16 St	(11) 1.8 ± 0.3	4.4 ± 0.3[b]	4.6 ± 0.5[b]	4.1 ± 0.7[b]
All rac-α-tocopherol-26 Br	(12) 1.8 ± 0.3	5.2 ± 0.4[c]	1.6 ± 0.2	1.7 ± 0.1
All rac-α-tocopherol-31 Br	(13) 1.8 ± 0.3	3.1 ± 0.1[b]	3.6 ± 0.7[b]	3.0 ± 0.2[b]
McHale's 4-side chain tocopherol	(15) 1.8 ± 0.3	7.3 ± 0.7[c]	8.6 ± 0.9[c]	8.2 ± 1.1[b]

[a] Results given are radioactivity of isolated PGE_2 (mean dpm $\times 10^{-4}/\mu g$ protein ± standard deviation). Experimental details are given in the text.
[b] $p > 0.01$.
[c] $p > 0.001$.

synthesis, but higher levels of inclusion failed to show the inhibitory effect of α-tocopherol.

ACKNOWLEDGMENTS

The authors are very grateful to Hoffmann-La Roche, Basle, Switzerland; the Henkel Corporation, Chicago; Dr. J. Pennock; Dr. K. U. Ingold; Dr. B. Kingsley; and Dr. D. McHale for generous gifts of tocopherols used in the present study.

REFERENCES

1. KASPAREK, S. 1980. *In* Vitamin E, a comprehensive treatise. L. J. Machlin, Ed.: 7-65. Marcel Dekker. New York & Basel.
2. DIPLOCK, A. T., H. BAUM & J. A. LUCY. 1971. Biochem. J. **123:** 721-729.
3. SCHWARZ, K. & C. M. FOLZ. 1957. J. Am. Chem. Soc. **79:** 3292-3296.
4. GIASUDDIN, A. S. M. & A. T. DIPLOCK. 1979. Arch. Biochem. Biophys. **196:** 270-280.
5. GIASUDDIN, A. S. M. & A. T. DIPLOCK. 1980. Arch. Biochem. Biophys. **210:** 348-362.
6. BUTTRISS, J. L. & A. T. DIPLOCK. 1984. Oxygen radicals in biological systems. Methods Enzymol. **105:** 131-138.
7. LOWRY, O. H., N. J. ROSEBROUGH, A. L. FARR & R. J. RANDALL. 1951. J. Biol. Chem. **193:** 265-275.
8. BUNYAN, J., A. T. DIPLOCK, E. E. EDWIN & J. GREEN. 1962. Br. J. Nutr. **16:** 519-530.
9. AMES, S. R., M. I. LUDWIG, D. R. NELAN & C. D. ROBESON. 1963. Biochemistry **2:** 188-190.
10. BENEDETTI, A., M. COMPORTI & H. ESTERBAUER. 1980. Biochim. Biophys. Acta **620:** 281-296.
11. HALLIWELL, B. & J. M. GUTTERIDGE. 1981. FEBS Lett. **128:** 347-354.
12. KITABCHI, A. E. 1981. *In* Vitamin E, a comprehensive treatise. L. J. Machlin, Ed.: 348-371. Marcel Dekker. New York & Basel.
13. PAPPU, A. S., P. FATHERPAKER & A. SREENIVASAN. 1979. Ind. J. Biochem. Biophys. **16:** 143-147.
14. DIPLOCK, A. T. & J. A. LUCY. 1973. FEBS. Lett. **29:** 205-210.

Tocopherol-Binding Proteins of Hepatic Cytosol

NEIL KAPLOWITZ, HARUHIKO YOSHIDA,
JOHN KUHLENKAMP, BARRY SLITSKY,
IRENE REN, AND ANDREW STOLZ

*Liver Research Laboratory
Wadsworth Branch, West Los Angeles Veterans Administration
Hospital Center and
The UCLA School of Medicine
Los Angeles, California 90073*

Tocopherol is a highly lipophilic substance. It is believed to travel in the circulation nonspecifically bound to lipoproteins. The liver is believed to play an important role in the processing of dietary α- and γ-tocopherol. The transfer of tocopherol between intracellular compartments in the hepatocyte is believed to involve cytosolic proteins that bind tocopherol.

Catignani in 1975 first described a molecular weight 31,000 fraction in gel filtration of rat liver cytosol that bound tocopherol. A void volume fraction was also noted to bind labeled α-tocopherol.[1] Excess α-tocopherol, however, displaced the labeled form only in the 31,000 molecular weight fraction. Subsequently it was shown by Catignani and Bieri that 400-fold excess α-tocopherol displaced 98% of the label, but γ-tocopherol displaced 60% of the label.[2] The binder was identified only in the liver and was found in mouse, guinea pig, rabbit, hamster, and chicken in addition to rat liver. Studies of specificity of binding revealed the need for free chroman hydroxyl group, intact chromanol ring, and side chain.[2] Three groups subsequently demonstrated the capacity of the crude cytosol fraction to transfer tocopherol. Murphy and Mavis demonstrated the activity of a 34,000 molecular weight gel filtration fraction from rat liver to transfer tocopherol from egg phosphatidylcholine liposomes to liver microsomes.[3] The activity was present only in liver and was absent in lung, heart, and brain of rats. Mowri *et al.* demonstrated the ability of this rat liver fraction to transfer α-tocopherol from liposomes to microsomes.[4] They showed that excess α-tocopherol could displace labeled α-tocopherol; γ-tocopherol also exhibited some inhibitory effect. They claimed to observe this activity in liver, spleen, heart, and lungs but not in kidney or brain cytosol of the rat. They also claimed that human liver possessed this activity but showed no data. Behrens and Madère showed that labeled tocopherol was associated with a high molecular weight peak and a 32,000 molecular weight fraction in gel filtration of hepatic cytosol after oral dosing *in vivo* with labeled α-tocopherol.[5] Subsequently they partially purified the fraction from rat liver, using ammonium sulfate fractionation, gel filtration, and ion exchange chromatography and showed transfer of labeled tocopherol from the binding protein to microsomes.[6] Their studies suggested that the molecular form of endogenous tocopherol associated with the void volume was predominantly γ-tocopherol, whereas the molecular form associated with the

32,000 molecular weight gel filtration fraction was mainly α-tocopherol.[5,7] The only report of another tocopherol transfer activity is that of Guarnieri *et al.*[8] These investigators identified only a void volume fraction in gel filtration of heart cytosol and observed transfer of tocopherol from this fraction to acidic non-histone proteins of isolated tocopherol-deficient nuclei.

Our laboratory has been involved in the identification, purification, and characterization of cytosolic proteins in rat and human liver, which bind organic anions, such as bilirubin and bile acids. In 1983, we identified and purified two bile acid-binding fractions in rat liver cytosol, one corresponding to the glutathione S-transferases (molecular weight 50,000), which is otherwise known as the Y fraction, and one corresponding to molecular weight 33,000, which we referred to as the Y' fraction.[9] Subsequently, we have shown that the bile acid binder in the Y' fraction is identical to 3α-hydroxysteroid dehydrogenase.[10] Among the bile acids that were bound with highest affinity by these fractions was the highly lipophilic lithocholic acid. In view of the reports of a 30,000-34,000 molecular weight tocopherol binding protein and the highly lipophilic nature of tocopherol, we were interested in its relationship to the bile acid binders. Therefore, we set out to purify the tocopherol binding protein from rat liver cytosol and to determine its relationship to the bile acid binder.

FIGURE 1 shows the molecular weight gel filtration chromatography of rat hepatic cytosol incubated with tracer [³H]D-α-tocopherol (8.3 Ci/mmol). [³H]α-Tocopherol was purified by isocratic reverse phase high-performance liquid chromatography (Ultrasil-ods C_{18} column) eluted with methanol/water (98:2) prior to use in all our work. Labeled α-tocopherol (300 pmol) was incubated for 1 hour at 4° C with 8 mL of 33% (w/v) hepatic cytosol prepared from Sprague-Dawley male rats and applied onto a 120 by 2.5 centimeter column of Sephadex G-75 superfine. Individual column fractions were assayed for protein absorbance, tocopherol radioactivity, and 3α-hydroxysteroid dehydrogenase activity. 3α-Hydroxysteroid dehydrogenase activity eluted as a single peak corresponding to the Y' fraction. Radioactive α-tocopherol eluted in two different molecular weight fractions. The high molecular weight peak of radioactive tocopherol appeared in the void volume of the column. The lower molecular weight peak of tocopherol binding nearly co-eluted with the 3α-hydroxysteroid dehydrogenase

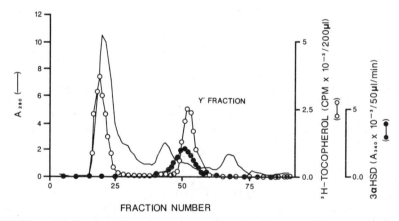

FIGURE NUMBER

FIGURE 1. Gel filtration of hepatic cytosol on Sephadex G75sf with [³H]α-tocopherol. 300 pmol of labeled material was added to 8 mL cytosol and eluted from a 2.5 × 120 cm Sephadex G75sf column with 10 mM sodium phosphate, pH 7.4.

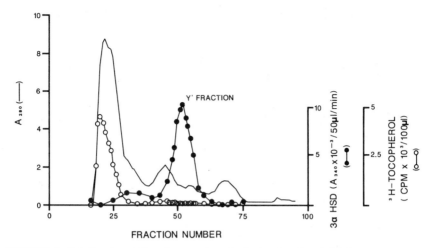

FIGURE 2. Gel filtration of hepatic cytosol on Sephadex G75sf with [^{3}H]α-tocopherol and excess unlabeled tocopherol. Conditions as in legend to FIGURE 1, but 100 nmol of unlabeled tocopherol was added.

activity in the Y' fraction. Thus, radio-labeled tocopherol eluted with two distinct molecular weight fractions, as has been previously reported.[1-8]

In order to determine which molecular weight fractions specifically bind tocopherol, another sample of hepatic cytosol was incubated with radiolabeled tocopherol in the presence of excess 100 nmol unlabeled tocopherol (FIG. 2). Again, 3α-hydroxysteroid dehydrogenase activity eluted as a single peak, identifying the Y' fraction. In the presence of excess, unlabeled α-tocopherol, only one peak of radioactive tocopherol binding was identified, which corresponded to the high molecular form appearing in the void volume. Therefore, the lower molecular weight tocopherol binding protein exhibited displacement of the labeled α-tocopherol, suggesting specific binding by the Y' tocopherol binder. By contrast, little displacement of tritiated tocopherol was found in the high molecular weight form, suggesting that this tocopherol is nonspecifically bound.

To provide a rapid and reproducible method for determining specific binding, we turned to gel filtration on Superose-12 using the fast protein liquid chromatography (FPLC) system. The elution of cytosol (0.2 mL) with labeled α-tocopherol is shown in FIGURE 3. This provided a convenient and highly reproducible means to examine the binding specificity and to identify binding activity in various organs and species.

To assess specific binding in this FPLC system, we incubated Y' fraction with labeled tocopherol (0.05 μM) and increasing concentrations of D-α-tocopherol as shown in FIGURE 4. Maximum displacement was seen at 5.0 μM α-tocopherol. Using 50 μM γ-tocopherol or δ-tocopherol, similar displacement was seen, as with 50 μM tocopherol, indicating no preference for α-tocopherol (FIG. 5). α-Tocopherol acetate, however, and quinone as well as bilirubin, estradiol, cholic acid, lithocholic acid, 3-methylcholanthrene, palmitate, and cholesterol at 50 μM exhibited no displacement (not shown), indicating specificity for tocopherol. More recently, we have found that at lower concentrations (0.1-10 μM), α-tocopherol is bound with an order of magnitude higher affinity than γ- or δ-tocopherol.

An important issue with respect to the Y' binder is whether it is found in human liver. We obtained four human liver samples from organ donors. The elution of labeled

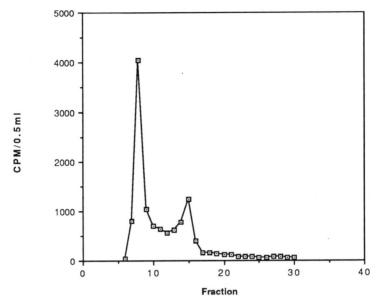

FIGURE 3. [³H]α-Tocopherol binding to rat liver cytosol proteins on Superose-12 FPLC: 0.2 mL of cytosol was incubated with ~2 pmol of labeled tocopherol for two hours at 4° and eluted from a 1.0 × 30 cm column with 50 mM sodium phosphate, pH 7.4.

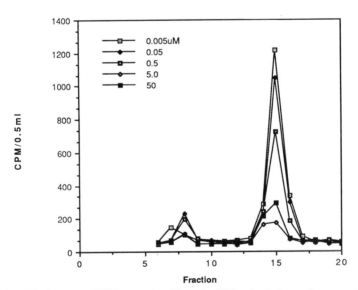

FIGURE 4. Displacement of [³H]α-tocopherol bound to Y' fraction by increasing concentrations of unlabeled α-tocopherol. Pooled Y' fraction was first prepared by open column gel filtration with [³H]α-tocopherol. Studies were conducted on Superose-12 FPLC as in FIGURE 3 after preincubations of 2 hours at 4° with increasing concentrations unlabeled α-tocopherol to displace the prelabeled Y' tocopherol fraction.

α-tocopherol with cytosol and its displacement by 50 μM unlabeled tocopherol with one liver sample in the Superose-12 FPLC system is shown in FIGURE 6. Similar results were obtained with the other three human liver samples. Thus, Y' α-tocopherol binder is present in human liver, and we are currently attempting to purify and further characterize it.

The bulk of our recent work has been to attempt to purify the rat Y' tocopherol binder. FIGURE 7 shows affigel blue chromatography of the pooled Y' fraction from gel filtration. We have previously used this chromatography in the purification of 3α-hydroxysteroid dehydrogenase. To our surprise and delight, this proved to be an invaluable step in the separation and purification of the Y' tocopherol binder. The tocopherol binding proteins eluted early in the salt gradient as two peaks that were completely separate from the 3α-hydroxysteroid dehydrogenase, which more avidly stuck to the column. We refer to these tocopherol binders as peaks I and II. The

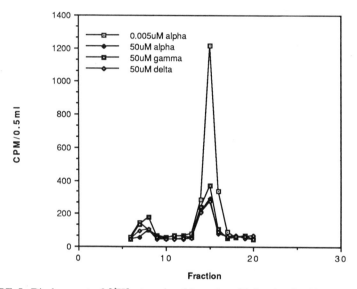

FIGURE 5. Displacement of [³H]α-tocopherol bound to Y' fraction by 50 μM α- and δ-tocopherol. See FIGURES 3 and 4 for conditions.

appearance of label in the void fractions was inconstant and represented nonspecific binding. The weak binding of the tocopherol binders to Affigel blue probably represents hydrophobic interaction.

FIGURE 8 demonstrates the next step in purification, namely chromatofocusing of pooled fractions from Affigel blue containing tocopherol binder I. The pooled peak I fractions from Affigel blue were preincubated with additional labeled tocopherol prior to chromatofocusing. Chromatofocusing permits proteins to be separated on the basis of their apparent isoelectric points due to a chemically generated pH gradient. [³H]α-Tocopherol eluted with a major peak in association with a protein peak at pH 5.1. Only small amounts of radioactive tocopherol were seen in other fractions. SDS-PAGE of the pooled fractions of the peak binding from chromatofocusing revealed a single 32 kDa band on silver staining (FIG. 9).

In subsequent work we have attempted to prepare additional quantities of the homogeneous preparation using modified techniques. We started by running rat liver cytosol on Sephacryl S-200, which is a more rapid technique for preparing pools of the Y' fraction (FIG. 10). Affigel blue chromatography, when run with smaller quantities of Y' fraction and a more shallow salt gradient than previously, was now able to resolve binder I into two peaks, referred to as I_a and I_b (FIG. 11). When aliquots of peaks I_a, I_b, and II were eluted on Superose-12 FPLC, the radioactivity eluted in the Y' fraction, indicating that these peaks on Affigel blue were Y' binders (FIG. 12). The pattern observed in FIGURE 11 was reproducible on three additional runs. Chromatofocusing of pooled I_a and I_b separately on mono-P FPLC defined a separate elution for each with I_a eluting at a lower pH than I_b (FIG. 13), although cross contamination was apparent. Our current view is that peak I_b represents the same

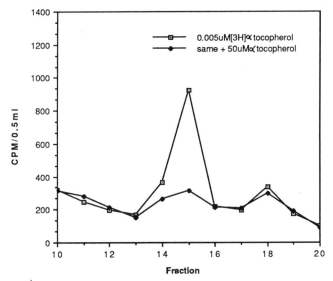

FIGURE 6. Binding of [³H]α-tocopherol in the Y' fraction of human cytosol and its displacement by 50 μM unlabeled α-tocopherol in Superose-12 FPLC. Conditions as in preceding FIGURES.

protein we purified as tocopherol I in the above experiments. Subsequently the peaks from mono-P corresponding to I_a and I_b were further purified on Sephadex G75 superfine where they eluted in the Y' fraction with [³H]α-tocopherol (not shown).

In conclusion, we have confirmed that a Y' molecular weight 32,000 tocopherol binding fraction is present in rat cytosol that specifically binds α-tocopherol; it also binds γ- and δ-tocopherol with lower affinity based on displacement studies but not other lipophilic molecules. Based on separation on Affigel blue, the tocopherol binder is distinct from bile acid binders. The tocopherol Y' binder is also found in human liver cytosol. Multiple, probably three, molecular forms of the Y' tocopherol binder have been identified. Further work is required to characterize the structural relationship between these forms.

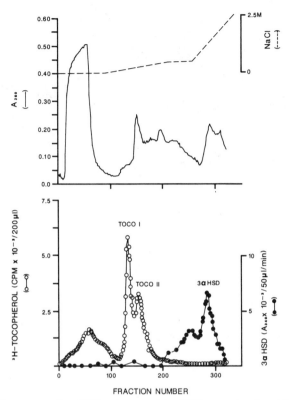

FIGURE 7. Chromatography of Y' fraction containing [^{3}H]α-tocopherol on Affigel blue. Affigel blue (2.5 × 50 cm) was eluted with a gradient of 10 mM sodium phosphate, pH 7.4 (250 mL), and also with 0.55 M sodium chloride (250 mL), followed by 2.5 M sodium chloride wash.

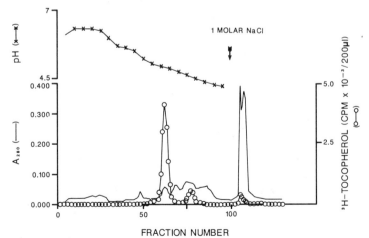

FIGURE 8. Chromatofocusing of peak I of [^{3}H]α-tocopherol binding from Affigel blue. A 1.0 × 50 cm column of PBE94 was eluted with 0.025 M bis-TRIS-HCl, pH 6.4, and then polybuffer 74, pH 4.0 (diluted 1:10).

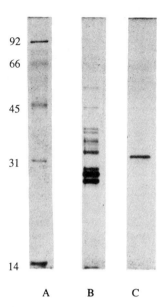

FIGURE 9. SDS-polyacrylamide gel electrophoresis. Lane A contains molecular weight standards as indicated by kilodaltons to the left. Lane B contains 6 μg of the crude Y' fraction from gel filtration. Lane C contains 3 μg tocopherol binding peak from chromatofocusing (FIG. 8). The protein was identified by silver stain after electrophoresis with 4% stacking and 12.5% running gel.

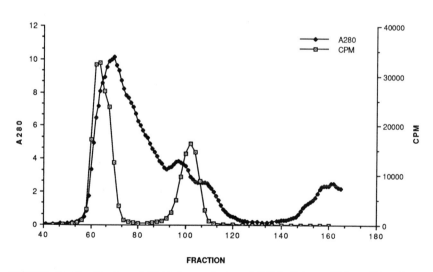

FIGURE 10. Identification of Y' binder on Sephacryl S-200. Column (5.0 × 100 cm) was eluted with 10 mM sodium phosphate, pH 7.4, at flow rate of 120 mL/h after loading 80 mL of 33% cytosol containing [³H]α-tocopherol.

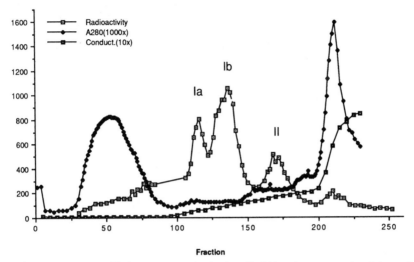

FIGURE 11. Elution of [³H]α-tocopherol binding in Affigel blue chromatography of the crude Y′ fraction. The pooled Y′ fraction from Sephacryl S200 was applied to a 2.5 × 50 cm column of Affigel blue and eluted with a gradient consisting of 500 mL of the same buffer and 500 mL also containing 0.55 M sodium chloride.

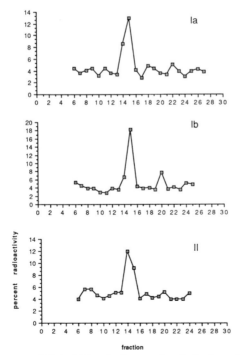

FIGURE 12. Superose-12 FPLC of 0.2 mL aliquots of peaks I$_a$, I$_b$, and II from FIGURE 11. Conditions are the same as in FIGURE 3.

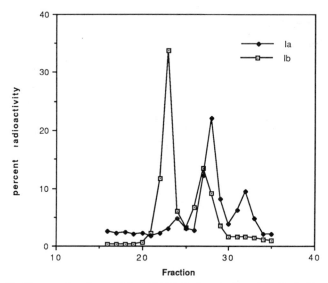

FIGURE 13. Chromatofocusing on Mono-P FPLC of peaks I_a and I_b. Peaks I_a and I_b from FIGURE 11 were pooled and applied to the column and eluted as in FIGURE 8. The data from the two separate runs are shown as a percentage of the radioactivity recovered from the column in each fraction.

REFERENCES

1. CATIGNANI, G. L. 1975. An α-tocopherol binding protein in rat liver cytoplasm. Biochem. Biophys. Res. Commun. **67:** 66-71.
2. CATIGNANI, G. L. & J. G. BIERI. 1977. Rat liver α-tocopherol binding protein. Biochim. Biophys. Acta **497:** 349-357.
3. MURPHY, D. J. & R. D. MAVIS. 1981. Membrane transfer of α-tocopherol—influence of soluble α-tocopherol-binding factors from the liver, lung, heart, and brain of the rat. J. Biol. Chem. **256:** 10464-10468.
4. MOWRI, H., Y. NAKAGAWA, K. INOUE & S. NOJIMA. 1981. Enhancement of the transfer of α-tocopherol between liposomes and mitochondria by rat-liver protein(s). Eur. J. Biochem. **117:** 537-542.
5. BEHRENS, W. A. & R. MADÈRE. 1982. Occurrence of a rat liver α-tocopherol binding protein *in vivo*. Nutr. Rep. Int. **25:** 107-112.
6. BEHRENS, W. A. & R. MADÈRE. 1982. Transfer of α-tocopherol to microsomes mediated by a partially purified liver α-tocopherol binding protein. Nutr. Res. **2:** 611-618.
7. BEHRENS, W. A. & R. MADÈRE. 1983. Interrelationship and competition of α and γ tocopherol at the level of intestinal absorption, plasma transport and liver uptake. Nutr. Res. **3:** 891-897.
8. GUARNIERI, C., P. FLAMIGNI & C. M. CALDARERA. 1980. A possible role of rabbit heart cytosol tocopherol binding in the transfer of tocopherol into nuclei. Biochem. J. **190:** 469-471.
9. SUGIYAMA, Y., T. YAMADA & N. KAPLOWITZ. 1983. Newly identified bile acid binders in rat liver cytosol: purification and comparison with glutathione S-transferases. J. Biol. Chem. **258:** 3602-3607.
10. STOLZ, A., H. TAKIKAWA, Y. SUGIYAMA, J. KUHLENKAMP & N. KAPLOWITZ. 1987. 3αHydroxysteroid dehydrogenase activity of the Y' bile acid binders in rat liver cytosol. Identification, kinetics and physiologic significance. J. Clin. Invest. **79:** 427-434.

α-Tocopherol as Compared with γ-Tocopherol Is Preferentially Secreted in Human Lipoproteins[a]

MARET G. TRABER AND HERBERT J. KAYDEN

Department of Medicine
New York University School of Medicine
New York, New York 10016

INTRODUCTION

α-Tocopherol is present in human plasma at concentrations several fold greater than is γ-tocopherol, in spite of the fact that the diet contains higher concentrations of γ-tocopherol.[1-3] Supplementation of the diet with vitamin E, either as *all-rac-α-*tocopheryl acetate or *RRR-α*-tocopheryl acetate, results in an increase of α-tocopherol, but a decrease in the plasma concentration of γ-tocopherol,[4-6] suggesting that there is a mechanism for preferentially increasing the α-tocopherol content of the plasma.

We have undertaken studies in humans to investigate the mechanisms by which α-tocopherol and γ-tocopherol are discriminated *in vivo*.

METHODS

Subjects

Studies were carried out both in normal human volunteers without metabolic abnormalities of lipid metabolism, and in patients with defined metabolic abnormalities. The subjects gave informed consent, and the study was carried out within the guidelines established by the Institutional Review Board of New York University School of Medicine. Except for the study shown in FIGURE 1, a standard protocol was followed. After an overnight fast (12 h), blood was drawn for a pretreatment sample. Then the subject ingested a single dose of either *all-rac-α*-tocopheryl acetate (Hoffmann-La Roche, Nutley, NJ) or equal amounts of both *all-rac-α*-tocopherol (Hoffmann-La Roche, Inc.) and *RRR-γ*-tocopherol (Eastman Kodak, Rochester, NY) along with breakfast.

The dose containing free tocopherols was prepared the day prior to the experiment. Accurately weighed amounts of the tocopherols were mixed with butter (10 g), and

[a] These studies were supported in part by Grants from the National Heart, Lung and Blood Institute, #HL30842, and Hoffmann-La Roche, Nutley, NJ.

the container was covered with foil and kept refrigerated overnight. Following ingestion of the vitamin E capsule or vitamin E/butter mixture with breakfast, the subjects carried out their usual activities and consumed food ad libitum. Blood was drawn at the indicated intervals into Vacutainer tubes containing 0.05 mL 15% EDTA (Becton Dickinson, Rutherford, NJ). Plasma was immediately separately from red cells by centrifugation and stored at 4°C. Plasma lipoproteins were isolated within 36 h of blood-drawing.

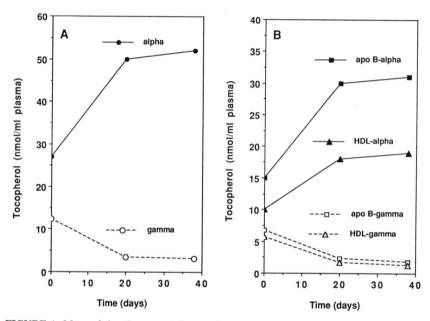

FIGURE 1. Mean of the plasma and lipoprotein tocopherol levels of 6 normal subjects after supplementation with 800 IU of *all-rac-*α-tocopheryl acetate for the indicated lengths of time. **A** shows the plasma α- and γ-tocopherol concentrations; **B** shows the α- and γ-tocopherol concentrations of apolipoprotein (apo) B-containing lipoproteins (chylomicrons, VLDL, and LDL) and HDL isolated by Mn-heparin precipitation.

Isolation of Lipoproteins by Ultracentrifugation

Plasma lipoproteins were isolated using a modification of the method of Havel *et al.,*[7] using the TL100 ultracentrifuge (Beckman Instruments, Inc. Palo Alto, CA), as previously described.[8] The density was adjusted with solid KBr such that lipoproteins were isolated at the following density intervals: chylomicrons + very low density lipoproteins (VLDL) ($d < 1.006$ g/mL), low density lipoproteins (LDL) ($1.019 < d < 1.063$ g/mL), and high density lipoproteins (HDL) ($d > 1.063$ g/mL). Upon isolation, the lipoprotein fractions were stored at 4°C for less than 2 days prior to analysis for tocopherol contents.

Casual samples of bile were obtained from random patients who had undergone gallbladder surgery with removal of the gallbladder and placement of an indwelling T-tube. Bile was collected from the T-tube by allowing the bile to drain into a sterile glass tube. One of these patients was studied following the administration of vitamin E according to the standard protocol.

Tocopherol Analysis

The tocopherols were quantitated as previously described[9] using high-pressure liquid chromatography (HPLC) with fluorescence detection (excitation 205, emission 340 nm) by comparison of peak heights to known quantities of authentic *all-rac-α*-tocopherol and *RRR-γ*-tocopherol. During the tocopherol extraction and quantitation procedures, the samples were protected from light. Recoveries of both tocopherols were in excess of 98 percent.

RESULTS

Administration of Vitamin E Supplements to Normal Subjects

Although administration of vitamin E supplements in the form of *all-rac-α*-tocopheryl acetate to normal subjects has been reported to decrease the levels of γ-tocopherol in plasma,[4,5] the effects on specific lipoprotein fractions has not been reported. To determine whether supplements of α-tocopherol specifically reduced the γ-tocopherol in any one lipoprotein fraction, the α- and γ-tocopherol contents of lipoproteins isolated from normal subjects given a twice daily (with breakfast and dinner) supplement of 400 IU of *all-rac-α*-tocopheryl acetate were estimated from the HPLC tracings of a previously reported study.[10] FIGURE 1A demonstrates that the plasma α-tocopherol at 20 days was nearly twice the presupplementation value, whereas the γ-tocopherol had decreased from 12.4 ± 4.1 nmol/mL to 3.5 ± 0.9. The increase in the α-tocopherol concentration along with the decrease in the γ-tocopherol concentration resulted in nearly a sevenfold increase in the α- /γ-ratio. These changes were maintained at the next time point of 38 days. In this study, plasma was separated by manganese-heparin precipitation into two lipoprotein fractions: apolipoprotein (apo) B-containing lipoproteins (*i.e.* chylomicrons, VLDL, LDL) and HDL. α- and γ-Tocopherols were similarly distributed into the two lipoprotein fractions for each subject (FIG. 1B).

The time course of the disappearance of γ-tocopherol from the plasma in response to supplemental vitamin E was studied in a subject given a single dose of *all-rac-α*-tocopheryl acetate (800 IU) with breakfast following an overnight fast. Blood samples were taken for 48 h at appropriate intervals and the tocopherol contents of plasma and lipoprotein fractions determined. By 24 h the plasma α-tocopherol concentration had increased more than one-third; the γ-tocopherol content decreased by one-third, resulting in an increase in the α- /γ-ratio by nearly sixfold (FIG. 2). The α-tocopherol content of the chylomicron + VLDL fraction reached a peak at 4 h, whereas the

LDL and HDL fractions reached peak values at 24 hours. By contrast, the γ-tocopherol decreased at 7 h in the chylomicron + VLDL fraction, and at 24 h in both LDL and HDL, suggesting that α- and γ-tocopherol are transported differently (data not shown).

To determine whether α- and γ-tocopherols compete with each other for absorption and transport in lipoproteins, two subjects were given equal doses (1 g) of α- and γ-tocopherol. The results of a representative experiment are shown in FIGURE 3. Plasma levels of both α- and γ-tocopherols increased up to 6 h; by 24 h the γ-tocopherol concentration decreased precipitously, while the α-tocopherol concentration remained elevated. During the peak in the absorption phase (6-12 h), the α-/γ-ratio decreased from 5.9 to 1.1, but returned to the time 0 values by 24 hours. FIGURE 4 shows that the chylomicron + VLDL fraction contained similar increases of both α- and γ-tocopherols up to 6 hours; then the γ-tocopherol decreased precipitously (FIG. 4B).

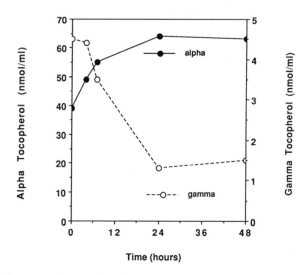

FIGURE 2. Plasma α- and γ-tocopherol concentrations of a normal subject supplemented with a single 800 IU dose of *all-rac-α-tocopheryl* acetate.

The α-tocopherol content of the LDL and HDL fractions increased at 24 h, whereas the γ-tocopherol content decreased. Taken together these data demonstrate that both tocopherols are equally well-absorbed, but following absorption and secretion in chylomicrons, the two tocopherols are transported differently.

Administration of Vitamin E Supplements to Subjects with Abnormalities of Lipid Metabolism

Chylomicrons are rapidly catabolized in the circulation by lipoprotein lipase[11] to remnants that are taken up by the liver. Lipoprotein lipase hydrolyzes triglycerides

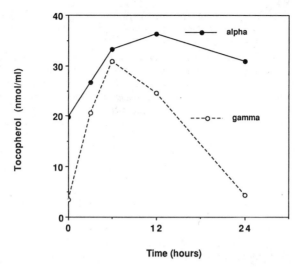

FIGURE 3. Plasma α- and γ-tocopherol concentrations of a normal subject following ingestion of a single dose (1 g each) of *all-rac*-α- and *RRR*-γ-tocopherols.

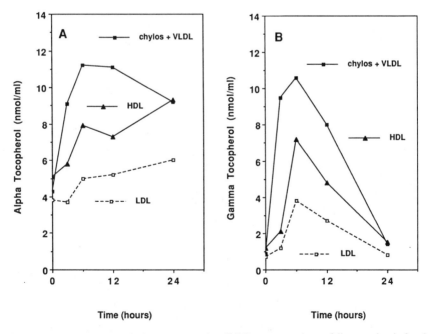

FIGURE 4. α-Tocopherol (**A**) and γ-tocopherol (**B**) concentrations of lipoproteins isolated from the plasma of the subject shown in FIGURE 3.

to free fatty acids and monoglycerides with transfer of fatty acids[11] and tocopherol[12] to tissues. Lipoprotein lipase-deficient patients, who catabolize chylomicrons very slowly,[13] have circulating plasma triglycerides in excess of 11 mmol/L (1000 mg/dL) with >90% of the circulating tocopherol in chylomicrons. Two such patients were given a single oral dose containing equal amounts (1 g) of α- and γ-tocopherols. Both tocopherols increased in the plasma at all time points up to 24 h (data not shown), and most of each tocopherol was contained within the chylomicron + VLDL fraction (FIG. 5). These data demonstrate that a deficiency of lipoprotein lipase results in the accumulation in the plasma of chylomicron particles containing equal increases of α- and γ-tocopherols in response to an oral supplementation of both.

In a patient with an acquired deficiency of lipoprotein lipase (due to pancreatitis[14]), supplementation with 800 IU *all-rac*-α-tocopheryl acetate resulted in a marked increase in the α-tocopherol content, but no alteration in the γ-tocopherol content of the plasma or the other lipoprotein fractions, with the exception of a slight decrease in the γ-tocopherol content of the chylomicron + VLDL fraction at 24 h (data not shown). These data suggest that the decrease in the γ-tocopherol content of the plasma of normal subjects following ingestion of α-tocopherol is a result of transport mechanisms for lipids subsequent to chylomicron secretion.

To test this hypothesis a patient with dysbetalipoproteinemia was given an oral dose containing 1 g each of α- and γ-tocopherols. In this patient, chylomicrons were hydrolyzed by lipoprotein lipase, VLDL was secreted by the liver, but the uptake of chylomicron remnants, especially VLDL remnants, by the liver was impaired due to

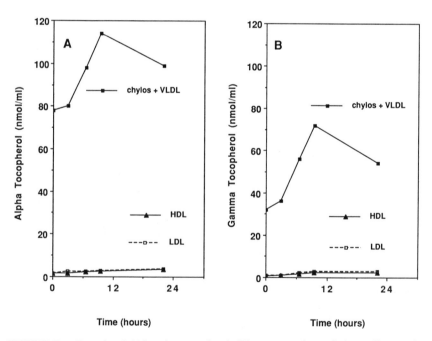

FIGURE 5. α-Tocopherol (**A**) and γ-tocopherol (**B**) concentrations of plasma lipoproteins following ingestion of a single dose of (1 g each) *all-rac* α- and *RRR*-γ-tocopherols by a patient with lipoprotein lipase deficiency.

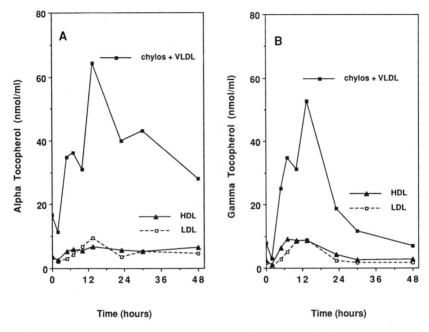

FIGURE 6. α-Tocopherol (A) and γ-tocopherol (B) concentrations of plasma lipoproteins following ingestion of a single dose (1 g each) of *all-rac* α- and *RRR*-γ-tocopherols by a patient with dysbetalipoproteinemia.

a genetically abnormal apolipoprotein E phenotype. Thus an abnormal VLDL particle accumulates in the plasma. Following ingestion of the two tocopherols, both tocopherols increased in the plasma up to 13.5 h, whereas the γ-tocopherol concentration decreased at 24 h (data not shown). FIGURE 6 demonstrates that the chylomicron + VLDL fraction contained increases in both α- and γ-tocopherols, but the γ-tocopherol concentration decreased more markedly at 23 hours. At 48 h the γ-tocopherol content had decreased to the time 0 value, whereas the α-tocopherol remained at nearly twice the initial value. These data support the hypothesis that the liver secretes VLDL particles preferentially enriched in α-tocopherol.

A group of patients has been described who have a rare defect that results in vitamin E deficiency in the absence of lipid malabsorption.[15] In collaborative studies carried out with Dr. Ron Sokol of the University of Colorado Health Science Center, Denver, CO, a male patient with this disorder was given a 1 g dose of each α- and γ-tocopherols. The plasma and lipoproteins were isolated according to the standard protocol. This subject absorbed both α- and γ-tocopherols, with equal increases of both forms in the plasma at 12 hours. Although the subject had deficient plasma levels of the vitamin at the outset of the experiment, by 12 hours the plasma levels were similar to those of normal subjects (data not shown). As shown in FIGURE 7 this subject has what appears to be a normal pattern for the transport of the two tocopherols up to 24 hours. As shown in FIGURE 8, however, the chylomicron + VLDL fraction in this patient was different from that of the normal subject, in that both α- and γ-tocopherols decreased precipitously at 24 h in the patient, but only the

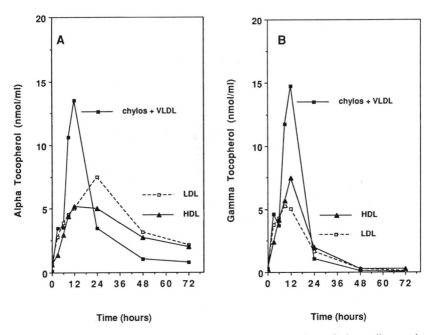

FIGURE 7. α-Tocopherol (**A**) and γ-tocopherol (**B**) concentrations of plasma lipoproteins following ingestion of a single dose (1 g each) of *all-rac* α- and *RRR*-γ-tocopherols by a patient with familial isolated vitamin E deficiency.

γ-tocopherol decreased rapidly at 24 h in the control subject. These data suggest that the defect in patients with familial vitamin E deficiency may result from an impaired secretion of α-tocopherol in VLDL. Studies are presently underway using deuterated tocopherols to assess the cause of familial vitamin E deficiency.

Effect of Vitamin E Supplements on Biliary Excretion of Tocopherols

Because the liver secretes bile containing tocopherol, it seemed possible that γ-tocopherol might be excreted in the bile and α-tocopherol incorporated into VLDL and secreted into the plasma. To test this hypothesis patients undergoing gallbladder surgery, who required the placement of a T-tube in the bile duct, were studied. Casual samples of both bile and plasma were obtained and the α- and γ-tocopherol contents determined. As seen in TABLE 1, the plasma contained higher concentrations of both tocopherols than did the bile. Furthermore, the α-/γ-ratio was not appreciably different between the bile samples and the plasma samples for each subject, but was slightly lower in the bile than in the plasma.

To evaluate whether there was a preferential excretion of γ-tocopherol in response to an oral dose of both tocopherols, a patient who had undergone gallbladder surgery participated following her release from the hospital, but prior to removal of the T-tube. Following administration of a single dose containing 300 mg each of α- and γ-

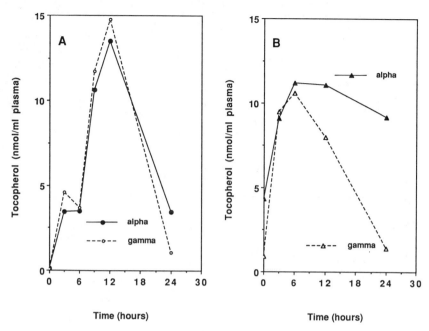

FIGURE 8. Comparison of the of α- and γ-tocopherol concentrations of the chylomicrons + VLDL fractions isolated from a subject with familial vitamin E deficiency (**A**) and a normal subject (**B**).

TABLE 1. The α- and γ-Tocopherol Concentrations in Plasma and Bile of Patients following Gallbladder Surgery

Subject	Plasma Tocopherol (nmol/mL)			Bile Tocopherol (nmol/mL)		
	α-	γ-	α- /γ-	α-	γ-	α- /γ-
1	13.0	0.8	15.5	20.9	0.4	58.2
2	18.4	3.8	4.8	28.1	8.2	3.5
3	18.6	0.3	59.7	21.6	0.4	60.1
4	18.8	2.9	6.5	16.5	2.2	7.5
5	19.8	2.1	9.5	36.0	4.1	8.8
6	20.2	2.9	7.0	6.3	1.2	5.3
7	20.2	3.6	5.6	18.4	4.1	4.5
8	22.8	4.3	5.3	36.7	10.1	3.6
9	25.3	3.6	7.0	10.2	1.8	5.8
10	29.3	4.1	7.2	25.3	5.0	5.0
11	33.0	0.7	45.9	1.0	0.1	14.2
12	34.2	1.0	33.9	1.3	0.1	18.4
13	36.3	5.5	6.6	14.6	3.4	4.3
14	46.1	6.0	7.7	10.9	1.9	5.7
Mean	25.4	3.0	15.9	17.7	3.1	14.6
SD	9.1	1.8	17.5	11.4	3.0	19.3

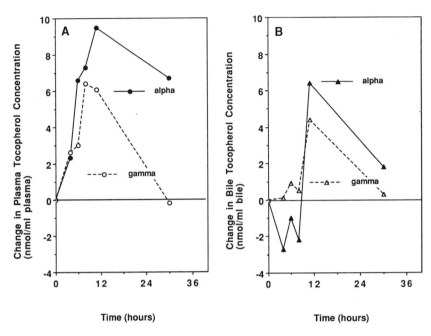

FIGURE 9. Change in the α- and γ-tocopherol concentrations of plasma (**A**) and bile (**B**) following ingestion of a single dose (300 mg each) of *all-rac*-α- and *RRR*-γ-tocopherols by a patient who had undergone gallbladder surgery.

tocopherols, the increments of the tocopherols in plasma and bile compared to their concentrations at the initiation of the experiment were measured and are shown in FIGURE 9. These data demonstrate that during the early time points of the experiment γ-tocopherol was increasing in the bile, whereas the concentration of α-tocopherol decreased (FIG. 9B). The peak in the bile α-tocopherol concentration took place at 11 h; simultaneously, both α- and γ-tocopherols increased markedly in the plasma (FIG. 9A). These data suggest that γ-tocopherol is excreted in the bile, whereas α-tocopherol is preferentially secreted in lipoproteins, until the mechanism for recognition is saturated. At that time, both tocopherols are indiscriminately excreted in the bile. This hypothesis is currently under investigation.

DISCUSSION

The purpose of these studies was to assess the mechanisms by which humans discriminate between α- and γ-tocopherols. We have demonstrated that supplementation with a single dose of *all-rac*-α-tocopheryl acetate, in as short a period of time as 24 h, results in an increase in the plasma α-tocopherol and a decrease in the γ-tocopherol concentrations. By contrast, administration of equal amounts of α- and γ-tocopherols results in similar increases in both tocopherols up to 12 h; then the γ-, but not the α-tocopherol, concentration decreases. Examination of the tocopherol contents of the lipoprotein fractions indicates that these changes appeared virtually simultaneously in all of the fractions isolated.

Studies were carried out in patients with defined metabolic abnormalities of lipoprotein metabolism to separate the various steps of de novo lipoprotein secretion. Patients with lipoprotein lipase deficiency, when given a dose containing equal amounts of α-tocopherol and γ-tocopherol, had equal increases of both tocopherols in their plasma and in the chylomicron + VLDL fraction up to 24 hours. Furthermore, a patient with an acquired lipoprotein lipase deficiency, who was given only α-tocopheryl acetate, had increases in the plasma α-tocopherol concentration, but no decrease in the γ-tocopherol concentration at 24 hours. Taken together, these data demonstrate that α- and γ-tocopherols do not compete for absorption in the intestinal cell during the secretion of tocopherols in chylomicrons, and both are secreted in chylomicrons. Similar conclusions have been obtained in studies using rats.[16,17]

The decrease in the γ-tocopherol concentration observed at 24 h in the normal subjects probably results from uptake of chylomicrons and chylomicron remnants by the liver, with the preferential incorporation of α-tocopherol in nascent VLDL and secretion of nascent VLDL particles by the liver, as indicated in the proposed mechanism for tocopherol transport shown in FIGURE 10. The subsequent catabolism of VLDL enriched in α-tocopherol in the plasma compartment would result in a marked

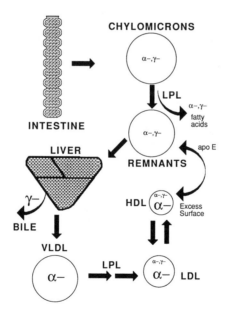

FIGURE 10. Proposed scheme for the transport of vitamin E in lipoproteins. Chylomicrons are secreted by the intestine containing both α- and γ-tocopherols. These particles are catabolized in the circulation by lipoprotein lipase (LPL) with transfer of fatty acids and tocopherols to the tissues and transfer of excess surface components including tocopherols to HDL with transfer of apo E from HDL to the chylomicrons to form remnants. The remnants are taken up by the liver, which preferentially secretes α-tocopherol in nascent VLDL containing the newly absorbed lipids. The catabolism of VLDL leads to the production of LDL and HDL containing α-tocopherol. It is proposed that the γ-tocopherol is excreted by the liver into the bile.

increase in plasma α-tocopherol, but not γ-tocopherol, in the postabsorptive phase. This mechanism is supported by the studies in the patients with hyperlipidemia. In subjects with lipoprotein lipase deficiency there was no decrease in the plasma γ-tocopherol content at 24 h, suggesting that the catabolism of chylomicrons and uptake of chylomicron remnants with secretion of VLDL by the liver are important for the "disappearance" of γ-tocopherol from the plasma. In the patient with dysbetalipoproteinemia the plasma levels of the tocopherols increased to concentrations similar to those observed in the lipase deficient subjects, but the catabolism of the chylomicrons and secretion of VLDL particles in this subject resulted in the decrease in the γ-tocopherol levels at 24 hours.

This mechanism fits with the known properties of the cytosolic liver tocopherol binding protein isolated in rats,[18-20] which recognizes γ-tocopherol with one-tenth the affinity of α-tocopherol. We suggest that it is the protein that determines the incorporation of α- or γ-tocopherol into nascent lipoprotein particles during their assembly and secretion from the liver. Studies directed to establish the role of the putative tocopherol binding protein in the transport of vitamin E in humans are in progress.

The γ-tocopherol present in the plasma appears to result from the catabolism of chylomicrons. As indicated in FIGURE 10, γ-tocopherol enters the plasma compartment in chylomicrons. During the catabolism of these particles at early time points the concentrations of both α- and γ-tocopherols increased in the LDL and HDL fractions. This phenomenon could occur during the transfer of excess surface components of chylomicrons to HDL during chylomicron catabolism by lipoprotein lipase.[21] It is well-known that HDL particles can rapidly exchange tocopherol with LDL particles.[22,23] By this mechanism, γ-tocopherol could be incorporated "simultaneously" into these lipoprotein particles.

The other aspect of liver tocopherol transport that was examined in this study was the excretion of tocopherols in the bile. We had anticipated that if the liver preferentially secreted α-tocopherol in the VLDL, then γ-tocopherol might be preferentially excreted in the bile. These data do not unequivocally demonstrate that this is so. Casual samples of bile contained both α- and γ-tocopherols at concentrations lower than in the plasma with only slightly lower α-/γ-ratios. Administration of equal amounts of α- and γ-tocopherols to a patient with an indwelling T-tube resulted in a small increase in the excretion of γ-tocopherol with a small decrease in the excretion of α-tocopherol at early time points; however, by 12 h post-dose the excretion of α-tocopherol far exceeded that of γ-tocopherol. It should be noted that the subjects for this aspect of the study were patients who had recently undergone surgery and were not necessarily consuming a normal diet. The excretion of large amounts of both tocopherols suggests that any specific mechanism for transport of α-tocopherol was saturated by the large dose. This latter point may explain the relative safety of vitamin E with respect to other fat soluble vitamins. It appears that vitamin E is rapidly excreted in the bile in response to ingestion of a large oral dose of the vitamin.

Behrens and Madere[24] have suggested, based on their studies in rats, that γ-tocopherol is more rapidly excreted from the tissues, and γ-tocopherol in the plasma reflects this more rapid tissue turnover. There is an alternative interpretation. We propose that less γ-tocopherol is actively secreted in VLDL, which leads to a lower plasma level of γ-tocopherol, which in turn leads to lower levels of γ-tocopherol in the tissues. Excretion of tocopherols from the body appears to be by way of the bile and the feces.

In conclusion, the data presented here illustrate that both α- and γ-tocopherols are similarly well-absorbed by humans, but by 24 h there are mechanisms that reduce the γ-tocopherol concentration in the plasma of normal human subjects. The studies carried out in the hyperlipidemic subjects indicate that the liver may secrete VLDL preferentially enriched in α-tocopherol, whereas the studies in the patients following gallbladder surgery suggest that γ-tocopherol may be preferentially excreted in the bile. The preliminary study in the patient with familial vitamin E deficiency suggests that these genetically affected patients may become vitamin E-deficient due to the absence of, or a defect in, the mechanism for the incorporation of α-tocopherol into nascent VLDL by the liver. To confirm the results of these studies they must be repeated using physiological amounts of tocopherols labeled with stable isotopes.

ACKNOWLEDGMENTS

Nora Lagmay and Cheryl Thellman provided excellent technical assistance.

REFERENCES

1. BIERI, J. G. & R. P. EVARTS. 1974. Gamma tocopherol: metabolism, biological activity and significance in human nutrition. Am. J. Clin. Nutr. **27:** 980-6.
2. CHOW, C. K. 1975. Distribution of tocopherols in human plasma and red blood cells. Am. J. Clin. Nutr. **28:** 756-60.
3. BEHRENS, W. A. & R. MADERE. 1986. Alpha- and gamma-tocopherol concentrations in human serum. J. Am. Coll. Nutr. **5:** 91-6.
4. BAKER, H., G. J. HANDELMAN, S. SHORT, L. J. MACHLIN, H. N. BHAGAVAN, E. A. DRATZ & O. FRANK. 1986. Comparison of plasma α- and γ-tocopherol levels following chronic oral administration of either all-rac-α-tocopherol acetate or RRR-α-tocopherol acetate in normal adult male subjects. Am. J. Clin. Nutr. **43:** 382-7.
5. HANDELMAN, G. J., L. J. MACHLIN, K. FITCH, J. J. WEITER & E. A. DRATZ. 1985. Oral α-tocopherol supplements decrease plasma γ-tocopherol levels in humans. J. Nutr. **115:** 807-13.
6. BEHRENS, W. A. & R. MADERE. 1985. Transport of α- and γ-tocopherol in human plasma lipoproteins. Nutr. Res. **5:** 167-74.
7. HAVEL, R. J., H. A. EDER & J. H. BRAGDON. 1955. The distribution and chemical composition of ultracentrifugally separated lipoproteins in human serum. J. Clin. Invest. **34:** 1345-53.
8. TRABER, M. G., H. J. KAYDEN & M. J. RINDLER. 1987. Polarized secretion of newly synthesized lipoproteins by the Caco-2 human intestinal cell line. J. Lipid Res. **28:** 1350-63.
9. HATAM, L. J. & H. J. KAYDEN. 1979. A high performance liquid chromatographic method for the determination of tocopherol in plasma and cellular elements of the blood. J. Lipid Res. **20:** 639-45.
10. HATAM, L. J. & H. J. KAYDEN. 1981. The failure of α-tocopherol supplementation to alter the distribution of lipoprotein cholesterol in normal and hyperlipoproteinemic persons. Am. J. Clin. Pathol. **76:** 122-4.
11. NELSSON-EHLE, P., A. S. GARFINKEL & M. C. SCHOTZ. 1980. Lipolytic enzymes and plasma lipoprotein metabolism. Annu. Rev. Biochem. **49:** 667-93.
12. TRABER, M. G., T. OLIVECRONA & H. J. KAYDEN. 1985. Bovine milk lipoprotein lipase transfers tocopherol to human fibroblasts during triglyceride hydrolysis *in vitro.* J. Clin. Invest. **75:** 1729-1734.
13. STALENHOEF, A. F. H., J. M. MALLOY, J. P. KANE & R. J. HAVEL. 1984. Metabolism of apolipoproteins B-48 and B-100 of triglyceride-rich lipoproteins in normal and lipoprotein lipase-deficient humans. Proc. Natl. Acad. Sci. USA **81:** 1839-43.

14. GOLDBERG, I. J., J. R. PATERNITI, G. H. FRANKLIN, H. N. GINSBERG, F. GINSBERG-FELLNER & W. V. BROWN. 1983. Transient lipoprotein lipase deficiency with hyperchylomicronemia. Am. J. Med. Sci. **286:** 28-31.
15. SOKOL, R. J., H. J. KAYDEN, D. B. BETTIS, M. G. TRABER, H. NEVILLE, S. RINGLE, W. B. WILSON & D. A. STUMP. 1988. Isolated vitamin E deficiency in the absence of fat malabsorption—familial and sporadic cases: Characterization and investigation of causes. J. Lab. Clin. Med. **111:** 548-59.
16. PEAKE, I. R. & J. G. BIERI. 1977. α- and γ-Tocopherol in the rat: *in vitro* and *in vivo* tissue uptake and metabolism. J. Nutr. **101:** 1615-22.
17. TRABER, M. G., H. J. KAYDEN, J. BALMER-GREEN & M. H. GREEN. 1986. Absorption of water-miscible forms of vitamin E in a patient with cholestasis and in thoracic duct-cannulated rats. Am. J. Clin. Nutr. **44:** 914-923.
18. CATIGNANI, G. L. & J. G. BIERI. 1977. Rat liver α-tocopherol binding protein. Biochim. Biophys. Acta **497:** 349-357.
19. MURPHY, D. J. & R. D. MAVIS. 1981. Membrane transfer of α-tocopherol. J. Biol. Chem. **256:** 10464-8.
20. BEHRENS, W. A. & R. MADERE. 1982. Transfer of α-tocopherol to microsomes mediated by a partially purified liver α-tocopherol binding protein. Nutr. Res. **2:** 611-8.
21. GOTTO, A. M., H. J. POWNALL & R. J. HAVEL. 1986. Introduction to the plasma lipoproteins. Methods Enzymol. **128:** 3-41.
22. BJORNSON, L. K., C. GNIEWKOWSKI & H. J. KAYDEN. 1975. A comparison of the exchange of α-tocopherol and free cholesterol between rat plasma lipoproteins and erythrocytes. J. Lipid Res. **16:** 39-53.
23. MASSEY, J. B. 1984. Kinetics of transfer of α-tocopherol between model and native plasma lipoproteins. Biochim. Biophys. Acta **193:** 387-392.
24. BEHRENS, W. A. & R. MADERE. 1987. Mechanisms of absorption, transport and tissue uptake of RRR-α-tocopherol and d-γ-tocopherol in the white rat. J. Nutr. **117:** 1562-1569.

Localization of α-Tocopherol in Membranes[a]

J. C. GOMEZ-FERNANDEZ,[b] J. VILLALAIN,[b]
F. J. ARANDA,[b] A. ORTIZ,[b] V. MICOL,[b]
A. COUTINHO,[c] M. N. BERBERAN-SANTOS,[c]
AND M. J. E. PRIETO[c]

[b] *Departamento de Bioquimica y Biologia Molecular*
Facultad de Veterinaria
Universidad de Murcia
E-30071, Murcia, Spain
[c] *Centro de Quimica Fisica Molecular*
Instituto Superior Técnico
1096 Lisboa Codex, Portugal

INTRODUCTION

Tocopherols have been shown to be very important components of biological membranes, where they act mainly as potent antioxidants[1] and contribute to membrane stabilization.[2] In order to understand better the molecular mechanism of tocopherols, it is important to study their interaction with membrane components and especially with lipids. In this way the localization and dynamics of tocopherols in membranes can be known. A number of studies have been done, mainly with α-tocopherol reconstituted in phospholipid vesicles, applying a wide variety of physical techniques. We will summarize in this paper our studies using DSC, FT-IR, and fluorescence spectroscopy.

PERTURBATION OF PHOSPHOLIPID PHASE TRANSITION BY TOCOPHEROLS

The inclusion of increasing concentrations of α-tocopherol in vesicles of fully saturated phospholipids has been shown to progressively broaden the temperature range of the phase transition of the phospholipid, with its onset temperature being

[a] This work was supported in part by Grant PA86-0211 from Dirección General de Investigación Científica y Technológica (Spain) to J. C. G.-F. and by Research Grant 27777 from Instituto Nacional de Investigação Científica (Portugal) to A. C.

lowered and the enthalpy of the gel to liquid-crystalline transition being reduced. This has been found in studies employing differential scanning calorimetry (DSC),[3-8] electron spin resonance (ESR),[9] [2]H nuclear magnetic resonance (^{2}H NMR),[8] and Fourier transform infrared (FT-IR) spectroscopy.[5]

It is interesting to note that α-tocopheryl acetate, when included in *dipalmitoylphosphatidylcholine* (DPPC), gave the same effect, but less marked, as in the case of α-tocopherol as shown by DSC (FIG. 1). The lowering and broadening of the phase transition induced by α-tocopherol may be expected from molecules that preferentially partition into fluid domains of the bilayer, decreasing the van der Waals interactions between the terminal methyl and methylene groups of the phospholipid hydrocarbon chain.[7]

FT-IR measurements were also employed, examining bands that report on interactions in the acyl chains (CH$_2$ stretching vibration) and in the interfacial region of

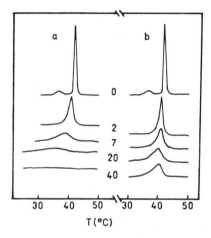

FIGURE 1. The DSC calorimetric curves for pure dipalmitoylphosphatidylcholine (DPPC) and DPPC/α-tocopherol systems. Molar percentages of α-tocopherol in DPPC are indicated on the curves. Results correspond to samples containing (a) α-tocopherol and (b) α-tocopheryl acetate. Samples were normalized to the same amount of lipid in each case. Measurements were carried out at 4 K/min in a Perkin-Elmer DSC-4 calorimeter.

the phospholipid (C=O stretching vibration). FIGURE 2 shows that the maximum of the C$_2$ antisymmetric stretching vibration band of pure DPPC is shifted from 2918 cm^{-1} to 2922.4 cm^{-1} during the main phase transition, this shift being associated with the change from all-*trans* to *gauche* conformers.[10-11] The incorporation of increasing concentrations of α-tocopherol produces a progressive broadening of the phase transition and a shift of the onset of this transition to lower temperatures. Both above and below the phospholipid phase transition there is a decrease in *gauche* isomers. α-Tocopheryl acetate broadens the phase transition, however, but does not appreciably affect the proportion of *gauche* conformers at the very high concentration (20 mole-percent) tested.

The perturbation of the membrane interfacial region, produced by α-tocopherol, can be fully appreciated by monitoring the frequency of the C = O stretching band of DPPC (FIG. 3). This band centered at 1735 cm^{-1} and is very broad because of

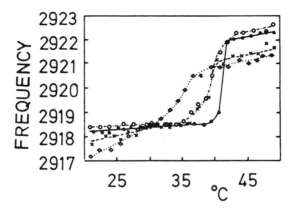

FIGURE 2. Temperature dependence of the CH_2 antisymmetric band of DPPC. (●——●) Pure DPPC, (○----○) 20 mole-percent of α-tocopheryl acetate, (x---x) 5 mole-percent of α-tocopherol, and (◇---◇) 20 mole-percent of α-tocopherol in DPPC. All infrared spectra have been obtained at 2 cm^{-1} resolution in a Nicolet MX-1 FT-IR spectrometer assisted by a Nicolet 1200-S computer.

the superposition of the bands corresponding to the *sn*-1 and *sn*-2 C = O groups of the fatty acid esters of DPPC, both in dehydrated and in hydrated forms.[12] Two bands can be resolved by different computational techniques, like second-derivative band decomposition, as shown in FIGURE 3, which belong to the dehydrated C = O groups (highest frequency, 1743 cm^{-1} for DPPC at 25°C) and hydrated C = O groups (lower frequency, 1729 cm^{-1} for DPPC at 25°C). As can be observed, the effect of α-tocopherol on the composite band is more pronounced than that of α-tocopheryl acetate. α-Tocopherol induces a decrease in the frequency of the maximum of this band at all temperatures. On the other hand, the effect on the frequency of the

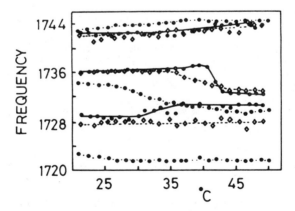

FIGURE 3. Temperature dependence of the C=O ester band of DPPC. (○——○) Pure DPPC, (◇---◇) 20 mole-percent of α-tocopheryl acetate, and (●----●) 20 mole-percent of α-tocopherol in DPPC. Upper and lower traces show the *sn*-1 and *sn*-2 components, respectively, and medium traces show the maximum frequency of the composite band.

dehydrated component is small, but, however, it is significant on the hydrated component. α-Tocopherol induced a decrease in frequency of the second component of about 7 cm^{-1}, whereas α-tocopheryl acetate induced a decrease of 1-2 cm^{-1} only.

The results shown above indicate that the effect of α-tocopherol is found both in the acyl chains and in the interfacial region of the phospholipid. This conclusion is compatible with the model proposed by Perly et al.,[13] where α-tocopherol is situated in both monolayers in an arrangement of phytyl tail to phytyl tail, with the phenolic hydroxyl group located in the lipid/water interfacial region of the membrane. The strong effect of α-tocopherol on the structure of the lipid/water interface of the membrane might be thought to be due to the formation of hydrogen bonding between the α-tocopherol hydroxyl group and the polar part of DPPC, as suggested by Srivastava et al.[9] We have not observed significant changes in the phosphate stretching band of DPPC induced by the presence of α-tocopherol; hence it seems that the hydroxyl group of α-tocopherol is hydrogen bonded to a C = O group of DPPC. It is clear that the hydroxyl group of α-tocopherol allows this molecule to be positioned in the bilayer in such a position that the van der Waals interactions with the acyl chains of the phospholipids can be maximized. Because α-tocopheryl acetate has this group blocked by the acetyl replacement, it may not give such a strong perturbation on the DPPC structure, and it would possibly be located in a more hydrophobic position than that of α-tocopherol. The importance of the hydroxyl group of α-tocopherol in determining its interaction with phospholipids has been also emphasized by Lai et al.,[14] working with a hemisuccinate ester of α-tocopherol that has a more remarkable lower effect on the phospholipid phase transition than the free α-tocopherol.

PREFERENCE OF TOCOPHEROL FOR FLUID DOMAINS IN THE MEMBRANE

The concentration of α-tocopherol in biological membranes is rather low. It has been estimated to be in the range of 0.1 to 1.0 mole-percent (of phospholipid).[6] The existence of domains in the membrane with heterogeneous lipid composition, however, could produce an accumulation of α-tocopherol in particular membrane regions. Lipid domains giving lipid heterogeneity in the lateral plane of the bilayer have been postulated for a number of biological membranes, including animal membranes and a plant plasma membrane.[15] These lipid domains, having different lipid composition, have also different degrees of fluidity.

In addition, the transverse asymmetry of plasma membrane phospholipids is a well-documented fact,[16] and evidence exists for differences in fluidity between bilayer halves of the plasma membrane.[17]

Keeping this in mind, we have investigated whether α-tocopherol has a preference for fluid or solid domains in phospholipid vesicles.[7] DSC measurements are presented in FIGURE 4, showing that when α-tocopherol is present in equimolar mixtures of dimyristoylphosphatidylcholine (DMPC) and distearoylphosphatidylcholine (DSPC), which show monotectic behavior, α-tocopherol preferentially partitions in the fluid phase. Experiments were also designed to investigate whether α-tocopherol has a preference for phosphatidylcholine (PC) or for phosphatidylethanolamine[7] (PE).

The interaction of α-tocopherol with PE is different than what is found with PC. FIGURE 5 shows DSC thermograms of DMPE/α-tocopherol mixtures, where it is

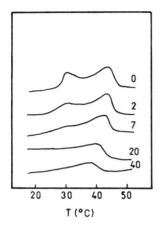

FIGURE 4. The DSC calorimetric curves for mixtures of dimyristoylphosphatidylcholine/distearoylphosphatidylcholine (DMPC/DSPC) in a 1:1 molar ratio, containing different amounts of α-tocopherol. Molar-percent contents in α-tocopherol are indicated on the curves.

evident that several peaks are present. It seems that α-tocopherol does not give a good mixing with DMPE, and lateral phase separations occur, probably producing phases with different contents in α-tocopherol and phospholipid, so that the transition temperature will be lower as more α-tocopherol is present in each particular phase. This complex effect may be thought to be due to the perturbation of the intermolecular hydrogen bonds present in vesicles made of this phospholipid.[18] We have confirmed that α-tocopherol can establish hydrogen bonds with DMPE by FT-IR spectroscopy. FIGURE 6 shows the spectra corresponding to the $C = O$ stretching band of pure DMPE: 10 mole-percent of α-tocopheryl acetate in DMPE, and 10 mole-percent of

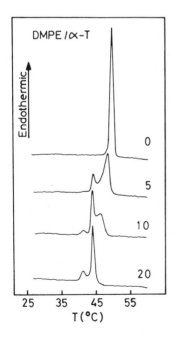

FIGURE 5. The DSC calorimetric curves for pure DMPE and systems containing different amounts of α-tocopherol. Molar-percent contents in α-tocopherol are indicated on the curves.

α-tocopherol in DMPE, all of them at 41°C, that is, below the phase transition temperature of pure DMPE (49°C). It can be seen that pure DMPE (FIG. 6A) presents a broad band from which two components may be recovered by spectral deconvolution, as mentioned before.

The inclusion of α-tocopheryl acetate does not produce any significant change in the pattern observed for the pure phospholipid (FIG. 6B). α-Tocopherol, however, produces a significant change in the pattern of this band (FIG. 6C), where it can be seen that the deconvoluted band has three components. The first one appears at 1742 cm^{-1}. This high frequency indicates that this group is not engaged in hydrogen bonding, either to water or to phospholipids.[19] The second one is centered at 1734 cm^{-1}, and the third component is located at 1718 cm^{-1}. Given the low frequency of this component, and by comparison with the spectrum of α-tocopheryl acetate/DMPE (FIG. 6B) where this component is absent, it can be assumed that it corresponds to the C = O ester groups of DMPE, hydrogen-bonded to the hydroxyl group of α-tocopherol.

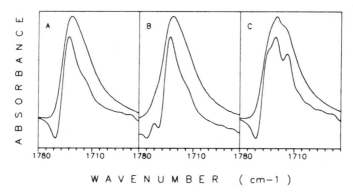

FIGURE 6. Infrared spectra of the C=O stretching region of DMPE. (A) Pure DMPE, (B) 10 mole-percent of α-tocopheryl acetate, and (C) 10 mole-percent α-tocopherol in DMPE at 41°C. Lower traces show the corresponding Fourier deconvoluted spectra using Gaussian lines of 20 cm^{-1} full-width at half-height and a resolution enhancement factor of 2.1.

Nevertheless α-tocopherol is shown to preferentially partition into the most fluid domains when it is included in mixtures of PE and PC, independent of whether most dipalmitoyl phosphatidy (ethanolamine (DPPE) fluid domains are richer in PE or in PC.[7] This was shown by DSC experiments in which α-tocopherol was included in vesicles made of equimolar mixtures of either DMPC/dipalmitoylphosphatidyl-ethanolamine (DPPE) or dilauroylphosphatidylethanolamine (DLPE)/DSPC, both mixtures showing monotectic behavior.[7] The preference of α-tocopherol for the more fluid component in these mixtures clearly distinguishes α-tocopherol from cholesterol, which was shown to prefer always PC over PE in phospholipid mixtures.[20]

In view of these observations, it is likely that α-tocopherol will not be homogeneously distributed in the membrane, but rather associated with the most fluid zones. Incidentally, this will cause α-tocopherol to be associated with the most unsaturated fatty acyl chains and hence will facilitate its peroxidation-protecting task.

TABLE 1. Fluorescence Parameters of α-Tocopherol in Solution and Incorporated into Phospholipid Vesicles

Medium	γ_{max} (nm)^a	$\phi_F{}^b$	τ_F (ns)^c
Methanol	316	0.43	ND
Ethanol	317	0.34	1.8
Acetonitrile	311	ND	1.0
Diethyl ether	312	ND	ND
Ethyl acetate	312	ND	ND
n-Hexane	312	0.11	ND
Cyclohexane	312	0.16	0.8
Dimethylformamide	311	ND	ND
DPPC (SUV),^{d} 25°C	316	ND	1.6
EYL^e (SUV), 25°C	316	ND	1.7

^{a} Emission fluorescence when excited at 295 nm, obtained from corrected spectra.
^{b} Quantum yields determinated considering ϕ_F of naphthalene in ethanol as 0.21.[30]
^{c} Fluorescence lifetimes determined by the single photon counting technique.
^{d} Small unilamellar vesicles of dipalmitoylphosphatidylcholine.
^{e} Egg yolk lecithin.

LOCALIZATION OF TOCOPHEROL IN PHOSPHOLIPID VESICLES AS SEEN BY ITS INTRINSIC FLUORESCENCE

α-Tocopherol has intrinsic fluorescence, and we have tried to exploit this property inasmuch as this is a very convenient means of directly observing the molecule. First of all, we determined some fluorescent parameters of α-tocopherol. TABLE 1 shows λ_{max} of the fluorescence emission spectra, quantum yield (ϕ_F), and fluorescence lifetime (τ_F), determined for α-tocopherol in a number of solvents and incorporated into phospholipid vesicles. It is interesting that the λ_{max} and the τ_F obtained for α-tocopherol in phospholipid vesicles are similar to those obtained in protic solvents (*e.g.* ethanol). This observation suggests that the chromanol moiety of α-tocopherol should be situated in a polar region of the model membrane, in agreement with previous suggestions.[9,18]

An important point when considering the intrinsic fluorescence of α-tocopherol in the membrane is to know whether all the molecules will be fluorescent or if nonfluorescent aggregates may be formed, as claimed recently.[21] To discern between these two possibilities, we have done the absorption spectra of α-tocopherol in an aprotic organic solvent like *n*-hexane. FIGURE 7 shows that the maximum of the

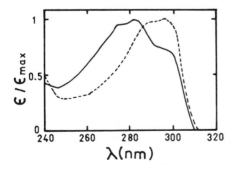

FIGURE 7. Absorption spectra of α-tocopherol in *n*-hexane at a concentration of (—) 4.4×10^{-5}M and (----) 1.42×10^{-4} M.

spectrum at low concentration of α-tocopherol in *n*-hexane is at 283 nm (predominance of the monomeric form), but it is shifted to 295 nm at a much higher concentration (predominance of the hydrogen bound dymer). Experiments made with α-tocopherol in phospholipid vesicles showed that α-tocopherol has a maximum near 295 nm within a wide range of concentrations (data not shown), indicating that most α-tocopherol molecules are associated. It could not be discerned from these data whether α-tocopherol molecules are associated, when present in membranes, (presumably through hydrogen bonding), between themselves or with phospholipid or water molecules.

The experiments of FIGURE 8, however, clearly show that although α-tocopherol molecules are associated, the aggregates formed are fluorescent, because linear relationships are found between fluorescent intensity and concentrations in a large range, both in *n*-hexane solution and incorporated into small unilamellar DPPC vesicles at 25°C (up to molar ratios 4:1 DPPC: α-tocopherol). A similar result was obtained with α-tocopherol incorporated into multibilayer vesicles of egg yolk lecithin at 25°C (not shown).

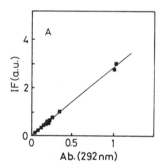 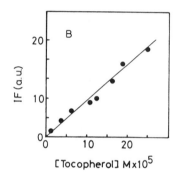

FIGURE 8. Fluorescence intensity (in arbitrary units) of α-tocopherol corrected for the inner filter effect versus concentration of α-tocopherol (**A**) in *n*-hexane (concentration expressed as absorbance in *n*-hexane) and (**B**) in small unilamellar vesicles (SUV) made of DPPC at 25°C (lipid concentration 10^{-3}M).

The localization of α-tocopherol in the bilayer has been also approached through the quenching of its intrinsic fluorescence by membrane probes like 5-doxylstearate (5-NS), which has its nitroxide group at carbon-5, and 16-doxylstearate (16-NS), with the nitroxoide group at carbon-16. These probes have been used before in a number of similar studies designed to study the localization of chromophores in membranes.[22] FIGURE 9 shows that 5-NS quenches α-tocopherol fluorescence much more effectively than 16-NS, as would be expected if the chromanol moiety is located near the lipid/water interface. The quenching process seems to follow a collisional mechanism as shown by the linearity of the Stern-Volmer plots.

Similarly we have also attempted to study the localization of α-tocopherol in egg yolk phosphatidylcholine multilamellar vesicles (MLV) by using a set of n-(9-anthroyloxy) stearic acid (*n*-AS) probes. The explicit distance dependence (r^{-6}) of electronic energy transfer (dipolar mechanism) has allowed its application as a spectroscopic ruler for determining distances in biological systems.[23,24] Energy transfer from α-tocopherol (donor), to the fluorescent probes *n*-AS (acceptor), is moderately efficient

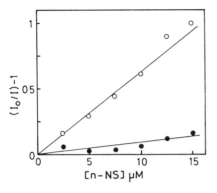

FIGURE 9. Stern-Volmer plots of quenching of α-tocopherol fluorescence in DPPC at 50°C by (○) 5-NS and (●) 16-NS. Lipid concentration was kept at 0.25 mM, and DPPC/α-tocopherol molar ratio was 100:1.

with a Förster critical radius, $R_o = 14$ Å. In egg yolk phosphatidylcholine MLV, different transfer efficiencies were obtained for the family of probes (FIG. 10).

The *n*-AS probes are known to be located at a graded series of depths from the surface, depending on their substitution position (n), in the aliphatic chain.[25] Considering that the R_o value is identical for all acceptors, it can be concluded that the chromophore group of α-tocopherol is situated in the membrane in a region between the 9-anthroyloxy located at carbon-7 and that at carbon-2, the former being the nearest one. This attribution is again compatible with other previous results we have already shown. Furthermore, we have found that acrylamide, which is a water-soluble fluorescence quencher, is a very inefficient quencher of α-tocopherol in fluid membranes (results not shown), acrylamide being an efficient quencher of α-tocopherol in ethanolic solution. This indicates that although α-tocopherol may have its chromanol group relatively close to the polar part of the membrane, it is not sufficiently exposed to allow acrylamide to reach it, acrylamide being known to have a very low capacity of penetration through phospholipid bilayers.[26] Hence the conclusion of these studies on the location of α-tocopherol in phospholipid vesicles is that its hydroxyl group may

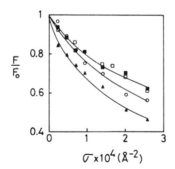

FIGURE 10. Relative yield of α-tocopherol fluorescence (F/F_o) versus σ (superficial concentration) of (○) 2-AS, (▲) 7-AS, (■) 9-AS, and (□) 12-AS in egg yolk lecithin (EYL) at 25°C. Samples were prepared by combination of chloroform solutions containing EYL and the appropriate amounts of donor and acceptor. After drying, multilamellar vesicles were formed by addition of aqueous buffer and careful mixing. Each point in the plot represents different experimental sets. Measurements were carried out in a Shimadzu RF-640 spectrofluorometer, the excitation and emission wavelengths being 295 and 329 nm, respectively.

be located at the lipid/water interface, forming a hydrogen bond with carbonyl or phosphate groups of phospholipids, and its chromanol moiety lies in a position close to that occupied by 7-AS and 5-NS. The situation of the hydroxyl group of α-tocopherol in the lipid/water interface is of interest in explaining its mechanism of action because any oxidizing agent approaching the membrane surface will find reducing protons. Hence the introduction of those agents in the membrane will be prevented.

LATERAL DIFFUSION COEFFICIENT OF α-TOCOPHEROL IN PHOSPHOLIPID VESICLES

In order to understand the mechanism of action of α-tocopherol in membranes and how it may be active at very low concentrations, it may be very illustrative to know the lateral diffusion coefficient of this molecule when incorporated into phospholipid vesicles. This can be approached through studies of the quenching of the intrinsic fluorescence of α-tocopherol by 5-NS. This quenching has been shown above to be effective (FIG. 9).

The extent of collisional quenching in a lipid bilayer depends upon the lipid/water partition coefficient and upon the rate of diffusion of the colliding species in the lipid bilayer.[27] Therefore the collisional quenching of fluorescence can be used for calculating the diffusion coefficients for α-tocopherol in lipid vesicles. In a membrane, where quenching occurs only in the lipid phase and where partition with the water phase may be significant, the Stern-Volmer relation for collisional quenching is modified, and the following relation applies:

$$1/\kappa app = am \ (1/\kappa m - 1/\kappa mP) + 1/\kappa mP$$

where κapp is the apparent (measured) bimolecular quenching constant in $M^{-1}s^{-1}$, am is the fractional volume of the membrane, κm is the bimolecular quenching constant in the membrane phase, and P is the partition coefficient, in units of (moles of quencher per liter of phospholipid)/(moles of quencher per liter of water). The partition coefficient is also expressed as a mole fractional ratio, that is, (moles of quencher per mole of phospholipid)/(moles of quencher per mole of water). A plot of $1/\kappa app$ as a function of am gives a straight line, with $1/\kappa mP$ as intercept and $(1/\kappa m - 1/\kappa mP)$ as slope.

FIGURE 11A shows Stern-Volmer plots for the quenching of α-tocopherol fluorescence when incorporated into egg yolk lecithin (EYL) MLV at 25°C, by 5-NS, at different lipid concentrations, keeping the molar ratio EYL/α-tocopherol as 100:1. From these plots, κapp values were calculated, and they were used for the plot shown in FIGURE 11B. From the last plot (FIG. 11B), κm was calculated to be 3.4×10^9 $M^{-1}s^{-1}$, and P was found to be 3.2×10^4 (moles of 5-NS per mole of EYL)/(moles of 5-NS per mole of water).

It is noteworthy that this value for the partition coefficient is very similar to that found by other authors for asolectin bilayers at 25°C,[28] which was 5.9×10^4 expressed in the same units. In order to calculate the lateral diffusion coefficient of α-tocopherol in the membrane, we have followed the Smoluchowski equation as modified for fluorescence quenching measured in the steady state including transient effects:[29]

$$\kappa_m = 4\pi N'R_{pq} \ \gamma \ (D_p+D_q)(1 + R_{pq}\gamma/\sqrt{(D_p+ D_q)\tau o})$$

where γ is the quenching efficiency of the fraction of collisional encounters that are effective in quenching; R_{pq} is the sum of the molecular radii of probe plus quencher; N' is Avogadro's number per millimole; D_p and D_q are the diffusion coefficients of the probe and the quencher, respectively, in the membrane, in units of cm^2s^{-1}; and τo is the fluorescence lifetime of the probe in the absence of quencher.

From the van der Waals radii we estimate a molecular radius of 4.25 Å for α-tocopherol and 4.55 Å for 5-NS. We have assumed γ to be 1, so that the calculated diffusion coefficient is the smallest possible and would be higher for $\gamma < 1$. See Fato *et al.*[28] for a discussion of the problems that can be found when trying to estimate γ for this type of system. τ_o was estimated to be 1.7 nanoseconds. Finally, we have assumed D_q to be 2.5×10^{-7} cm^2 according to Fato *et al.*,[28] which found this value for a similar fluid membrane.

All of this leads to a D_p value of 4.8×10^{-6} cm^2s^{-1}. This means that α-tocopherol has a very high mobility in a fluid bilayer, and hence it will be quite efficient in order

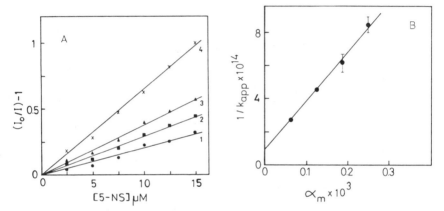

FIGURE 11. **A:** Stern-Volmer plots of quenching of α-tocopherol fluorescence by 5-NS at 25°C in egg yolk lecithin vesicles at different membrane fractional volumes (α_m) : (1) 0.25×10^{-3}; (2) 0.1875×10^{-3}; (3) 0.125×10^{-3}; (4) 0.0625×10^{-3}. The α-tocopherol to phospholipid ratio was kept 1:100 (mol:mol). Experimental procedures are as described in the legend of FIGURE 10. **B:** Plot of $1/\kappa app$ versus membrane fractional volumes (α_m) using values from panel **A**. Each point represents the average value $\pm$ SE of three different experiments.

to act wherever it is needed. This value is very similar to the one calculated by other authors[28] for ubiquinone-3 (5.8×10^{-6} cm^2s^{-1}), which is a molecule very similar in structure to α-tocopherol.

It appears then, that there might be, at least, two mechanisms to compensate for the low concentration of α-tocopherol in the membrane, its preferential partitioning in most of the fluid domains, and its high lateral mobility in the plane of the bilayer.

CONCLUSIONS

The hydroxyl group of α-tocopherol is essential in determining its effect on phospholipid membranes where it disrupts the lipid/water interface and weakens the van der Waals interaction between the fatty acyl chains. Hydrogen bonds are established between the hydroxyl group of α-tocopherol and a C = O group of DPPC or DMPE. α-Tocopherol favorably partitions into the most fluid domains when included in mixtures of phospholipids with monotectic behavior. The study of the intrinsic fluorescence of α-tocopherol reveals that its chromophore group is situated in the membrane in a relatively polar position but not readily accessible to the water domain. This is confirmed by resonance energy transfer studies using a series of probes located at graded depths in the membrane.

The lateral diffusion coefficient of α-tocopherol in fluid phospholipid vesicles was calculated through quenching of its intrinsic fluorescence by a spin probe. A value of 4.8×10^{-6} cm^{2}s^{-1} was calculated, indicating a very high lateral diffusion of α-tocopherol.

REFERENCES

1. BURTON, G. W., K. H. CHEESEMAN, T. DOBA, K. U. INGOLD & T. F. SLATER. 1983. *In* Biology of Vitamin E (Ciba Foundation Symposium 101): 4-18. Pitman. London.
2. TAPPEL, A. L. 1972. Ann. N. Y. Acad. Sci. **205:** 12-28.
3. MASSEY, J. B., H. S. SHE & H. J. POWNALL. 1982. Biochem. Biophys. Res. Commun. **106:** 842-847.
4. LAI, M. Z., N. DUZGUNES & F. C. SZOKA. 1985. Biochemistry **24:** 1646-1653.
5. VILLALAIN, J., F. J. ARANDA & J. C. GOMEZ-FERNANDEZ. 1986. Eur. J. Biochem. **158:** 141-147.
6. MCMURCHIE, E. J. & G. H. MCINTOSH. 1986. J. Nutr. Sci. Vitaminol. **32:** 551-558.
7. ORTIZ, A., F. J. ARANDA & J. C. GOMEZ-FERNANDEZ. 1987. Biochim. Biophys. Acta **898:** 214-222.
8. WASSALL, S. R., J. L. THEWALT, L. WONG, H. GORRISEN & R. J. CUSHLEY. 1986. Biochemistry **25:** 319-326.
9. SRIVASTAVA, S., R. S. PHADKE, G. GOUIL & C. N. R. RAO. 1983. Biochim. Biophys. Acta **734:** 353-362.
10. ASHER, I. M. & I. W. LEVIN. 1977. Biochim. Biophys. Acta **468:** 63-72.
11. CAMERON, D. G., H. L. CASAL & H. H. MANTSCH. 1980. Biochemistry **19:** 3665-3672.
12. BLUME, A., W. HUBNER & G. MESSNER. 1988. Biochemistry **27:** 8239-8249.
13. PERLY, B., I. C. P. SMITH, L. HUGHES, G. W. BURTON & K. U. INGOLD. 1985. Biochim. Biophys. Acta **734:** 353-362.
14. LAI, M. Z., N. DUZGUNES & F. C. SZOKA. 1985. Biochemistry **24:** 1646-1653.
15. STORCH, J. & A. M. KLEINFELD. 1985. Trends Biochem. Sci. **10:** 418-421.
16. BERGELSON, L. D. & L. I. BARSUKOV. 1977. Science **197:** 224-230.
17. DIPLOCK, A. & J. A. LUCY. 1973. FEBS Lett. **29:** 205-210.
18. HITCHCOCK, P. B., R. MASON & G. G. SHIPLEY. 1975. J. Mol. Biol. **94:** 297-299.
19. WONG, P. T. T. & H. H. MANTSCH. 1988. Chem. Phys. Lipids **46:** 213-224.
20. VAN DIJCK, P. W. M., B. DE KRUIJFF, L. L. M. VAN DEENEN, J. DE GIER & R. A. DEMEL. 1976. Biochim. Biophys. Acta **455:** 576-587.
21. KAGAN, V. E. & P. J. QUINN. 1988. Eur. J. Biochem. **171:** 661-667.
22. BLATT, E. & W. H. SAWYER. 1985. Biochim. Biophys. Acta **822:** 43-62.
23. STRYER, L. 1978. Ann. Rev. Biochem. **47:** 819-846.
24. ENNG, B. K. K. & L. STRYER. 1978. Biochemistry **17:** 5241-5248.
25. THULBORN, K. R. & W. H. SAWYER. 1978. Biochim. Biophys. Acta **511:** 125-140.
26. CHALPIN, D. B. & A. M. KLEINFELD. 1983. Biochim. Biophys. Acta **731:** 465-474.
27. LAKOWICZ, J. R. & D. HOGEN. 1980. Chem. Phys. Lipids **26:** 1-40.
28. FATO, R., M. BATTINO, M. DEGLI ESPOSTI, G. PARENTI CASTELLI & G. LENAZ. 1986. Biochemistry **25:** 3378-3390.
29. UMBERGER, J. Q. & V. K. LAMER. 1945. J. Am. Chem. Soc. **67:** 1099-1109.
30. PARKER, C. A. 1968. *In* Photoluminescence of solutions. 266-267. Elsevier. Amsterdam.

Tocopherol Stabilizes Membrane against Phospholipase A, Free Fatty Acids, and Lysophospholipids[a]

VALERIAN E. KAGAN

Institute of Physiology
Bulgarian Academy of Sciences
Sofia 1113, Bulgaria

INTRODUCTION

Tocopherols (vitamin E) are indispensable components of the lipid bilayer of biological membranes; a decrease in their content brings about structural and functional damage of the membranes.[1-3] It is generally known that vitamin E is a lipid-soluble antioxidant in cell membranes, functioning as a free radical scavenger to prevent lipid peroxidation.[4,5] In addition to its antioxidant function, tocopherols are capable of quenching singlet molecular oxygen, thus protecting membranes against light-induced oxidative damage.[3,6] Besides this antioxidative role, vitamin E may become incorporated into biological membranes through a physicochemical association of the tocopherol side chain with polyenoic fatty acid residues in membrane phospholipids, that is, by way of van der Waals interactions.[7,8] These molecular mechanisms underlying the biological effects of tocopherols have been studied in great detail and are generally accepted (FIG. 1).

Recently it has been demonstrated that in addition to its antioxidant and physicochemical stabilizing effects in biological membranes, vitamin E can protect biological membranes against the damaging action of phospholipases, especially phospholipase A, as well as against the phospholipid hydrolysis products by phospholipase A, namely, free fatty acids and lysophospholipids.[9,10]

The aim of the present paper is to analyze the molecular mechanisms underlying protective effects of vitamin E in lipid bilayers as well as in natural membranes in which modification of physical properties or damage was due to the presence of free fatty acids, lysophospholipids, or both. It is noteworthy that sharp elevation of concentrations of the phospholipid hydrolysis products is a characteristic feature of many pathological processes, such as ischemia, stress damages, and hypoxia.[11,12]

FORMATION OF ALPHA-TOCOPHEROL COMPLEXES WITH FREE FATTY ACIDS AND LYSOPHOSPHOLIPIDS IN SOLUTIONS

Using UV absorption, fluorescence, and [^{1}H]NMR measurements, we have shown that alpha-tocopherol could form complexes with both free fatty acids and lysophos-

[a] The author thanks the Committee for Science of Bulgaria for financial support of this work.

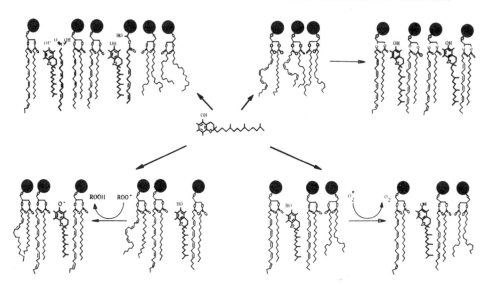

FIGURE 1. Principal mechanisms of the stabilizing effects of alpha-tocopherol in biomembranes.

pholipids in organic solvents.[10,13] To identify the functional groups involved in the formation of alpha-tocopherol fatty acid complexes, [¹H]NMR high resolution spectroscopy was used. A [¹H]NMR spectrum of alpha-tocopherol solution in C^2HCl_3 is shown in FIGURE 2.

The line with δ = 4.31 parts per million (ppm) corresponds to the chromanol hydroxyl proton; the lines with δ = 2.10-2.15 ppm correspond to chromanol methyl protons; the line with δ = 1.21 ppm corresponds to the phytol chain methylene protons; and the multiple signal at 0.82 ppm corresponds to methyl protons of the phytol chain.[10,13] In the presence of fatty acid (arachidonic), the [¹H]NMR spectrum was changed. The lines corresponding to hydroxyl protons (4.31), chromanol methyl protons at positions 5, 7, and 8 (2.10-2.15), and much less phytol chain methylene protons (1.21) were broadened. The broadening of the chromanol methyl protons signal was found to be strongly dependent on the number of double bonds when a series of fatty acids was examined (palmitic, oleic, linoleic, arachidonic), whereas the broadening of the hydroxyl line was always well-pronounced both for saturated and unsaturated fatty acids. The broadening of the phytol chain methylene protons signals occurred upon alpha-tocopherol interaction with only unsaturated fatty acids. Addition of lysophosphatidylcholine to alpha-tocopherol solution in C^2HCl_3 resulted in similar changes in the [¹H]NMR spectrum, that is, broadening of chromanol OH-group and CH₃-group signals.

All of these findings led us to suggest a model of alpha-tocopherol complex formation with either free fatty acids or lysophospholipids in solution through two types of interaction, namely: formation of a hydrogen bond between the alpha-tocopherol chromanol nucleus hydroxyl group and the C-O group of the fatty acid or lysophospholipid; and interaction of the acyl chains of fatty acids or lysophospholipids with the chromanol nucleus methyl groups of alpha-tocopherol. The latter interaction was markedly enhanced with an increase in the number of double bonds in the acyl chain. Thus the phytol chain of alpha-tocopherol is not essential for the complex formation in the solutions. In other words, the complexes would also be formed upon fatty acids or lysophospholipid interactions with 2,2,5,7,8-pentamethyl-6-hydroxy-chromane (PMC), in which the phytol chain is substituted by the methyl group. Indeed, the formation of complexes between PMC and free fatty acids was confirmed by [¹H]NMR, UV absorbance, and fluorescence measurements.

The hypothetical structure of the complexes of alpha-tocopherol with phospholipid hydrolysis products could be illustrated by the use of the Pauling-Corey molecular models. FIGURE 3 shows the formation of such a complex between alpha-tocopherol and linoleic acid: a hydrogen bond between the linoleic acid carboxyl group and the alpha-tocopherol hydroxyl group. The 9,10- and 12,13-cis-double bonds of fatty acids form a structure that is complementary to the chromanol nucleus methyl groups.

Can the suggested complexes of chromanols with free fatty acids and lysophospholipids be formed in the membranes thereby diminishing the disordering effects of phospholipid hydrolysis products? If the answer is positive, then both alpha-tocopherol and PMC should protect membranes against damage induced by free fatty acids and lysophospholipids; if negative, then only alpha-tocopherol (but not PMC) should protect membranes against damage induced by phospholipase A and phospholipid hydrolysis products.

EFFECTS OF ALPHA-TOCOPHEROL AND PMC ON THE PHASE TRANSITIONS OF PHOSPHOLIPIDS IN LIPOSOMES IN THE PRESENCE OF FREE FATTY ACIDS

Phase transitions of phospholipids in monolayer liposomes were studied using spin-probe electron spin resonance (ESR) and [¹H]NMR techniques. FIGURE 4 shows the

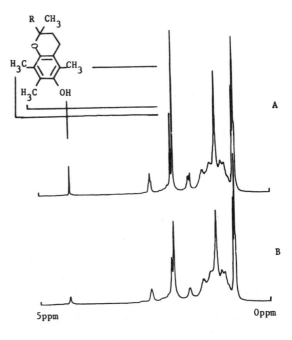

FIGURE 2. [¹H]NMR high resolution spectra of C^2HCl_3 solutions containing 5×10^{-2} M alpha-tocopherol (A) and alpha-tocopherol + 5×10^{-3} M arachidonic acid (B). Temperature, 243° K; number of scans, 20; pulse delay, 15 seconds.

5ppm   0ppm

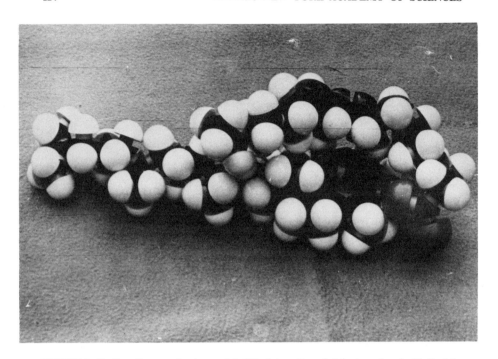

FIGURE 3. Pauling-Corey molecular model of the interaction of alpha-tocopherol with linoleic acid.

temperature dependence of incorporation of a spin-probe, 12-imoxylstearate, into monolayer liposomes prepared from oleoylpalmitoylphosphatidylcholine (OPPC). Spin-labeled fatty acid (12-imoxylstearate) could be incorporated into the phospholipid bilayer only when the latter was in the liquid-crystalline state.[14,15] Thus, partition of the spin-probe between liposomes and aqueous phase (A/A_o) could be used for registering phase transitions of phospholipids. One can see the phase transition of OPPC at 15° C. Addition of arachidonic acid to the incubation medium (up to a concentration of 5 mole-percent) resulted in a drastic disordering effect: no phase transition was observed in the temperature interval from 0 to 40° C, and phospholipids in liposomes were in a liquid-crystalline state. Subsequent addition of alpha-tocopherol (5 mole-percent) completely abolished the chaotropic effect of the fatty acid and also shifted the phase transition to higher temperatures. The tocopherol homologue devoid of the phytol chain, PMC, exerted no stabilizing effect on the membrane microviscosity despite its ability to form complexes with free fatty acids in organic solvents. In the presence of PMC, the temperature dependence of spin-probe incorporation into liposomes was the same as in the presence of fatty acids.

Similar data were obtained using [¹H]NMR measurements, taking into account that signals from protons of molecules in the gel state are so broadened that they could not be distinguished from the baseline. The resolved signals originate from molecules in the liquid-crystalline state.[16] The temperature dependence of these resolved signals gives information about the gel liquid-crystalline state transition of

lipids in liposomes. FIGURE 5 shows the [¹H]NMR high-resolution spectra of liposomal suspensions from dipalmitoylphosphatidylcholine (DPPC) in D_2O in the temperature range of 30° to 50° C, which is in agreement with the data in the literature.[16]
After addition of linoleic acid (up to a concentration of 5 mole-percent), the phase
transition was broadened and shifted to lower temperatures. A similar effect was
produced by alpha-tocopherol (5 mole-percent). When linoleic acid and alpha-tocopherol were added together, the temperature dependence of [¹H]NMR spectra did
not differ significantly from the control one (phospholipid liposomes without additions). The temperature dependence of the relative intensities of signals (*i.e.* the ratio
of the signal intensity at a given temperature to its intensity at 50° C) for choline and
methylene groups of DPPC is presented in FIGURE 6. The dotted lines show the
expected curves if the chaotropic effects of alpha-tocopherol and linoleic acid were
additive. It is clear that alpha-tocopherol substantially diminished the disordering
effect of linoleic acid, thus stabilizing the microviscosity of the lipid bilayer. Taking
into consideration that alpha-tocopherol itself exerted a disordering effect, one might
suggest that the stabilizing action of alpha-tocopherol is due to the formation of a
complex with linoleic acid.

Summarizing these data, we conclude that alpha-tocopherol can prevent or even
abolish the disordering effects of free fatty acids on phospholipid bilayers due to the
formation of complexes within the membrane core. The alpha-tocopherol homologue,
devoid of phytol chain PMC, possesses no protective effect on lipid bilayers, modified
by fatty acids.

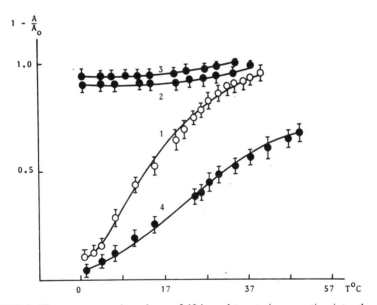

FIGURE 4. The temperature dependence of 12-imoxylstearate incorporation into oleoylpalmitoylphosphatidylcholine (OPPC) liposomes. 1, OPPC; 2, OPPC + arachidonic acid (15 mole-
percent); 3, OPPC + arachidonic acid (15 mole-percent) + 2,2,5,7,8-pentamethyl-6-hydroxy-
chromane (5 mole-percent); 4, OPPC + arachidonic acid (15 mole-percent) + alpha-tocopherol
(5 mole-percent).

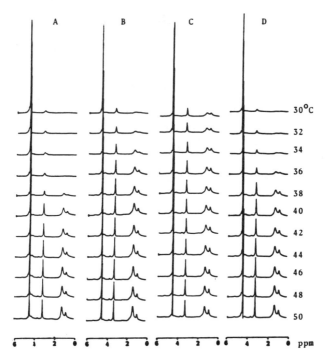

FIGURE 5. [^{1}H]NMR spectra of dipalmitoylphosphatidylcholine (DPPC) in the temperature range of 30° to 50° C. A, DPPC liposomes; B, DPPC liposomes + alpha-tocopherol (5 mole-percent); C, DPPC liposomes + linoleic acid (20 mole-percent); D, DPPC liposomes + linoleic acid (20 mole-percent) + alpha-tocopherol (5 mole-percent).

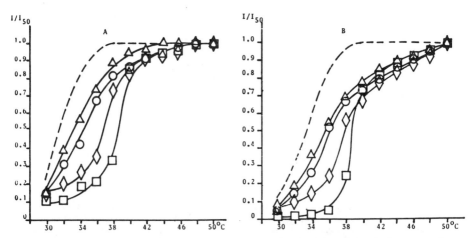

FIGURE 6. Graphs of temperature dependence of relative intensity of signal of protons of choline (A) and methylene (B) groups in DPPC liposomes (see legend to FIG. 5).

EFFECTS OF ALPHA-TOCOPHEROL AND PMC ON THE
PERMEABILITY OF NATURAL MEMBRANES

One of the earliest functional manifestations of the disordering effects of phospholipid hydrolysis products on lipid bilayers and lipid-protein interactions in biomembranes is a sharp increase of their permeability.[17] Obviously the formation of complexes of alpha-tocopherol with either free fatty acids or lysophospholipids should result in a decrease of permeability, induced by phospholipid hydrolysis products, if the complexes themselves do not disturb the membrane organization. In this section the effects of alpha-tocopherol and PMC on the permeability of membranes of skeletal muscle sarcoplasmic reticulum, rat liver mitochondria, and rat brain synaptosomes in the presence of free fatty acids or phospholipase A_2 are described.

It is known that the efficiency of Ca^{2+} transport by sarcoplasmic reticulum vesicles can be characterized by the Ca^{2+}/ATP ratio.[17] The decrease of the Ca^{2+}/ATP ratio is indicative of the increase of sarcoplasmic reticulum membrane permeability to Ca^{2+}

TABLE 1. Effects of Alpha-Tocopherol (alpha-T) and 2,2,5,7,8-Pentamethyl-6-Hydroxychromane (PMC) on Linoleic Acid (LA)-Induced Inhibition of Ca^{2+}-Transport in Sarcoplasmic Reticulum Vesicules from Rabbit Skeletal Muscles[a]

Additions	Efficiency of Ca^{2+}-Transport (Ca^{2+}/ATP)
Control	1.7
+ LA (30 μM)	0.7
+ PMC (100 μM)	1.2
+ Alpha-T (100 μM)	1.7
LA (30 μM) + PMC (100 μM)	0.3
LA (30 μM) + Alpha-T (100 μM)	1.5

[a] Incubation medium contained 100 mM NaCl, 2 mM MgCl$_2$, 1.9 mM ATP, 5 mM Na-oxalate, 42 μM CaCl$_2$, 10 mM Tris-HCl; pH = 7.2 (37° C); 100 μg protein/mL.

ions. The data in TABLE 1 show that addition of linoleic acid to a suspension of sarcoplasmic reticulum membranes resulted in a decrease of Ca^{2+}/ATP. When the fatty acid was added after preliminary treatment of membranes with alpha-tocopherol, its damaging effect greatly decreased. PMC exerted no protection against the fatty acid-induced permeability; on the contrary, it caused an increase of permeability.

In mitochondria, the modifying effect of oleic acid was manifested in a concentration-dependent stimulation of respiration (succinate oxidase activity). FIGURE 7 shows that here again alpha-tocopherol produced a concentration-dependent protection (decrease in the rate of oxygen consumption), whereas PMC stimulated succinate oxidase activity.

The transmembrane potential in synaptosomes can be measured using fluorescent probe 3,3-propyl-2,2-thiocarbocyanide (Di-S-C$_3$-/5/5): the decrease of transmembrane potential is accompanied by an increase of the fluorescence intensity of Di-S-C$_3$-(5) incorporated into the membrane.[18] The effect of phospholipase A_2 and chromanols on the transmembrane potential of rat brain synaptosomes is illustrated on FIGURE 8. Addition of phospholipase A_2 to synaptosomal suspension led to an increase

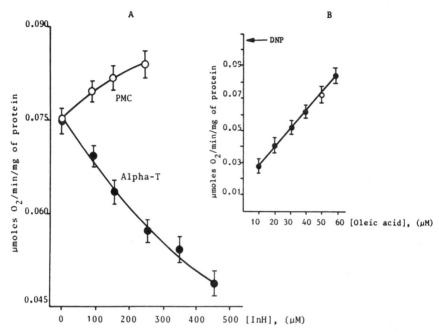

FIGURE 7. Effect of alpha-tocopherol and 2,2,5,7,8-pentamethyl-6-hydroxychromane (PMC) on oleic acid-stimulated oxygen consumption (succinate-oxidase activity) of isolated rat liver mitochondria. Incubation medium: 0.25 M sucrose, 5 mM phosphate buffer (pH 7.5 at 20° C), 10 mM KCl, 100 mM EDTA, 5 mM succinate, 0.9 mg protein/mL, and 50 μM oleic acid. Insert: Effect of oleic acid on the oxygen consumption of isolated rat liver mitochondria. DNP, dinitrophenol (50 μM).

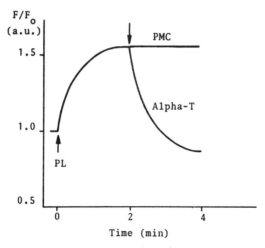

FIGURE 8. Kinetics of changes in Di-S-C$_3$-(5) (10^{-8}M) fluorescence in a synaptosome suspension (300 μg/mL) in the presence of phospholipase A$_2$ (10 μg/mL) and alpha-tocopherol (100 μM) or PMC (100 μM). Fluorescence excitation at 650 nm; emission at 688 nm.

of Di-S-C$_3$-(5) fluorescence, the effect being reversed by alpha-tocopherol. PMC was ineffective in eliminating the drop of transmembrane potential induced by phospholipase A$_2$. Similar results were obtained when the effects of fatty acids were examined, that is, alpha-tocopherol prevented or even abolished the damaging effects of linoleic or arachidonic acid, whereas its homologue, devoid of the phytol chain, had no protective action.

We can conclude that only alpha-tocopherol (but not PMC) can form complexes within the membranes that are able to eliminate the disordering effects of phospholipid hydrolysis products, thus preventing damage of the membrane permeability barrier (FIG. 9).

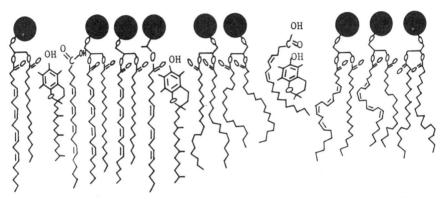

FIGURE 9. A scheme of alpha-tocopherol and PMC complexes with fatty acids in lipid bilayer.

EFFECTS OF ALPHA-TOCOPHEROL ON THE FLEXIBILITY OF INTRINSIC MEMBRANE PROTEINS

The increase of the molecular mobility of phospholipid molecules within the bilayer creates the necessary prerequisites for the increase in the motions of the segments of the polypeptide chain of intrinsic membrane proteins. This in turn should result in a decreased thermal stability of membrane proteins.[15] Two examples of this kind of effect are given below, illustrating the increased flexibility of Ca^{2+}-ATPase and rhodopsin after addition of free fatty acids to the membranes, as well as a stabilizing action of alpha-tocopherol.

In FIGURE 10, semilogarithmic plots of rhodopsin thermal denaturation at 69° C in bovine rod outer segments are presented. Both oleic and arachidonic acids, added to a suspension of photoreceptor membranes, caused a significant increase in the rate of rhodopsin thermal denaturation. Alpha-tocopherol completely abolished this action of fatty acids, whereas PMC was without effect. Differential scanning microcalorimetric data confirm these effects of alpha-tocopherol: the shifts in the transition temperatures for opsin and rhodopsin thermal denaturation, appearing in the presence of arachidonic acid, were diminished by alpha-tocopherol (FIG. 11, TABLE 2).

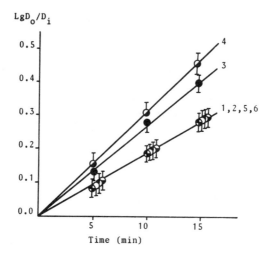

FIGURE 10. Kinetics of rhodopsin thermal denaturation in rod outer segment membranes (ROSM) at 69° C. 1, ROSM; 2, + alpha-tocopherol (5 mole-percent); 3, + oleic acid (2 mole-percent); 4, + arachidonic acid (2 mole-percent); 5, + oleic acid + alpha-tocopherol; 6, + arachidonic acid + alpha-tocopherol.

Thermograms of sarcoplasmic reticulum membranes have two characteristic transition temperatures upon Ca^{2+}-ATPase denaturation (FIG. 12). Treatment of sarcoplasmic reticulum vesicle suspension with arachidonic acid caused a shift of transition temperatures to lower values, whereas alpha-tocopherol, added subsequently, produced an opposite effect, that is, it restored the original positions of transition temperatures (TABLE 3).

These data suggest that alpha-tocopherol is able to eliminate the modifying effects of free fatty acids on intrinsic membrane proteins.

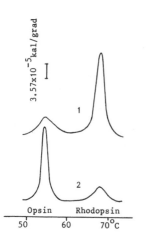

FIGURE 11. The differential scanning calorimetric curves of bovine ROSM. 1, dark adapted; 2, after bleaching.

TABLE 2. Transition Temperatures for Opsin and Rhodopsin Thermal Denaturation in Bovine Rod Outer Segments

	Opsin		Rhodopsin	
	T° C	$t_{1/2}$° C	T° C	$t_{1/2}$° C
Control	55.2 ± 0.2	3.6 ± 0.1	69.5 ± 0.2	2.8 ± 0.1
+ Arachidonic acid (2.5 mole-percent)	53.3 ± 0.2	3.6 ± 0.1	68.5 ± 0.2	2.8 ± 0.1
+ Arachidonic acid (2.5 mole-percent) + alpha-tocopherol (5 mole-percent)	54.2 ± 0.2	3.4 ± 0.1	69.0 ± 0.2	3.0 ± 0.1

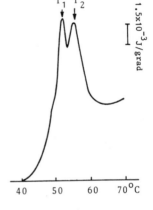

FIGURE 12. The differential scanning calorimetric curve of sarcoplasmic reticulum membranes.

TABLE 3. Transition Temperatures for Ca^{2+}-ATPase in Sarcoplasmic Reticulum Membranes

	T_1° C	T_2° C
Control	52.0	55.5
+ Alpha-tocopherol (30 μg/mg protein)	52.6	56.0
+ Arachidonic acid (20 μg/mg protein)	50.0	52.9
+ Arachidonic acid (20 μg/mg protein) + alpha-tocopherol (30 μg/mg protein)	51.5	55.2

EFFECTS OF ALPHA-TOCOPHEROL AND PMC ON PHOSPHOLIPASE A$_2$ and LYSOPHOSPHOLIPID-INDUCED INHIBITION OF CYTOCHROME P-450-DEPENDENT MONOOXYGENASE ACTIVITY IN LIVER MICROSOMES

The cytochrome P-450-dependent multienzyme monooxygenase complex in microsomal membranes is extremely sensitive to modifications of its lipid microenvironment, and particularly to phospholipase A[19]. In our experiments, 7-ethoxycoumarin deethylase (7-ECDase) activity was substantially decreased after treatment of rat liver microsomes with phospholipase A^2 (TABLE 4). Of the two phospholipid hydrolysis products formed, only lysophospholipids were effective as inhibitors of 7-ECDase because only gamma-myristoyl-lysophosphatidylcholine (but not fatty acids) could mimic the effect of phospholipase A$_2$.[20] When combinations of phospholipase A$_2$ plus alpha-tocopherol or lysophosphatidylcholine plus alpha-tocopherol were used, the protective effect of vitamin E was observed. PMC exerted protection neither in combination with phospholipase A$_2$, nor with lysophosphatidylcholine (TABLE 4).

Thus, intramembranous complexes of phospholipid hydrolysis products with alpha-tocopherol exert protection of membranes against these damaging species, whereas the complexes with PMC (if formed) are not able to make free fatty acids and lysophospholipids harmless.

EFFECTS OF PHOSPHOLIPASE A$_2$, FREE FATTY ACIDS, AND LYSOPHOSPHOLIPIDS ON MEMBRANE FRACTIONS FROM VITAMIN E-DEFICIENT ANIMALS

Suggesting that one of the physiological functions of vitamin E is protection of membranes against damage caused by phospholipid hydrolysis products, it is reason-

TABLE 4. Inhibition of 7-Ethoxycoumarin Deethylase (7-ECDase) in Rat Liver Microsomes by Phospholipase A$_2$ and Phospholipid Hydrolysis Products

Conditions	7-ECDase Activity	
	Control	Vitamin E-deficiency
Control	100.0	100.0
Phospholipase A$_2$ (0.65 U)	46.2	13.6
Phospholipase A$_2$ (0.65 U) + alpha-tocopherol (25 g/mg protein)	77.0	56.0
Phospholipase A$_2$ (0.65 U) + 6-PMC (10 μM)	46.2	30.0
γ-myristoyl-lyso-PC (10 μg/ mg protein)	40.9	27.2
γ-myristoyl-lyso-PC + alpha-tocopherol (25 μg/mg protein)	73.6	72.7
Oleic acid (10 μg/mg protein)	100.0	72.7

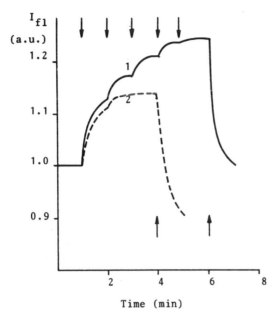

FIGURE 13. Changes of potential-dependent fluorescence of probe Di-S-C$_3$-(5) in synaptosomal membranes. 1, controls; 2, vitamin E-deficient animals. Arrows down, additions of linoleic acid (10 μM); arrows up, additions of alpha-tocopherol (50 μM).

able to expect a higher sensitivity of membrane fraction from vitamin E-deficient animals to phospholipase A$_2$, free fatty acids, and lysophospholipids.

Comparison of the sensitivity of synaptosomes, obtained from control and vitamin E-deficient rats (the vitamin E content in plasma of control and vitamin E-deficient animals was 9.1 ± 0.1 and 0.8 ± 0.2 mg/mL, respectively) to exogenous free fatty acids is presented in FIGURE 13. Four portions of arachidonic acid (10 nmol in each) were necessary to induce complete disappearance of transmembrane potential in controls, whereas the same effect was achieved after addition of half the amount of arachidonic acid in the experimental group. Introduction of exogenous alpha-tocopherol resulted in restoration of the membrane potential both in control and vitamin E-deficient preparations.

In rat liver microsomes from vitamin E-deficient animals, the content of cytochrome P-450 and the activity of 7-ECDase were substantially decreased in comparison with controls (TABLE 5). The inhibitory effects of either phospholipase A$_2$ or gamma-myristoyl-lysophosphatidylcholine on deethylase activity was also much more pronounced than that in controls. Exogenous alpha-tocopherol possessed a strong protective effect both in control and in vitamin E-deficient preparations (TABLE 4), whereas PMC did not restore the enzymic activity.

In skeletal muscle, sarcoplasmic reticulum membranes from rats kept on a diet enriched with vitamin E (for 3 weeks 50 mg of alpha-tocopherol per 1 kg of body weight daily) Ca^{2+}-ATPase were more resistant to thermal inactivation both in the presence and in the absence of exogenous free fatty acids as compared to the control group (FIG. 14).

TABLE 5. Monooxygenase Activity in Vitamin E-deficient Rat Liver Microsomes

	Control	Vitamin E-deficiency
Vitamin E content in rat liver (μg alpha-T/mg tissue)	35.1 ± 3.3	8.3 ± 0.4
Cytochrome P-450 (nmol/mg of protein)	0.94	0.63
Activity of 7-ECDase (nmol 7-hydroxycoumarin/mg of protein/min)	0.126 ± 0.001	0.072 ± 0.001

Thus, *in vivo* vitamin E deficiency causes an increase in the sensitivity of membrane structures to phospholipid hydrolysis products, which can be overcome by addition of exogenous tocopherol. Enrichment of the diet with vitamin E leads to a higher stability of membranes to the deleterious effects of free fatty acids.

Summarizing all the data presented, we can conclude that protection of membranes against the damaging effects of fatty acids and lysophospholipids is one of the physiological functions of vitamin E, which is realized through formation of stable complexes. The structure of these complexes within the membranes should be studied in detail.[21-23]

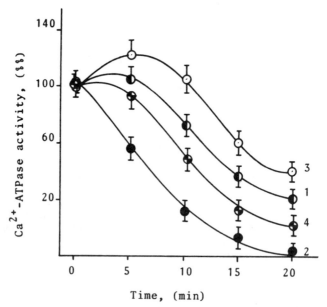

FIGURE 14. Effects of arachidonic acid on thermal inactivation of Ca^{2+}-dependent ATPase in rat skeletal muscle sarcoplasmic reticulum. 1-2, controls; 3-4, vitamin E-enriched diet (50 mg of alpha-tocopherol per 1 kg of body weight daily for 3 weeks); 2 and 4, addition of arachidonic acid (20 μg/mg of protein).

REFERENCES

1. MACHLIN, L. J., ED. 1984. Vitamin E. Marcel Dekker, Inc. New York.
2. HORWITT, M. K. 1980. Therapeutic uses of vitamin E in medicine. Nutr. Rev. **38:** 105-113.
3. DE DUVE, C. & O. HAYAISHI, EDS. 1978. Tocopherol, oxygen and biomembranes. Elsevier. North Holland Biomedical Press. Amsterdam.
4. TAPPEL, A. L. 1962. Vitamin E is the biological lipid antioxidant. Vitam. Horm. **20:** 493-502.
5. WITTING, L. A. 1980. Vitamin E and lipid antioxidants in free radical-initiated reactions. *In* Free Radicals in Biology. W. A. Pryor, Ed. Vol. 4: 295-327.
6. GRAMS, Y. W. & K. ESKINS. 1972. Dye-sensitized photoperoxidation of tocopherols. Correlation between singlet oxygen reactivity and vitamin E activity. Biochemistry **11:** 606-644.
7. DIPLOCK, A. T. & J. A. LUCY. 1973. The biochemical models of action of vitamin E and selenium: a hypothesis. FEBS Lett. **29:** 205-210.
8. LUCY, J. A. 1972. Functional and structural aspects of biological membranes: a suggested structural role of vitamin E in the control of membrane permeability and stability. Ann. N.Y. Acad. Sci. **203:** 3-16.
9. KAGAN, V. E., YU. V. ARKHIPENKO, S. K. DOBRINA, YU. P. KOZLOV & V. B. RITOV. 1977. Stabilizing effects of vitamin E on biomembranes exposed to lipid peroxidation. Biochemistry USSR. **42:** 1194-1199 (in Russian).
10. ERIN, A. N., M. M. SPIRIN, L. V. TABIDZE & V. E. KAGAN. 1984. Formation of α-tocopherol complexes with fatty acids. A hypothetical mechanism of stabilization of biomembranes by vitamin E. Biochim. Biophys. Acta **774:** 96-103.
11. MEERSON, F. Z., V. E. KAGAN, YU. P. KOZLOV, L. M. BELKINA & YU. V. ARKHIPENKO. 1982. The role of lipid peroxidation in pathogenesis of ischemic damage and the antioxidant protection of the heart. Basic. Res. Cardiol. **77:** 465-476.
12. MEERSON, F. Z. 1984. Adaptation, Stress and Prophylaxis. 1-329. Springer-Verlag. Berlin.
13. ERIN, A. N., V. I. SKRYPIN & V. E. KAGAN. 1985. Formation of α-tocopherol complexes with fatty acids. Nature of complexes. Biochim. Biophys. Acta **815:** 209-216.
14. PONTUS, S. M. & M. DELMELLE. 1975. Fluid lipid fraction in rod outer segment membrane. Biochim. Biophys. Acta **401:** 221-228.
15. TYURIN, V. A., V. E. KAGAN, S. A. SHUKOLJUKOV, N. K. KLAAN & O. A. AZIZOVA. 1979. Thermal stability of rhodopsin and lipid-protein interactions in the photoreceptor membranes. J. Therm. Biol. **4:** 203-208.
16. RESTALL, C. J. & D. CHAPMAN. 1986. Spectroscopic and calorimetric studies of lipids and biomembranes. *In* Lipids and Membranes: Past, Present and Future. J. A. Op den Kamp & B. Roelofsen, Eds.: 61-89. Elsevier Science Publishers, B. V. Amsterdam.
17. HASSELBACH, W. & H. OETLIKER. 1983. Energetics and electrogenicity of the sarcoplasmic reticulum calcium pump. Annu. Rev. Physiol. **45:** 325-347.
18. ERIN, A. N., V. I. SKRYPIN, L. L. PRILIPKO & V. E. KAGAN. 1986. Stabilizing effect of α-tocopherol on synaptosomes treated with phospholipase A₂. Bull. Exp. Bio. Med. (USSR) **102:** 25-28 (in Russian).
19. VERECZKEY, L. & K. MAGYAR. 1985. Cytochrome P-450, Biochemistry, Biophysics and Induction. 1-561. Akademiai Kiado. Budapest.
20. VINER, R. I., K. N. NOVIKOV, YU. V. ARKHIPENKO, V. B. SPIRICHEV & V. E. KAGAN. 1986. Non-antioxidant stabilization of cytochrome P-450 by α-tocopherol. Effectiveness under vitamin E-deficiency. Biochemistry USSR **51:** 1549-1554 (in Russian).
21. URANO, S., K. YANO & M. MATSUO. 1988. Membrane-stabilizing effect of vitamin E: effect of α-tocopherol and its model compounds on fluidity of lecithin liposomes. Biochem. Biophys. Res. Commun. **150:** 469-475.
22. URANO, S., M. IDA, I. OTANI & M. MATSUO. 1987. Membrane stabilization of vitamin E: interaction of α-tocopherol with phospholipids in bilayer liposomes. Biochem. Biophys. Res. Commun. **146:** 1413-1418.
23. KAGAN, V. E. & P. J. QUINN. 1988. The interaction of α-tocopherol and homologues with shorter hydrocarbon chains with phospholipid bilayer dispersions. Eur. J. Biochem. **171:** 661-667.

The Role of Vitamin E and Selenium on Arachidonic Acid Oxidation by way of the 5-Lipoxygenase Pathway

PALLU REDDANNA, JAY WHELAN,
JOHN R. BURGESS, MARY L. ESKEW,
GEORGE HILDENBRANDT, ARIAN ZARKOWER,
RICHARD W. SCHOLZ, AND C. CHANNA REDDY[a]

*Department of Veterinary Science and
Environmental Resources Research Institute
The Pennsylvania State University
University Park, Pennsylvania 16802*

THE ARACHIDONIC ACID CASCADE

Arachidonic acid, the most abundant C_{20} polyunsaturated fatty acid found in the phospholipids of mammalian tissues, is a biosynthetic precursor of several families of compounds that exert diverse biological effects. Once the action of phospholipases releases arachidonic acid from phospholipids, it is metabolized by one of the two pathways shown in FIGURE 1. The cyclooxygenase pathway produces prostaglandins (PG), thromboxanes (TX), and prostacyclins (PGI), whereas the lipoxygenase pathway leads to the formation of leukotrienes (LT) and lipoxins. The enzymic oxidation of arachidonic acid by way of the cyclooxygenase and lipoxygenase pathways to produce a spectrum of biologically active compounds is collectively referred to as the arachidonic acid cascade. Recent attention has focused on those factors that can regulate the concentration of these biologically active eicosanoids, especially in relation to their possible role in several pathological conditions including arteriosclerosis, arthritis, asthma, and anaphylactic reactions.[1-3] One area of particular interest has been the effect of fatty acid hydroperoxides (FAHP) on lipoxygenase and cyclooxygenase activities. For example, both cyclooxygenase and lipoxygenase exhibit an obligatory requirement for FAHP (< 1 μM) as an activator; however, these enzymes are inhibited by higher concentrations (> 10 μM) of FAHP.[4-7] The interest in FAHP, as modulators of the arachidonic acid cascade, probably reflects the implication of lipid peroxidation, one of the possible sources of FAHP formation, in many pathological and nonpathological *in vivo* processes.

[a] Address all correspondence to C. Channa Reddy, 226 Fenske Laboratory, Penn State University, University Park, PA 16802.

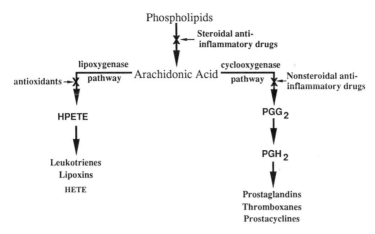

FIGURE 1. A simplified scheme for the enzymatic oxidation of arachidonic acid.

PROPOSED MODULATORY FUNCTIONS OF VITAMIN E AND SELENIUM

Researchers generally agree that vitamin E and selenium (Se) function synergistically in animal tissues to constitute an important antioxidant defense mechanism against free radical-mediated lipid peroxidation of cell membranes. As an essential component of selenium-dependent glutathione peroxidase (Se-GSH-Px), Se is involved in cellular antioxidant defense by reducing semistable hydroperoxides to less reactive alcohols.[8-10] On the other hand, vitamin E, as an integral part of cell membranes, functions to scavenge the free radicals that promote peroxidative chain reactions.[11-13] Thus, they both control cellular lipid peroxide levels by related but independent mechanisms.

In addition to their general antioxidant defense role, vitamin E and Se-GSH-Px could play the more specific role of modulating the enzymatic oxidation of arachidonic acid by way of the cyclooxygenase and lipoxygenase pathways. This hypothesis arises from the mechanistic similarities between the nonenzymatic and enzymatic oxidation of arachidonic acid. The potential roles that vitamin E and Se-GSH-Px could play in modulating the arachidonic acid cascade appears schematically in FIGURE 2. The immediate oxygenation products of the enzymatic and nonenzymatic oxidation of arachidonic acid include hydroperoxyeicosatetraenoic acids (HPETE) and cyclic endoperoxides. As described earlier, these products both serve as precursors for the biosynthesis of PG and LT, and have significant influence on the enzymes associated with the arachidonic acid cascade. Thus, an enzyme system that can reduce these reactive HPETE has the potential for modulating the arachidonic acid cascade. The Se-GSH-Px system has a capacity for reducing potentially reactive FAHP and thus influencing both the enzyme activities and the product profiles of the arachidonic acid cascade.

As FIGURE 3 shows, free radicals are an integral part of both the lipoxygenase-catalyzed reaction and leukotriene A_4 (LTA$_4$) biosynthesis. Therefore, vitamin E could

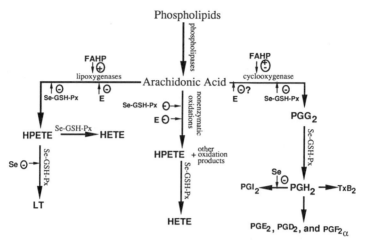

FIGURE 2. The proposed role of vitamin E and selenium in the arachidonic acid cascade. E, vitamin E; Se, selenium; Se-GSH-Px, selenium-dependent glutathione peroxidase; ⊖, inhibition; ⊕, activation; ⊖?, controversial reports; ±, activates at low concentration and inhibits at high concentration.

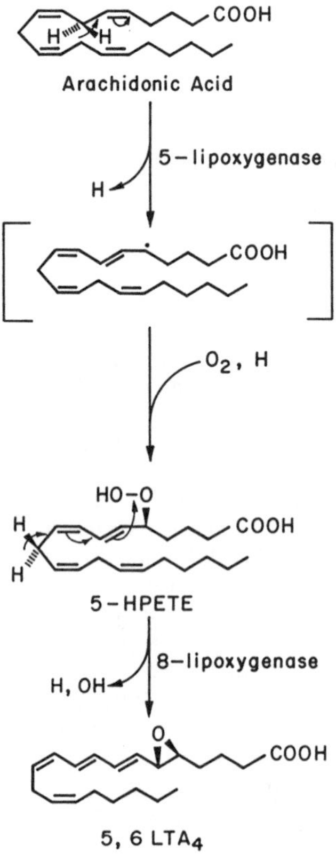

FIGURE 3. Mechanism of synthesis of 5,6-LTA₄ from arachidonic acid by sequential action of 5- and 8-lipoxygenases.

interfere with the essential radicals involved with the catalytic cycles of the lipoxygenase reaction, thus influencing product formation. By contrast, vitamin E can protect these enzymes from errant free radicals generated during catalysis, which are known to cause the self-catalyzed inactivation of these enzymes. Similarly, vitamin E could also modulate the cyclooxygenase-catalyzed reaction in which the essential role of free radicals has been well-established.[1,5] Thus, by removing FAHP activators and essential radicals, Se-GSH-Px and vitamin E could play a major role in regulating the biosynthesis of PG and LT. The role of vitamin E and Se in the arachidonic acid cascade has been recently reviewed.[3,14,15] This article briefly discusses the results of both *in vitro* and *in vivo* experiments conducted in our laboratory to examine the role of vitamin E and Se-GSH-Px in the enzymatic transformation of arachidonic acid into LT through the 5-lipoxygenase pathway.

INHIBITION OF 5-LIPOXYGENASE ACTIVITY BY VITAMIN E AND ITS ANALOGUES

We set out to investigate the effects of vitamin E and its analogues on the enzyme activity of an electrophoretically pure 5-lipoxygenase from potato tubers.[16] By measuring oxygen uptake polarographically, we determined that D-α-tocopherol strongly inhibited lipoxygenase activity (TABLE 1). This inhibition was concentration-dependent with an IC_{50} value of 5 μM. The inhibition by D-α-tocopherol was found to be irreversible and noncompetitive with respect to the arachidonic acid substrate (FIG. 4). A similar inhibitory response was observed with D-γ-tocopherol. Interestingly, D-α-tocopherol acetate and D-α-tocopherol quinone also exhibited an inhibitory effect on 5-lipoxygenase, although to a lesser extent. This is somewhat surprising because the latter two vitamin E analogues are known to be poor antioxidants. The data indicate that the inhibition is not specific for a natural isomer of vitamin E. Also, these results suggest that the inhibition of 5-lipoxygenase by vitamin E and its analogues is probably unrelated to their antioxidant function.

Our observations with potato 5-lipoxygenase agree with the findings of Grossman and Waksman for soybean 15-lipoxygenase.[17] Our results differ from theirs, however, in that D-α-tocopherol acetate does not inhibit 5-lipoxygenase to the same extent observed with D-α-tocopherol, whereas Grossman and Waksman found them to be equipotent on 15-lipoxygenase. As expected, classical antioxidants like butylated hydroxytoluene (BHT) and nordihydroguaiaretic acid (NDGA) inhibited 5-lipoxygenase potently, but the interesting aspect of our study is that the concentrations of D-α-tocopherol required to inhibit the enzyme are comparable to that of BHT and NDGA. Furthermore, these values appear to be within the physiological range of cellular vitamin E levels. For example, in certain tissues like lung, heart, testes, and liver, the local concentrations of vitamin E within subcellular organelles of cells are reported to be in the micromolar range.[18] Therefore, it is quite conceivable that the 5-lipoxygenase in those tissues, especially lung, might well be under check by vitamin E. Thus, by modulating the enzyme activity of 5-lipoxygenase, tissue vitamin E levels may exert a profound influence on the formation of LT and other biologically active compounds formed from arachidonic acid. Indeed, our data on the elevated levels of LTB_4 and 5-HETE in macrophages during vitamin E-deficient states support this hypothesis.[19]

Inasmuch as the inhibition of 5-lipoxygenase by vitamin E appears to be unrelated to its antioxidant function, we investigated the possibility that vitamin E might be inhibiting the enzyme activity by a specific interaction with the protein itself. We

TABLE 1. Effects of Vitamin E and Its Analogues on 5-Lipoxygenase Activity[a]

Inhibitor	Concentration (μM)	Specific Activity[b]	Percent Inhibition
None	—	11.0	0
D-α-Tocopherol	5	6.1	45.0
	10	3.9	65.0
	100	0.6	95.0
D-α-Tocopherol acetate	5	9.2	17.0
	10	8.3	25.0
	100	5.7	48.0
D-γ-Tocopherol	5	3.5	68.0
	10	3.1	72.0
	100	0.8	92.0
D-α-Tocopherol quinone	5	8.4	23.0
	10	8.3	25.0
	100	4.8	57.0
BHT	5	3.0	73.0
	10	2.9	73.0
	100	2.0	82.0
NDGA	5	2.2	80.0
	10	1.7	85.0
	100	0.7	93.0

[a] Values given for specific activity are the averages of 3 separate experiments. Individual values among the 3 experiments were within 5% variation.
[b] Specific activity is expressed as μmoles of oxygen consumed per min per mg protein.

tested this possibility by incubating ^{14}C-labeled D-α-tocopherol with the purified potato 5-lipoxygenase and separating the unbound radioactive D-α-tocopherol by gel filtration. A radioactivity peak coeluted with the lipoxygenase protein peak in the void volume of G-15 column, indicating a possible complex formation between protein and D-α-tocopherol. We investigated the nature of the binding of D-α-tocopherol to the enzyme protein further by repeatedly extracting the protein/D-α-tocopherol complex with ethylacetate. Greater than 90% of the radioactivity was still associated with the protein, suggesting that vitamin E binds strongly to 5-lipoxygenase. The binding pattern of vitamin E with 5-lipoxygenase was further analyzed by subjecting the D-α-tocopherol/protein complex to tryptic digestion. When we analyzed the resulting peptide mixture with HPLC, we found that D-α-tocopherol was associated mainly with a single peptide that was slightly larger in size and relatively hydrophobic in nature. (Information on the exact amino acid composition of this peptide is so far unavailable.) Interestingly the vitamin E/5-lipoxygenase complex did not cross-react with the antiserum raised against pure 5-lipoxygenase from potato tubers, indicating that vitamin E might be binding to the same sites recognized by antibodies.

INHIBITION OF 5-LIPOXYGENASE BY Se-GSH-Px

To gain additional insight into the fundamental processes involved in or responsible for regulating LT biosynthesis, we have systematically analyzed the effects of Se-GSH-

Px on the catalytic activities of the purified 5-lipoxygenase. Inhibition of 5-lipoxygenase by the addition of Se-GSH-Px from bovine erythrocytes at various time points, following initiation of the reaction with arachidonic acid, is shown in FIGURE 5. As measured by O_2 consumption using the Clark type electrode, enzyme activity was completely inhibited in the presence of both Se-GSH-Px and GSH. Omitting either Se-GSH-Px or GSH had no effect on the lipoxygenase activity. Also, no inhibition was observed in the presence of heat-denatured Se-GSH-Px. The data shown in FIGURE 5 suggest that the longer the time interval before the addition of Se-GSH-Px, the greater the time required to inhibit the reaction. The Se-GSH-Px-mediated inhibition of 5-lipoxygenase activity was reversed by the addition of 5-HPETE; no significant reversal of inhibition was observed with 5-hydroxyeicosatetraenoic acid (5-HETE); the reversal of the Se-GSH-Px inhibition by 5-HPETE was transient and was soon followed by a significant decline in oxygen consumption, most likely attributable to the rapid reduction of HPETE by Se-GSH-Px. To determine the specificity of FAHP activation, we tested the effects of 8-, 9-, 11-, 12-, and 15-HPETE on the Se-GSH-Px inhibition of 5-lipoxygenase individually. It should be noted that potato lipoxygenase catalyzes the insertion of molecular oxygen at all six possible positions in arachidonic acid to yield 5-, 8-, 9-, 11-, 12-, and 15-HPETE as primary oxygenation products.[20,21] All these HPETE reversed the inhibition by Se-GSH-Px, but not their corresponding hydroxy fatty acids. Also, non-FAHP like H_2O_2, cumene hydroperoxide, and *t*-butyl hydroperoxide failed to reverse the inhibition.

To determine that Se-GSH-Px inhibits 5-lipoxygenase by effectively removing FAHP, an obligatory requirement for the lipoxygenase reaction, we investigated the

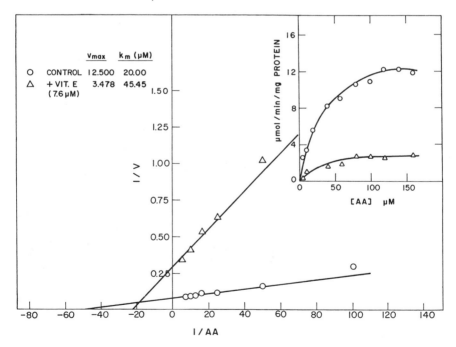

FIGURE 4. Double reciprocal plots of 5-lipoxygenase in the presence and absence of D-α-tocopherol.

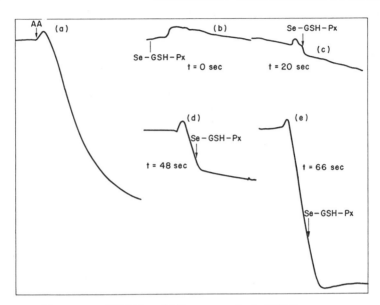

FIGURE 5. Time course of inhibition of 5-lipoxygenase by Se-GSH-Px.

catalytic efficiency of Se-GSH-Px towards 5-, 8-, 9-, 11-, 12-, and 15-HPETE. We found all HPETE to be equally good substrates with an apparent K_m of $\sim$ 10 μM and an apparent V_{max} of $\sim$ 100 μmol per min per mg of protein estimated for each of them. These kinetic constants are comparable to those determined for H_2O_2, a classical substrate for Se-GSH-Px. Also, FAHP derived from dihomo-γ-linoleic acid and eicosapentaenoic acid were found to be good substrates for this enzyme, indicating that Se-GSH-Px inhibits 5-lipoxygenase by scavenging the FAHP activator. To confirm that the inhibition of Se-GSH-Px is attributable to its catalytic efficiency in reducing FAHP rather than to any protein-protein interaction between the two enzymes, we substituted a structurally different GSH-Px—in this case non-Se-GSH-Px associated with the GSH-S-transferases from rat liver—for Se-GSH-Px in the reaction mixture. Non-Se-GSH-Px inhibited 5-lipoxygenase activity; however, we needed a large amount of this enzyme to achieve an inhibition of lipoxygenase activity comparable to that obtained with Se-GSH-Px. This observation is understandable because Se-GSH-Px is approximately 50 times more efficient than non-Se-GSH-Px in reducing FAHP.[10] Nevertheless, these data provide evidence to support the contention that FAHP is continuously required for the lipoxygenase reaction. These observations are consistent with those of Hemler and Lands,[4,5] reported for cyclooxygenase, and Rouzer and Samuelsson, for human neutrophil lipoxygenase.[6] Thus, LT biosynthesis by way of the 5-lipoxygenase pathway may be partly controlled by the cellular FAHP levels, which is in turn under the influence of Se-GSH-Px and non-Se-GSH-Px. There is, however, only limited *in vivo* experimental evidence to support this hypothesis.

INFLUENCE OF DIETARY VITAMIN E AND Se ON THE PRODUCTS OF THE 5-LIPOXYGENASE PATHWAY

We have investigated the effects of altered vitamin E and Se nutrition on the secretion of arachidonic acid metabolites by zymogen-stimulated pulmonary alveolar macrophages. The cells were obtained by lung lavage from male Long-Evans hooded rats fed torula yeast-based diets either supplemented with or deficient in vitamin E or Se or both. Neither vitamin E nor Se deficiency had any effect on the number of harvested alveolar macrophages or the composition of the cell types recovered from pulmonary airways. The most interesting observation, shown in TABLE 2, was that the levels of 5-HETE and LTB_4 increased significantly only in the group fed the diet adequate in Se but deficient in vitamin E—approximately a 60% increase in 5-HETE production and a 90% increase in LTB_4 formation when compared to the control group (+E, +Se). This result contrasts with the effects of vitamin E and Se deficiency on the formation of cyclooxygenase products. We observed that the levels of TXB_2 and PGE_2 increased significantly in macrophages obtained from rats fed on diets deficient in Se, vitamin E, and both.

The specific effects of vitamin E deficiency on the 5-lipoxygenase pathway are intriguing. It is well-established, however, that maximal 5-lipoxygenase activity requires Ca^{2+},[22] and vitamin E has been reported to inhibit Ca^{2+} release from the storage vesicles.[23] Therefore, enhanced Ca^{2+} flux under a vitamin E-deficient state could lead to an increase in 5-lipoxygenase activity. Also important to this discussion is the fact that cytosolic 5-lipoxygenase is translocated to the membrane site by elevated Ca^{2+} levels,[24] thus bringing this enzyme into close proximity with the phospholipase A_2, which one would also expect to be activated by Ca^{2+}. Therefore, an increased availability of arachidonic acid might lead to an increase in 5-HPETE production, a precursor for both 5-HETE and LTB_4 formation. Also, one can speculate that the Ca^{2+}-activated 5-lipoxygenase might effectively transform 5-HPETE into 5,6-LTA_4 through its intrinsic 8-lipoxygenase activity.[20,25] The data is, however, too preliminary to warrant absolute confidence in such conclusions as these.

In our research, Se deficiency did not have any significant effect on the LTB_4 production by alveolar macrophages (TABLE 2); however, in a similar study, Gairola and Tai found that macrophage LTB_4 production was significantly reduced in Se-deficient states.[26,27] These differences might be, in part, attributable to differences in rat strains. Gairola and Tai employed Fisher 344 rats, whereas we used Long-Evans hooded rats. Furthermore, they fed their animals on the Se-deficient diet for 38 weeks compared to the nine weeks our animals consumed the Se-deficient diets. Also, Gairola and Tai recovered five times more alveolar macrophages than we did.

At least five reports indicate a loss of chemotactic properties of polymorphonuclear leukocytes (PMNL) from Se-deficient animals.[26-30] The loss in chemotactic properties of PMNL has been reported to be consistent with decreased LTB_4 production.[30] Reduced LTB_4 might also result in a reduced stimulation for the release of granule-bound enzymes in PMNL.[31] These findings indicate a possible role for Se in the

TABLE 2. Effects of Vitamin E and Se Deficiency on the Release of LTB_4 and 5-HETE in alveolar macrophages[a]

| Treatment | Metabolite (ng/5 × 10^5 cells) | |
	LTB_4	5-HETE
+E, +Se	1.32 ± 0.20^c	1.20 ± 0.11^c
−E, +Se	2.46 ± 0.37^b	1.96 ± 0.24^b
+E, −Se	1.47 ± 0.11^c	1.29 ± 0.11^c
−E, −Se	1.46 ± 0.11^c	1.30 ± 0.29^c

[a] Values are means ± SE of observations from 8-12 animals. Means with the same superscript letters within the vertical columns are not significantly different ($p > 0.05$).

modulation of the 5-lipoxygenase pathway. Also, Bryant and Baily demonstrated the importance of Se in the lipoxygenase pathway of platelets.[32] More specifically they found that platelets from Se-deficient rats synthesize less 12-HETE than those of Se-adequate rats.

There is, in short, no question that PG and LT are involved in such disease processes as inflammation, allergies, and cardiovascular dysfunctions. Indeed there may be no known disease in which these compounds are not implicated. The body employs several lines of defense against the overproduction of these biologically active compounds, and the fact that Se and vitamin E are approved as anti-inflammatory agents for use in human and veterinary medicine indicates their importance in controlling the inflammatory response, perhaps through their modulatory function on the arachidonic acid cascade.

REFERENCES

1. LANDS, W. E. M., R. J. KULMACZ & P. J. MARSHALL. 1984. *In* Free Radicals in Biology. W. A. Pryor, Ed.: VI: 39-61. Academic Press. New York.
2. NEEDLEMAN, P., J. TURK, B. A. JAKSCHIK, A. R. MORRISON & J. B. LIFKOWITH. 1986. Annu. Rev. Biochem. 55: 69-102.
3. REDDY, C. CHANNA, J. WHELAN & R. W. SCHOLZ. 1988. *In* Cellular Antioxidant Defense Mechanisms. C. K. Chow, Ed.: Vol. 1: 139-149. CRC Press.
4. HEMLER, M. E., H. W. COOK & W. E. M. LANDS. 1976. Arch. Biochem. Biophys. 193: 340-345.
5. HEMLER, M. E. & W. E. M. LANDS. 1980. J. Biol. Chem. 255: 6253-6261.
6. ROUZER, C. A. & B. SAMUELSSON. 1986. FEBS Letters 204: 293-296.
7. WHELAN, J., P. REDDANNA, J. R. BURGESS & C. CHANNA REDDY. 1986. Fed. Proc. Fed. Am. Soc. Exp. Biol. 45: 1935.
8. TAPPEL, A. L. 1980. Ann. N.Y. Acad. Sci. 355: 18-31.
9. REDDY, C. CHANNA, C. E. THOMAS & R. W. SCHOLZ. 1985. *In* Xenobiotic Metabolism: Nutritional Effects. J. W. Finley & D. E. Schwals, Eds.: 277: 253-265. ACS Symposium Series.
10. HONG, Y., C.-H. LI, J. R. BURGESS, M. CHANG, A. ZISMAN, K. SRIKUMAR & C. CHANNA REDDY. 1989. J. Biol. Chem. 264: 13793-13800.
11. LUCY, J. A. 1972. Ann. N.Y. Acad. Sci. 203: 4-11.
12. DIPLOCK, A. T. & J. A. LUCY. 1973. FEBS Letters 29: 205-210.
13. MCCAY, P. B. & M. M. KING. 1980. *In* Vitamin E: A Comprehensive Treatise. L. J. Machlin, Ed.: 289-317. Marcel Dekker. New York.
14. WHELAN, J., J. R. BURGESS, G. HILDENBRANDT, R. W. SCHOLZ & C. CHANNA REDDY. 1989. Free Radicals Biol. Med. In press.
15. PANGANAMALA, R. V. & D. G. CORNWELL. 1980. Ann. N.Y. Acad. Sci. 393: 376-391.
16. REDDANNA, P., K. R. MADDIPATI & C. C. REDDY. 1985. FEBS Lett. 193: 39-43.
17. GROSSMAN, S. & E. G. WAKSMAN. 1984. Eur. J. Biochem. 16: 281-289.
18. KORNBURST, D. J. & R. D. DAVIS. 1980. Lipids 15: 315-322.
19. ESKEW, M. L., A. ZARKOWER, W. J. SCHEUCHENZUBER, J. R. BURGESS, R. W. SCHOLZ, G. HILDENBRANDT & C. CHANNA REDDY. 1989. Prostaglandins 38: 79-89.
20. WHELAN, J., P. REDDANNA, G. PRASAD & C. CHANNA REDDY. 1987. *In* Proceedings of the Short Course on Polyunsaturated Fatty Acids and Eicosanoids. W. E. M. Lands, Ed: 468-471. AOCS Press. Champaign, IL.
21. WHELAN, J., P. REDDANNA, G. PRASAD, K. R. MADDIPATI & C. CHANNA REDDY. 1988. Ann. N.Y. Acad. Sci. 524: 391-392.
22. JAKSCHIK, B. A. & L. H. LEE. 1980. Nature 287: 51-52.
23. BUTLER, A. M., J. M. GERRARD, J. PELLER, P. F. STODDARD, G. H. R. RAO & J. G. WHITE. 1979. Prostaglandins, Leukotrienes Med. 2: 203-216.

24. ROUZER, C. A. & B. SAMUELSSON. 1987. Proc. Natl. Acad. Sci. USA **84:** 7393-7397.
25. SHIMIZU, T., O. RADMARK & B. SAMUELSSON. 1984. Proc. Natl. Acad. Sci. USA **81:** 689-693.
26. GAIROLA, C. & H. H. TAI. 1985. Biochem. Biophys. Res. Commun. **132:** 397-403.
27. GAIROLA, C. & H. H. TAI. 1986. Biochem. Pharmacol. **35:** 2423-2428.
28. AZIZ, E. S. & P. H. KLESIUS. 1985. Vet. Immunol. Immunopathol. **10:** 381-390.
29. AZIZ, E. S. & P. H. KLESIUS. 1986. Am. J. Vet. Res. **47:** 148-151.
30. AZIZ, E. S. & P. H. KLESIUS. 1986. Am. J. Vet. Res. **47:** 426-428.
31. BORGEAT, P., P. SIROIS, P. BRAQUET & M. ROLA-PLEZCZYNSKI. 1985. *In* Biological Protection with Prostaglandins. M. M. Chen, Ed.: Vol. I: 13-26. CRC Press.
32. BRYANT, R. W. & J. M. BAILEY. 1980. Biochem. Biophys. Res. Commun. **92:** 268-276.

Role of Vitamin E in Neural Tissue[a]

DAVID P. R. MULLER AND
MARK A. GOSS-SAMPSON

Institute of Child Health
London WC1N 1EH
United Kingdom

INTRODUCTION

It is now well-established that vitamin E (alpha-tocopherol) is important for the maintenance of normal neurological structure and function in humans and experimental animals. In humans, a severe and prolonged deficiency of the vitamin results in a characteristic and progressive neurological syndrome characterized by ataxia of limbs and gait, areflexia, proprioceptive loss, ophthalmoplegia, retinal pigmentation, and general muscle weakness.[1] The neuropathological lesions associated with vitamin E deficiency are similar in humans and experimental animals (*e.g.* rat and monkey) and are characterized by a degeneration of the axons of the gracile and cuneate nuclei in the brainstem, the posterior columns of the spinal cord, and in the peripheral nerves, with a selective loss of large caliber myelinated fibers.[2]

Alpha-tocopherol appears to be the only significant lipid soluble chain-breaking antioxidant *in vivo,*[3] and this is presumed to be its principal role. It is, however, not known why the nervous system should be particularly susceptible to a deficiency of this vitamin. In order to further understand the role of alpha-tocopherol in neurological tissue, aspects of the neurobiology of vitamin E and some other antioxidant systems have been studied and correlated with functional studies of axonal transport and neuroelectrophysiology.

MATERIAL AND METHODS

One hundred eighty weanling male Wistar rats were obtained from Charles River Ltd., UK. Half of the rats were placed on a vitamin E-deficient diet (Machlin/Draper-HLR 814), supplied by Dyets, Pennsylvania, USA. The remainder (controls) received the same diet to which alpha-tocopheryl acetate (100 mg/kg) had been added. Rats from each group were killed at fixed times over a period of 55 weeks for the different investigations. The various tissues and neuroanatomical regions were obtained following perfusion with ice-cold saline, as previously described.[4]

[a]We thank Hoffmann-La Roche and Co. and the Friedreich's Ataxia Group for financial support.

Alpha-tocopherol concentrations were determined by high-performance liquid chromatography/fluorometry using a modification[5] of the method of Buttriss and Diplock.[6] Concentrations of alpha-tocopherol were routinely expressed as $\mu g/g$ lipid. Total lipid concentrations were determined by the hydroxamic acid method of Snyder and Stevens[7] after extraction with 2:1 chloroform-methanol.[8] The activities of superoxide dismutase and glutathione peroxidase were determined by the method of Crapo et al.[9] and Beutler et al.,[10] respectively, and expressed as units/mg protein. Protein concentrations were determined by the method of Lowry et al.[11] The uptake of radiolabeled alpha-tocopherol (dl-3,4-[³H]alpha-tocopherol, 0.3 mCi/mg, supplied by Hoffmann-La Roche) by the various tissues, following its injection into the tail vein of anesthetized rats, was carried out as previously described.[4] The axonal transport (fast anterograde and retrograde) of acetylcholinesterase was measured in the sciatic nerve by a double ligature technique essentially as described by Oikarinen and Kalimo.[12] The activity of acetylcholinesterase was estimated in 2 mm sections of nerve by a radiometric assay,[13] which measures the 1-[¹⁴C]acetate released from 1-[¹⁴C]acetylcholine chloride (Amersham International, 305 Ci/mg). Results are expressed as the percentage increase of acetylcholinesterase activity at the relevant ligature site after 3 hours accumulation.

The lumbar and cortical somatosensory evoked potentials; their respective conduction velocities and the electromyographic recordings were determined, as previously described.[14] The right tibial nerve was stimulated electrically (20-25 V, frequency 2.5 Hz) such that a moderate paw twitch was obtained. Lumbar somatosensory-evoked potentials were recorded from between the fifth and sixth lumbar vertebral spines and cortical somatosensory-evoked potentials from over the left somatosensory cortex. Electromyographic activity was recorded from four well-separated sites on the gastrocnemius muscle of the right limb. All recordings were made using a Medelec MS6 electrophysiological recorder set to a recording band pass of 8 Hz to 8 kHz. Results are expressed as the mean ± 1 SD or the mean with range, and the significance of difference between mean values was calculated by the Student's t test.

RESULTS

Alpha-Tocopherol Status

The concentrations of alpha-tocopherol ($\mu g/g$ lipid) in deficient animals from weaning to 52 weeks (expressed as a percentage of control values) in non-neurological (serum, liver, and adipose tissue) and neurological (brain, spinal cord, and nerve) tissues are shown in FIGURE 1. Concentrations declined rapidly in serum, liver, and adipose tissue and after 16 weeks of deficiency were undetectable in serum and only just detectable in liver and adipose tissue (< 2 % of control values). Concentrations in brain, cord, and nerve declined more slowly with the loss of alpha-tocopherol from the nerve during the first 20 weeks of deficiency being intermediate between that of the non-neurological tissues and the brain and cord. After 36 weeks of deficiency, the concentration of alpha-tocopherol in the neurological tissues was 4-7% of control values and thereafter remained relatively constant.

The concentrations of alpha-tocopherol in the various regions of brain and spinal cord of control and deficient animals at 52 weeks are shown in FIGURE 2. In the

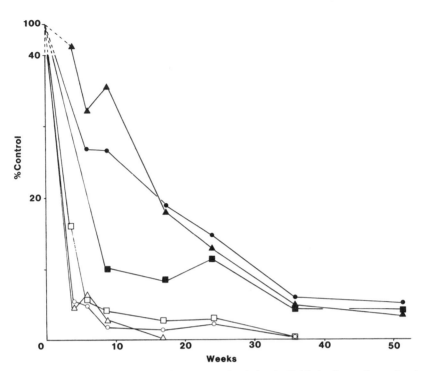

FIGURE 1. Mean concentrations of alpha-tocopherol (μg/g lipid) in tissues from vitamin E-deficient rats (expressed as a percentage of control values) from weaning to 52 weeks (n = 3). Brain, ▲; Cord, ●; Nerve, ■; Serum, △; Liver, ○; and Adipose tissue □. (M. A. Goss-Sampson et al.[28] With permission from the *Journal of the Neurological Sciences.*)

brains of control rats the cortex consistently had the highest and the cerebellum the lowest concentration (1032 : 807-1184 and 704 : 664-784 μg/g lipid, respectively). Within the spinal cord, the lumbar 4-6 region had the highest concentration (949 : 743-1158 μg/g lipid). Alpha-tocopherol concentrations in the peripheral nerve (sciatic and tibial) were 775 : 670-842 μg/g lipid. After 52 weeks of deficiency the mean concentration of alpha-tocopherol was similar (20-26 μg/g lipid) in all the brain regions with no region exhibiting selective retention or loss of the vitamin. The concentration of alpha-tocopherol in the various regions of the spinal cord was, with the exception of the lumbar 4-6 region, approximately twice that found in the brain (44-50 μg/g lipid) and was similar in the peripheral nerve with a mean of 36 μg/g lipid.

Antioxidant Enzyme Activities

The specific activities of superoxide dismutase and glutathione peroxidase were estimated longitudinally in the brains of control and deficient animals. At no time was there any significant difference between the activity of either enzyme in the two groups of animals. The activities found in whole brains at 52 weeks are shown in FIGURE 3. There were also no significant differences in the activities of the two enzymes in the various brain regions, either within or between the two groups of rats.

Uptake of Radiolabeled Alpha-Tocopherol

In previous studies, the uptake of radiolabeled alpha-tocopherol into neurological tissue was shown to be maximal 6 hours after injection of the radiolabel into the tail vein of rats.[4] This time point was, therefore, used in the current study. FIGURE 4 shows the uptake (expressed as a percentage of control values) of radiolabeled alpha-tocopherol by neurological tissues of vitamin E-deficient rats from 11 to 55 weeks. The whole sciatic and tibial nerves of deficient animals showed a significant increase in uptake after 11 weeks (150% of controls), which increased to 181% by 55 weeks. The whole brain and spinal cord of deficient animals did not show any increase in uptake until 26 weeks, and it was not until 36 weeks, when loss of endogenous tocopherol was maximal in all the neurological tissues, that uptake was similar to that seen in the peripheral nerve. Uptake by specific regions of the brain, cord, and nerve was also investigated over the same time period, but no evidence of selective uptake was found.

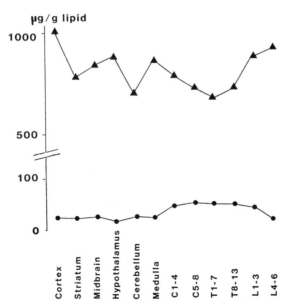

FIGURE 2. Mean concentrations of alpha-tocopherol in regions of brain and spinal cord of control (▲) and deficient (●) rats after 55 weeks (n = 3). C, cervical; T, thoracic; L, lumbar regions of spinal cord.

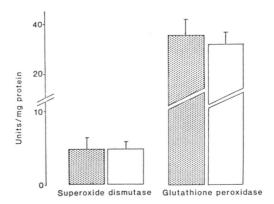

FIGURE 3. Activities of superoxide dismutase and glutathione peroxidase (mean ± 1 SD) in whole brains of control ▨ and deficient ☐ rats after 55 weeks (n = 6).

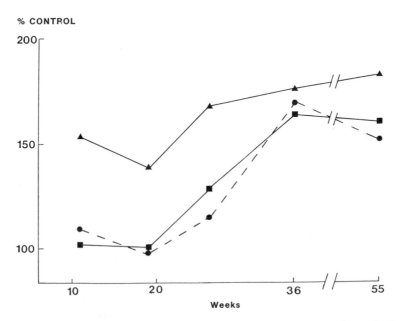

FIGURE 4. Mean uptake of [³H]alpha-tocopherol (expressed as a percentage of control values) by neurological tissues of vitamin E-deficient rats from weaning to 55 weeks (n = 3). Brain, ●; Cord, ■; and Nerve, ▲. (M. A. Goss-Sampson et al.[28] With permission from the *Journal of the Neurological Sciences.*)

Axonal Transport

Anterograde and retrograde fast axonal transport of acetylcholinesterase was determined from 8-52 weeks. The results at 52 weeks are shown in FIGURE 5. The deficient animals exhibited a 25% reduction in anterograde accumulation ($p < 0.02$) and a 20% reduction in retrograde accumulation ($p < 0.05$). No significant differences in either anterograde or retrograde transport were found at earlier time points (9-36 weeks).

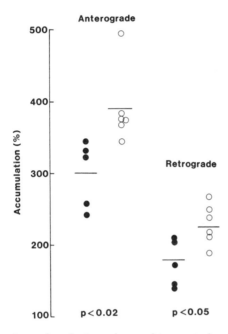

FIGURE 5. Fast anterograde and retrograde axonal transport of acetylcholinesterase in sciatic nerves of vitamin E-deficient (●) and control (○) rats after 52 weeks. —— denotes mean.

Neuroelectrophysiology

The results of the electrophysiological studies have been described in detail elsewhere[14] and are only summarized here. No differences in peripheral conduction velocities (lumbar somatosensory evoked potentials) were observed between the deficient (n = 12) and control (n = 8) animals after 40-42 weeks of deficiency (44.08 ± 2.44 and 45.10 ± 2.33 ms^{-1}, respectively), whereas central conduction velocities (cortical somatosensory evoked potentials) were significantly slowed ($p < 0.001$) in the same deficient animals (14.04 ± 1.13 compared with 16.71 ± 0.96 ms^{-1}, see FIGURE 6). Electromyographic studies of distal muscle (gastrocnemius) showed abnormalities (presence of spontaneous fibrillation, positive sharp waves or polyphasic

m/sec

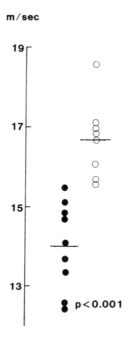

FIGURE 6. Conduction velocity of cortical somatosensory-evoked potentials in vitamin E-deficient (●) and control (○) rats at 40-42 weeks. —— denotes mean.

groups) in all the deficient animals (n = 12). None of these abnormalities were found in any control rat (n = 8).

DISCUSSION

There have been a number of studies on the effects of chronic vitamin E deficiency in the rat,[15,16] and the concentration of alpha-tocopherol in various non-neurological tissues throughout the deficiency has been documented.[17,18] There have not, however, been any previous detailed longitudinal studies on the neurobiology of alpha-tocopherol and other antioxidant systems during long-term deficiency in the rat, although there is some information on the vitamin E-deficient mouse.[19] This is also the first study that has attempted to correlate the concentrations of antioxidants with neurological function during vitamin E deficiency.

The rapid decrease in alpha-tocopherol concentrations in serum, liver, and adipose tissue observed in this study has been reported by others.[17,18] The decrease in concentration in brain, cord, and nerve was less rapid, and the nervous tissues still retained 4-5% of the control concentrations after 52 weeks of deficiency. Similar observations have been reported in the vitamin E-deficient mouse.[19] These findings, together with those of Ingold *et al.*,[20] who showed, using deuterated tocopheryl acetate, that the half-life of alpha-tocopherol was increased in the brain and spinal cord compared to other tissues, strongly suggest that neurological tissues preferentially conserve vitamin E and that its turnover may be reduced. These results also demonstrate that circulating concentrations of alpha-tocopherol do not always accurately reflect concentrations in neurological tissues, and this is particularly the case during the course of vitamin E depletion.

All tissues appear to show two phases of depletion: an initial rapid loss during the first 4-8 weeks of deficiency, followed by a second phase of slow prolonged depletion. Bieri[17] suggested that the first phase corresponded to a rapidly mobilized pool of labile vitamin E and that the second represented vitamin E bound to subcellular or membranous structures. It is possible that this latter phase relates to the loss of the functional and more critical component of tissue vitamin E. It may, therefore, be significant that the neurological tissues appear to maintain a greater proportion of alpha-tocopherol in the second, less labile pool.

The distribution of alpha-tocopherol in the various regions of brain and cord of control rats is similar to that previously reported,[4,21] with the lowest concentrations being found in the cerebellum and the rostral end of the spinal cord. This is of interest, because in humans a severe deficiency of vitamin E results in a characteristic spino-cerebellar syndrome.[1] After 52 weeks of deficiency, the concentrations of alpha-tocopherol were similar in the various brain regions and along the cord.

After 55 weeks, no differences in the activities of either glutathione peroxidase or superoxide dismutase were observed between the vitamin E-deficient and control groups. This indicates that these two water-soluble antioxidant enzyme systems do not compensate for the reduced concentrations of the lipid-soluble antioxidant alpha-tocopherol. In a recent study by Nelson,[22] the effects of the water-soluble free radical scavengers, ethoxyquin and promethazine, on the neuropathology of vitamin E deficiency in rats were studied. It was found that the rats that received vitamin E-deficient diets supplemented with either ethoxyquin or promethazine for 36-39 weeks had no evidence of the neuropathological lesions that were present in the unsupplemented deficient rats. There was also no evidence that alpha-tocopherol was spared in the rats receiving the ethoxyquin or promethazine. This study therefore provides support for the assumption that free radical damage is involved in the pathogenesis of the neurological lesions resulting from a deficiency of vitamin E.

The uptake of intravenously injected labeled tocopherol by peripheral nerve was much more rapid than that of the cord or brain. This suggests that in deficiency states the nerve may preferentially take up any circulating tocopherol at the expense of other tissues. Over the 55 weeks of deficiency no particular region of brain, cord, and nerve showed a preferential uptake. The distribution of radiolabel in the various brain regions was similar to that described by Vatassery et al.[21]

The characteristic pathological features of the neurological lesions are a progressive primary axonopathy with a secondary demyelination that predominantly affects the centrally directed primary sensory neurons.[2] This is consistent with the electrophysiological findings after 40-42 weeks of deficiency that showed a significantly slowed conduction within the central somatosensory pathway but normal conduction in the peripheral sensory pathway of the hind limbs. These findings are similar to those previously reported in humans with severe vitamin E deficiency.[23,24]

A reduction in anterograde and retrograde fast axonal transport of acetylcholinesterase was observed after 52 weeks of deficiency, but not before. This is in agreement with the finding that if alterations in axonal transport occur they generally arise late in the course of nerve degeneration. Ultrastructural studies of sensory nerve endings show an accumulation of organelles, multivesicular bodies, and tubulovesicular structures.[16,25] These observations, along with the reduced axonal transport, suggest there may be a defect in "turnaround" at the axon terminal.

Histological changes compatible with a necrotizing myopathy are observed in vitamin E-deficient rats from as early as 12 weeks of deficiency.[26] The abnormal electromyographic results obtained in the deficient animals after 40-42 weeks indicate, however, that a process of chronic partial denervation is also occurring. Similar abnormalities in an electromyogram have been reported in vitamin E-deficient states in humans.[23,27] Further studies are therefore required to delineate the precise effect of vitamin E deficiency on nerve-muscle interaction.

The presence of hind-limb weakness and ataxia was evident in the vitamin E-deficient rats by 36 weeks, at which time alpha-tocopherol concentrations were undetectable in non-neurological tissues and were less than 10% of control values in neurological tissues. At this same time point, the uptake of radiolabeled vitamin E was found to be maximal in all neurological tissues. Electrophysiological abnormalities were evident at 40-42 weeks, but longitudinal studies were not carried out and therefore their precise time of onset remains to be established. Although abnormalities of axonal transport did not occur until 52 weeks of deficiency, it is possible that more sensitive and selective methods of studying axonal transport may have detected alterations earlier. It therefore appears that a concentration of alpha-tocopherol in neurological tissues of at least 10% of control values is critical in order to presumably prevent peroxidation of neurological membranes and thereby protect against the neurological sequelae of vitamin E deficiency.

ACKNOWLEDGMENTS

We thank Mr. C. J. MacEvilly for technical assistance, and Professor P. K. Thomas (Royal Free Hospital School of Medicine, London) and Dr. A. Kriss (The Hospitals for Sick Children, Great Ormond Street, London) for help with the electrophysiological studies.

REFERENCES

1. MULLER, D. P. R., J. K. LLOYD & O. H. WOLFF. 1983. Vitamin E and neurological function. Lancet i: 225-227.
2. NELSON, J. S., C. D. FITCH, V. W. FISCHER, G. O. BROUN & A. C. CHOU. 1981. Progressive neuropathologic lesions in vitamin E deficient Rhesus monkeys. J. Neuropathol. Exp. Neurol. 40: 166-186.
3. BURTON, G. W., A. JOYCE & K. U. INGOLD. 1983. Is vitamin E the only lipid-soluble, chain-breaking antioxidant in human blood plasma and erythrocyte membranes? Arch. Biochem. Biophys. 221: 281-290.
4. GOSS-SAMPSON, M.A. & D. P. R. MULLER. 1987. Studies on the neurobiology of vitamin E (alpha-tocopherol) and some other antioxidant systems in the rat. Neuropath. Appl. Neurobiol. 13: 289-296.
5. METCALFE, T., D. P. R. MULLER & B. W. L. BROOKSBANK. 1984. Vitamin E concentrations in brains from foetuses with Down's Syndrome. IRCS. Med. Sci. 12: 121.
6. BUTTRISS, J. L. & A. T. DIPLOCK. 1983. High performance liquid chromatography methods for vitamin E in tissues. Methods Enzymol. 105: 131-138.
7. SNYDER, F. & N. A. STEVENS. 1958. A simplified spectrophotometric determination of ester groups in lipids. Biochim. Biophys. Acta 34: 244-245.

8. FOLCH, J., M. LEES & S. G. M. SLOANE. 1957. A simple method for the isolation and purification of total lipids from animal tissues. J. Biol. Chem. 226: 497-507.

9. CRAPO, J. D., J. M. McCORD & I. FRIDOVICH. 1978. Preparation and assay of superoxide dismutases. Methods Enzymol. 52: 382-393.

10. BEUTLER, E., K. G. BLUME, J. C. KAPLAN, G. W. LOHR, B. RAMOT & W. N. VALENTINE. 1977. International committee for standardization in haematology: Recommended methods for red cell enzyme analysis. Br. J. Haematol. 35: 331-340.

11. LOWRY, O. H., N. J. ROSEBROUGH, A. L. FARR & R. J. RANDALL. 1951. Protein measurement with the folin phenol reagent. J. Biol. Chem. 193: 265-275.

12. OIKARINEN, R. & H. KALIMO. 1984. Acetylcholinesterase activity and its fast axonal transport in rabbit sciatic nerves during the recovery phase of experimental allergic neuritis. Neuropathol. Appl. Neurobiol. 10: 163-171.

13. TUCEK, R. R. 1974. Transport and changes of activity of choline acetyltransferase in the peripheral stump of an interrupted nerve. Brain Res. 82: 249-269.

14. GOSS-SAMPSON, M. A., A. KRISS, J. R. MUDDLE, P. K. THOMAS & D. P. R. MULLER. 1988. Lumbar and cortical evoked potentials in rats with vitamin E deficiency. J. Neurol. Neurosurg. Psychiatry 51: 432-435.

15. MACHLIN, L. J., R. FILIPSKI, J. S. NELSON, L. R. HORN & M. BRIN. 1977. Effects of a prolonged vitamin E deficiency. J. Nutr. 107: 1200-1208.

16. TOWFIGHI, J. 1981. Effects of chronic vitamin E deficiency on the nervous system of the rat. Acta Neuropathol. 54: 261-268.

17. BIERI, J. G. 1972. Kinetics of tissue alpha-tocopherol depletion and repletion. Ann. N.Y. Acad. Sci. 203: 181-191.

18. MACHLIN, L. J. 1980. Vitamin E: A Comprehensive Treatise. Dekker. New York.

19. VATASSERY, G. T., C. K. ANGERHOFER & F. J. PETERSON. 1984. Vitamin E concentrations in the brains and some selected peripheral tissues of selenium-deficient and vitamin E-deficient mice. J. Neurochem. 42: 554-558.

20. INGOLD, K. U., G. W. BURTON, D. O. FOSTER, L. HUGHES, D. A. LINDSAY & A. WEBB. 1987. Biokinetics of and discrimination between dietary RRR- and SRR-α-tocopherols in the male rat. Lipids 22: 163-172.

21. VATASSERY, G. T., C. K. ANGERHOFER, C. A. KNOX & D. S. DESHMUKH. 1984. Concentrations of vitamin E in various neuroanatomical regions and subcellular fractions, and the uptake of vitamin E by specific areas of rat brain. Biochim. Biophys. Acta 792: 118-122.

22. NELSON, J. S. 1987. Effects of free radical scavengers on the neuropathology of mammalian vitamin E deficiency. In Clinical and Nutritional Aspects of Vitamin E. O. Hayaishi & M. Mino, Eds.: 157-159. Elsevier. Amsterdam, New York, Oxford.

23. BRIN, M. F., T. A. PEDLEY, R. E. LOVELACE, R. G. EMERSON, P. GOURAS, C. MACKAY, H. J. KAYDEN, J. LEVY & H. BAKER. 1986. Electrophysiologic features of abetalipoproteinemia. Neurology 36: 669-673.

24. SATYA-MURTI, S., L. HOWARD, G. KROHEL & B. WOLFF. 1986. The spectrum of neurologic disorder from vitamin E deficiency. Neurology 36: 917-921.

25. BRADLEY, D. J., J. R. MUDDLE, E. SOUTHAM & P. K. THOMAS. 1986. Morphological and neurophysiological studies on experimental vitamin E deficiency in rats. J. Physiol. (London) 376: 34P.

26. NELSON, J. S., L. J. MACHLIN & R. WELSH. 1978. Resolution of necrotizing myopathy in vitamin E deficient rats fed tocopherol. Fed. Proc. 37: 758.

27. WICHMAN, A., F. BUCHTHAL, G. H. PEZESHKPOUR & R. E. GREGG. 1985. Peripheral neuropathy in abetalipoproteinemia. Neurology 35: 1279-1289.

28. GOSS-SAMPSON, M. A., C. J. MACEVILLY & D. P. R. MULLER. 1988. Longitudinal studies of the neurobiology of vitamin E and other antioxidant systems, and neurological function in the vitamin E deficient rat. J. Neurol. Sci. 87: 25-35.

Vitamin E Deficiency Neuropathy in Children with Fat Malabsorption

Studies in Cystic Fibrosis and Chronic Cholestasis[a]

RONALD J. SOKOL,[b,j] NANCY BUTLER-SIMON,[b]
JAMES E. HEUBI,[c] SUSAN T. IANNACCONE,[c]
H. JUHLING McCLUNG,[d] FRANK ACCURSO,[b]
KEITH HAMMOND,[b] MELVIN HEYMAN,[e]
FRANK SINATRA,[f] CAROLINE RIELY,[g]
JEAN PERRAULT,[h] JOSEPH LEVY,[i] AND
ARNOLD SILVERMAN[b]

[b] *University of Colorado School of Medicine*
Denver, Colorado 80262

[c] *Children's Hospital Research Foundation*
Cincinnati, Ohio

[d] *Children's Hospital Medical Center*
Columbus, Ohio

[e] *University of California at San Francisco School of Medicine*
San Francisco, California

[f] *Children's Hospital Medical Center*
Los Angeles, California

[g] *Yale University School of Medicine*
New Haven, Connecticut

[h] *Mayo Clinic*
Rochester, Minnesota

[i] *Columbia University College of Physicians and Surgeons*
New York, New York

[a] This work was supported in part by U.S. Public Health Service Grants RR00069, RR00123, and RR01271 from the General Clinical Research Branch, Division of Research Resources, National Institutes of Health; a Grant from the Bureau of Maternal and Child Health and Crippled Children's Services (MCJ-080508-03); the Cystic Fibrosis Foundation; a Grant from Eastman Chemical Products, Inc., Kingsport, TN; and the Abby Bennett Liver Research Fund.

[j] Send correspondence to Ronald J. Sokol, M.D., Department of Pediatrics, Section of Pediatric Gastroenterology and Nutrition, University of Colorado School of Medicine, Box C228, 4200 East Ninth Avenue, Denver, Colorado 80262.

Over the past decade, investigators from several centers have documented the association between a biochemical deficiency of vitamin E and the development of a distinctive degenerative neuromuscular disorder in children and adults with various forms of chronic fat malabsorption, including chronic cholestatic hepatobiliary disorders,[1-7] abetalipoproteinemia,[8-10] cystic fibrosis,[11-13] and other malabsorptive conditions.[14-18] Common to these patients was an impairment in intestinal absorption of vitamin E caused by defective intraluminal lipid digestion (e.g., cystic fibrosis), micellar solubilization (e.g., chronic cholestasis), mucosal absorption (e.g., short bowel syndrome), or lymphatic transport (e.g., abetalipoproteinemia and intestinal lymphangiectasia). The resulting secondary deficiency of vitamin E results in low vitamin E content in neuromuscular tissues,[4,19] predisposing selective areas of the brain, spinal cord, and peripheral nerves[1,6] to degeneration, most likely mediated by free radical-induced lipid peroxidation. Verification of the pathogenetic role of vitamin E deficiency in this neuromuscular disorder was provided by the consistent stabilization or improvement in neurologic symptomatology[20,21] and peripheral nerve electrophysiology[2] following correction of the vitamin E deficiency state. In addition, histological lesions of brain,[1] spinal cord,[1] peripheral nerve,[6,22] and muscle in affected patients resembled lesions observed in animal models of pure dietary vitamin E deficiency.[23]

In this report we describe recent efforts at a) prospectively evaluating for, and treating, vitamin E deficiency in very young infants with cystic fibrosis, identified by a newborn screening test; and b) treatment of vitamin E-deficient children with chronic cholestasis, who were unresponsive to conventional vitamin E therapy, with a novel water-soluble form of vitamin E, D-alpha tocopheryl polyethylene glycol-1000 succinate (TPGS) (Eastman Chemical Products, Inc., Kingsport, TN).

VITAMIN E DEFICIENCY IN INFANTS WITH CYSTIC FIBROSIS

Biochemical deficiency of vitamin E uniformly occurs in children and adults with pancreatic insufficiency caused by cystic fibrosis (CF) if supplemental vitamin E is not provided.[24,25] Clinically significant abnormalities in neurologic function appear to occur only when hepatic involvement by CF is also present;[11-13] however, peripheral nerve electrophysiologic function may be impaired[26] and histologic spinal cord lesions may be observed[27-29] prior to clinical abnormalities.

Methods

The purpose of this investigation was to prospectively evaluate vitamin E status in a group of infants diagnosed with CF prior to age 3 months (by sweat test) following identification by the CF newborn screening program in Colorado.[30] The CF newborn screen consists of analysis of immunoreactive trypsinogen (IRT) in the dried blood spot obtained in the first few days of life for metabolic disease screening. If the initial IRT is elevated (> 140 ng/mL), a repeat blood spot is requested and, if again elevated (> 80 ng/mL), a sweat test is performed on the infant. This two-tiered approach results in a predictive value of 50% after two positive IRT blood spot tests.[30] Thirty-six infants with CF, detected between 1984 and 1987, were entered into a prospective multidisciplinary study of gastrointestinal function, nutritional status, growth and development, and pulmonary status. Vitamin E status was evaluated at initial diagnosis (mean age of 51.0 ± 26.7 days), and at 6 and 12 months of age. Vitamin E status was evaluated by measurement of serum alpha- and gamma-tocopherol concentrations by high-performance liquid chromatography[31] and calculation of the ratio of total tocopherols (alpha and gamma): total serum lipid concentration, measured by a colorimetric technique.[32] For purposes of this study, very conservative thresholds for definition of vitamin E deficiency were used: serum alpha-tocopherol below 3 μg/mL and ratio of total tocopherols:total lipids below 0.6 mg/g.[33]

Following diagnosis, all infants received 1.0 mL per day of a multiple vitamin supplement (Poly-Vi-Sol, Mead-Johnson) that contained 5 IU of DL-alpha tocopheryl acetate, an additional supplement of DL-alpha tocopheryl acetate (25 IU at 6 weeks, 50 IU at 6 months, and 100 IU at 12 months of age), and pancreatic enzyme supplements. Thus each child received approximately 5-10 IU/kg/day of supplemental vitamin E. Choice of continued breast-feeding or infant formulas (excluding soy-based formulas) was left to parental discretion until 1985, when all infants were randomized to receive standard cow's milk formula versus Pregestamil (Mead-Johnson, Evansville, IN) at weaning from the breast or at time of diagnosis if not breast-fed. Seventy-two hour fecal fat excretion was analyzed in a random subset of patients in a metabolic inpatient unit and expressed as the coefficient of excretion ((g fat excreted ÷ g fat ingested) × 100%).

Results

Vitamin E deficiency was present in 38% of infants at time of diagnosis (FIG. 1). Hypoalbuminemia was more prevalent in vitamin E-deficient compared to vitamin E-sufficient patients (FIG. 1) and in breast versus formula-fed infants at time of

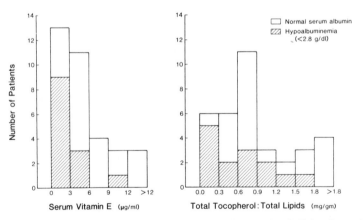

FIGURE 1. Serum vitamin E concentrations and the ratio of serum vitamin E (total tocopherols) to total serum lipid concentrations in 36 infants with cystic fibrosis identified by newborn screening. Serum levels < 3 μg/mL and ratios < 0.6 mg/g are considered deficient.

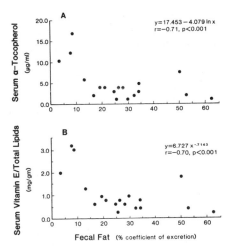

FIGURE 2. Relationships between serum vitamin E concentrations (A) or ratio of serum vitamin E to total serum lipids (B) and fecal fat coefficient of excretion at time of diagnosis in infants with cystic fibrosis.

diagnosis ($^{11}/_{22}$ versus $^{2}/_{14}$, p < 0.05). Vitamin E deficiency tended to be more common in breast- versus formula-fed infants ($^{9}/_{21}$ versus $^{3}/_{13}$); however, this difference did not reach statistical significance. Despite therapy with supplemental vitamin E throughout the first year of life, approximately 10% of patients remained vitamin E-deficient. Serum vitamin E concentrations and the ratios of serum vitamin E:total lipids at diagnosis were inversely related to fecal fat excretion, supporting the presumed mechanism of vitamin E malabsorption in producing the low serum values (FIG. 2). No clinical abnormalities were detected by standard neurologic examination during the first year of life in any of the vitamin E-deficient infants.

Conclusions

Vitamin E deficiency was relatively common in the first two to three months of life in infants with CF, responding to previously recommended doses of vitamin E for CF[34] in most infants. The treatment failures may have been caused by poor compliance or excessive malabsorption of vitamin E in selected patients. The impact of reversing vitamin E deficiency at this young age is unknown; however, prospective continued observation of these patients is currently in progress.

VITAMIN E DEFICIENCY IN CHRONIC CHILDHOOD CHOLESTASIS

Biochemical evidence of vitamin E deficiency has been observed in approximately 50 to 75% of infants and children with chronic forms of cholestatic hepatobiliary disorders,[35-38] including extrahepatic biliary atresia, Alagille syndrome (arteriohepatic dysplasia), familial forms of intrahepatic cholestasis, and neonatal hepatitis. Treatment of the deficiency is hampered by the extremely poor intestinal absorption of orally administered vitamin E during severe cholestasis, inasmuch as inadequate secretion of bile produces bile acid concentrations in the duodenal lumen insufficient for the solubilization of dietary fat.[4] Oral coadministration of conjugated bile acids improves vitamin E absorption during cholestasis;[4] however, chronic oral bile acid therapy is currently not recommended in children. When treated with even extraordinary doses (100-200 IU/kg/day) of available preparations of oral vitamin E (alpha-tocopherol, alpha-tocopheryl acetate, alpha-tocopheryl succinate), many children with severe cholestasis fail to absorb adequate vitamin E, resulting in persistent vitamin E deficiency and neurologic degeneration as early as the second year of life.[2,22,38] Previously we have successfully administered intramuscular injections of vitamin E to such children, with resultant improved neurologic function.[20] Unfortunately, the parenteral form of vitamin E (Ephynal,[R] Hoffmann-La Roche, Nutley, NJ) is still an investigational drug and not readily available in the United States; treatment requires repeated intramuscular injections for several years.

Over the past four years, we have evaluated intestinal absorption, efficacy, and safety of a water-soluble form of vitamin E, TPGS, in children with severe cholestasis. Because of the amphipathic structure of TPGS (FIG. 3), it forms micelles in the absence of bile acids (critical micellar concentration of 0.04 to 0.06 mmol/L),[39] allowing TPGS to traverse the unstirred water layer covering the intestinal mucosa. Recent evidence suggests that the TPGS molecule may be absorbed intact into the enterocyte and then hydrolyzed;[40] however, in the intact animal, intraluminal or brush border hydrolysis of TPGS is also plausible. We have previously reported our initial studies using TPGS in twenty-two children with chronic cholestasis who failed to absorb other forms of vitamin E.[41,42] In this report we will extend these observations to include 38 patients for up to 4 years of observation on TPGS treatment.

Methods

Thirty-eight children (0.5 to 20 years old, mean 6.4 ± 5.8 years; 15 boys, 23 girls) with chronic forms of neonatal cholestatic hepatobiliary disorders and with well-documented vitamin E deficiency were studied for greater than six months at seven centers in the United States (TABLE 1). Diagnoses of underlying liver disease included arteriohepatic dysplasia (Alagille syndrome) in 15 patients, extrahepatic biliary atresia in 8, nonsyndromatic paucity of interlobular bile ducts in 6, progressive intrahepatic cholestasis in 3, familial progressive intrahepatic cholestasis (Byler's disease) in 3, and neonatal hepatitis in three. Each child developed cholestatic liver disease within

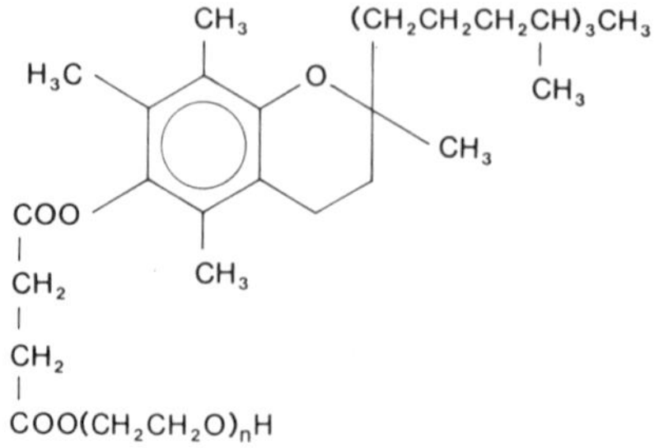

FIGURE 3. Chemical structure of D-alpha-tocopheryl polyethylene glycol-1000 succinate (TPGS).

the first three months of life. Four additional children with extrahepatic biliary atresia who did not complete a 6-month trial of TPGS were excluded from this analysis: two died from liver failure (ages 6 and 13 months) and two underwent orthotopic liver transplantation (ages 2 years and 5 $\frac{1}{12}$ years). Vitamin E deficiency was established by low serum vitamin E concentrations (fluorometric[43] or high-performance liquid chromatography method[31]), low ratios of serum vitamin E (alpha and gamma-tocopherol) to total serum lipid concentrations,[33] elevated hydrogen peroxide hemolysis when measured,[44] low fat and muscle vitamin E content when measured,[4,6] and the presence of characteristic neurologic findings previously associated with vitamin E deficiency[1-7] in children older than age 18-24 months. All subjects had failed to show normalization of the indices of vitamin E status after treatment with up to 70 to 212 IU/kg/day of oral alpha-tocopherol or alpha-tocopheryl acetate. Nine patients had been receiving intramuscular injections of DL-alpha-tocopherol up to the time of this study for correction of the vitamin E-deficiency state. Oral supplements of vitamin D_2, K, and A and a multiple vitamin were administered to most children. Phenobarbital or bile acid-binding resins were prescribed for those patients with intrahepatic disorders requiring treatment for hypercholesterolemia or pruritus or for the induction of choleresis.

TPGS was administered as a 10 to 20% solution (37 to 75 IU/mL of D-alpha-tocopheryl succinate). At each study center, TPGS solution was formulated from pure TPGS in the hospital pharmacy. Solid TPGS was melted into a liquid state by heating to above 40°C and stirring to ensure homogeneity. Weighed portions were slowly poured into measured volumes of boiling sterile water causing the TPGS to initially form a stiff gel that dissolved with subsequent stirring for 1-3 hours while cooling to room temperature. The TPGS was bottled, stored at room temperature or refrigerated and dispensed to patients within 3 months of preparation. The final solution was clear amber in color and virtually tasteless.

After enrollment into this trial, baseline studies were obtained, and TPGS treatment was initiated. The initial patients received a brief course (2-4 weeks) of 50 IU/kg/day; however, serum vitamin E concentrations rose above the normal range. Thereafter, the starting dose of TPGS was lowered to 25 IU/kg/day in all subsequent patients. TPGS was administered as one daily dose given with breakfast at least 2 hours before the first daily dose of bile acid-binding resin. Each subject was monitored 2 weeks, 4 weeks, 2 months, and 4 months after starting TPGS therapy and every 3-4 months thereafter. Blood was obtained for complete blood count, differential, platelet count, serum electrolytes, urea nitrogen, creatinine, aspartate and alanine amino transferases, alkaline phosphatase, direct and total bilirubin, osmolality, vitamin E, and total lipid concentrations. A urinalysis was performed. General physical examinations were performed every 3-4 months and neurologic examinations a minimum of every 6-12 months. Parents and subjects were questioned for the presence of gastrointestinal symptoms or other adverse reactions possibly related to the TPGS therapy. The dose of TPGS was adjusted to maintain a ratio of serum vitamin E to total serum lipid concentration above 0.8 mg/g for children 12 years or older, and well above 0.6 mg/g for those under age 12 years, while attempting to keep the serum vitamin E concentration below 20-25 µg/mL. If severe hyperlipidemia was present, the ratio of serum vitamin E:total lipids was normalized despite serum vitamin E concentrations above 25 µg/mL.

In order to quantify changes in neurologic function during this study, a neurologic score[20,42] was assigned for each examination by rating each of 12 neurologic signs from 0 (normal) to 3+ (severely abnormal), based on specific criteria for each sign (a complete summary of the neurologic scoring system is available from the authors on request). The neurologic signs evaluated were hyporeflexia and areflexia, truncal

TABLE 1. Clinical and Neurologic Data

Patient Number	Diagnosis of Liver Disease	Age at Entry (years)	Sex	Most Recent TPGS Dose IU/kg/day	Duration of TPGS Therapy (years)	Total Neurologic Score Before TPGS	Total Neurologic Score After TPGS
1	EHBA[a]	2.0	F	25	1.0	3	1
2	Neonatal Hepatitis	1.8	F	14	2.3	0	0
3	PIBD[b]	4.2	F	25	0.5	2	1
4	EHBA	0.8	M	18.2	0.8	0	0
5	AHD[c]	2.7	F	25	4.0	4.5	0
6	AHD	5.3	F	23.1	1.0	5	5
7	EHBA	0.5	M	21	0.4	0	0
8	AHD	19.3	M	10	2.0	11	8
9	EHBA	9.2	M	22.5	1.0	4	4
10	EHBA	5.5	F	21.9	2.3	3	1
11	EHBA	1.3	F	18	1.0	2.5	0
12	AHD	12.0	F	22.5	1.0	9.5	8.5
13	AHD	0.6	M	15	4.0	0	0
14	PIC[d]	3.8	M	26.3	4.0	3	2
15	AHD	1.1	F	20	4.0	0	0
16	PIC	14.0	F	25.9	3.0	14	13
17	Neonatal Hepatitis	2.8	M	15.2	2.0	4	3
18	AHD	6.3	M	25	0.8	6	6

19	AHD	13.8	F	25	1.0	11	11
20	AHD	2.4	F	24.4	3.0	3	1
21	PIBD	10.8	M	25	0.5	16	17
22	AHD	3.9	F	25	3.0	0	0
23	EHBA	0.5	F	25	0.8	0	0
24	PIBD	15.8	M	37.6	3.0	17	19
25	FPIC[e]	15.5	F	16.3	3.0	5	5
26	PIBD	5.2	F	25	3.0	0	0
27	PIBD, α1 Antitrypsin Deficiency	16.1	F	25	1.2	18	18
28	FPIC	9.8	F	25	1.5	5	3
29	AHD	20.0	F	24	1.0	20	20
30	Neonatal Hepatitis	3.2	M	25	2.0	2	3
31	AHD	1.9	F	25	1.0	2	1
32	EHBA	3.2	F	12.5	2.0	4	2.5
33	PIBD	7.2	F	25	0.5	3	3
34	AHD	0.5	M	20.6	1.0	0	0
35	FPIC	18.0	M	22.5	2.0	7	6
36	PIC	9.5	M	25	1.5	9	6
37	AHD	1.2	M	25	0.5	0	0
38	AHD	7.0	M	25	1.0	13	9

[a] EHBA = extrahepatic biliary atresia.
[b] PIBD = nonsyndromatic paucity of interlobular bile ducts.
[c] AHD = arteriohepatic dysplasia.
[d] PIC = progressive intrahepatic cholestasis.
[e] FPIC = familial progressive intrahepatic cholestasis.

and limb ataxia, impaired position and vibratory senses, loss of light touch and pain sensation, ophthalmoplegia, dysarthria, proximal muscle weakness, scoliosis, and pes cavus. If the neurologic abnormality was unilateral, only half of the numerical value was assigned. The specific neurologic signs were chosen for this scoring system because they have been reported in patients with vitamin E deficiency and neuromuscular degeneration.[1-7]

Intestinal absorption of polyethylene glycol-1000 (PEG-1000) released from the TPGS was assessed in a subgroup of patients and four control adults. Because of possible absorption of PEG-1000 hydrolyzed off the TPGS molecule and concern over its potential toxicity in children with chronic liver disease, urine was collected from 13 patients and 4 normal adults for 24 hours after an oral loading dose of 100 IU/kg of TPGS up to a maximum dose of 2000 IU. The urine was stored at 4°C for up to 2 months, shipped on dry ice, and analyzed for PEG size and content by high-pressure liquid chromatography and gas chromatography as previously described.[41] Because PEG is not metabolized and is rapidly excreted in the urine, the percentage of the ingested dose that was absorbed was calculated by dividing the quantity of PEG excreted in the urine by the ingested dose and multiplying by 100.

This study was approved by the Human Subjects Committee at the University of Colorado School of Medicine and the Institutional Review Boards for Human Investigation at the other participating institutions. The use of TPGS in this study was under Investigational New Drug status as approved by the Food and Drug Administration. Informed written consent was obtained from parents of subjects under age 18 years and directly from the subject older than age 18 years.

Statistical Analysis

Statistical analysis of laboratory data was performed by the paired Student's t test comparing baseline values to those obtained at 6 months, 1, 2, 3, or 4 years of TPGS therapy. PEG excretion data were compared by unpaired t tests.

Results

An initial dose of 25 IU/kg/day of TPGS effectively normalized the biochemical indices of vitamin E status in all patients. Over the course of therapy, doses (IU/kg) were reduced as serum vitamin E concentrations rose to near 20-25 μg/mL or as patients gained weight, resulting in a final dose of 22.6 ± 4.9 IU/kg/day after a mean of 1.8 ± 1.5 years of treatment (TABLE 1). There were no gastrointestinal complaints related to the TPGS use in any subject. One patient (no. 16) during the study developed an acute worsening of cholestasis. TPGS was temporarily discontinued and the cholestasis gradually resolved, and, when TPGS therapy was resumed, there was no subsequent exacerbation of cholestasis. Therefore, it was unlikely that the TPGS caused hepatotoxicity in this patient. In another patient (no. 35), a pruritic rash developed; however, this resolved while TPGS therapy was continued.

Monitoring for hematologic, hepatic, renal, or metabolic toxicity failed to reveal significant changes in laboratory variables out of the normal ranges for up to four years of TPGS therapy (TABLE 2). A small portion of the administered PEG-1000

TABLE 2. Laboratory Tests Monitored during TPGS Therapy

Laboratory Parameter	Years of TPGS Therapy						Normal Values
	0 (n = 34)	0.5 (n = 28)	1.0 (n = 28)	2.0 (n = 15)	3.0 (n = 10)	4.0 (n = 2)	
Sodium	138.5 ± 3.7	139.8 ± 3.4[a]	139.7 ± 2.8	140.5 ± 3.5	139.8 ± 2.6	140	135-148 mmol/L
Potassium	4.5 ± 0.6	4.3 ± 0.6	4.2 ± 0.5[a]	4.5 ± 0.4	4.6 ± 0.5	4.5	3.5-5.8 mmol/L
Chloride	106 ± 3	107 ± 4	107 ± 4	106 ± 4	108 ± 3	110	98-105 mmol/L
Carbon Dioxide	20.0 ± 2.8	19.6 ± 3.3	20.3 ± 3.4	20.6 ± 4.1	20.3 ± 3.8	19.8	18-27 mmol/L
Urea Nitrogen	13.7 ± 7.1	12.8 ± 4.6	11.0 ± 4.7	13.4 ± 5.2	13.9 ± 2.7	18.5	10-20 mg/dL
Creatinine	0.4 ± 0.2	0.6 ± 0.7	0.5 ± 0.6	0.4 ± 0.2	0.4 ± 0.1	0.4	0.2-1.0 mg/dL
Osmolality	289 ± 12	288 ± 9	293 ± 15	293 ± 8	287 ± 4	294	270-290 mOsm/kg
AST[b]	232 ± 164	213 ± 110	234 ± 136	194 ± 120	207 ± 158	209	8-45 IU/L
ALT[c]	179.3 ± 106.2	186 ± 107	226 ± 177	129 ± 95	141 ± 103	156	7-46 IU/L
Bilirubin	8.4 ± 5.7	8.8 ± 5.7	9.1 ± 4.9	7.5 ± 4.2	8.3 ± 6.4	8.0	0.1-1.0 mg/dL
Hematocrit	33.8 ± 4.1	35.1 ± 3.8	33.4 ± 3.4	33.5 ± 3.5	34.7 ± 3.7	34.8	31-43%
Hemoglobin	11.5 ± 1.6	11.9 ± 1.3	11.3 ± 1.2	11.5 ± 1.2	11.9 ± 1.4	12.1	11.0-14.5 g/dL
Vitamin E	3.8 ± 3.7	12.5 ± 5.9[a]	13.7 ± 6.4[a]	12.9 ± 6.6[a]	11.8 ± 6.5[a]	11.1	5-20 μg/mL
Vitamin E/Lipids	0.48 ± 0.41	1.37 ± 0.56[a]	1.40 ± 0.60[a]	1.49 ± 0.56[a]	1.13 ± 0.60[a]	0.76	>0.6 mg/g[d] >0.8 mg/g[e]

[a] $p < 0.05$ versus values at 0 years of therapy
[b] aspartate aminotransferase
[c] alanine aminotransferase
[d] for ages <12 years
[e] for 12 years or older

was absorbed during the 24 hours after an oral loading dose of TPGS (FIG. 4), as previously reported.[41] An average of 1.7 ± 1.6% (mean ± SD) of the orally administered PEG-1000 was absorbed in the 13 study subjects analyzed. Compared with the 4 adult control subjects who received the same 3360 mg dose of PEG-1000, the older study subjects absorbed significantly less of the PEG-1000 (3.0 ± 1.3% versus 0.8 ± 0.7%, $p < 0.02$). There were no significant differences in mean molecular weight of the excreted PEG between the patients and the normal adults (925 ± 125 versus 914 ± 46), and no low molecular weight PEG, ethylene glycol, or diethylene glycol was detected in the urine of any patient or normal adult.

The neurologic score data (TABLE 1) indicated that 16 patients showed improvement in neurologic function, 18 showed stabilization of function despite progressive worsening prior to TPGS therapy, and 3 showed slight worsening of function. Patients younger than age 3 years without neurologic dysfunction remained normal during the TPGS trial. Patients younger than age 3 years with neurologic dysfunction tended to show a prompt response to TPGS therapy with reversal of abnormalities in 6 to 12 months. Older patients, however, particularly those with severe, handicapping symptomatology, had a more limited, gradual improvement or only a stabilization of dysfunction. Patients studied in Denver had previously undergone serial neurologic examinations and were assigned neurologic scores for several years prior to TPGS therapy. When the neurologic scores were plotted versus age of the patients,[42] there was a statistically significant change ($p < 0.05$) in slope (calculated by linear regression), comparing the posttreatment to the pretreatment total neurologic scores by the Wilcoxon signed-rank test.

Discussion

The extreme hydrophobic nature of vitamin E is responsible for an absolute requirement of micellar solubilization by intraluminal bile acids before intestinal absorption of ingested vitamin E.[4,45] Children with protracted, severe cholestasis fail to secrete adequate concentrations of bile acids into the intestine, producing an environment in which vitamin E is unable to traverse the unstirred water layer that covers the luminal surface of the intestinal epithelium. TPGS is a unique form of vitamin E, incorporating a molecule of water-soluble PEG-1000 by ester linkage onto the end of alpha-tocopheryl succinate, creating an amphipathic structure capable of forming micelles. Previous studies[39,41] demonstrated that TPGS can be adequately absorbed in vitamin E-deficient children with severe cholestasis. This study extends those observations to include 38 children, all of whom responded to TPGS therapy with normalization of the biochemical indices of vitamin E status. Even though a small amount of the PEG-1000 contained in TPGS was absorbed, there was no apparent clinical or biochemical evidence of toxicity detected during prospective monitoring. Furthermore, neurologic function, that had been deteriorating in most patients because of a prolonged deficiency of vitamin E, was stabilized or improved in the vast majority of patients. Eight young vitamin E-deficient children who had not yet developed neurologic dysfunction remained normal throughout the TPGS trial, confirming that correcting vitamin E deficiency early in its course can prevent the expected neurologic injury.

A word of caution must be emphasized. Because up to 5.2% of the administered PEG-1000 in TPGS may be absorbed and because of the complete reliance for PEG excretion on glomerular filtration and urinary excretion, induction of a hyperosmolar state is possible if TPGS is administered during renal insufficiency or dehydration.

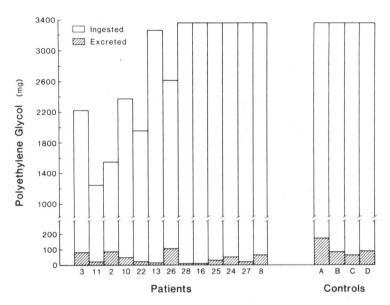

FIGURE 4. Polyethylene glycol excretion in urine for 24 hours after oral dose of TPGS in 13 patients with chronic cholestasis and in 4 normal adult controls.

Therefore, TPGS should not be administered to individuals with significant renal compromise. Because renal abnormalities have been observed in patients with arteriohepatic dysplasia and other cholestatic disorders,[46-48] renal function and serum osmolality should be evaluated and monitored in such patients if TPGS therapy is to be considered.

In conclusion, our study has shown that an oral dose of 15 to 25 IU/kg/day of TPGS appears to be a safe and effective means of treating vitamin E deficiency in children with chronic cholestasis who fail to absorb massive doses of available preparations of vitamin E. Although no significant toxicity of TPGS has been observed, the number of patients studied is still relatively small. Thus further studies are needed to confirm the safety of TPGS in children with chronic cholestasis.

REFERENCES

1. ROSENBLUM, J. L., J. P. KEATING, A. L. PRENSKY & J. S. NELSON. 1981. A progressive neurologic syndrome in children with chronic liver disease. N. Engl. J. Med. **304:** 503-508.
2. GUGGENHEIM, M. A., S. P. RINGEL, A. SILVERMAN *et al.* 1982. Progressive neuromuscular disease in children with chronic cholestasis and vitamin E deficiency: diagnosis and treatment with alpha-tocopherol. J. Pediatr. **100:** 51-58.
3. ALVAREZ, F., P. LANDRIEU, P. LAGET, F. LEMONNIER, M. ODIEVRE & D. ALAGILLE. 1983. Nervous and ocular disorders in children with cholestasis and vitamin A and E deficiencies. Hepatology **3:** 410-414.
4. SOKOL, R. J., J. E. HEUBI, S. T. IANNACCONE, K. E. BOVE & W. F. BALISTRERI. 1983. Mechanism causing vitamin E deficiency during chronic childhood cholestasis. Gastroenterology **85:** 1172-1182.

5. GUGGENHEIM, M. A., V. JACKSON, J. LILLY & A. SILVERMAN. 1983. Vitamin E deficiency and neurologic disease in children with cholestasis: a prospective study. J. Pediatr. 102: 577-579.
6. SOKOL, R. J., J. E. HEUBI, S. T. IANNACCONE, K. E. BOVE & W. F. BALISTRERI. 1984. Vitamin E deficiency with normal serum vitamin E concentrations in children with chronic cholestasis. N. Engl. J. Med. 310: 1209-1212.
7. NAKAGAWA, M., Y. TAZAWA, Y. KOBAYASHI et al. 1984. Familial intrahepatic cholestasis associated with progressive neuromuscular disease and vitamin E deficiency. J. Pediatr. Gastroenterol. Nutr. 3: 385-389.
8. AZIZI, E., J. L. ZAIDMAN, J. ESHCHAR & A. SZEINBERG. 1978. Abetalipoproteinemia treated with parenteral and oral vitamin A and E and with medium chain tryglycerides. Acta Pediatr. Scand. 67: 797-801.
9. MULLER, D. P. R., J. K. LLOYD & A. BIRD. 1977. Long-term management of abetalipoproteinemia. Possible role for vitamin E. Arch. Dis. Child. 52: 209-214.
10. MULLER, D. P. R., J. K. LLOYD & O. H. WOLFF. 1983. Vitamin E and neurological function. Lancet i: 225-228.
11. STEAD, R. J., D. P. R. MULLER, S. MATTHEWS, M. E. HODSON & J. C. BATTEN. 1986. Effect of abnormal liver function on vitamin E status and supplementation in adults with cystic fibrosis. Gut 27: 714-718.
12. ELIAS, E., D. P. R. MULLER & J. SCOTT. 1981. Association of spinocerebellar disorders with cystic fibrosis or chronic childhood cholestasis and very low serum vitamin E. Lancet ii: 1319-1321.
13. BYE, A. M., D. P. R. MULLER, J. WILSON et al. 1985. Symptomatic vitamin E deficiency in cystic fibrosis. Arch. Dis. Child. 60: 162-164.
14. HARDING, A. E., D. P. R. MULLER, P. K. THOMAS & H. J. WILLISON. 1982. Spinocerebellar degeneration secondary to chronic intestinal malabsorption: a vitamin E deficiency syndrome. Ann. Neurol. 12: 419-424.
15. SATYA-MURTI, S., L. HOWARD, G. KROHEL & B. WOLF. 1986. The spectrum of neurologic disorder from vitamin E deficiency. Neurology 36: 917-921.
16. WEDER, B., O. MEIENBERG, E. WILDI & C. MEIER. 1984. Neurologic disorder of vitamin E deficiency in acquired intestinal malabsorption. Neurology 34: 1561-1565.
17. HOWARD, L., L. OVESEN, S. SATYA-MURTI & R. CHU. 1982. Reversible neurological symptoms caused by vitamin E deficiency in a patient with short bowel syndrome. Am. J. Clin. Nutr. 36: 1243-1249.
18. BERTONI, J. M., F. A. ABRAHAM, H. F. FALLS & H. H. ITABASHI. 1984. Small bowel resection with vitamin E deficiency and progressive spinocerebellar syndrome. Neurology 34: 1046-1052.
19. TRABER, M., R. J. SOKOL, S. P. RINGEL, H. E. NEVILLE et al. 1987. Lack of tocopherol in peripheral nerves of vitamin E-deficient patients with peripheral neuropathy. N. Engl. J. Med. 317: 262-265.
20. SOKOL, R. J., M. A. GUGGENHEIM, S. T. IANNACCONE, C. A. MILLER, A. SILVERMAN, W. F. BALISTRERI & J. E. HEUBI. 1985. Improved neurologic function following correction of vitamin E deficiency in children with chronic cholestasis. N. Engl. J. Med. 313: 1580-1586.
21. ALAGILLE, D. 1985. Vitamin E deficiency is responsible for neurologic abnormalities in cholestatic children. J. Pediatr. 107: 422-425.
22. SOKOL, R. J., K. E. BOVE, J. E. HEUBI & S. T. IANNACCONE. 1983. Vitamin E deficiency during chronic childhood cholestasis: presence of sural nerve lesion prior to 2 ½ years of age. J. Pediatr. 103: 197-204.
23. NELSON, J. S. 1980. Pathology of vitamin E deficiency. In Vitamin E—A Comprehensive Treatise. L. J. Machlin, Ed.: 397-428. Marcel-Dekker. New York.
24. FARRELL, P. M., J. G. BIERI, J. F. FRATONONI et al. 1977. The occurrence and effects of human vitamin E deficiency—a study in patients with cystic fibrosis. J. Clin. Invest. 60: 233-241.
25. FARRELL, P. M., E. H. MISCHLER & G. GUTCHER. 1982. Evaluation of vitamin E deficiency in children with lung disease. Ann. N.Y. Acad. Sci. 393: 96-106.
26. CYNAMON, H. A., D. E. MILOV, E. VALENSTEIN & M. WAGNER. 1988. Effect of vitamin E deficiency on neurologic function in patients with cystic fibrosis. J. Pediatr. 113: 637-640.

27. SUNG, J. H. 1964. Neuroaxonal dystrophy in mucoviscidosis. J. Neuropathol. Exp. Neurol. 23: 567-583.
28. GELLER, A., F. GILLES & H. SHWACHMAN. 1977. Degeneration of fasciculus gracilis in cystic fibrosis. Neurology 27: 185-187.
29. CAVALIER, S. J. & P. GAMBETTI. 1981. Dystrophic axons and spinal cord demyelination in cystic fibrosis. Neurology 31: 714-718.
30. HAMMOND, K. B., M. C. REARDON, F. J. ACCURSO et al. 1986. Early detection and follow-up of cystic fibrosis in newborns: the Colorado experience. In Genetic Disease: screening and management. 81-101. Alan R. Liss, Inc. New York.
31. BIERI, J. G., T. J. TOLLIVER & G. L. CATIGNANI. 1979. Simultaneous determination of alpha tocopherol and retinol in plasma and red cells by high pressure liquid chromatography. Am. J. Clin. Nutr. 32: 2143-2149.
32. ZOELLNER, N. & K. KIRSCH. 1962. A micromethod for lipids using sulpho oxanillin reaction. Z. Ges. Exp. Med. 135: 545.
33. FARRELL, P. M., S. L. LEVINE, D. MURPHY et al. 1978. Plasma tocopherol levels and tocopherol-lipid relationships in a normal population of children as compared to healthy adults. Am. J. Clin. Nutr. 31: 1720-1726.
34. SOKOL, R. J. 1988. Vitamin E deficiency and neurologic disease. Annu. Rev. Nutr. 8: 351-373.
35. GUGGENHEIM, M. A., V. JACKSON, J. LILLY & A. SILVERMAN. 1983. Vitamin E deficiency and neurologic disease in children with cholestasis: a prospective study. J. Pediatr. 102: 577-579.
36. ALVAREZ, F., D. CRESTEIL, F. LEMMONIER, A. LEMMONIER & D. ALAGILLE. 1984. Plasma vitamin E levels in children with cholestasis. J. Pediatr. Gastroenterol. Nutr. 3: 390-393.
37. TAZAWA, Y., M. NAKAGAWA, M. YAMADA et al. 1984. Serum vitamin E levels in children with corrected biliary atresia. Am. J. Clin. Nutr. 40: 246-250.
38. SOKOL, R. J., M. A. GUGGENHEIM, J. E. HEUBI et al. 1986. Frequency and clinical progression of the vitamin E deficiency neurologic disorder in children with prolonged neonatal cholestasis. Am. J. Dis. Child. 139: 1211-1215.
39. TRABER, M. G., H. J. KAYDEN, J. B. GREEN & M. H. GREEN. 1986. Absorption of water-miscible forms of vitamin E in a patient with cholestasis and in thoracic duct cannulated rats. Am. J. Clin. Nutr. 44: 914-923.
40. TRABER, M. G., C. A. THELLMAN, M. J. RINDLER & H. J. KAYDEN. 1988. Uptake of intact TPGS (D-alpha-tocopheryl polyethylene glycol 1000 succinate) a water-miscible form of vitamin E by human cells in vitro. Am. J. Clin. Nutr. 48: 605-611.
41. SOKOL, R. J., J. E. HEUBI, N. BUTLER-SIMON, H. J. McCLUNG, J. R. LILLY & A. SILVERMAN. 1987. Treatment of vitamin E deficiency during chronic childhood cholestasis with oral D-alpha-tocopheryl polyethylene glycol-1000 succinate. Gastroenterology 93: 975-985.
42. SOKOL, R. J., N. A. BUTLER-SIMON, D. BETTIS, D. J. SMITH & A. SILVERMAN. 1987. Tocopheryl polyethylene glycol 1000 succinate therapy for vitamin E deficiency during chronic childhood cholestasis: neurologic outcome. J. Pediatr. 111: 830-836.
43. HANSEN, L. G. & W. J. WARWICK. 1969. A fluorometric micromethod for serum vitamins A and E. Am. J. Clin. Pathol. 51: 538-541.
44. GORDON, H. H., H. M. NITOWSKI & M. CORNBLATH. 1955. Studies of tocopherol deficiency in infants and children. I. Hemolysis of erythrocytes in hydrogen peroxide. Am. J. Dis. Child. 90: 669-681.
45. GALLO-TORRES, H. E. 1970. Obligatory role of bile for the intestinal absorption of vitamin E. Lipids 5: 379-384.
46. ALAGILLE, D., A. ESTRADA, M. HADCHOUEL, M. GAUTIER et al. 1987. Syndromic paucity of interlobular bile ducts (Alagille syndrome or arteriohepatic dysplasia): review of 80 cases. J. Pediatr. 110: 195-200.
47. CHUNG-PARK, M., M. PETRELLI, A. S. TAVILL et al. 1982. Renal lipidosis associated with arteriohepatic dysplasia (Alagille's syndrome). Clin. Nephrol. 18: 314-320.
48. OESTREICH, A. E., R. J. SOKOL, F. J. SUCHY & J. E. HEUBI. 1983. Renal abnormalities in arteriohepatic dysplasia and nonsyndromic intrahepatic biliary hypoplasia. Ann. Radiol. 26: 203-209.

Neuropathies in Adults with or without Fat Malabsorption

HERBERT J. KAYDEN AND MARET G. TRABER

Department of Medicine
New York University School of Medicine
New York, New York 10016

Although a variety of pathologic syndromes were described in different species as a consequence of experimental vitamin E deficiency, observations in humans were virtually nonexistent until the mid 1960s. The genetic disorder abetalipoproteinemia (ABL) was intensively studied during that decade, and I postulated that the neurologic components of the ABL syndrome were the effects of a nutritional deficiency, rather than a direct consequence of the genetic abnormality.[1] The most likely candidate to be considered responsible for the neurologic defect was vitamin E—or rather the deficiency of vitamin E.[1] The evidence marshaled originally included the following: (a) Vitamin E appeared to be absorbed virtually solely by incorporation into chylomicrons. Patients with ABL did not form chylomicrons. (b) Vitamin E in normal subjects was transported predominantly in association with apolipoprotein B lipoproteins. These were entirely absent in patients with ABL, and plasma levels of vitamin E in ABL patients were undetectable by the then available methodology. (c) Vitamin E deficiency in some species had been characterized by anemia. An additional indication of vitamin E deficiency was the red blood cell content of vitamin E. It was sharply reduced—so low in fact that autohemolysis could be demonstrated in the red blood cells of ABL patients. The observations on autohemolysis were particularly important, because we showed that parenteral administration of vitamin E reversed the abnormality in a short time, although plasma levels of vitamin E remained low.[2]

In adult patients with ABL the neurologic abnormalities were so severe that there were accompanying musculoskeletal abnormalities, which confined the patients to wheelchairs or beds. We therefore began supplementing children with vitamin E before the pathology was severe or established. Although we initially used parenteral administration of the vitamin, it became apparent that absorption of finite amounts occurred when higher doses of vitamin E were given orally (> 150 mg/kg body weight). The proof that absorption occurred was demonstrated by the reversal of the abnormal autohemolysis test,[2] and more particularly by following adipose tissue concentrations of α-tocopherol by methods established by our laboratory.[3] The sensitivity of this analytical method is such that needle biopsy aspirations are adequate for quantitation of adipose tissue levels of α-tocopherol. We have analyzed more than 100 adipose tissue needle aspiration biopsies, in addition to many surgical specimens.

The results of our treatment program have been most gratifying and can be summarized as follows: (a) In those patients in whom neurologic abnormalities were present (ataxia, absent reflexes, poor muscular coordination), adequate therapy resulted in a halt in the progression of the neurologic abnormalities. (b) In those patients with early or minimal neurologic pathology (abnormal conduction time), therapy in a good proportion resulted in improvement in both coordination and the objective measurements of conduction time and amplitudes. (c) In infants in whom the diagnosis of ABL was made prior to the development of any neurologic defects, prophylactic. treatment with vitamin E prevented the appearance of any abnormal neurologic findings.[4] These series of observations establish most securely that the neurologic syndrome seen in patients with ABL is a consequence of malabsorption of the fat soluble vitamin E. The data on the nervous tissue content of α-tocopherol, which provides conclusive proof of the role of tocopherol in nervous tissue, will be shown later in this paper.

The specific neurologic lesion due to tocopherol deficiency has been demonstrated in the postmortem examinations of patients with ABL.[5] Lesions in both the brain and spinal cord are similar to the neuropathology found in experimental animals who are made vitamin E-deficient by dietary manipulations for extended periods of time. In both the rat and the monkey, as well as in humans, degeneration of the posterior column and spinocerebellar tracts are evident in sections of the spinal cord. The lesion is an axonopathy affecting particularly the large caliber myelinated fibers in the dorsal columns, sensory roots, and peripheral nerves. In the brain, spheroid formation is apparent, particularly in the cuneate and gracilis nucleus, and changes in the cerebellum are also noted. The nature of the process has been described as a peripheral neuropathy with a dying back of the axon. The precipitating cause of the pathologic process is less well-defined. The suggestion has frequently been made that the degeneration is a consequence of free radical generation and injury occurring in the nervous tissue that is deficient in the putative major antioxidant—namely tocopherol. But confirmation of the proposed sequence of events has not yet been obtained. Perhaps the studies by David P. R. Muller, James S. Nelson, and K. U. Ingold, using deuterated tocopherol in vitamin E-deficient rats, will provide adequate information on this subject.

The previous presentations have detailed changes occurring in children with malabsorption—in particular children with cholestasis due to a variety of syndromes. In adults, recognized cases of neurologic disease as a consequence of fat malabsorption have been described in patients with cystic fibrosis,[6] blind-loop,[7] and short bowel[8] syndrome, as well as in patients with cholestasis.

The documentation of low plasma vitamin E levels in the subjects with malabsorption has prompted the study of the effects of supplementation with vitamin E. There are a number of reports that indicate the beneficial effect of such treatment: interruption in the progress of the disease, and also improvement in coordination and stabilization, with a decrease in ataxia. In the patients with ABL plasma, and even erythrocyte, levels of tocopherol are an inadequate representation of the response to therapy. As noted, the measurement of tocopherol from needle aspiration biopsies of adipose tissue obtained in patients with ABL has provided a guide to the level of oral supplementation with tocopherol and led to our recommendation of a dose of 150 mg/kg/day for such subjects. Examples of the response to such therapy are presented in TABLE 1.

Over the past 7 years a new syndrome has been identified in nine adult subjects, which we have called familial isolated vitamin E deficiency. In these patients the characteristic neurologic syndrome of vitamin E deficiency is present, although its manifestations have varied from patient to patient. The first case report of the syndrome was from Germany[9] and published in 1981. The patient was a 12-year-old boy, born of a consanguineous marriage (first degree cousins, once removed), who had ataxia, sensory neuropathy hypotrophic musculature, and a low serum vitamin E. Two of his relatives (paternal aunt and uncle) had died of a clinically similar disorder in their late adolescence (18 and 23 years of age, respectively). Their parents had also been first degree cousins. Studies of biopsies of skeletal muscle and of sural nerve revealed changes similar to those described in patients with ABL. The strikingly low

TABLE 1. Restoration of Adipose Tissue Tocopherol to Normal Levels in Two ABL Patients

Patient	Adipose Tissue Tocopherol (ng tocopherol/mg triglyceride)		Plasma Tocopherol (μg/mL)	
	pre-vitamin E	post-vitamin E	pre-vitamin E	post-vitamin E
AMV	31	378	0.58	0.20
LL	39	558	1.60	1.00
Controls	262 ± 33		8.8 ± 3.4	

serum vitamin E level, 0.45 μg/mL, suggested that the pathologic state was a reflection of tocopherol deficiency, although no abnormality in fat absorption was evident. Supplementation with 1.5 g of vitamin E daily for a year resulted in clinical improvement and normal serum tocopherol levels. A follow-up publication in 1988[10] documented the improvement in the patient who is now 19 years of age and noted that interruption of the daily supplementation for a period as short as one week resulted in a sharp decline in the serum level of vitamin E to values characteristic of the deficiency state, that is, <3 μg/mL.

The second report was published in 1984 from Canada and described a 10-year-old boy, born of a consanguineous marriage (parents were first cousins), whose major symptoms were of diffuse muscle weakness (most prominent distally in the lower limbs), generalized areflexia, a decrease in proprioception and vibration sense, and slight limb and gait ataxia.[11] His serum vitamin E was <1 μg/mL. He was given supplemental vitamin E, and when examined nine months later his serum vitamin E level was normal and his muscular weakness had markedly decreased so that he could walk without crutches. The neurologic deficits, however, were unchanged.

The third case report was published in 1985 from England and described a 23-year-old woman, who had developed a progressive neurologic disorder comprising ataxia, areflexia, and marked loss of proprioception at age 13.[12] Her level of serum vitamin E was below levels of detection. When given 2 g of tocopheryl acetate, the serum tocopherol level rose to the lower level of normal values at the end of 4 hours and remained at this level for 24 hours. The patient had elevated serum cholesterol and low density lipoprotein levels. She was treated with daily doses of 800 mg of tocopheryl acetate for 15 months, with maintenance of normal serum vitamin E levels. The progression of the neurologic disorder was halted and there was modest improvement in vibration and position sense. The patient became pregnant, but the pregnancy was terminated at 18 weeks.

The fourth case was reported in 1987 from North Carolina and described a 19-year-old man who had severe manifestations of the neuromuscular component of vitamin E deficiency, but in addition had dystonic posturing and bradykinesia.[13] His illness apparently began at age 7 when he developed gait difficulty, clumsiness, and dysarthria. By age 17 he was bedridden. When seen at age 19, he was oriented and could carry out calculations; however, his speech was unintelligible, his mouth was open, and he drooled constantly. The striking feature was bradykinesia with dystonic posturing of neck, hands, and feet. The neurologic examination was difficult to evaluate because of the dyskinesia, but there was no tremor; tendon reflexes were absent, and plantar responses were extensor. There was a moderate diminution in position and vibratory sense in the legs. The vitamin E level in serum was 0.7 μg/mL, 1.1 μg/mL, and nondetectable on three separate occasions. In response to supplemental vitamin E the plasma tocopherol level rose to 3.5 μg/mL on a daily dose of 1800 IU, and to 5.3 μg/mL on 3600 IU daily. After 5 months of treatment there appeared to be no progression of the disorder, and although the objective findings had not changed, the patient and his parents thought some improvement had occurred.

This report[14] stresses that pathologic alterations have been noted in the extrapyramidal system of patients with vitamin E deficiency due to cystic fibrosis, biliary atresia, and malabsorption due to abdominal radiation. These have included axonal swellings in the globus pallidus and zona reticularis of the substantia nigra, inadequate pigmentation of the substantia nigra, and lipofuscin-like pigment deposits in the glia of the globus pallidus, substantia nigra, and inferior putamen.

The fifth case was reported in 1987 from Japan and described a 62-year-old man who had a progressive neurologic disorder, comprising ataxia, areflexia, and loss of proprioception; he dated the onset of his symptoms to age 52.[14] The patient's maternal uncle in his seventh decade had areflexia, ataxia, and diminished sense of vibration and proprioception. Serum vitamin E levels in the patient and the uncle were 1.1 and 3.2 μg/mL, respectively.

Biopsy of the quadriceps muscle showed numerous fluorescent inclusions and strong acid phosphatase activity in the muscle fibres. By electron microscopy, oval or round deposits were apparent between myofibrils, corresponding to autofluorescent inclusions. Sural nerve biopsy showed moderate loss of large myelinated axons.

The response to a 2 g oral dose of tocopheryl acetate resulted in a prompt rise in plasma level, equal to that seen in normal control subjects. At 48 h, however, the level was much lower (69% and 56% of the peak value in patient and uncle, respectively, whereas in control subjects it was only 36%). It was noted that even after 4 months of supplementation with 800 mg/day of α-tocopheryl acetate, the fall in plasma levels from the peak concentration after a 2 g oral dose was again 70% in the proband. The response to 7 months of therapy was only a slight improvement in position sense and a negative Romberg sign.

Four additional patients with familial isolated vitamin E deficiency have been reported in 1988 by R. J. Sokol et al.[15] Three of the patients are siblings (two sisters and their brother), and one unrelated woman is the fourth patient. The clinical features of these patients are presented in TABLE 2 and show the variations in symptomatology,

TABLE 2. Clinical Features of Four Patients with Familial Isolated Vitamin E Deficiency[a]

	Patient			
	1	2	3	4
Age (years)	23	27	21	30
Hyporeflexia	−	−	−	+ + +
Truncal ataxia	+ +	−	−	+ + +
Limb ataxia	+ +	−	+	+ +
Head titubation	+ +	−	−	+ + +
Vibratory sense loss	+ + +	+ +	+ +	+ + +
Position sense loss	−	+	−	+ + +
Ophthalmoplegia	−	−	−	−
Dysarthria	−	−	−	+ +
Pes cavus	+	−	−	+ +
Scoliosis	−	−	−	+
Weakness	−	−	−	+
Optic Fundus	Normal	Normal	Normal	Normal

[a] +, mild; + +, moderate; + + +, severely abnormal; −, abnormality not present.

with the 30-year-old woman (patient 4) being the most severely affected. Details of the nerve conduction studies are presented in reference 15; they can be summarized by stating that there were slight motor and sensory nerve conduction delays and decreased amplitude of sensory nerve action potentials in two of the four patients. Somatosensory-evoked response was performed only in patient 3 and demonstrated a symmetric prolongation between Erb's point and the cortical wave potential, compatible with bilateral large sensory fiber dysfunction in the posterior column pathway.

Serum vitamin E levels were strikingly reduced with values of 1.8, 1.8, 1.2, and 1.0 μg/mL in the four patients. As noted in other patients, an oral vitamin E tolerance test (OVETT) supported the observations that absorption of the pharmacologic dose (100 IU/kg body wt) was within normal levels, but the decrease in the plasma tocopherol was greater in each of the four patients at 24, 36, 48, and 72 hours than was found in control subjects. Further evidence of decreased tocopherol levels in the patients was provided by adipose tissue biopsies that gave values of 128, 29, 28, and 143 ng tocopherol/mg triglyceride in the four patients in contrast to the normal expected range of 150-400. Lastly, we obtained small segments of sural nerve in three patients and reported values of 2.9, 1.5, and 0.8 ng tocopherol/μg cholesterol, a value well below the mean of 20 ± 16 found in 34 patients with peripheral neuropathy unrelated to vitamin E deficiency.[16]

The description of these nine patients emphasizes that vitamin E deficiency results in a reasonably specific neurologic syndrome. In these patients the problem of contributory deficiency states that may have complicated the vitamin E-deficiency syndrome in patients with malabsorption is eliminated as absorption of all fats, minerals, and vitamins is normal, and the deficiency syndrome is exclusively related to vitamin E.

There appears to be little question that the abnormal handling of tocopherol in these patients is a genetic abnormality as evidenced by the occurrence in three siblings, the presence of affected members in two generations, and the high incidence of consanguinity in parents. The nature of the autosomal recessive abnormality awaits future research and investigation.

Once again, it becomes apparent that physicians, and especially neurologists in motion disorder clinics, should consider vitamin E deficiency in the differential diagnosis of the etiology of patients with peripheral neuropathies or spinocerebellar ataxia. We would hope that more frequent measurements of plasma tocopherol levels would identify additional patients with vitamin E deficiency, for this is a disorder that can be treated with beneficial results.

REFERENCES

1. KAYDEN, H. J. 1969. Vitamin E deficiency in patients with abetalipoproteinemia. *In* Vitamins A, E and K. Clinical, physiological and chemical problems. H. F. von Kress and F. U. Blum, Eds.: 301-308. Schattauer Verlag. New York.
2. KAYDEN, H. J. & R. SILBER. 1965. The role of vitamin E deficiency in the abnormal autohemolysis of acanthrocytosis. Trans. Assoc. Am. Physicians **78**: 334-342.
3. KAYDEN, H. J., L. H. HATAM & M. G. TRABER. 1983. The measurement of nanograms of tocopherol from needle aspiration biopsies of adipose tissue: normal and abetalipoproteinemic subjects. J. Lipid Res. **24**: 652-6.
4. BRIN, M. F., T. A. PEDLEY, R. E. LOVELACE, R. G. EMERSON, P. GOURAS, C. MACKAY, H. J. KAYDEN, J. LEVY & H. BAKER. 1986. Electrophysiologic features of abetalipoproteinemia: Functional consequences of vitamin E deficiency. Neurology **36**: 669-673.
5. NEWMAN, R. P., E. J. SCHAEFER, C. B. THOMAS & E. H. OLDFIED. 1984. Abetalipoproteinemia and metastatic spinal cord glioblastoma. Arch. Neurol. **41**: 554-556.

6. ELIAS, E., D. P. R. MULLER & J. SCOTT. 1981. Association of spinocerebellar disorders with cystic fibrosis or chronic childhood cholestasis and very low serum vitamin E. Lancet ii: 1319-21.
7. BRIN, M., M. R. FETELL, P. H. A. GREEN, H. J. KAYDEN, A. P. HAYS, M. N. BEHRINS & H. BAKER. 1985. Blind loop syndrome, vitamin E malabsorption and spinocerebellar degeneration. Neurology 35: 338-342.
8. HOWARD, L., L. OVESEN, S. SATYA-MURTI & R. CHU. 1982. Reversible neurological symptoms caused by vitamin E deficiency in a patient with short bowel syndrome. Am. J. Clin. Nutr. 36: 1243-9.
9. BURCK, U., H. H. GOEBEL, H. D. KUHLENDAHL, C. MEIER & K. M. GOEBEL. 1981. Neuromyopathy and vitamin E deficiency in man. Neuropediatrics 12: 267-78.
10. KOHLSCHUTTER, A., C. HUBNER, W. JANSEN & S. G. LINDNER. 1988. A treatable familial neuromyopathy with vitamin E deficiency, normal absorption, and evidence of increased consumption of vitamin E. J. Inher. Metab. Dis. 11: 149-52.
11. LAPLANTE, P., M. VANASSE, J. MICHAUD, G. GEOFFROY & P. BROCHU. 1984. A progressive neurological syndrome associated with an isolated vitamin E deficiency. Can. J. Neurol. Sci. 11: 561-4.
12. HARDING, A. E., S. MATTHEWS, S. JONES, C. J. K. ELLIS, I. W. BOOTH & D. P. R. MULLER. 1985. Spinocerebellar degeneration associated with a selective defect of vitamin E absorption. N. Engl. J. Med. 313: 32-5.
13. KRENDEL, D. A., J. M. GILCHREST, A. O. JOHNSON & E. H. BOSSEN. 1987. Isolated deficiency of vitamin E with progressive neurologic deterioration. Neurology 37: 538-40.
14. YOKOTA, T., Y. WADA, T. FURUKAWA, H. TSUKAGOSHI, T. UCHIHARA & S. WATABIKI. 1987. Adult-onset spinocerebellar syndrome with idiopathic vitamin E deficiency. Ann. Neurol. 22: 84-7.
15. SOKOL, R. J., H. J. KAYDEN, D. B. BETTIS, M. G. TRABER, H. NEVILLE, S. RINGEL, W. B. WILSON & D. A. STUMPF. 1988. Isolated vitamin E deficiency in the absence of fat malabsorption—familial and sporadic cases: Characterization and investigation of causes. J. Lab. Clin. Med. 111: 548-59.
16. TRABER, M. G., R. J. SOKOL, S. P. RINGEL, H. E. NEVILLE, C. A. THELLMAN & H. J. KAYDEN. 1987. Lack of tocopherol in peripheral nerves of vitamin E-deficient patients with peripheral neuropathy. N. Engl. J. Med. 317: 262-265.

Possible Involvement of Free Radicals in Neuroleptic-Induced Movement Disorders

Evidence from Treatment of Tardive Dyskinesia with Vitamin E

JEAN LUD CADET[a] AND JAMES B. LOHR[b]

Neurological Institute
Columbia University
New York, New York 10032
and
[b] *Department of Psychiatry*
University of California at San Diego
San Diego, California 92093

INTRODUCTION

Defined phenomenologically, tardive dyskinesia (TD) is a sign complex characterized by certain types of abnormal movements that are secondary to prolonged use of neuroleptic drugs.[1-5] In recent years, TD has acquired greater importance to practitioners because of its occurrence in almost epidemic proportion and the evidence that its prevalence may be increasing.[3,4] TD was originally described as a "dyskinesie facio-bucco-lingui-masticatrice" (BLM or orofacial syndrome).[2] The concept has evolved to include nonrepetitive choreic and choreoathetoid movements of fingers, hands, and feet. It also includes choreoathetoid movements of the legs and trunk. Tardive dystonia[6] and tardive akathisia[7] may also be related to the TD complex.

Tardive dyskinesia must be differentiated from other neurological disorders such as Huntington's chorea, Sydenham's chorea, drug-induced chorea, levodopa-induced dyskinesias, and the idiopathic and symptomatic dystonias. History of chronic use of neuroleptics is necessary before a diagnosis of TD can be made.

EFFECTS OF NEUROLEPTICS ON SOME NEUROTRANSMITTER SYSTEMS

The first evidence that neurotransmitters were involved in the action of neuroleptics came with the demonstration by Carlsson and Linquist that both haloperidol and

---

[a] Address correspondence to Jean Lud Cadet, Columbia University, Department of Neurology, 630 W. 168th Street, Black Building, #307, New York, New York 10032.

chlorpromazine, when given acutely, cause an increase in the levels of metabolites of dopamine and norepinephrine.[8] It was proposed that the drugs, by blocking dopamine receptors in the brain, led to an increased firing of the presynaptic neuron, with resulting increase in the synthesis and release of the neurotransmitter.[8-10] The biochemical changes are associated with electrophysiological evidence of increase in the firing rate of dopamine (DA) neurons in the nigrostriatal DA system.[11,12]

Both biochemical and physiological studies on the chronic effects of neuroleptics have shown that they are different from those observed after acute treatment with these drugs. Acute administration of neuroleptics causes increased firing of dopamine neurons, whereas chronic treatment leads to a decrease in the firing rate.[12] Furthermore, in the rat caudate-putamen, the levels of the metabolites return to normal after a few months of neuroleptic treatment.[13-15] Bird and Anton have reported that one year of treatment with a phenothiazine neuroleptic actually causes a significant decrease in homovanillic acid (HVA) in the caudate-putamen of subhuman primates.[16] Saller and Salama have also shown that chronic administration of haloperidol causes reduction of the basal levels of the metabolites of DA in the striatum.[17]

In addition to perturbing the DA system, neuroleptics influence several other neurotransmitters. Although neurochemical changes seen in these systems do not correlate with the clinical potencies of neuroleptics, neuroleptics can block alpha-adrenergic receptors.[18] The level of glutamic acid decarboxylase (GAD), the enzyme that catalyzes the formation of gamma-aminobutyric acid (GABA) from glutamate, is decreased in the substantia nigra of rats treated with haloperidol.[19] It was also reported that similar decreases occurred in the substantia nigra, the globus pallidus, and the subthalamic nucleus of subhuman primates and that these abnormalities correlated with the presence of orofacial dyskinesias in these animals.[20] An important observation of this study was that animals without dyskinesia did not show the decrease in GAD activity.

FREE RADICAL PRODUCTION BY NEUROLEPTICS

Although these properties of phenothiazines have been neglected in recent studies of their effects on the brain, these drugs form free radical intermediates during their metabolism.[21-31] Using potentiometric titration, Michaels and associates were able to show that phenothiazine-derived dyes form intermediates between their oxidized and reduced states that were similar to the semiquinone intermediate seen during the oxidation of hydroquinone.[21] Later on, they observed a red-colored free radical of an N-substituted phenothiazine following oxidation by Br_2 in 80% acetic acid.[22] Subsequently, other authors have been able to clearly demonstrate the existence of free radical intermediates of phenothiazines by using electroparamagnetic resonance studies.[23-29] The oxidation reaction has been produced in the presence of metal ion, and concentrated acidic and alkaline solutions.[21-29] Of clinical importance is the finding of these intermediates in the urine samples of patients who are being treated with neuroleptics.[30-31]

The phenothiazine chlorpromazine can inhibit pyruvate and glutamate oxidation, oxidative phosphorylation, and the enzyme cytochrome oxidase.[32,33] Moreover, chlorpromazine inhibited catalase but not ascorbic acid oxidase.[33] It is of interest that ascorbic acid can act as a trap for the phenothiazine radical.[28] The possibility exists that the inhibitory effects on these enzymatic systems may be secondary to the production of free radical intermediates, inasmuch as Cavannaugh has shown them to be substrates for oxidative enzymes such as peroxidase-H_2O_2.[34]

NEUROPATHOLOGICAL FINDINGS AFTER CHRONIC NEUROLEPTIC TREATMENT

Chronic treatment with neuroleptics has been reported to cause significant abnormalities in the CNS in the few studies in which such adverse effects were sought[35-51] (TABLE 1). Most studies, however, have concentrated on neurotransmitter alterations associated with chronic administration of these drugs.

TABLE 1. Neuropathological Effects of Long-Term Neuroleptic Administration in Animals

Investigators	Findings
Aksel (1956)	Chromatolysis, degeneration of cytoplasm after acute administration of chlorpromazine.
Roizin et al. (1959)	Chromatolysis, satellitosis, and neuronophagia in cerebral cortex, lenticular nuclei, diencephalon, and cerebellum of monkeys given 1-15 mg/kg chlorpromazine im 5 times a week for 8 months.
Mackiewicz and Gershon (1964)	Diffuse neuronal damage in various brain areas of guinea pigs given 0.05 mg/kg reserpine ip or chlorpromazine im q.d. for 4-12 weeks.
Dom (1967)	Glial changes in limbic system of rats given 0.16 mg/kg haloperidol po q.d. for 4 months.
Sommer and Quandt (1970)	Cell alterations and necrosis in brain stem of rabbits given 3.3 mg/kg chlorpromazine q.d. for 6 months.
Pakkenberg et al. (1973 and 1974)	20% cell loss in the basal ganglia of rats given 3.4 mg/kg perphenazine sc every 2 weeks for 1 year, but no significant cell loss in cortex or basal ganglia of rats treated similarly for only 1-2 months.
Hackenberg and Lange (1975)	Increased glia/neuron ratio in brain stem and cerebellum of rats given 10 or 15 mg/kg chlorpromazine po q.d. for 6 months.
Gerlach (1975)	No significant difference in number of neurons in substantia nigra of rats given 3.4 mg/kg perphenazine sc every 2 weeks for 1 year or 40 mg/kg perphenezine sc every 2 weeks for 6 months.
Nielsen and Lyon (1978)	10% neuron loss in ventrolateral but not dorsomedial striatum of rats given 4 mg/kg flupenthixol im q.d. for 36 weeks.
Benes et al. (1983 and 1985)	Axon-collateral sprouting in substantia nigra and increase in the striatum of (1) size of neurons, (2) dendritic calibers, and (3) number of associated synaptic vesicles in rats given 3 mg/kg haloperidol injections q.d. for 16 weeks.

TABLE 2. Neuropathological Findings in Patients with Tardive Dyskinesia (TD)

Investigators	Findings in TD Brains
Grunthal and Walther-Buhl (1960)	Inferior olive damage.
Hunter et al. (1968)	No specific changes.
Gross and Kaltenbach (1969)	Caudate lesions in all 3 patients; substantia nigra lesions in one.
Christensen et al. (1970)	Degenerative changes in substantia nigra, and brainstem gliosis.
Jellinger (1977)	Swelling of large neurons and satellitosis in caudate.
Campbell et al. (1985)	Excess iron and mild gliosis in substantia nigra and basal ganglia.

Aksel[35] reported that chlorpromazine causes chromatolysis, degeneration of the cytoplasm and of the nuclei, and accumulation of chromatin around the nuclear membrane of cells in the caudate-putamen, the thalamus, and the cerebellum of cats. Roizin and his collaborators undertook similar studies using rats or rhesus monkeys.[36] There were moderate chromatolytic changes, increased satellitosis, and neuronophagia in the cortex, the lenticular nuclei, the thalamus, and the hypothalamus. Other areas of the brain such as the pons, the medulla, and the cerebellum were also affected. Electronmicroscopy revealed increased osmiophilia and reduction in the size of the mitochondria, and of the cytoplasm of neurons and their processes. Chronic administration of these drugs causes nonspecific neuronal loss and gliosis in the brainstem, the limbic system, and the cerebral cortex.[43] Both chlorpromazine and haloperidol cause significant alterations in the synaptic areas of the basal ganglia and the hypothalamus.[45–48] Chronic treatment with haloperidol leads to the deposition of granular and fibrillary material in the postsynaptic dendrites and vacuolization of presynaptic axon terminals.[47] Pakkenberg and colleagues found a 20% neuronal loss in the basal ganglia of rats treated with perphenazine enanthate.[41,42] Nielsen and Lyon confirmed those findings by showing a 10% cell loss in the ventrolateral striatum.[49] More recently, Benes and her co-workers have demonstrated that there was a significant shift in the distribution of axon terminals in the brains of rats chronically treated with haloperidol.[50,51] These investigators were also able to show increases in the size of striatal terminals that were associated with increases in the number of vesicles at those synapses.[51]

Very few studies on human postmortem tissues have been carried out to evaluate the possible neuropathological effects of neuroleptics on the brain and their possible relation to the development of drug-induced persistent dyskinesia[52–57] (TABLE 2). Roizin and co-workers had found varying degrees of chromatolysis in the basal ganglia, thalamus, hypothalamus, cerebellum, and cerebral cortex of six patients who had been treated with neuroleptics.[36] Lipid degeneration of neurons, cell disorganization, decreases in Purkinje cell number, satellitosis, and neuronophagia were also present in some of the cases. Christensen and colleagues studied 28 brains of patients with persistent dyskinesias and compared them to 28 controls.[55] The patients had received an average of 24 months of treatment with various neuroleptics, and the duration of the dyskinetic syndrome varied from four months to seven years. The authors reported that the most important differences between the two groups were found in the mesencephalon. For example, there was more gliosis in the midbrain and in the brain stem and more cell degeneration in the substantia nigra in the cases with dyskinesia than in the control brains. Confounding factors were gender differences between the groups and the older age of both the patient and control groups. Older patients might be more susceptible to the effects of neuroleptics. Jellinger reported on the findings in 28 brains of patients who had been treated chronically with similar drugs including chlorpromazine, trifluoperazine, and thioridazine.[56] Fourteen of these patients had suffered from persistent extrapyramidal symptoms. The neuropathological changes were seen mainly in the caudate nucleus. Forty-six percent of the cases showed swelling of large neurons, glial satellitosis, and proliferation of astroglia. Small striatal neurons were not affected. There were fewer marked changes in the putamen and globus pallidus in which there was some evidence of central chromatolysis and ballooning of the cytoplasm. These abnormalities were seen in 57% of the cases who had suffered from movement disorders before death, in only 7% of the patients without these disorders, and in only 4% of age-matched psychotics who had no history of long-term neuroleptic treatment. Although the mechanisms by which chronic neuroleptic treatment may cause pathological abnormalities in selective areas of the brain are not known, the possible involvement of reactive species in these processes is suggested by the finding of increased iron deposit in the brain of a patient who suffered from tardive dyskinesia.[57]

NEUROTRANSMITTER MODELS OF TARDIVE DYSKINESIA

Several models have been put forward to explain the development and persistence of TD. The most popular model is that of postsynaptic dopamine receptor supersensitivity. This hypothesis suggests that, because of chronic blockade of the receptors by antagonists, there develops a compensatory increase in the number of binding sites for dopamine in the basal ganglia. It has also been shown that neuroleptic-treated animals develop a behavioral supersensitivity to dopamine agonists such as apomorphine and amphetamine.[58-62] Because of the increased responsiveness to DA agonists after chronic use of neuroleptics, the development of TD is thought to be related to enhancement of dopaminergic mechanisms secondary to the increased number of DA receptors. One of the problems with the dopamine receptor hypothesis has to do with the fact that these binding sites increase in number within days of starting treatment with the neuroleptics, whereas TD develops several months to years after initiation of drug treatment. Moreover, the dopamine receptor hypothesis does not explain the persistence of TD over several years, for it is known that, after withdrawal of neuroleptics, the number of dopamine receptors returns to normal in animals that have been treated with these agents. Moreover, it does not address the issues related to risk factors that are known to be associated with TD (see below for further discussion).

It has also been suggested that the increased levels of norepinephrine may be important in the etiology of TD. This proposition was based on the findings of increased activity of dopamine-β-hydroxylase (DBH), the enzyme that catalyzes the synthesis of norepinephrine from dopamine.[63,64] It has also been shown that cerebrospinal fluid (CSF) norepinephrine is increased in a subset of patients who suffer from TD.[64] More recently, Fibiger and Lloyd have reviewed the evidence that suggests that the GABAergic system may be involved in the pathogenesis of TD and suggested that there might be a degenerative process that causes the abnormalities seen in the GABA system.[65] We agree with the suggestion that these drugs may be responsible for degenerative changes in the basal ganglia and have suggested the following model, which may help reconcile some of the findings discussed above.[66]

FREE RADICAL HYPOTHESIS OF TARDIVE DYSKINESIA

Because neuroleptics cause increases in the turnover of catecholamines, more monoamines will be available for their catabolism during treatment with these drugs. Both enzymatic and nonenzymatic catabolism of catecholamines can lead to the formation of cytotoxic compounds that might have damaging effects on cellular viability and neurotransmission. These active species would affect not only the dopamine or norepinephrine systems but also surrounding GABAergic, cholinergic, or peptidergic neurons. In addition, these compounds can produce free radicals in a more direct way inasmuch as chronic treatment with chlopromazine causes an increase in the levels of manganese in the central nervous system[67,68] and because the interaction of phenothiazine derivatives with trace metals can also generate free radicals.[25–27]

In addition to possible free radical-induced cell death, other processes may serve as substrates for the development of TD. The production of cytotoxic species during chronic usage of neuroleptics may lead to the initiation of membrane lipid peroxidation. Such a process, once started, would lead to the destabilization of the cell membrane. This proposition is in accord with the recent work of Cohen and Zubenko who were able to demonstrate that *in vitro* exposure of normal human platelets to psychotropic drugs resulted in changes in the structural order of the cell membranes.[69,70] Cohen and Zubenko subsequently demonstrated that striatal cells of rats treated with neuroleptics also showed abnormal physicochemical properties.[71] More recently, these researchers have reported that patients who suffer from TD after chronic neuroleptic treatment showed these abnormalities whereas those patients without TD did not.[72] It is thus conceivable that subgroups of patients who develop TD may have started with low levels of some free scavenging mechanisms and thus were not able to protect themselves from the damaging effects of the toxins produced during treatment with neuroleptics.

This hypothesis allowed us to make certain predictions that are discussed below. For example, these patients may be more at risk to develop parkinsonian symptoms during their treatment and to deteriorate to the schizophrenic "burn-out" state. Some studies have reported such an occurrence.[73–77] In these studies, the investigators have commented on the fact that the coexistence of parkinsonism and TD occurs more frequently than is generally believed. Crane reported that 12.5% of 180 patients had both neuroleptic-induced parkinsonism and TD.[74] The report by Wojcik and others indicated that patients with TD demonstrated more parkinsonian signs when examined.[75] Richardson and Craig also reported 26.7% of 86 patients, who suffered from neuroleptic-induced abnormalities, had both parkinsonism and tardive dyskinesia.[76] In a more recent study, it was reported that the presence of severe or worsening parkinsonism was associated with the development of TD.[77]

Another prediction is that poor prognosis schizophrenic patients who show poor response to neuroleptic treatment would be at high risk to develop TD. One complicating factor with this group of patients has to do with the reports that spontaneous involuntary movements may be seen in chronic schizophrenic patients who have not been treated with neuroleptics.[78] Although the number of nontreated patients in the study of Crow and colleagues was small (47 patients) in comparison to the treated group (411 patients), that report raised a very important point about the existence of abnormal movements in severe schizophrenia and their relationship to chronic neuroleptic use. In the absence of any diagnosable medical diathesis, the free radical hypothesis of dyskinesia may help to explain the occurrence of these movement abnormalities in severe chronic schizophrenics. Thus, idiopathic movements in schizophrenia (spontaneous dyskinesias), the progression of the schizophrenic illness, and tardive dyskinesia may share a similar free radical-based pathogenic molecular mechanism.[79]

TREATMENT OF TARDIVE DYSKINESIA WITH VITAMIN E

In order to test the free radical hypothesis, it was decided to evaluate the possibility that vitamin E might be an effective treatment of TD in some patients.[80] Subjects were chosen from among consenting inpatients and outpatients at Saint Elizabeths Hospital in Washington, DC. Patients were maintained on constant doses of neuroleptic and anticholinergic medications throughout the study.

The patients underwent an initial two-week stabilization period during which they were placed on placebo in order to obtain baseline ratings. They were then treated for a four-week period with either α-tocopherol or placebo (chosen on a random basis). The starting dose was 400 IU in the morning; this was raised to 400 IU twice a day during the second week, and finally to 400 IU three times a day during the third and fourth weeks. At the end of that time, they were then crossed-over to either active α-tocopherol or placebo depending on the previous treatment in the preceding four weeks.

Patients were evaluated on a biweekly basis, using the Brief Psychiatric Rating Scale (BPRS), a modified version of the Abnormal Involuntary Movement Scale (AIMS) with a score range of 0 to 36, and a modified version of the Simpson-Angus Scale for Extrapyramidal Side Effects (SAS) with a score range of 0 to 24. All ratings were performed blind to the patients' medications status.

Fifteen patients with the diagnosis of chronic schizophrenia (n = 9) or schizoaffective disorder (n = 6), by specific criteria, and persistent TD for at least one year participated in the study. TD was diagnosed by two independent raters. The sample consisted of 11 men and 4 women with a mean age of 44 ± 18 (range 19-71), a mean age at onset of illness of 24 ± 7 years (range 17-34), and a mean duration of movement disorder of 2.6 ± 19 years (range 1-6 years). Three patients had movements that were primarily dystonic in nature. No patients reported side effects of α-tocopherol.

There was a significant overall reduction in the AIMS score after treatment with α-tocopherol, but not after placebo (7.5 ± 4.8 versus 13.5 ± 6.4, $p < .0001$). The mean reduction in the AIMS score with α-tocopherol was 43%, with seven patients showing a greater than 50% reduction in their dyskinesia. There was no difference in SAS score after α-tocopherol compared with placebo (5.3 ± 5.5 versus 4.5 ± 4.7, NS). In a subset of 10 patients who had blood drawn for α-tocopherol concentrations, the mean serum α-tocopherol level rose from 11.8 ± 4.8 $\mu g/mL$ to 23.7 $\mu g/mL$ (normal range, 5-20 $\mu g/mL$).

When the BPRS score was divided according to subscores (anxiety, depression, aggression, mania, positive or productive symptoms, and negative or withdrawal symptoms), the α-tocopherol score was significantly less than the placebo score on the anxiety subscale (1.1 ± 1.9 versus 2.4 ± 2.5, $p < .005$) and the depression subscale (1.4 ± 2.4 versus 3.1 ± 3.2, $p < .005$).

A group of 12 patients completed a second cross-over phase. Again, there was a significant overall reduction in the AIMS score after treatment with α-tocopherol but not placebo (6.2 ± 3.3 versus 11.1 ± 5.1, $p < .005$), and no difference in the SAS score (3.7 ± 4.8 versus 4.1 ± 4.0, NS). There was no significant difference between mean AIMS scores after the two placebo periods (13.5 ± 6.4 versus 11.1 ± 5.1, NS).

Patients were then divided into two groups according to whether they had a greater than 50% improvement after α-tocopherol (n = 7) or less than 50% improvement (n = 8). The former group had a significantly shorter duration of TD (1.13 ± 0.35 versus 3.29 ± 2.06 years, $p < .02$) and a significantly later age of onset of psychiatric illness (27.1 ± 7.3 versus 19.7 ± 1.7 years, $p < .03$) than the latter group. The two groups did not differ on other clinical variables.

DISCUSSION AND CONCLUSIONS

The purpose of this paper has been to present some of the ideas that have been developed over the past few years in an attempt to reconcile certain biochemical and neuropathological data in the literature concerning use of neuroleptics and the development of persistent tardive dyskinesia (TD) in some patients. It has been reported that TD is more prevalent in chronic schizophrenics who show a deteriorating course, in aged individuals, and in patients who suffer from parkinsonian side effects of neuroleptics. The free radical hypothesis was invoked in order to develop a unifying hypothesis that would explain the existence of these risk factors. The treatment study with vitamin E provides some indirect evidence that this theoretical approach to TD may be partially correct. Nevertheless, more experiments are needed, and studies such as large-scale collaborative epidemiological and treatment efforts similar to the one that is being carried out for Parkinson's disease will be necessary to answer questions related to prevention of TD and to the free radical burden in patients treated with neuroleptics.

In the final analysis, however, it must be pointed out that the significance of a hypothesis does not rest only on its correctness, but also on its heuristic value. One of the most important aspects of the free radical hypothesis is that many of its predictions are eminently testable. Even if incorrect, studies of free radical mechanisms in neuropsychiatric illnesses may help to elucidate certain fundamental mechanisms involved in both normal and abnormal processes of the CNS. In the case of TD, we have demonstrated a significant improvement with vitamin E in a subset of patients. The answer to whether the positive response is related to the invoked mechanisms will have to await further studies.

REFERENCES

1. JESTE, D. V. & R. J. WYATT. 1982. Understanding and Treating Tardive Dyskinesia. Guilford Press. New York.
2. SIGWALD, J., D. BOUTTIER, C. RAYMONDEAUD & C. PIOT. 1959. Rev. Neurol. 100: 751-755.

3. KANE, J. M. & J. M. SMITH. 1982. Arch. Gen. Psychiatry **39:** 473-481.
4. LIEBERMAN, J., J. M. KANE, M. WOERNER, P. WEINHOLD, N. BASAVARAJU, J. KURUCZ & K. BERGMANN. 1984. Psychopharm. Bull. **20:** 382-386.
5. KANE, J. M., M. WOERNER, P. WEINHOLD, J. WEGNER, B. KINON & M. BORENSTEIN. 1984. Psychopharm. Bull. **20:** 387-389.
6. BURKE, R. E., S. FAHN, J. JANKOVIC, C. D. MARSDEN, A. E. LANG, S. GOLLOMP & J. ILSON. 1982. Neurology **32:** 1335-1346.
7. WEINER, W. J. & E. D. LUBY. 1983. Ann. Neurol. **13:** 466-467.
8. CARLSSON, A. & M. LINDQUIST. 1963. Acta Pharmacol. Toxicol. **20:** 140-143.
9. WIESEL, F. A. & G. SEDVALL. 1975. Eur. J. Pharmacol. **30:** 364-367.
10. CARLSSON, A. 1978. Am. J. Psychiatry **135:** 164-173.
11. BUNNEY, B. S., J. R. WALTERS, R. H. ROTH & G. K. AGHAJANIAN. 1973. J. Pharmacol. Exp. Ther. **185:** 560-571.
12. BUNNEY, B. S. & A. A. GRACE. 1978. Life Sci. **23:** 1715-1728.
13. SCATTON, B., C. GARRET & L. JULOU. 1975. Naunyn-Schmiedeberg's Arch. Pharmakol. **289:** 419-434.
14. SCATTON, B., J. GLOWINSKI & L. JOULOU. 1976. Brain Res. **109:** 184-189.
15. SCATTON, B. 1980. Adv. Biochem. Psychopharmacol. **24:** 31-36.
16. BIRD, E. D. & A. H. ANTON. 1982. Psychiatry Res. **6:** 1-6.
17. SALLER, C. F. & A. I. SALAMA. 1985. Neuropharmacology **24:** 123-129.
18. SCHELKUNOV, E. L. 1967. Nature **214:** 1210-1212.
19. GUNNE, L. M. & J. E. HAGGSTROM. 1983. Psychopharmacology **81:** 191-194.
20. GUNNE, L. M., J. E. HAGGSTROM & G. SJOQUIST. 1984. Nature **309:** 347-349.
21. MICHAELIS, L., M. P. SCHUBERT & S. GRANICK. 1940. J. Am. Chem. Soc. **62:** 204-211.
22. MICHAELIS, L., S. GRANICK & P. SCHUBERT. 1941. J. Am. Chem. Soc. **63:** 351-355.
23. FORREST, I. S., F. M. FORREST & M. BERGEN. 1958. Biochim. Biophys. Acta **29:** 441-442.
24. LAGERCRANTZ, C. 1961. Acta Chem. Scand. **15:** 1545-1556.
25. BORG, D. C. & G. C. COTZIAS. 1962. Proc. Natl. Acad. Sci. USA **48:** 617-622.
26. BORG, D. C. & G. C. COTZIAS. 1962. Proc. Natl. Acad. Sci. USA **48:** 623-642.
27. BORG, D. C. & G. C. COTZIAS. 1962. Proc. Natl. Acad. Sci. USA **48:** 643-651.
28. PIETTE, L. H., G. BULOW & I. YAMAZAKI. 1964. Biochim. Biophys. Acta **88:** 120-129.
29. HEINEKEN, F. W., M. BRUIN & F. BRUIN. 1962. J. Chem. Phys. **37:** 1479-1482.
30. FORREST, F. M. & I. S. FORREST. 1957. Am. J. Psychiatry **113:** 931-932.
31. FORREST, F. M., I. S. FORREST & A. S. MASON. 1957. Am. J. Psychiatry **114:** 931-932.
32. YAMAMOTO, I., A. TSUJIMOTO, Y. TSUJIMURA, M. MINAMI & Y. KUROGOCHI. 1957. Jap. J. Pharmacol. **6:** 138-146.
33. YAMAMOTO, I., N. ADACHI, Y. KUROGOCHI & A. TSYJIMOTO. 1960. Jpn. J. Pharmacol. **10:** 38-46.
34. CAVANAUGH, D. J. 1957. Science **125:** 1040-1041.
35. AKSEL, J. S. 1956. Encephale **45:** 566.
36. ROIZIN, L., C. TRUE & M. KNIGHT. 1959. Res. Publ. Assoc. Res. Nerv. Ment. Dis. **37:** 285-324.
37. MACKIEWICZ, J. & S. GERSHON. 1964. J. Neuropsychiatry **5:** 159-169.
38. CAZULLO, C. L., G. F. GOLDWURM & F. VANNI. 1965. *In* Proceedings of the Fifth International Congress of Neuropathology. F. Luthy & A. Bischoff, Eds.: 842-853. Exerpta Medica. Amsterdam.
39. DOM, R. 1967. Acta Neurol. Belg. **67:** 755-762.
40. SOMMER, H. & J. QUANDT. 1970. *In* Proceedings of the Sixth International Congress of Neuropathology. 466-491. Masson & Cie. Paris.
41. PAKKENBERG, H., R. FOG & B. NILAKANTAN. 1973. Psychopharmagologia (Berlin) **29:** 329-336.
42. PAKKENBERG, H. & R. FOG. 1974. Psychopharmacologia (Berlin) **40:** 165-169.
43. HACKENBERG, P. & E. LANGE. 1975. Exp. Pathol. Bd. (Suppl) **:** 132-142.
44. GERLACH, J. 1975. Psychopharmacologia (Berlin) **45:** 51-54.
45. KOIZUMI, J. & H. SHIRAISHI. 1970. J. Electron Microsc. **19:** 182-187.
46. KOIZUMI, J. & H. SHIRAISHI. 1972. Folia Psychiatr. Neurol. Jpn. **23:** 319-326.
47. KOIZUMI, J. & H. SHIRAISHI. 1973. Folia Psychiatr. Neurol. Jpn. **27:** 51-57.
48. KOIZUMI, J. & H. SHIRAISHI. 1973. Folia Psychiatr. Neurol. Jpn. **27:** 59-67.

49. NIELSEN, E. B. & M. LYON. 1978. Psychopharmacology **59:** 85-87.
50. BENES, F. M., P. A. PASKEVICH & V. B. DOMESICK. 1983. Science **221:** 969-971.
51. BENES, F. M., P. A. PASKEVICH, J. DAVIDSON & V. B. DOMESICK. 1985. Brain Res. **329:** 265-274.
52. GRUNTHAL, V. E. & H. WALTHER-BUHL. 1960. Psychiatr. Neurol. (Basel) **140:** 249-257.
53. HUNTER, R., W. BLACKWOOD, M. C. SMITH & J. N. CUMINGS. 1968. J. Neurol. Sci. **7:** 263-273.
54. GROSS, H. & E. KALTENBACH. 1969. *In* The Present Status of Psychotropic Drugs. A. Cerletti & F. J. Bove, Eds.: Excerpta Medica. Amsterdam.
55. CHRISTENSEN, E., J. D. MOLLER & A. FAURBYE. 1970. Acta Psychiatr. Scand. **46:** 14-23.
56. JELLINGER, K. 1977. *In* Neurotoxicology. L. Roizin, H. Shiraki & N. Grcevic, Eds.: 25-42. Raven Press. New York.
57. CAMPBELL, W. G., M. A. RASKIND, T. GORDON & C. M. SHAW. 1985. Am. J. Psychiatry **142:** 364-365.
58. CLOW, A., A. THEODOROU, P. JENNER & C. D. MARSDEN. 1980. Eur. J. Pharmacol. **63:** 135-144.
59. WADDINGTON, J. L. & S. J. GAMBLE. 1980. Eur. J. Pharmacol. **67:** 363-369.
60. WADDINGTON, J. L. & S. J. GAMBLE. 1980. Psychopharmacology **71:** 75-77.
61. WADDINGTON, J. L., S. J. GAMBLE & R. C. BOLURNE. 1981. Eur. J. Pharmacol. **69:** 511-513.
62. WADDINGTON, J. L. & S. J. GAMBLE. 1982. Eur. J. Pharmacol. **68:** 387-393.
63. JESTE, D. V., B. H. PHELPS, R. L. WAGNER, C. D. WISE & R. J. WYATT. 1979. Lancet **ii:** 850-851.
64. JESTE, D. V., D. R. DOONGAJI & M. LINNOILA. 1984. Br. J. Psychiatry **144:** 177-180.
65. FIBIGER, H. C. & K. G. LLOYD. 1984. Trends Neurosci. **7:** 462-464.
66. CADET, J. L., J. B. LOHR & D. V. JESTE. 1986. Trends Neurosci. **9:** 107-108.
67. BIRD, E. D., G. H. COLLINS, M. H. DODSON & L. G. GRANT. 1967. *In* Progress in Neurogenetics. A. Barbeau & J. R. Burnette, Eds.: 600-605. Excerpta Medica. Montreal/Amsterdam.
68. WEINER, W. J., P. A. NAUSIEDA & H. L. KLAWANS. 1980. *In* Tardive Dyskinesia: Research and Treatment. W. E. Fann, R. C. Smith, J. M. Davis & E. F. Domino, Eds.: 159-163. SP Medical and Scientific Books. New York.
69. ZUBENKO, G. S. & B. M. COHEN. 1984. Psychopharmacology **84:** 289-292.
70. ZUBENKO, G. S. & B. M. COHEN. 1985. Biol. Psychiatry **20:** 384-396.
71. COHEN, B. M. & G. S. ZUBENKO. 1985. Psychopharmacology **86:** 365-368.
72. ZUBENKO, G. S. & B. M. COHEN. 1986. Psychopharmacology **88:** 230-236.
73. CRANE, G. E. 1971. Am. J. Psychiatry **127:** 1407-1410.
74. CRANE, G. E. 1972. Arch. Neurol. **27:** 426-430.
75. WOJCIK, J. D., A. J. GELENBERG, R. A. LABRIE & M. MIESKE. 1980. Compr. Psychiatry **21:** 370-380.
76. RICHARDSON, M. A. & T. J. CRAIG. 1982. Am. J. Psychiatry **139:** 341-343.
77. CHOUINARD, G., L. ANNABLE, P. MERCIER & A. ROSS-CHOUINARD. 1986. Psychopharmacol. Bull. **22:** 259-263.
78. CROW, T. J., S. R. BLOOM, A. J. CROSS, I. N. FERRIER, E. C. JOHNSTONE, F. OWEN, D. G. C. OWENS & G. W. ROBERTS. 1984. *In* Catecholamines: Neuropharmacology and Central Nervous System—Therapeutic Aspects. 61-67. Alan R. Liss. New York.
79. CADET, J. L. 1988. Medical Hypotheses **27:** 59-63.
80. LOHR, J. B., J. L. CADET, M. A. LOHR, L. LARSON, E. WASLI, L. WADE, R. HYLTON, C. VIDONI, D. V. JESTE & R. J. WYATT. 1988. Schizophr. Bull. **14:** 291-296.

The Endogenous Toxin Hypothesis of the Etiology of Parkinson's Disease and a Pilot Trial of High-Dosage Antioxidants in an Attempt to Slow the Progression of the Illness

STANLEY FAHN

Department of Neurology
Columbia University College of Physicians and Surgeons
and
The Neurological Institute of New York
Columbia Presbyterian Medical Center
New York, New York 10032

INTRODUCTION

Parkinsonism is a neurological syndrome manifested by any combination of tremor at rest, rigidity, bradykinesia, and loss of postural reflexes.[1] At least two of these four cardinal features should be present before the diagnosis of parkinsonism is made. Parkinsonism of unknown etiology is known both as Parkinson's disease (PD) and also as idiopathic parkinsonism. PD is a progressive degenerative disorder of the central nervous system in which there is loss of monoamine neurons in the brain stem nuclei (predominantly the substantia nigra and the locus ceruleus) associated with eosinophilic cytoplasmic inclusion bodies (Lewy bodies) in these neurons. Accompanying this loss of cells is a marked reduction of monoamines in the brain. The most important monoaminergic loss is that of dopamine located in the nigrostriatal fibers. Replacement of dopamine deficiency by levodopa therapy is the most effective treatment for reversing parkinsonian symptoms. This symptomatic therapy, however, does not prevent worsening of the disease over time with less response to treatment.

Without knowing the etiology of PD, an approach to slow or prevent its progressive worsening has not been feasible. If there were a plausible hypothesis, however, then attempts to slow the progression of PD could be carried out. Two decades ago, one suggestion for the etiology of PD was that the illness may be due to a slow virus.[2] The disease has not been transmitted to animals, however, and this hypothesis is not supported. The concept of an infectious etiology is often resurrected, most recently that an intrauterine influenza could be the mechanism.[3] Hereditary factors seemed to be ruled out by a study in twins showing little concordance for PD among monozygotic twins.[4] This low concordance rate in twins was used as the basis for proposing that there may be an essential intrauterine factor that is unevenly distributed between the twins so that the one receiving the smaller amount would develop PD.[5]

Duvoisin,[6] in his review on the possible causes of PD, discarded the idea of an environmental toxin on the basis that there has been no change in the occurrence of the disease over time. In support of this view, Eldridge and Rocca[7] emphasized that the age-specific incidence rates have changed little over time.[8] The discovery, however, that the chemical agent, 1-methyl-4-phenyl-1,2,3,6-tetrahydropyridine (MPTP), can cause parkinsonism that appears to be clinially identical to that of PD[9] raised the concept once again that PD could be due to an environmental toxin. Calne and Langston[10] proposed that a combination of an environmental insult plus normal aging could be the basis leading to degeneration of monoamine neurons resulting in PD. The concept that normal metabolic processes in brain could lead to loss of monoamine-containing neurons is another hypothesis that seems plausible to this author and is considered in this paper; I shall call it the "endogenous toxin" hypothesis of Parkinson's disease.

THE ENDOGENOUS TOXIN HYPOTHESIS

Brody[11] counted the neurons in the locus ceruleus (norepinephrine-containing) and in the cerebral cortex and discovered that only the former is continually lost in normal humans with aging. He found that in youth there are approximately 19,000 cells, and for people in their 80s, only 10,000 cells. A similar study was carried out in the substantia nigra (dopamine-containing).[12] At birth the nigra contains approximately 400,000 cells; at age 60, approximately 250,000. The loss of nigral neurons with increased age was also found to take place in animals as well as humans. In addition to loss of these dopaminergic cells, there is a parallel loss of dopamine in the striatum, the destination of dopaminergic nerve fibers, with age. Carlsson and Winblad[13] measured dopamine and its metabolite, 3-O-methyldopamine, in the caudate and putamen postmortem in neurologically normal individuals between the ages 28 and 91 years and found statistically significant linear regression of these amines over this time span.

Supporting the results of cell counts showing a loss of these catecholaminergic neurons[11,12] is the reduction in the activities of the enzymes catalyzing the synthesis of dopamine in the substantia nigra and striatum[14,15] with aging. When the cell population or dopamine content reaches approximately 20% of youthful levels, symptoms of parkinsonism appear.[16] In contrast to the decline of synthesizing enzymes, the activities of the catabolic enzymes, monoamine oxidase types A and B, increase with age.[14] This finding suggests an increased rate of formation of homovanillic acid and hydrogen peroxide with aging, and this information adds to the importance in considering the endogenous toxin hypothesis of PD.

The loss of catecholaminergic neurons over time in normal individuals suggests the possibility that some metabolic process unique to these cells is responsible for its own self-destruction over time. One can link this loss of cells with the development of Parkinson's disease by at least three different scenarios (FIG. 1). In the first possibility (FIG. 1A), an individual who develops PD would have a faster rate of loss of these nigral neurons. The schematic diagram (purely hypothetical) suggests that whereas the average decline of these neurons would ultimately lead to parkinsonism if one lived to an age of approximately 110, the PD patient reaches threshold for symptoms at half that age.

The second scheme (FIG. 1B) assumes that the individual destined to develop PD has a normal rate of loss of nigral neurons, but was born with about half the number of such neurons, thus reaching threshold for symptoms also at about age 55. This scenario would be compatible with the hypothesis of Eldridge and Ince,[5] who postulated an intrauterine factor being required to support the growth of embryonic nigral neurons. This model is supported by the finding that certain strains of mice are born with different numbers of dopamine-containing neurons, and this influences their behavior.[17]

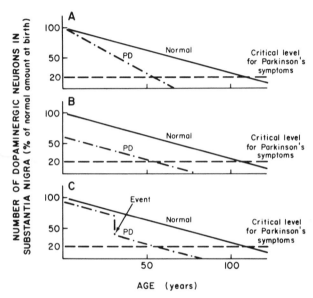

FIGURE 1. Hypothetical rates of neuronal loss in the substantia nigra and their possible linkage to the pathogenesis of Parkinson's disease. The average normal rate of cell loss is schematically drawn based on the results obtained by McGeer et al.[12] In all three scenarios, parkinsonian symptoms begin when the nigral population is approximately 20% of normal.[16] A: The rate of cell loss in individuals destined to develop Parkinson's disease proceeds at approximately twice the normal rate. Possibilities for such an increased rate are discussed in the text. B: The rate of cell loss in those who develop PD is the same as in normal individuals, but the number of neurons in the nigra are approximately 50% of that found in normal individuals. C: The rate of cell loss and the number of cells at birth are identical in the two populations, but those who eventually develop PD lost neurons due to some environmental event.

The third scenario (FIG. 1C) represents those individuals who are born with the normal amount of dopamine neurons and who have a decline of these cells at the normal rate, but who suffer some cerebral insult in their lifetime, leading to a loss of some of these neurons, so that they develop parkinsonism. This cerebral insult could be from a multitude of factors including infection, trauma, or exposure to subthreshold doses of environmental toxins, such as MPTP. This last scenario represents the proposal put forth by Calne and Langston.[10]

All three scenarios on the pathogenesis of Parkinson's disease have in common an underlying background of normal loss of monoaminergic neurons. Any single one

$$\text{Dopamine} + H_2O + O_2 \xrightarrow{\text{MAO}} 3,4-\text{Dihydroxyphenylacetaldehyde} + NH_3 + H_2O_2$$

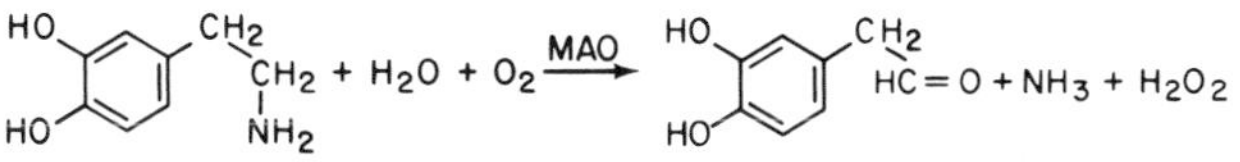

FIGURE 2. Oxidation of dopamine. Monoamine oxidase stoichiometrically generates hydrogen peroxide from the oxidation of dopamine and other monoamines.

or any combination of the three scenarios in FIGURE 1 could play a role in causing PD. If this linkage with normal nigral loss is correct, then by understanding the mechanism of this normal decline of dopamine neurons, we should be better able to understand the etiology of PD and perhaps even find a means to slow down the progression of the disease.

The fact that such neuronal loss occurs in all animal species studied would favor a common endogenous mechanism for such a loss, particularly one selective for these specific types of neurons. There are two well-recognized specific chemical features of these cells: they synthesize and degrade monoamines, and they form and store neuromelanin (at least in primates). The biochemical process of enzymatic oxidation of monoamines leads to the formation of one mole of hydrogen peroxide for each mole of amine that is oxidized.[18] The nonenzymatic oxidation of the catecholamines leads to the formation of cytotoxic quinones as well as hydrogen peroxide.[19–22] Hydrogen peroxide, of course, can be converted to the superoxide and hydroxyl radicals, which are toxic to cells.

In their review of Parkinson's disease in 1977, Fahn and Duffy[23] had concluded that the disorder appears to be a system degeneration, in which the neuromelanin-containing neurons in the brain are selectively lost. They suggested that an intermediate metabolite in the synthesis of neuromelanin might be toxic to the neuron, leading to its demise. This concept has been emphasized by Graham[19,20] and by Mann and Yates.[21,22] Cohen,[18] meanwhile, proposed that the free radicals derived from hydrogen peroxide generated from oxidation of dopamine contribute to the pathobiology of PD (FIG. 2). In turn, hydrogen peroxide is linked by way of one electron transfer reaction with the superoxide and hydroxyl radicals (FIG. 3).

In brain, the major pathway for scavenging hydrogen peroxide is through glutathione peroxidase, which is reduced in the substantia nigra, putamen, and globus pallidus in patients with Parkinson's disease.[24] In addition, reduced glutathione[25] and peroxidase and catalase activities[26] are also reduced in the substantia nigra of PD patients. Dexter et al.[27] found that malondialdehyde, an intermediate in the lipid peroxidation process, was increased in the substantia nigra in PD. Thus, the post-mortem pathological biochemistry of PD supports the notion that oxyradicals may be playing a role in the destruction of neurons in this disorder.

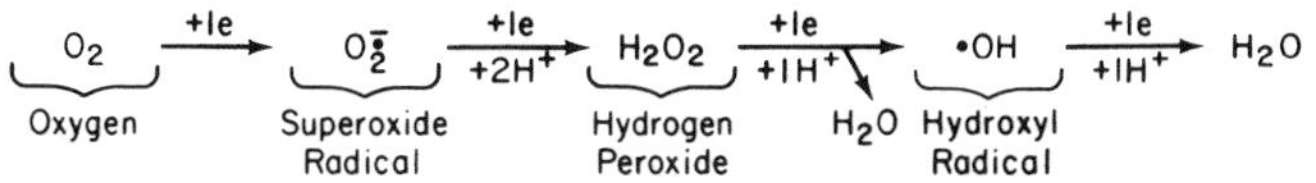

FIGURE 3. One electron transfer reaction, depicting the relationship between hydrogen peroxide and the oxyradicals.

Even so, we must explain the mechanism whereby excessive accumulation of free radicals occurs in patients with PD, leading to a possible increased rate of neuronal loss in scenario A of FIGURE 1. One possibility is that there is an increased production of free radicals due to increased turnover of dopamine, which can occur as a compensatory mechanism associated with reduction of dopamine-containing neurons,[28] and that the normal scavenging system is inadequate to handle this increased load. Another possibility is that an increased accumulation of oxyradicals results from a deficiency of scavengers, possibly on a genetic or environmental basis. The finding that nigral neuronal loss in patients with PD is most pronounced in specific regions of the nigra, rather than being uniform throughout the nigra (Gibb and Lees, personal communication), suggests that the microenvironment in this sensitive region may not allow sufficient scavenging of oxyradicals that are being generated. The absence of a parkinsonian state in individuals who have a total body deficiency of tocopherol (vitamin E deficiency) does not negate the endogenous toxin hypothesis because the local microenvironment of the substantia nigra in such individuals is still intact and capable of sustaining a relatively preserved level of tocopherol in such individuals.

PILOT STUDY OF HIGH-DOSAGE ANTIOXIDANTS

If the endogenous toxin hypothesis on the etiology of PD is correct, then it is theoretically possible to slow the progression of the disease by reducing the formation of oxyradicals or by increasing the scavenging of oxyradicals in the brain. In 1979, when I first considered this hypothesis as a plausible mechanism for the causation of Parkinson's disease, the nigral toxicity of MPTP was still unknown. My approach at that time was to attempt to increase the level of lipid and water-soluble antioxidants in brain by recommending to patients with early PD that they take high dosage of DL-alpha-tocopherol (vitamin E) and ascorbate (vitamin C). Because it was not certain that such an approach would be effective, and in order to follow the patients' course without masking the symptoms of parkinsonism, I made this suggestion only to patients not yet on levodopa therapy. Levodopa is such an effective symptomatic treatment, that once a patient is on this drug, it is difficult to measure the severity of the disease. My patients with mild PD were not on levodopa, because I follow the therapeutic principle of delaying the introduction of levodopa therapy as a means of delaying the complications of long-term treatment with this drug. I prescribe levodopa only when the symptoms become a threat to occupational, physical, or social disability.[29,30] This approach in therapeutics also provided a means to follow the progressive worsening of the illness in those placed on antioxidants by measuring the severity of the disease using the Columbia PD Rating Scale[31] and the Schwab-England Activities of Daily Living Scale.[32]

Starting on June 29, 1979, I suggested to all patients not yet receiving levodopa therapy that it would be reasonable for them to take high dosages of vitamins E and C. All qualified patients were handed a written protocol explaining how to gradually increase vitamins E and C to 3200 units/day and 3000 mg/day, respectively, in four divided doses. From June 1979 until December 1986, a total of 76 patients were given this recommendation, and all but one adopted this suggestion. The dates patients were placed on these antioxidants are presented in TABLE 1.

Many patients with early and mild PD were seen by me only once on consultation, and they were subsequently followed by their local physicians. Of the 49 patients

TABLE 1. Initiation of Antioxidants in Patients with Early Parkinson's Disease[a]

Antioxidants Initiated	
Year	No.
1979	11
1980	14
1981	6
1982	8
1983	6
1984	4
1985	17
1986	9
Total =	75

[a] By the end of 1986, 75 patients had been placed on tocopherol and ascorbic acid. Forty-nine of them had been started by the end of 1984. The duration of treatment of these 49 subjects would be sufficient to allow for analysis of their results.

starting antioxidants before 1985, 18 continued to be followed by me regularly, so that the date that levodopa was started is known for certain. Fifteen of these 18 began taking antioxidants when the duration of their PD was less than 4 years, and only these patients are analyzed (TABLE 2). There were 6 men and 9 women. The mean age (± SEM) at onset of PD was 50.7 ± 2.3 with a range of 34-71 years.

The end point for analysis is the time that levodopa is required, when symptoms are severe enough to become a threat to employment or to social or physical disability. Although my standard treatment regimen for all patients with mild PD does not include levodopa until symptoms are severe enough to warrant this medication, patients can receive anticholinergics and amantadine in an effort to delay the start of dopaminergics. All these patients were taking these other drugs. A similar therapeutic strategy has been used by Tanner.[33] Inasmuch as her patients were managed in a manner similar to my patients, except that they did not receive antioxidants, they can serve as a control population to compare the effects of antioxidants.

Of the 15 carefully followed patients with early PD who were treated with antioxidants, all but four have eventually required the administration of levodopa (Sinemet) or bromocriptine. The duration of PD before these dopaminergics were required ranged from 31 to 106 months, with four patients not yet requiring these medications. The mean ± SEM duration of PD before starting dopaminergics to the present time is 69.6 ± 4.9 months.

Because Tanner divided her patients according to age at onset, I have used the same format to allow a direct comparison of the two populations. The mean duration of PD before starting dopaminergics was 72 ± 6.5 months for the 11 patients whose PD started before they were 54 years old (TABLE 3), and 63 ± 3.9 months for the four patients who were age 54 or more (TABLE 4) at the onset of PD. These durations are 2.5 to 3 years longer than those reported by Tanner (TABLES 3 and 4), and thereby suggest that antioxidants may be useful in slowing down the progression of PD.

Adverse effects from 3200 units/day of tocopherol and 3000 mg/day of ascorbate were almost nonexistent. A few patients complained of some mild indigestion from tocopherol, and one complained of thinning of hair. They reduced the dosage to 2000 units/day.

TABLE 2. Description of Patients Placed on High-Dosage Antioxidants and the Duration of Time when Levodopa Therapy Was Required to Treat Their Parkinsonism. Cases Are Arranged According to Patients' Entry into the Study.

Patient	Sex	PD Onset Date	Age	Initial visit	Vit. E started	Months of PD before Vit. E	Sinemet[a] started	Months on Vit. E before Sinemet	Months of PD before Sinemet
1	M	4/77	47	4/77	6/79	26	3/82	33	59
2	F	10/77	52	3/79	7/79	21	5/80	10	31
3	F	3/78	56	5/78	9/79	18	6/83	45	63
4	F	2/79	54	1/80	1/80	11	2/84	49	60
5	F	7/76	38	3/80	3/80	44	9/81	18	62
6	F	9/79	71	6/80	6/80	9	5/84	47	56
7	F	9/79	46	10/80	10/80	13	12/83	38	51
8	M	7/77	52	11/80	11/80	40	12/84	49	89
9	M	4/79	46	11/80	12/80	19	12/84	48	67
10	M	7/80	51	11/81	11/81	16	NYS[b]	>89	>106
11	M	3/79	34	4/82	4/82	37	9/84	29	66
12	M	9/82	52	11/82	11/82	2	NYS	>77	>80
13	F	1/82	53	12/82	12/82	11	NYS	>76	>88
14	F	7/81	47	8/83	8/83	25	1/89	67	92
15	F	6/83	61	6/84	6/84	0	NYS	>72	>74
					Mean:	19.5		49.8	69.6
					SEM	3.4		5.9	5.9

[a] Sinemet is the trade name for carbidopa/levodopa.
[b] Not yet started on Sinemet.

TABLE 3. Results of Antioxidants according to Duration of Disease when Levodopa Was Required for Patients with Onset of Parkinson's Disease before the Age of 54 Years[a]

Patient	Results of Antioxidant Therapy Age at Onset < 54 Age at onset	Months of PD before Sinemet
11	34	66
5	38	62
7	46	51
9	46	67
1	47	59
14	47	92
10	51	>106
8	52	89
12	52	>80
2	52	31
13	53	>88
N = 11		
Mean	47.1	71.9
SEM	1.9	6.5

[a] Tanner: mean = 40 months.

DISCUSSION OF THE PILOT STUDY

The pilot study contained no control group, inasmuch as it was not designed as a definitive study, but as one to obtain preliminary experience using high dosages of tocopherol and ascorbate. Fortunately, Tanner[33] uses the identical therapeutic principle in managing her patients, that is, delaying levodopa therapy until there is a threat of social, physical, or occupational disability. Because she did not use antioxidants, we can compare the results of the patients treated in this pilot study and those treated by her. By such a comparison we find that the antioxidants appear to have delayed the end point when levodopa is required to treat the disease. It is important to point out that this does not make this pilot study a controlled study. Because the patients in the two protocols were not managed by the same investigator in a double-blind, randomly assigned fashion, the determination as to whether the antioxidants actually slowed the progression of the disease cannot be adequately evaluated in this pilot

TABLE 4. Results of Antioxidants according to Duration of Disease when Levodopa Was Required for Patients with Onset of Parkinson's Disease Older than Age 53 Years[a]

| | Results of Antioxidant Therapy Age at Onset > 53 | |
Patient	Age at onset	Months of PD before Sinemet
4	54	60
3	56	63
6	71	56
15	61	> 74
N = 4		
Mean:	60.5	63.3
SEM	3.8	3.9

[a] Tanner: mean = 24 months.

study. On the other hand, inasmuch as the comparison with Tanner's data suggests that antioxidants may extend the time before Sinemet therapy is required, a large double-blind trial is warranted. Such a controlled clinical trial is currently underway in the large, North American multicenter, controlled trial known as DATATOP (Deprenyl and Tocopherol Antioxidant Therapy of Parkinsonism), which is evaluating 2000 units/day tocopherol and 10 mg/day deprenyl in 800 subjects with early Parkinson's disease. The differences between the DATATOP study and the pilot study are presented in TABLE 5.

DATATOP uses tocopherol as the only antioxidant, based on data indicating it is the preferred antioxidant for protection against oxyradicals.[34] DATATOP also tests deprenyl, an inhibitor of monamine oxidase type B. The two drugs are used in a 2 × 2 factorial design, with the primary response variable being the duration of time between randomization and when levodopa is required. Deprenyl can act to reduce the quantity of oxyradicals in the catecholamine pathways by inhibiting monoamine oxidase, and thus reducing the synthesis of hydrogen peroxide; it also prevents the

TABLE 5. Comparison of This Pilot Study with DATATOP

Parameters	This Study	DATATOP
Number	15	800
Drugs used	Vitamin E + Vitamin C	Vitamin E and Deprenyl
Blind?	No	Yes
Controls?	No	Randomized
Presence of other drugs?	Other anti-PD drugs allowed	No
End point	Need for Sinemet	Need for anti-PD medications
Time to end point	From onset of PD symptoms	From time of randomization

conversion of MPTP to MPP+. The schematic diagram illustrating the sites of action of the two treatment drugs is presented in FIGURE 4.

CONCLUSION

Currently, the two leading theories on the etiology of Parkinson's disease (idiopathic parkinsonism) are the exogenous toxin hypothesis and the endogenous toxin hypothesis. The former is spearheaded by the knowledge that the chemical MPTP can cause loss of cells in the substantia nigra and produce parkinsonism in animals and humans. The latter is based on the concept that there is a loss of catecholamine-containing cells in the brain in normal individuals and animals with aging, and that such a loss is more pronounced in subjects with Parkinson's disease. The endogenous

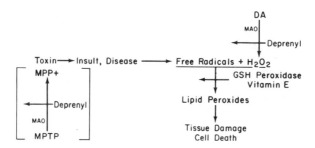

FIGURE 4. Diagram displaying the sites of action of deprenyl and tocopherol in preventing or scavenging oxyradicals. These two drugs are currently being tested in a large 2 × 2 factorial, double-blind, multicenter, placebo-controlled, clinical trial in 800 subjects with early and mild Parkinson's disease.

toxin hypothesis is analyzed in this paper. An attempt to slow down the progression of Parkinson's disease based on the endogenous toxin hypothesis has led to a pilot study using high-dosage antioxidants (tocopherol and ascorbate) in patients with early disease. The results of this noncontrolled pilot study suggest that the point in time when it is necessary to treat patients with levodopa therapy is delayed. This finding is one basis for conducting a large multicenter, controlled clinical trial analyzing antioxidants; this study is currently underway and is evaluating tocopherol and deprenyl in slowing the progression of Parkinson's disease.

REFERENCES

1. FAHN, S. 1988. The extrapyramidal disorders. *In* Cecil Textbook of Medicine, 18th edition. J. B. Wyngaarden & L. H. Smith, Jr., Eds.: 2143-2152. Saunders. Philadelphia.
2. POSKANZER, D. C. & R. S. SCHWAB. 1963. Cohort analysis of Parkinson's syndrome. Evidence for a single etiology related to subclinical infection about 1920. J. Chronic Dis. **16:** 961-973.
3. MATTOCK, C., M. MARMOT & G. STERN. 1988. Could Parkinson's disease follow intrauterine influenza?: a speculative hypothesis. J. Neurol. Neurosurg. Psychiatry **51:** 753-756.
4. WARD, C. D., R. C. DUVOISIN, S. E. INCE, J. D. NUTT, R. ELDRIDGE & D. B. CALNE. 1983. Parkinson's disease in 65 pairs of twins and in a set of quadruplets. Neurology **33:** 815-824.
5. ELDRIDGE, R. & S. E. INCE. 1984. The low concordance rate for Parkinson's disease in twins: A possible explanation. Neurology **34:** 1354-1356.
6. DUVOISIN, R. C. 1982. The cause of Parkinson's disease. *In* Movement Disorders. C. D. Marsden & S. Fahn, Eds.: 8-24. Butterworth Scientific. London.
7. ELDRIDGE, R. & W. A. ROCCA. 1985. The clinical syndrome of striatal dopamine deficiency: parkinsonism induced by MPTP. N. Engl. J. Med. **313:** 1159-1160.
8. RAJPUT, A. H., K. P. OFFORD, C. M. BEARD & L. T. KURLAND. 1984. Epidemiology of parkinsonism: Incidence, classification, and mortality. Ann. Neurol. **16:** 278-282.
9. BALLARD, P. A., J. W. TETRUD & J. W. LANGSTON. 1985. Permanent human parkinsonism due to 1-methyl-4-phenyl-1,2,3,6-tetrahydropyridine (MPTP): seven cases. Neurology **35:** 949-956.
10. CALNE, D. B. & J. W. LANGSTON. 1983. Aetiology of Parkinson's disease. Lancet **2:** 1457-1459.
11. BRODY, H. 1976. An examination of cerebral cortex and brainstem aging. *In* Neurobiology of Aging. R. D. Terry & S. Gershon, Eds.: 177-181. Raven Press. New York.
12. MCGEER, P. L., E. G. MCGEER & J. S. SUZUKI. 1977. Aging and extrapyramidal function. Arch. Neurol. **34:** 33-35.
13. CARLSSON, A. & B. WINBLAD. 1976. Influence of age and time interval between death and autopsy on dopamine and 3-methoxytyramine levels in human basal ganglia. J. Neural Transm. **38:** 271-276.
14. COTE, L. J. & L. T. KREMZNER. 1983. Biochemical changes in normal aging in human brain. Adv. Neurol. **38:** 19-30.
15. MCGEER, E. G. 1978. Aging and neurotransmitter metabolism in the human brain. *In* Alzheimer's Disease: Senile Dementia and Related Disorders. R. Katzman, R. D. Terry & K. L. Bick, Eds.: **7:** 427-440. Raven Press. New York.
16. BERNHEIMER, H., W. BIRKMAYER, O. HORNYKIEWICZ, K. JELLINGER & F. SEITELBERGER. 1973. Brain dopamine and the syndromes of Parkinson and Huntington. J. Neurol. Sci. **20:** 415-455.
17. REIS, D. J., J. S. FINK & H. BAKER. 1983. Genetic control of the number of dopamine neurons in the brain: relationship to behavior and responses to psychoactive drugs. *In* Genetics of Neurological and Psychiatric Disorders. S. S. Kety, L. P. Rowland, R. L. Sidman & S. W. Matthysse, Eds.: 55-75. Raven Press. New York.

18. COHEN, G. 1983. The pathobiology of Parkinson's disease: biochemical aspects of dopamine neuron senescence. J. Neural. Transm. Suppl. **19:** 89-103.
19. GRAHAM, D. G. 1978. Oxidative pathways for catecholamines in the genesis of neuromelanin and cytotoxic quinones. Mol. Pharmacol. **14:** 633-643.
20. GRAHAM, D. G. 1979. On the origin and significance of neuromelanin. Arch. Pathol. Lab. Med. **103:** 359-362.
21. MANN, D. M. A. & P. O. YATES. 1982. Pathogenesis of Parkinson's disease. Arch. Neurol. **39:** 545-549.
22. MANN, D. M. A. & P. O. YATES. 1983. Possible role of neuromelanin in the pathogenesis of Parkinson's disease. Mech. Ageing Dev. **21:** 193-203.
23. FAHN, S. & P. DUFFY. 1977. Parkinson's disease. *In* Scientific Approaches to Clinical Neurology. E. S. Goldensohn & S. H. Appel, Eds.: 1119-1158. Lea & Febiger. Philadelphia.
24. KISH, S. J., C. MORITO & O. HORNYKIEWICZ. 1985. Glutathione peroxidase activity in Parkinson's disease brain. Neurosci. Lett. **58:** 343-346.
25. PERRY, T. L., D. V. GODIN & S. HANSEN. 1982. Parkinson's disease: a disorder due to nigral glutathione deficiency? Neurosci. Lett. **33:** 305-310.
26. AMBANI, L. M., M. H. VAN WOERT & S. MURPHY. 1975. Brain peroxidase and catalase in Parkinson's disease. Arch. Neurol. **32:** 114-118.
27. DEXTER, D. T., C. J. CARTER, F. R. WELLS, F. JAVOY-AGID, Y. AGID, A. LEES, P. JENNER & C. D. MARSDEN. 1989. Basal lipid peroxidation in substantia nigra is increased in Parkinson's disease. J. Neurochem. **52:** 381-389.
28. HORNYKIEWICZ, O. 1982. Brain neurotransmitter changes in Parkinson's disease. *In* Movement Disorders. C. D. Marsden & S. Fahn, Eds.: 41-58. Butterworth Scientific. London.
29. FAHN, S. & D. B. CALNE. 1978. Considerations in the management of parkinsonism. Neurology **28:** 5-7.
30. LESSER, R. P., S. FAHN, S. R. SNIDER, L. J. COTE, W. P. ISGREEN & R. E. BARRETT. 1979. Analysis of the clinical problems in parkinsonism and the complications of long-term levodopa therapy. Neurology **29:** 1253-1260.
31. DUVOISIN, R. C. 1971. The evaluation of extrapyramidal disease. *In* Monoamines noyaux Gris Centraux et Syndrome de Parkinson. Symposium Bel-Air IV. J. de Ajuriaguerra & G. Gauthier, Eds.: 313-325. Georg & Cie. Geneva.
32. SCHWAB, R. W. & A. C. ENGLAND, JR. 1969. Projection technique for evaluating surgery in Parkinson's disease. *In* Third Symposium on Parkinson's Disease. F. J. Gillingham & M. C. Donaldson, Eds.: 152-157. E & S Livingstone. Edinburgh.
33. TANNER, C. 1986. Data submitted as part of the NIH grant application NS 24778. I. Shoulson, principal investigator.
34. WILLSON, R. L. 1983. Free radical protection: why vitamin E, not vitamin C, beta-carotene or glutathione? *In* Biology of Vitamin E. (Ciba Foundation Symposium 101). 19-44. Pitman Books. London.

Prophylaxis of Periventricular Hemorrhage in Preterm Babies by Vitamin E Supplementation

MALCOLM CHISWICK, GORDON GLADMAN,
SUNHIL SINHA, NANCY TONER,
AND JACQELINE DAVIES[a]

Neonatal Medical Unit and [a] Department of Radiology
North Western Regional Perinatal Centre
St. Mary's Hospital
Manchester M14 0JH, England

INTRODUCTION

Ultrasound imaging of the brain in preterm babies during the first week of life reveals hemorrhage in and around the lateral ventricles (periventricular hemorrhage) in about 40% of babies born with a gestation time of less than 33 weeks.[1-3] Serial scanning shows that these lesions usually occur within the first 3 days of life, with 50% occurring on the first day.[4] Blood clot is visible as an echodense lesion, and among babies who die, there is good anatomical agreement between the ultrasound appearance and observations at necropsy.[5] For simplicity, three grades of hemorrhage, in increasing order of severity, can be recognized by ultrasound: *Grade 1:* hemorrhage within the germinal matrix in the floor of the lateral ventricles (subependymal hemorrhage, SEH); *Grade 2:* hemorrhage within the cavity of the lateral ventricles (intraventricular hemorrhage, IVH); and *Grade 3:* hemorrhage within brain parenchyma, adjacent to the lateral ventricles (parenchymal hemorrhage) and contiguous with intraventricular echodensity.

The strongest association of periventricular hemorrhage is with preterm birth, and the risk increases with decreasing gestational age. Certain clinical factors increase the risk of periventricular hemorrhage,[6] including respiratory distress syndrome, the need for assisted ventilation, and pneumothorax. These disturbances are thought to cause fluctuations in systemic blood pressure and cerebral perfusion, which are transmitted to the primitive and friable vasculature of the subependymal region, the site of origin of hemorrhage.[7]

Babies with isolated subependymal or a small IVH have a favorable outcome. Very large IVH, and particularly parenchymal hemorrhage, carries a high risk of death or major long-term neurological sequelae, such as cerebral palsy. Posthemorrhagic ventricular dilatation occurs, a complication of IVH, and also increases the risk of neurodevelopmental sequelae. We have been studying the role of vitamin E supplementation as a prophylaxis against periventricular hemorrhage.

Vitamin E

Vitamin E is an antioxidant, and one of its functions is to protect cell membranes against lipid peroxidation. Newborn babies, particularly those born prematurely, have low circulating levels of vitamin E compared with older infants, children, and adults.[8] *In vitro* hydrogen peroxide hemolysis is enhanced in newborn babies, and this can be corrected by vitamin E supplementation.[9] Probably the only clinical disorder attributable to vitamin E deficiency in early infancy is a hemolytic anemia in preterm babies aged 6-10 weeks fed proprietary formulas.[10] This is now rarely seen.

Our interest in vitamin E in relation to periventricular hemorrhage was stimulated by a fortuitous observation made by us in 1980. During the course of a small study in preterm babies designed to assess the appropriate dose of intramuscular vitamin E required to increase their plasma levels to adult values, we observed that IVH was seen less frequently at necropsy in supplemented babies than in controls.[11] Following the introduction of ultrasound brain scanning to our unit, we conducted a randomized controlled pilot study that showed that babies < 32 weeks gestation who were supplemented with three daily doses (20 mg/kg) of intramuscular vitamin E from birth had a lower incidence of IVH (18.8%) than controls (56.3%).[12]

In this article, we summarize the results of our definitive randomized controlled trial of vitamin E (DL-alpha-tocopherol acetate supplementation)[13] and our experience since then of single dose intramuscular vitamin E supplementation given soon after birth.

RANDOMIZED CONTROLLED TRIAL OF VITAMIN E IN THE PREVENTION OF PERIVENTRICULAR HEMORRHAGE

Patients and Methods

From January 1984 to September 1985 we enrolled into the trial 231 preterm babies of < 33 weeks gestation. One hundred and fifty were born at this hospital, and 81 were referred from other maternity hospitals in the North Western Region of England. The study was approved by the hospital ethics committee.

Babies were randomized to a vitamin E supplementation or control group, without stratification for place of birth, according to directions contained in a sealed envelope that was opened just before or immediately after birth (inborn babies) or soon after transfer to the unit (referred babies). Supplemented babies received three daily doses of intramuscular vitamin E (Ephynal, Hoffmann-La Roche, Basel), 20 mg/kg, within 2 hours of randomization (day 0) and 24 and 48 hours later (days 1 and 2). We considered it unethical to give the control group intramuscular placebo injections.

Plasma vitamin E concentration, plasma total lipids,[14] and susceptibility of red blood cells to hydrogen peroxide hemolysis[15] were measured in a sample of arterial or venous blood drawn from each baby immediately before the first dose of vitamin E and at comparable times in each control baby. Measurements were repeated 24, 48, and 72 hours later (days 1, 2, and 3). Plasma vitamin E (total tocopherol) was measured by a colorimetric method in which ferrous iron (produced by the reduction of ferric iron by vitamin E) was used as an index of vitamin E concentration.[16]

Babies were scanned through the anterior fontanelle, using a 7.5 MHz probe with a Technicaire mechanical sector scanner. Inborn babies had their first scan within two hours of birth, and referred babies were scanned on admission to the unit (median 10 h; range 4-26 h). Thereafter babies were scanned daily for the first week, and at least twice weekly until discharge from the unit. Scans were recorded on videotape and reviewed at the completion of the study. The definitions of various grades of hemorrhage were as outlined in the introduction to this article. The medical and nursing care of the babies was according to our ward protocol. Clinical information relevant to the occurrence of periventricular hemorrhage was collected prospectively in each baby. Unless otherwise stated, statistical significance was tested by the Chi square or Student's *t* test, as appropriate.

Results

Lethal malformations were present in three inborn babies who were randomized before birth, and these were immediately excluded from the trial for ethical considerations. The mean $\pm$ SD plasma vitamin E concentration was identical in supplemented and control groups on day 0 (0.43 $\pm$ 0.21 mg/dL). Thereafter there was a progressive rise in plasma vitamin E levels in supplemented babies, reaching 2.98 $\pm$ 0.92 mg/dL on day 3. On each day, supplemented babies had a higher mean level compared with controls ($p < 0.001$) (FIGURE 1). On day 0, the mean $\pm$ SD vitamin E:plasma lipid ratio was also similar in supplemented (1.4 $\pm$ 0.89 mg/g) and control groups (1.39 $\pm$ 0.68 mg/g), and the trend of mean values thereafter was identical to the plasma vitamin E trends.

An abnormal hydrogen peroxide hemolysis test was defined as hemolysis of more than 10% of the red blood cells in the hydrogen peroxide solution. On day 0, the same proportion of supplemented and control babies (52.7%) had an abnormal result. On each of the days, 1 to 3, less than 5% of supplemented babies had abnormal hemolysis, whereas the proportion of control babies with an abnormal test on these days remained high (40-55%).

Among the 228 babies who entered the trial, 107 (46.9%) developed hemorrhages, and in most (n = 82), this was first observed within 48 hours of birth. Randomization ensured that small differences in the incidence of clinical risk factors for periventricular hemorrhage between supplemented and control groups were due to chance, and we confirmed that any difference was not statistically significant. There were 18 babies who had hemorrhages on the initial scan, and these babies were excluded from the following analysis, which compares the incidence of hemorrhage in supplemented and control groups.

As shown in TABLE 1, the incidence of IVH and the combined incidence of IVH and parenchymal hemorrhage were lower in the supplemented group (8.8% and 10.8%) than in the control group (34.3% and 40.7%) ($p < 0.0001$). The 95% confidence interval for the difference in the combined incidence of IVH and parenchymal hemorrhage between the two groups was 18.9%-41.0%.

The combined incidence of IVH and parenchymal hemorrhage was also lower in supplemented babies compared with controls when inborn and referred babies were considered separately (95% confidence interval for difference in incidence; inborn 18.0%-43.0%; referred 10.5%-55.5%). These differences were largely due to a much lower incidence of IVH in the supplemented babies.

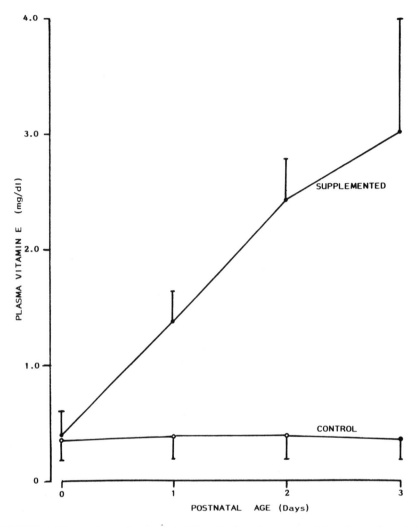

FIGURE 1. Plasma vitamin E (mean ± SD) in the first three postnatal days in supplemented and control babies.

A multivariate analysis (binomial logit model) which adjusted for a variety of clinical factors other than vitamin E that might influence the occurrence of hemorrhage, confirmed that vitamin E had an independent protective effect against all grades of hemorrhage combined ($p < 0.001$).

There were 89 babies whose initial scan was normal, but who later developed hemorrhages. When supplemented (n=31) and control groups (n=58) were compared, there was a striking difference in the distribution of hemorrhages on the first abnormal scan in these babies. Subependymal hemorrhage predominated in the supplemented group, with an incidence of 74.2% (versus 31.0% in controls), whereas

IVH or parenchymal hemorrhage predominated in controls, with an incidence of 69.0% (versus 25.8% in supplemented babies)(p < 0.0001).

The survival rate of inborn and referred babies was 85.7% and 71.6%, respectively, and there was no significant effect of vitamin E on the survival rate in either group.

SINGLE-DOSE VITAMIN E PROPHYLAXIS AGAINST PERIVENTRICULAR HEMORRHAGE

Pending further trials by other investigators, we felt it appropriate to introduce vitamin E prophylaxis into our routine clinical practice. Although our trial did not reveal important harmful effects definitely attributable to vitamin E, we were aware that plasma vitamin E levels were monitored regularly until only 72 hours after birth. The "peak" level at this time might not represent the true maximum level in individual babies.

Following the trial, we were not in a position to conduct a further randomized study addressing the question of different dosage regimens. Bearing in mind that the protective effect of vitamin E was already apparent on the first abnormal scan, and that in about 75% of babies the first abnormal scan occurred within 48 hours of birth, we thought it a reasonable compromise to offer all babies of < 33 weeks gestation a single intramuscular dose of vitamin E (20 mg/kg) soon after birth (inborn babies) or on admission to the unit (referred babies). We agreed to analyze the results of this policy after one year and compare them with the results of the three-dose randomized controlled trial.

We recognized from the outset the potential disadvantages of using historical controls from the previous randomized controlled trial (referred to below as unsupplemented babies). The purpose of the study was to provide a critical evaluation of our clinical practice.

TABLE 1. Number (%) of Different Grades of Periventricular Hemorrhage in Vitamin E-Supplemented (Three-Dose or One-Dose) and Control Group[a]

	SEH[b]	IVH[c]	Parenchymal	IVH or Parenchymal
Three dose (n = 102)	20 (19.6)	9 (8.8)	2 (2.0)	11 (10.8)
Control (n = 108)	14 (13.0)	37 (34.3)	7 (6.5)	44 (40.7)
One dose (n = 121)	23 (19.0)	16 (13.2)	9 (7.4)	25 (20.7)

[a] 95% confidence intervals for difference in incidence: IVH, three-dose versus control, 15.0%-36.0%; one-dose versus control, 10.2%-31.8%. IVH or parenchymal, three-dose versus control, 18.9%-41.0%; one-dose versus control, 8.3%-31.8%.
[b] SEH = subependymal hemorrhage.
[c] IVH = intraventricular hemorrhage.

Patients and Methods

During the 13-month period following the original randomized controlled trial, 121 consecutively admitted babies, of < 33 weeks gestation, received a single intramuscular dose of vitamin E (20 mg/kg) within two hours after birth (inborn) or on admission to the unit (referred). Plasma vitamin E was measured in randomly selected babies (n = 39) 12 hours after dosage and at intervals during the first 10 days. The analyst and the method used were the same as in the randomized controlled trial.

In keeping with our routine clinical practice, babies had brain scans several times during the first week, and further scans were carried out as indicated until the baby was discharged. No new personnel carried out the scans and the method used, and grading of hemorrhage was the same as in the randomized controlled trial. Clinical information relevant to the occurrence of hemorrhage was recorded prospectively in each baby.

Results

The mean ± SD plasma vitamin E level at 12 hours was 0.73 ± .35 mg/dL, rising to a peak at 48 hours (day 2) of 1.42 ± 0.58 mg/dL and falling by day 10 to 0.7 ± 0.3 mg/dL. On days 1, 2, and 3, the mean plasma level was significantly higher in three-dose supplemented babies compared with single-dose supplemented.

Compared with the original unsupplemented babies, the single-dose supplemented group were a sicker population (TABLE 2). Although a similar proportion was referred in the two groups (27.3% versus 23.1%), a greater proportion of single-dose supplemented babies suffered respiratory distress ($p < 0.05$), received assisted ventilation ($p < 0.005$), and had pneumothoraces ($p < 0.025$).

Nonetheless, the combined incidence of IVH and parenchymal hemorrhage was lower in single-dose supplemented babies (20.7%) than in unsupplemented babies (40.7%)(95% confidence interval for difference 8.3% to 31.8%). This was solely due to a reduced incidence of IVH (13.2% versus 34.3%)(TABLE 1).

The survival rate among the single-dose supplemented babies (74.7%) did not

TABLE 2. Comparison of Risk Factors for Periventricular Hemorrhage in Single-Dose Supplemented and Unsupplemented Babies[a]

	Single-dose Vitamin E (n = 121)	Unsupplemented (n = 108)
Gestational age (weeks)	28.5 ± 2.2	28.5 ± 2.2
Birth weight (g)	1194 ± 431	1185 ± 427
Referred	33 (27.3)	25 (23.1)
Respiratory distress	86 (71.1)*	62 (57.4)
Assisted ventilation	95 (78.5)***	64 (59.3)
Pneumothorax	30 (24.8)**	13 (12.0)

[a] The mean ± SD is shown for gestational age and birth weight. Percentages are shown in parentheses.
***$p < 0.005$; **$p < 0.025$; *$p < 0.05$.

differ significantly from babies who received three-dose supplementation (80.7%), and as in the randomized controlled trial, no effect of vitamin E on survival rate was observed.

Discussion

Our findings confirmed that vitamin E supplementation was associated with increased resistance to hydrogen peroxide hemolysis. In babies who were supplemented with three doses of vitamin E, their mean plasma vitamin E level rose progressively until day 3 and was not measured after that. By contrast, following single-dose supplementation, a peak plasma level was observed on day 2, and the mean plasma level was significantly lower in these babies on days 1, 2, and 3 compared with three-dose supplementation.

The randomized controlled trial showed a protective effect of three-dose supplementation predominately against IVH. Although there appeared to be a protective effect against parenchymal hemorrhage, the number of babies who suffered these hemorrhages was too small to draw any conclusions. IVH and parenchymal hemorrhage are of potential clinical importance, whereas isolated subependymal hemorrhages do not influence outcome. This was the justification for measuring the effect of supplementation on the combined incidence of IVH and parenchymal hemorrhage.

Single-dose supplementation, among the whole population, was associated with a significant reduction in the combined incidence of IVH and parenchymal hemorrhage. This was solely due to a reduced incidence of IVH. In contrast to the randomized controlled study, there was no suggestion of a protective effect against parenchymal hemorrhage. Furthermore, protection against IVH appeared less complete with single-dose prophylaxis, as shown by comparing the 95% confidence intervals for the difference in incidence of IVH (versus control) in the two supplementation regimens (see TABLE 1).

The problem of using historical controls is nicely illustrated in our single-dose supplementation study insofar as the supplemented population was at greater risk for hemorrhage than the historical controls. This biased the study against finding a protective effect of single-dose supplementation; yet a protective effect was still observed. We cannot determine, however, whether the seemingly lesser protection with our single-dose regimen was a result of the population being at greater risk for hemorrhage or insufficient vitamin E reaching its site of action.

It is likely that the subependymal region is an area of poor perfusion.[17] We speculate that the protective effect of vitamin E against periventricular hemorrhage is based on its ability to trap free radicals generated during ischemic injury of the subependymal layer, so limiting progression of tissue damage and the extent of hemorrhage during reperfusion.

Progression of hemorrhage cannot be defined accurately without continuous brain scanning. In our randomized controlled trial, apparent progression of hemorrhage, based on scanning at 24-hour intervals, was uncommon and seemingly uninfluenced by supplementation. A comparison of the findings on the first abnormal brain scan in supplemented babies and the control group is in keeping with the suggestion that vitamin E protects by rapidly limiting the extent and progression of subependymal hemorrhage within 24 hours of its occurrence and that very early supplementation is important.

REFERENCES

1. LEVENE, M. I., J. S. WIGGLESWORTH & V. DUBOWITZ. 1981. Cerebral structure and intraventricular hemorrhage in the neonate: A real-time ultrasound study. Arch. Dis. Child. **56:** 416-424.

2. LIPSCOMB, A. Q., R. J. THORBURN, E. O. R. REYNOLDS et al. 1981. Pneumothorax and cerebral hemorrhage in preterm infants. Lancet **i:** 414-416.

3. MCMENAMIN, J. B., G. D. SHACKELFORD & J. J. VOLPE. 1984. Outcome of neonatal intraventricular hemorrhage with periventricular echodense lesions. Ann. Neurol. **15:** 285.

4. VOLPE, J. J. 1987. Neurology of the Newborn. 2nd edit. W. B. Saunders Company. Philadelphia. p. 331.

5. PAPE, K., E. S. BENNETT-BRITTON, W. SZMONOWICZ, D. J. MARTIN, C. R. FITZ & L. BECKER. 1983. Diagnostic accuracy of neonatal brain imaging: a postmortem correlation of computed tomography and ultrasound scans. J. Pediatr. **102:** 275-280.

6. LEVENE, M. I., C-L. FAWER & R. F. LAMONT. 1982. Risk factors in the development of intraventricular hemorrhage in the preterm neonate. Arch. Dis. Child. **8:** 410-417.

7. PERLMAN, J. M., J. B. MCMENAMIN & J. J. VOLPE. 1983. Fluctuating cerebral blood flow velocity in respiratory distress syndrome: relationship to the development of intraventricular hemorrhage. N. Engl. J. Med. **309:** 209-213.

8. MOYER, W. T. 1950. Vitamin E levels in term and preterm newborn infants. Pediatrics **6:** 893-896.

9. GYORGY, P., G. COGAN & C. S. ROSE. 1952. Availability of vitamin E in the newborn infant. Proc. Soc. Exp. Biol. Med. **81:** 536-538.

10. OSKI, F. A. & L. A. BARNESS. 1967. Vitamin E deficiency: a previously unrecognized cause of hemolytic anemia in the premature infant. J. Pediatr. **70:** 211-220.

11. CHISWICK, M. L., J. WYNN & N. TONER. 1982. Vitamin E and intraventricular hemorrhage in the newborn. Ann. N.Y. Acad. Sci. **393:** 109-118.

12. CHISWICK, M. L., W. JOHNSON & C. WOODHALL et al. 1983. Protective effect of vitamin E (DL-alpha tocopherol acetate) against intraventricular hemorrhage in premature babies. Br. Med. J. **287:** 81-84.

13. SINHA, S., J. DAVIES, N. TONER, S. BOGLE & M. L. CHISWICK. 1987. Vitamin E supplementation reduces frequency of periventricular hemorrhage in very preterm babies. Lancet **i:** 466-471.

14. FARRELL, P. M. S., S. L. LEVINE, M. D. MURPHY & A. J. ADAMS. 1978. Plasma tocopherol levels and tocopherol-lipid relationships in a normal population of children as compared to healthy adults. Am. J. Clin. Nutr. **31:** 1720-1726.

15. ROSE, C. S. & P. GYORGY. 1952. Specificity of hemolytic reaction in vitamin E deficient erythrocytes. Am. J. Physiol. **168:** 414-420.

16. MARTINELL, R. G. 1964. Method of determination of vitamin E [total tocopherols] in serum. Clin. Chem. **10:** 1078-1086.

17. PASTERNACK, J. F., D. R. GROOTHUIS & D. P. FISCHER. 1982. Regional cerebral blood flow in the newborn beagle pup: the germinal matrix is a low flow structure. Pediatr. Res. **16:** 499-503.

Discussion

HELEN MINTZ-HITTNER

Department of Ophthalmology and Pediatrics
Baylor College of Medicine
Houston, Texas 77030

"Children are not just small adults" is a favorite quotation among pediatricians. Likewise, "preterm infants are not just small adults," and further, "preterm infants are not just small children." This must be realized in discussing vitamin E deficiency and toxicity. In adults and children, unless an unusual state exists, such as insufficient supplementation in association with a disorder related to fat malabsorption, vitamin E deficiency does not occur. In adults and children, unless an unusual state exists, such as excessive supplementation in association with a disorder requiring anticoagulant therapy, vitamin E toxicity is not a clinical problem. In the unsupplemented preterm infant, however, "vitamin E deficiency" is present at birth (≤ 0.5 mg% plasma vitamin E levels),[1] and in the parenterally supplemented preterm infant, "vitamin E toxicity" has been documented in the neonatal period (≥ 6 mg% plasma vitamin E levels).[2,3] Thus, elevation of plasma vitamin E levels to "vitamin E sufficiency" in the neonatal period (1.2-3.0 mg% plasma vitamin E levels) is felt by many to be appropriate, but careful monitoring of plasma vitamin E levels is mandatory.

Chiswick *et al.* have reviewed the data of the controlled, randomized, masked clinical trial of triple dose im vitamin E to prevent the occurrence of periventricular hemorrhage (subependymal, intraventricular, and parenchymal hemorrhage) in preterm infants published by his group.[4] These data are supported by those of Speer *et al.* in which early multiple dose im vitamin E decreased the incidence and severity of periventricular hemorrhage.[5] Additionally, Chiswick *et al.* have presented new data using historical controls to substantiate the efficacy of single dose im vitamin E.[6] These data emphasize that efficacy of parenteral vitamin E can be demonstrated at low plasma vitamin E levels (1.4 mg%) when administered early (within two hours following birth).

Despite these favorable results, most neonatologists are hesitant to introduce vitamin E supplementation protocols to prevent the occurrence of periventricular hemorrhage[4-6] or to suppress the development of retinopathy of prematurity.[7-9] This reluctance is based upon multiple published reports of vitamin E toxicities that are all avoidable.

The route of administration is critical for obtaining efficacy without toxicity. Usage of parenteral vitamin E to prevent the occurrence of periventricular hemorrhage has been discouraged by data published by Rosenbaum *et al.*[3] In this trial, rapid iv vitamin E (over 30 to 60 minutes) was used. When vitamin E levels ≥ 6 mg% were measured, there was an increased incidence of early retinal hemorrhages and intraventricular hemorrhage. This vitamin E toxicity is felt to be due to a vitamin E competition with vitamin K and creation of a bleeding diathesis in the first 72 hours following birth (which coincides with the occurrence of 85% of all intraventricular hemorrhages in preterm infants).

205

The dose, as reflected in the targeted level of vitamin E, is also critical for obtaining efficacy without toxicity. In the clinical trial of Johnson et al.,[2] im and slow iv vitamin E (over 4 to 8 hours) were used to target a minimal vitamin E level of 5 mg%. When vitamin E levels ≥ 5 mg% were maintained for prolonged periods, there was an increased incidence of sepsis and necrotizing enterocolitis. This vitamin E toxicity is felt to be due to a vitamin E effect on macrophages.

All other reported vitamin E toxicities are related to product composition: oral Aquasol E (hyperosmolality and/or toxicity of propylene glycol resulted in necrotizing enterocolitis);[10] im E-Vicotrat (toxicity of polysorbate 80 produced transient calcification of thigh muscle);[11,12] iv E-Ferol (toxicity of polysorbates 80 and 20 resulted in hepatic failure, renal failure, and death);[13,14] and iv MVI-Pediatric (toxicity of polysorbates 80 and 20 requires the reduction of the daily dose in infants weighing ≤ 1000 grams at birth).[15]

When all of the reported toxicities of vitamin E in the preterm infant are understood to be preventable, an appropriately formulated vitamin E preparation can be employed as a useful adjunct to decrease the incidence and severity of intraventricular hemorrhage and retinopathy of prematurity.

REFERENCES

1. FARRELL, P. M. 1979. Vitamin E deficiency in preterm infants. J. Pediatr. **95:** 869-872.
2. JOHNSON, L., F. W. BOWEN, S. ABBASI et al. 1985. Relationship of prolonged pharmacologic serum levels of vitamin E to incidence of sepsis and necrotizing enterocolitis in infants with birth weight 1,500 grams or less. Pediatrics **75:** 619-638.
3. ROSENBAUM, A. L., D. L. PHELPS, S. J. ISENBERG, R. D. LEAKE & F. DOREY. 1985. Retinal hemorrhage in retinopathy of prematurity associated with tocopherol treatment. Ophthalmology **92:** 1012-1014.
4. SINHA, S. K., D. G. SIMS, J. M. DAVIES & M. L. CHISWICK. 1985. Relation between periventricular hemorrhage and ischemic brain lesions diagnosed by ultrasound in very pre-term infants. Lancet **2:** 1154-1156.
5. CHISWICK, M., G. GLADMAN, S. SINHA, T. TONER & J. DAVIES. 1989. Prophylaxis of periventricular hemorrhage in preterm babies by vitamin E supplementation. This volume.
6. SPEER, M. E., C. BLIFELD, A. J. RUDOLPH, P. CHADDA, M. E. B. HOLBEIN & H. M. HITTNER. 1984. Intraventricular hemorrhage and vitamin E in the very low birth weight infant: Evidence for efficacy of early intramuscular administration. Pediatrics **74:** 1107-1112.
7. HITTNER, H. M., L. B. GODIO, A. J. RUDOLPH et al. 1981. Retrolental fibroplasia: Efficacy of vitamin E in a double-blind clinical study of preterm infants. N. Eng. J. Med. **305:** 1365-1371.
8. FINER, N. N., G. GRANT, R. F. SCHINDLER, G. B. HILL & K. L. PETERS. 1982. Effect of intramuscular vitamin E on frequency and severity of retrolental fibroplasia: a controlled trial. Lancet **1:** 1087-1091.
9. JOHNSON, L., G. E. QUINN, S. ABBASI et al. 1989. Effect of sustained pharmacologic vitamin E levels on incidence and severity of retinopathy of prematurity: A controlled clinical trial. J. Pediatr. **114:** 827-838.
10. FINER, N. N., K. L. PETERS, Z. HAYEK & C. L. MERKEL. 1984. Vitamin E and necrotizing enterocolitis. Pediatrics **73:** 387-393.
11. SCHRODER, H., M. SCHULZ & K. AEISSEN. 1984. Muscular calcification following injection of vitamin E in newborn infants. Eur. J. Pediatr. **142:** 145-146.
12. SMITH, I. J., M. F. G. BUCHANAN, I. GOSS & P. J. CONGDON. 1983. Correspondence: Vitamin E in retrolental fibroplasia. N. Eng. J. Med. **309:** 669.

13. BOVE, K. E., N. KOSMETATOS, K. E. WEDIG *et al.* 1985. Vasculopathic hepatotoxicity associated with E-Ferol syndrome in low-birth-weight infants. J. Am. Med. Assoc. **254:** 2422-2430.
14. ALADE, S. L., R. E. BROWN & A. PAQUET. 1986. Polysorbate 80 and E-Ferol toxicity. Pediatrics **77:** 593-597.
15. HITTNER, H. M. & F. L. KRETZER. 1986. Toxicity of vitamin E in preterm infants. *In* Retinopathy of Prematurity: Current Concepts and Controversies. A. R. McPherson, H. M. Hittner & F. L. Kretzer, Eds.: **11:** 111-116. B. C. Decker, Inc. Toronto.

The Protective Effect of Administered α-Tocopherol against Hepatic Damage Caused by Ischemia-Reperfusion or Endotoxemia

SEIJI MARUBAYASHI,[a,b] KIYOHIKO DOHI,[a]
KEIZO SUGINO,[a,b] AND TAKASHI KAWASAKI[b,c]

[a] *Department of Surgery*
[b] *Department of Biochemistry*
Hiroshima University School of Medicine
1-2-3 Kasumi
Hiroshima 734, Japan

Metabolic events occurring in shock have been regarded as secondary effects due to decreased tissue perfusion leading to generalized cellular hypoxia, ischemia, and, finally, organ damage. Ischemia-reperfusion causes functional and structural damage to liver and kidney cells.[1-7] Among the various functional disorders, the status of energy metabolism is important for predicting the viability of ischemic organs. Defective energy metabolism in the liver has been also implicated in the development of the irreversible stage of shock.[6] Our recent studies[3,7] have provided evidence showing that the ability of rat liver cells to reverse the mitochondrial dysfunction caused by ischemia-reperfusion is correlated with the ability of the tissue to reverse the cell injury. This finding was obtained from experiments in which coenzyme Q_{10} (CoQ_{10}) pretreatment of ischemic rats was able to completely reverse impaired mitochondrial function by suppressing the increase in lipid peroxide, in both the mitochondria and tissue after reperfusion. The treatment was accompanied by a marked increase in the survival rate of ischemic rats. A similar protective effect of CoQ_{10} was also found in our laboratory in model experiments using rat kidney ischemia-reperfusion[5] and experimental endotoxin shock (endotoxemia) in mice.[8,9] These results suggested that cellular damage caused by either ischemia-reperfusion or endotoxemia may be explained by lipid peroxide formation, and may support the assumption that both preservation for transplantation and endotoxin-induced cell injury would be improved by modifying free radical metabolism and subsequent lipid peroxidation. The antioxidant activity of administered CoQ_{10} was demonstrated *in vivo* for the first time in these experiments.[3-9]

α-Tocopherol (α-Toc) functions *in vivo* as a chain-breaking antioxidant.[10,11] α-Toc has been reported to protect ischemic myocardium and is effective in lessening acute pathologic changes observed in mouse and rat heart.[12] No evidence has been obtained,

[c]To whom correspondence should be addressed.

however, to evaluate the effect of α-Toc treatment on cellular damage caused by ischemia of the liver and kidney, or endotoxemia. In our recent studies,[9,13,14] evidence was presented showing that α-Toc modified cellular free radical metabolism to prevent cellular injury in the case of ischemia-reperfusion or endotoxemia. This was supported by analysis of the levels of cellular antioxidants, α-Toc, CoQ homologues, and reduced glutathione (GSH), and of the protective effect of α-Toc treatment on these levels.[9,13,14]

MATERIAL AND METHODS

Preparation of Ischemic Rat Kidney

The kidneys of male Wistar rats weighing 300-350 g were skeletonized, and the left and right renal arteries, veins, and ureters were clamped.[5] At the end of the ischemic period, the clamps on the left kidney were released to start blood reperfusion, and then the right kidney was removed. α-Toc was administered intraperitoneal at a dose of 10 mg/kg body weight/day for 7 days before the operation, resulting in an approximate twofold increase in the tissue α-Toc content. As a placebo, solvent was injected in the same volume as that of the reagent.

Preparation of Ischemic Rat Liver

The livers of male Wistar rats weighing 250-300 g were made ischemic, and blood reperfusion was effected after various ischemic periods. Total hepatic ischemia was induced by clamping the hepatic artery, portal vein, and bile duct. A portafemoral shunt was made by connecting a branch of the portal vein to the left femoral vein with a polyethylene tube before ischemia, as described previously.[4,7,13,14] α-Toc was administered intraperitoneally by injection at 10 mg/kg body weight per day for 3 days before induction of ischemia. This resulted in a 2.74- and 1.82-fold increase in the content of α-Toc in the liver tissue and mitochondria, respectively. The solvent of the agent was also injected in the same manner as a placebo.

Preparation of Experimental Endotoxemia in Mice

Lipopolysaccharide (LPS; Difco, *E. coli* 055-B5) was administered intraperitoneally to ICR mice at a dose of 30 mg/kg body weight. α-Toc at a dose of 20 mg/kg body weight was injected intravenously just after LPS administration.

Measurement of Adenine Nucleotides

Adenine nucleotides were determined either enzymatically[4,5,7] in the experimental ischemia of rat kidney and liver or by high-performance liquid chromatography[8,9] in the case of endotoxemia in mice.

Assay of Lipid Peroxide

The measurement of lipid peroxide by a colorimetric reaction with thiobarbituric acid was carried out as previously described.[6,7,13]

Determination of α-Toc, CoQ_{10} and CoQ_9

Simultaneous determination of α-Toc and of oxidized and reduced CoQ homologue (CoQ_9 and CoQ_{10}) in liver tissue and mitochondria was carried out according to the method of Takada et al.[15]

Determination of Glutathione

Total glutathione, reduced glutathione (GSH), plus oxidized glutathione (GSSG) was measured using the method of Tietze,[16] as modified by Griffith.[17] Determination of GSSG was carried out by the recirculating assay method described by Griffith after GSH had been allowed to react with 2-vinylpyridine.[17]

Chemicals

α-Toc, CoQ_{10}, CoQ_9, and their solvents were obtained from the Eisai Co., Tokyo. Other chemicals were of analytical grade.

RESULTS AND DISCUSSION

Kidney Ischemia and Reperfusion

A preliminary experiment on ischemic damage in rat kidney had revealed that the rate and extent of adenosine triphosphate (ATP) resynthesis after reperfusion following ischemia determines the viability of the organ and is directly correlated with the survival rate.[18] This was confirmed by the present experiment and further supported by the protective effect of α-Toc pretreatment on the reperfusion injury in rat kidney ischemia.

Although ischemia of the rat kidney for 120 min did not permit survival of the animals (0/14), approximately one-half of the ischemic rats survived in the group administered α-Toc (7/15). Ischemia itself reduced the ATP level in the kidney tissue without any protective effect of α-Toc administration, whereas administration of α-Toc increased ATP resynthesis after 120 min of ischemia and reperfusion (FIG. 1). It should be emphasized that the effect of α-Toc was observed only after restoration of blood flow following ischemia for 120 min but not after ischemia itself.

Liver Ischemia and Reperfusion

Survival Rate and the Levels of Adenine Nucleotide and Lipid Peroxide after Hepatic Ischemia

In the case of liver, total ischemia for 90 min did not permit survival of the animals in the placebo group, whereas pretreatment with α-Toc increased the survival rate to 45.5% (5/11). When ischemia was prolonged to 120 min, no survival was observed even in the α-Toc-treated group (0/8).

The ability of α-Toc administration to restore the decreased hepatic energy metabolism after 90 min of ischemia and reperfusion is shown in FIGURE 2, in which α-Toc pretreatment enhanced the ATP level markedly without affecting the reduced level of ATP during ischemia or the rate and extent of ATP recovery after reflow

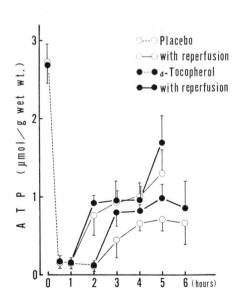

FIGURE 1. Effect of α-tocopherol pretreatment on renal ATP level after ischemia and reperfusion. In the placebo rats, solvent for α-Toc preparation was injected into control rats in the same volume and manner as α-Toc. Renal blood flow was started 1 and 2 h after ischemia, and ATP level was determined. Values are mean ± SD of five to eight samples.

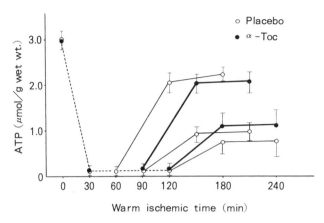

FIGURE 2. Effect of α-tocopherol pretreatment on hepatic ATP level after ischemia and subsequent reperfusion. In the placebo rats, solvent for α-Toc preparation was injected into control rats in the same volume and manner as α-Toc. Hepatic blood flow was started 60, 90, and 120 min after ischemia, and ATP level was determined. Solid line indicates ATP levels after reperfusion after ischemia; dashed line indicates ATP levels after ischemia. Each point represents mean ± SD of five separate experiments.

following 60 min of ischemia. The administration of α-Toc failed to improve the greatly decreased resynthesis of ATP after reflow following 2 h of ischemia.

The restorative effect of α-Toc on energy metabolism in the liver subjected to ischemia-reperfusion is explained by its antioxidant action. Although the level of malondialdehyde (MDA), which is derived from lipid peroxides, in the liver tissue remained relatively steady during the ischemic period, reperfusion following 90 min of ischemia resulted in a twofold increase in the MDA level, and α-Toc treatment completely suppressed this marked MDA elevation (TABLE 1). It should be emphasized that the protective effect of α-Toc treatment was obtained with rats not subjected to α-Toc deficiency, because it has been reported in review that the effect of α-Toc

TABLE 1. Effect of α-Tocopherol Administration on the Level of Liver Tissue Malondialdehyde (MDA)

Ischemia (min)	Reflow (min)	MDA (nmol/mg protein)
Placebo (n = 5)		
0[a]		0.76 ± 0.22
90	—	0.90 ± 0.20[b]
90	60	1.79 ± 0.27[b,c]
α-Toc-treated (n = 5)		
0		0.55 ± 0.11
90	—	0.82 ± 0.21
90	60	0.74 ± 0.19[c]

[a] Rats underwent sham operation.
[b,c] $p < 0.001$.

and other antioxidants on oxidative cellular damage usually gives disappointing results, and is seen only when tissue α-Toc levels are low.[19]

Changes in the Levels of α-Toc, CoQ Homologs, and GSH in Hepatic Ischemia and Reperfusion

The levels of endogenous antioxidants, α-Toc, CoQ homologues, and GSH were measured to examine the assumption that cellular damage caused by hepatic ischemia-reperfusion is due to formation of free radicals and subsequently produced lipid peroxides.

Liver tissue and mitochondrial α-Toc were decreased by 19% and 27%, respec-

TABLE 2. α-Tocopherol and CoQ Homologues in Liver Mitochondria during Ischemia and Reperfusion and the Effect of Pretreatment with α-Tocopherol

Treatment		α-Tocopherol (ng/mg protein)	$CoQ_9{}^a$ (ng/mg protein)	$CoQ_{10}{}^a$ (ng/mg protein)
Ischemia (min)	Reflow (min)			
Placebo (n = 5)				
0^b		187 ± 12.6^c	939 ± 93.5	129 ± 9.39
90	—	$136 \pm 21.7^{c,d}$	899 ± 84.5^e	133 ± 14.5^f
90	60	82.3 ± 22.4^d	$606 \pm 97.4^{e,g}$	$95.1 \pm 5.41^{f,h}$
α-Toc-treated (n = 6)				
0		340 ± 23.0	1036 ± 61.3	127 ± 15.2
90	—	308 ± 28.4	987 ± 77.9	123 ± 14.2
90	60	306 ± 23.8	962 ± 79.0^g	132 ± 6.65^h

^{a} CoQ_9 and CoQ_{10} represent total (oxidized and reduced) content of each CoQ homologue.
^{b} Rats received sham operation.
^{c,d,f,g,h} $p < 0.001$.
^{e} $p < 0.01$.

tively, during 90 min of ischemia, together with a 20% reduction in tissue GSH content, whereas tissue and mitochondrial total CoQ homologues remained constant during the same period. After reperfusion, all these antioxidants, including CoQ homologues were decreased by more than 30 percent. Pretreatment with α-Toc maintained the levels of liver mitochondrial α-Toc 1.8-fold higher than the basal level and prevented any decrease in CoQ homologues in the tissue and mitochondria and also any decrease of GSH during the reperfusion period (TABLES 2 and 3).

Based on these results, it is proposed that the decreases in cellular α-Toc and GSH in the process of ischemia, followed by marked decreases in cellular antioxidants tested during the reperfusion period, may indicate that free radical reactions are initiated in the process of ischemia and subsequent peroxidative processes occurring after reperfusion. The cooperative action of these endogenous antioxidants to scavenge free radicals and lipid peroxides, however, seems to be overwhelmed by stimulation of lipid peroxidation, so that the tissue and mitochondrial lipid peroxides are increased

TABLE 3. Concentration of Total and Oxidized Glutathione in Liver Tissue during Hepatic Ischemia and Reperfusion and the Effect of α-Tocopherol Administration

Treatment			
Ischemia (min)	Reflow (min)	GSH + GSSG (μmol/g liver)	GSSG (μmol/g liver)
Placebo (n = 5)			
0^a		7.17 ± 0.48^b	0.103 ± 0.007^c
90	—	$5.86 \pm 0.55^{b,d}$	0.116 ± 0.006^c
90	60	$4.24 \pm 0.51^{d,g}$	0.109 ± 0.011
α-Toc-treated (n = 5)			
0		6.93 ± 0.59^e	0.103 ± 0.008^f
90	—	5.91 ± 0.62^e	0.128 ± 0.011^f
90	60	5.50 ± 0.52^g	0.122 ± 0.014

[a] Rats received sham operation.
[b,d,f,g] $p < 0.001$.
[c] $p < 0.01$.
[e] $p < 0.05$.

only after blood restoration. This assumption was supported by Adkinson et al.[20] The observed reduction in GSH during ischemia-reperfusion was not accompanied by a reciprocal increase in GSSG (TABLE 3), suggesting that glutathione peroxidase, an important cellular antioxidant, is not involved in the prevention of cell damage. It is noteworthy that the protective effect of α-Toc pretreatment was quite similar to that of CoQ_{10}.[3,7,13,14] Administration of exogenous α-Toc and CoQ_{10} reversed the increase in lipid peroxidation, which lowered the consumption of lipid-soluble antioxidants as well as that of the water-soluble antioxidant, GSH, during reperfusion (TABLES 2 and 3).

Restoration of blood flow to previously ischemic organs causes a rapid increase in tissue oxygen tension, which promotes lipid peroxidation after initiation of free radical reactions during ischemia (FIG. 3). The mechanism leading to cellular damage caused by hepatic ischemia-reperfusion is tentatively presented in FIGURE 3.

Experimental Endotoxin Shock: Endotoxemia

The Survival Rate, and Levels of Hepatic Lipid Peroxide and ATP in Mice Subjected to Endotoxemia

Endotoxin shock results from toxication due to bacterial LPS, which leads to hypotension, decreased tissue blood perfusion, cellular hypoxia, that is, an incomplete ischemia, and finally cell damage. Cellular injury caused by endotoxin shock is therefore considered to be at least partly similar to that occurring in hepatic ischemia-reperfusion. Experimental endotoxin shock or, more correctly, endotoxemia, was induced in mice to determine whether lipid peroxidation plays an important role in the mechanism of cellular damage and whether α-Toc treatment protects the liver from endotoxemic damage.

No survival was found 48 h after LPS (30 mg/kg body weight) administration, although a survival rate of 43% (9/12) was found at 24 hours. Simultaneous administration of α-Toc with LPS restored the survival rates of the affected mice to 91.4% (32/35) and 42.9% (15/35), respectively, 24 and 48 h after administration.

The hepatic ATP level decreased gradually to 65% that of the control 24 h after LPS administration in the placebo group, and administration of α-Toc restored the level of ATP to the control level.

The level of lipid peroxide, which was determined as MDA, was increased 3.4-fold in the liver 8 h after LPS administration, and then gradually decreased to the control level in the next 16 hours. Treatment with α-Toc suppressed the hepatic MDA level completely to within the normal range up to 24 hours.

These results suggest that the transient stimulation of lipid peroxidation observed after injection of LPS may be a trigger for inducing cellular damage, resulting in a decrease in ATP synthesis and, finally, a decrease in the survival rate.

Changes in α-Toc, CoQ₉, and Glutathione in the Liver of Mice Given LPS

The contents of CoQ homologues and α-Toc in normal mouse liver are (in ng/mg protein): CoQ_9 (oxidized), 126; CoQ_9H_2 (reduced), 184; CoQ_{10}, 4.0; $CoQ_{10}H_2$, not detectable; α-Toc, 43.6. This indicates that the predominant homologue in mouse liver is CoQ_9 and that 60% of CoQ_9 exists in the reduced form.

The levels of endogenous α-Toc and CoQ_9H_2 were decreased to half of the control levels 8 h after LPS injection, when a maximal increase in hepatic MDA level was detected in the placebo group (TABLE 4), suggesting consumption of these antioxidants for the scavenging of free radicals or peroxy radicals. The content of α-Toc in the

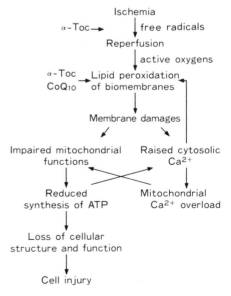

FIGURE 3. Schematic representation of the sequence of the events leading to ischemic cell injury.

TABLE 4. Effect of α-Tocopherol on Reduced CoQ_9 and α-Tocopherol Levels in Endotoxemic Liver

Treatment (h)	Reduced CoQ_9 (ng/mg protein)	α-Tocopherol (ng/mg protein)
Control	275 ± 39.8	52.7 ± 8.9
Placebo-treated		
8	126 ± 18.6[a]	33.0 ± 7.5[b]
16	149 ± 23.8[a]	19.0 ± 3.4[b]
24	128 ± 31.6[a]	18.9 ± 5.0[b]
α-Toc-treated		
8	268 ± 21.5[c]	4464 ± 568
16	247 ± 55.2[c]	782 ± 373
24	232 ± 80.7[c]	475 ± 62

[a,b] Significantly different from control ($p < 0.01$).
[c] Significantly different from placebo-treated group ($p < 0.01$). Results are mean ± SD of five to seven determinations.

liver was increased 84-fold after intravenous injection of α-Toc (20 mg/kg body weight) and then decreased rapidly. The high level of administered α-Toc provided protection against a decrease of endogenous CoQ_9H_2 in the endotoxemic liver. Endogenous GSH was decreased for up to 8 h, with a reciprocal increase of GSSG in the placebo group. Total glutathione, therefore, remained constant, suggesting the involvement of a GSH-GSH peroxidase system for maintaining the level of total glutathione during this period. Total glutathione, however, was decreased at 16 and 24 h due to a decrease in GSSG, suggesting possible inactivation of the peroxidase system during this period. α-Toc treatment gave significant protection against the decrease in total and reduced glutathione levels at 16 and 24 h (TABLE 5). The mechanism of LPS action leading to cellular damage is tentatively postulated in FIGURE 4.

TABLE 5. Effect of α-Tocopherol on Glutathione Levels in Endotoxemic Liver

Treatment (h)	GSH + GSSG	GSH (nmol/mg protein)	GSSG
Control	30.0 ± 3.5	28.2 ± 3.2	1.8 ± 0.7
Placebo-treated			
4	26.7 ± 5.4	15.4 ± 3.9[a]	11.3 ± 2.2[a]
8	23.2 ± 2.4	12.9 ± 2.5[a]	10.3 ± 2.8[a]
16	16.9 ± 1.9[a]	13.3 ± 1.7[a]	3.6 ± 0.9
24	17.2 ± 3.4[a]	14.6 ± 2.8[a]	2.6 ± 0.8
α-Toc-treated			
4	25.5 ± 4.0	16.0 ± 2.3[b]	9.5 ± 2.1[b]
8	25.1 ± 4.1	12.4 ± 3.9[b]	12.7 ± 3.4[b]
16	26.8 ± 7.9[c]	22.4 ± 7.4[d]	4.4 ± 1.5
24	24.8 ± 5.4[c]	21.6 ± 5.3[d]	3.2 ± 0.3

[a,b] Significantly different from control ($p < 0.01$).
[c,d] Significantly different from placebo-treated group ($p < 0.01$). Results are mean ± SD of at least 6 experiments.

The mechanism of α-Toc inhibition of peroxidative damage to membrane lipids *in vitro* has been suggested to be scavenging of lipid peroxyl radicals,[10] and another postulated a role of cellular α-Toc in the maintenance of intracellular GSH as a mechanism of prevention of cell injury *in vitro*.[21] It has been proposed that hydroxyl radicals induce cellular damage under oxidative stress through direct action on proteins, lipids, and nucleic acids,[19,22] and lipid peroxidation as a cause of oxidative cellular injury has been explained as a late event occurring only at the point of cell death.[19] The results described in this paper clearly demonstrate that cellular or organ viability remains at least partially reversible under conditions in which an increase in lipid peroxidation is detectable in both hepatic ischemia-reperfusion and endotoxemia in experimental animals. Although the effect of cellular antioxidants, α-Toc or CoQ₁₀, on oxidative cellular injury has been questioned,[19] our results showing the protective

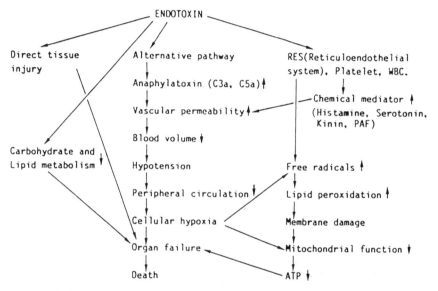

FIGURE 4. A scheme postulated for the mechanism of endotoxin shock, especially in the relation to lipid peroxidation. WBC = white blood cells; PAF = platelet-activating factor.

effect of α-Toc and CoQ₁₀ pretreatment against both postischemic and endotoxemic damage emphasize the usefulness of these antioxidants for clinical applications such as protection against organ damage during transplantation.

REFERENCES

1. McCord, J. M. 1985. Oxygen-derived free radicals in postischemic tissue injury. N. Engl. J. Med. **312:** 159-163.
2. Chien, K. R., J. Abrams, A. Serroni, J. T. Martin & J. L. Farber. 1978. Accelerated phospholipid degradation and associated membrane dysfunction in irreversible, ischemic liver cell injury. J. Biol. Chem. **253:** 4809-4817.

3. KAWASAKI, T., K. HAYASHI, S. MARUBAYASHI & K. DOHI. 1981. Preservation of mitochondrial functions, energy metabolism and viability of ischemic liver by coenzyme Q_{10} pretreatment. *In* Biomedical and Clinical Aspects of Coenzyme Q_{10}. K. Folkers & Y. Yamamura, Eds.: Vol. 3: 337-348. Elsevier. Amsterdam.

4. MARUBAYASHI, S., M. TAKENAKA, K. DOHI, H. EZAKI & T. KAWASAKI. 1980. Adenine nucleotide metabolism during hepatic ischemia and subsequent blood reflow periods and its relation to organ viability. Transplantation **30:** 294-296.

5. TAKENAKA, M., Y. TATSUKAWA, K. DOHI, H. EZAKI, K. MATSUKAWA & T. KAWASAKI. 1981. Protective effects of α-tocopherol and coenzyme Q_{10} on warm ischemic damages of the rat kidney. Transplantation **32:** 137-141.

6. KAWASAKI, T. & S. MARUBAYASHI. 1986. Liver in shock. *In* Treatment of Shock. J. M. Barrett & L. M. Nyhus, Eds.: 2nd Ed.: 151-162. Lea & Febiger. Philadelphia.

7. MARUBAYASHI, S., K. DOHI, H. EZAKI, K. HAYASHI & T. KAWASAKI. 1982. Preservation of ischemic rat liver mitochondrial functions and liver viability with CoQ_{10}. Surgery **91:** 631-637.

8. SUGINO, K., K. DOHI, K. YAMADA & T. KAWASAKI. 1987. The role of lipid peroxidation in endotoxin-induced hepatic damage and the protective effect of antioxidants. Surgery **101:** 746-752.

9. SUGINO, K., K. DOHI, K. YAMADA & T. KAWASAKI. 1989. Changes in the levels of endogenous antioxidants in the liver of mice with experimental endotoxemia and the protective effects of the antioxidants. Surgery. **105:** 200-206.

10. NIKI, E. 1987. Antioxidants in relation to lipid peroxidation. Chem. Phys. Lipids **44:** 227-253.

11. MACAY, P. B. & M. M. KING. 1980. Vitamin E: Its role as a biologic free radical scavenger and its relationship to the microsomal mixed-function oxidase system. *In* Vitamin E. L. J. Machlin, Ed.: 289-317. Marcel Dekker Inc. New York.

12. SONNEVELD, P. 1978. Effect of α-tocopherol on the cardiotoxicity of Adriamycin in the rat. Cancer Treat. Rep. **62:** 1033-1036.

13. MARUBAYASHI, S., K. DOHI, K. OCHI & T. KAWASAKI. 1986. Role of free radicals in ischemic rat liver cell injury. Prevention of damage by α-tocopherol administration. Surgery **99:** 184-191.

14. MARUBAYASHI, S., K. DOHI, K. YAMADA & T. KAWASAKI. 1984. Changes in the levels of endogenous coenzyme Q homologs, α-tocopherol, and glutathione in rat liver after hepatic ischemia and reperfusion, and the effect of pretreatment with coenzyme Q_{10}. Biochim. Biophys. Acta **797:** 1-9.

15. TAKADA, M., S. IKENOYA, T. YUZURIHA & K. KATAYAMA. 1982. Studies on reduced and oxidized coenzyme Q (ubiquinones). Biochim. Biophys. Acta **679:** 308-314.

16. TIETZE, F. 1969. Enzymic method for quantitative determination of nanogram amounts of total and oxidized glutathione. Anal. Biochem. **27:** 502-522.

17. GRIFFITH, O. W. 1980. Determination of glutathione and glutathione disulfide using glutathione reductase and 2-vinylpyridine. Anal. Biochem. **106:** 207-212.

18. TATSUKAWA, Y., K. DOHI, K. YAMADA & T. KAWASAKI. 1979. The role of CoQ_{10} for the preservation of the rat kidney. Life Sci. **24:** 1309-1314.

19. HALLIWELL, B. 1987. Oxidants and human disease: some new concepts. FASEB J. **1:** 358-364.

20. ADKINSON, D., M. E. HOLLWARTH, J. N. BENOIT, D. A. PARKS, J. M. MCCORD & D. N. GRANGER. 1986. Role of free radicals in ischemia-reperfusion injury to the liver. Acta Physiol. Scand. **548:** 101-107.

21. PASCOE, G. A., M. W. FARISS, K. OLAFSDOTTIR & D. J. REED. 1987. A role of vitamin E in protection against cell injury. Maintenance of intracellular glutathione precursors and biosynthesis. Eur. J. Biochem. **166:** 241-247.

22. HALLIWELL, B. & J. M. C. GUTTERIDGE. 1986. Iron and free radical reactions: two aspects of antioxidant protection. Trends Biochem. Sci. **11:** 372-375.

Brain Injury after Ischemia and Trauma

The Role of Vitamin E

SHINICHI YOSHIDA[a]

Department of Neurosurgery
Kanto Rosai Hospital
Kawasaki, Japan

INTRODUCTION

The abrupt interruption of the circulation to the brain (acute cerebral ischemia) produces an impairment of function, metabolism, and structure in a time-dependent manner. It is currently thought that the progression of metabolic and structural derangements during an ischemic period are the primary factors influencing the course of postischemic events. Thus, the shorter the ischemic duration, the better the brain recovers. It has become increasingly evident in more recent literature, however, that brain injury caused by transient global ischemia is incurred, in part, during the period of subsequent recirculation.[1] The role played by postischemic events in affecting outcome is of clinical significance inasmuch as most patients with acute cerebral ischemia do not receive medical attention within the first few hours of their insult. The mechanisms by which the ischemic insult perpetuates itself during the recirculation period, however, are largely unknown.

Lipid peroxidation by free radical reactions has been considered as a basic deteriorative process in a variety of chronic pathological conditions, such as aging, atherosclerosis, and the irradiation syndrome. In the central nervous system, however, it was relatively recent that free radical mechanisms were incriminated in the causation of acute damage. In 1977, Demopoulos, Flamm, and their collaborators[2-4] have proposed that free radical damage occurs in regional cerebral ischemia and spinal cord trauma. Their proposal was based on the following experimental findings: (1) Ischemia due to sustained middle cerebral artery occlusion as well as spinal cord trauma results in a gradual decrease in the tissue levels of ascorbic acid and cholesterol (consumption of endogenous antioxidants), together with a decrease in the tissue levels of phospholipid-bound polyunsaturated fatty acids (PUFA) (the main target of free radicals). (2) Methohexital, a barbiturate, prevents these changes, presumably, by acting as a free radical scavenger.

[a]Address correspondence to Shinichi Yoshida, Department of Neurosurgery, Kanto Rosai Hospital, Kizuki Sumiyoshi-cho 2035, Nakahara-ku, Kawasaki-shi, 211, Japan.

INTRAISCHEMIC VERSUS POSTISCHEMIC LIPID PEROXIDATION

Several groups that were inspired by the hypothesis quoted pursued the issue. We studied the effect of temporary forebrain ischemia on levels of free fatty acids, lipid peroxides, and phospholipids in the brain.[5] During ischemia, both saturated and unsaturated free fatty acids increased strikingly to approximately 11-fold in total by 30 minutes (FIG. 1). During recirculation, a rapid decrement occurred in free arachidonic acid, whereas saturated and monounsaturated free fatty acids slowly decreased to their basal levels in 180 minutes. The peroxide level, estimated by a thiobarbituric acid (TBA) test, did not change during ischemia, but was elevated transiently during reperfusion (FIG. 2). Phosphatidylethanolamine content decreased by 10-16% and phosphatidylcholine did not change significantly throughout the periods examined

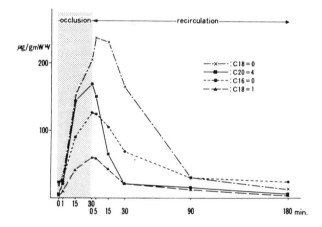

FIGURE 1. The effects of bilateral carotid occlusion and reperfusion on individual free fatty acids in gerbil brain. The mean values of six animals are presented at each time period. C18=0: stearic acid; C20=4: arachidonic acid; C16=0: palmitic acid; C18=1: oleic acid. (Yoshida *et al.*[5] With permission from the *Journal of Neurosurgery.*)

(FIG. 3). Our results indicated that diffuse cerebral ischemia disintegrates membrane phospholipids, probably by the action of phospholipases, and that peroxidative reactions take place during reflow by means of restoration of oxygen supply. Demopoulos, Flamm, and their collaborators considered that free radicals (coenzyme Q radical) are dislocated due to the lack of oxygen at the terminus of the mitochondrial respiratory chain and initiate the radical reaction. They postulated that oxygen molecules required for the chain propagation of peroxidative processes are sufficiently present in regional ischemia (intraischemic lipid peroxidation). By contrast, our results suggested that reperfusion following ischemia could favor formation of free radicals and active oxygen species, owing to incomplete reduction of oxygen molecules at a time when tissue oxygen tension rises to a level higher than normal (FIG. 4).[6] This postischemic lipid peroxidation was originally hypothesized by Siesjö[7] and Kogure and his collaborators.[8]

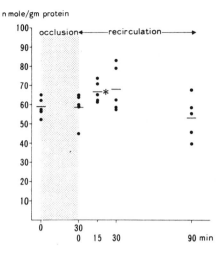

FIGURE 2. The effects of bilateral carotid occlusion and reperfusion on the levels of malonyldialdehyde precursors measured by a thiobarbituric acid test in gerbil brain. Each point represent one animal. The mean values are shown by horizontal lines. The symbol * indicates statistically significant differences from the control values, $p < 0.05$. (Yoshida et al.[5] With permission from the *Journal of Neurosurgery*.)

ORIGIN AND FATE OF FREE ARACHIDONIC ACID

Polyphosphoinositides in the brain, uniquely rich in arachidonate and stearate, decrease in amount after decapitation.[9] Brain free fatty acids, arachidonic acid, and stearic acid, in particular, increase rapidly after decapitation.[10] Brain diacylglycerols enriched in arachidonate and stearate also increase after decapitation.[11] We have recently found that the decrease in polyphosphoinositides is sufficient to account for the increase in arachidonate and stearate in the pools of diacylglycerol and free fatty

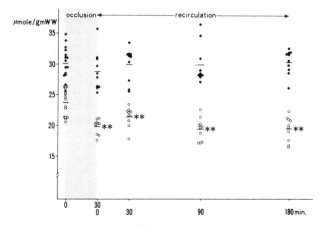

FIGURE 3. The effects of bilateral carotid occlusion and reperfusion on brain phosphatidylcholine (black circle) and phosphatidylethanolamine (white circle) in gerbils. Each point represents one animal. The mean values are shown by horizontal lines. The symbol ** indicates significant differences from the control values, $p < 0.01$. (Yoshida et al.[5] With permission from the *Journal of Neurosurgery*.)

acid during the early periods of *in vivo* ischemia as well as of decapitation ischemia.[12,13] Thus, it is very likely that polyphosphoinositides are degraded by the action of phospholipase C to yield diacylglycerols and inositol phosphates, and the diacylglycerols, thus produced, are further hydrolized by lipases to release free arachidonic acid and stearic acid. Other possible sources of free arachidonic acid in ischemia include phosphatidylcholine,[14,15] phosphatidylethanolamine,[16] and phosphatidylinositol.[14] Because energy failure incapacitates the resynthesis of phospholipids, free fatty acids accumulate during ischemia.

As soon as reperfusion provides oxygen to the brain tissue, a portion of free arachidonic acid undergoes enzymatic peroxidation. It has been shown that the tissue levels of cyclooxygenase products, such as prostaglandins and thromboxanes increase markedly upon cerebral recirculation, but not during ischemia.[17,18] Similarly, lipoxygenase products, such as leukotriene C_4 and D_4, increase strikingly in the brain tissue during postischemic reperfusion.[19] Thus, there is unequivocal evidence that cerebral

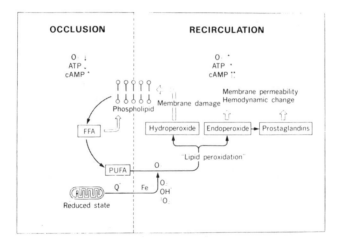

FIGURE 4. Schematic presentation of degradative processes of membrane phospholipids during ischemia and subsequent reperfusion. (Yoshida *et al.*[6] With permission from Igaku-shoin Ltd.)

reperfusion induces enzymatic peroxidation of liberated arachidonic acids to yield biologically active compounds, which may in turn change the permeability of blood vessels and may produce adverse effects. Oxygen radicals are generated at certain steps in the enzymatic, oxidative metabolism of free arachidonic acids.[20] The remaining portion of free arachidonic acid is used in the resynthesis of phospholipids and also incorporated into the acyl residues of triacylglycerol during reflow as the tissue energy state improves.[12] This reacylation seems to be the major fate of free PUFA during reperfusion.

CONTROVERSIES OF FREE RADICAL FORMATION IN CEREBRAL ISCHEMIA

The existence of free radical-mediated lipid peroxidation (nonenzymatic lipid peroxidation) in cerebral ischemia followed by reperfusion has not been unequivocally established and is still questioned. Although several reports[5,21-23] have shown an increased tissue level of lipid peroxides during postischemic reperfusion as measured by a TBA test or conjugated diene formation, the magnitude of increment is often small. Moreover, a failure to observe any change in the tissue level of TBA reactants during and following forebrain ischemia was also documented.[24] In sustained, regional cerebral ischemia, there are no confirmatory reports that have indicated the occurrence of pathological free radical reactions.

Brain parenchymal cells possess nonenzymatic as well as enzymatic defense against free radicals. The alteration of the defense line, if it occurs, will provide the indirect evidence for free radical reactions. The studies of the glutathione system in temporary forebrain ischemia, however, revealed no rise in the tissue level of the oxidized form (GSSG) despite that the level of the reduced form (GSH) fell steadily throughout ischemia and reperfusion.[25,26] Because there was no increase in GSSG, these studies failed to find the evidence for peroxidation. The decrease in GSH during severe ischemia may well be a reflection of anaerobic degradation of the glutathione pool (GSH + GSSG), which is unmatched by the corresponding, energy-dependent re-synthesis. The results on GSH-GSSG are inconclusive, however, because the glutathione reductase reaction coupled with the operation of the phosphogluconate pathway might, at least in theory, achieve instantaneous re-reduction of GSSG when the oxygen supply has been restored.[1] The reason for the continuous decrease in GSH during reperfusion in the face of a rapid recovery of the tissue energy state[27] remains unclear. It is possible that a portion of GSH may have been consumed during reperfusion in the synthesis of leukotrienes that contain a glutathione moiety. In contrast to the results in sustained, regional ischemia reported by Demopoulos, Flamm, and their collaborators,[2,3,4] Cooper and his collaborators[26] found no alteration of the tissue levels of total and reduced ascorbate in temporary forebrain ischemia.

When several barbiturates were tested for the ability to suppress lipid peroxidation *in vitro,* thiopental showed a definite effect, but methohexital had only a small effect, and pentobarbital, as well as phenobarbital, none.[28]

Inasmuch as lipid peroxidation is primarily a membrane phenomenon, it may not be reflected in the behavior of ascorbate and GSH-GSSG that scavenge free radicals or lipid peroxides in hydrophilic intracellular compartments. For this reason, we measured a lipid-soluble antioxidant, namely alpha-tocopherol, in temporary forebrain ischemia.[29] The brain level of alpha-tocopherol tended to decrease during ischemia and decreased further during early recirculation (FIG. 5). Because no mechanisms other than free radical reactions are known to cause a decrease in this vitamin, it is tempting to conclude that free radical chain propagation leading to accumulation of lipid peroxides in levels detectable by currently available methods becomes manifest after circulation is reinstituted (see FIG. 2). Our study, however, is also inconclusive for the occurrence of postischemic peroxidation, because metabolites of alpha-tocopherol, that is, polymers and tocopherol quinone, which would be expected to increase reciprocally, were not measured. We found the decrease in brain alpha-tocopherol even after decapitation-induced complete ischemia.[30,31] It is difficult to explain the decrease in alpha-tocopherol during ischemia at a time when little oxygen should be present in the tissue. Nonetheless, our data suggest that a low level of oxygen radicals may be present in the ischemic brain tissue.

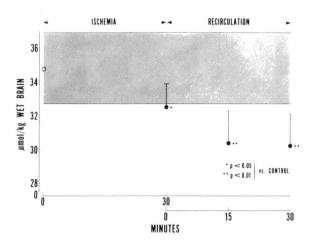

FIGURE 5. The effect of four-vessel occlusion and reperfusion on the levels of alpha-tocopherol in rat brain. Values are means ± standard deviation, and the number of animals is 5-6 at each time period. (Yoshida *et al.*[29] With permission from *Brain Research.*)

CEREBRAL LIPID PEROXIDATION *IN VITRO*

Lipid peroxidation in brain homogenates, in which radical reactions were enhanced by adding ferrous ions and ascorbic acid, was characterized by Rehncrona and his collaborators.[32] Incubation of the homogenate with 5% oxygen caused formation of TBA reactants, diene conjugation, accumulation of fluorescent products, and a loss of phospholipid-bound PUFA. Analysis of phospholipids revealed a decrease in the contents of phosphatidylethanolamine and phosphatidylserine and phosphatidylinositol, but not in phosphatidylcholine. Free radical reactions were accompanied by a fall in GSH and a rise in GSSG content. Incubation with 100% nitrogen resulted in no changes in the indices of lipid peroxidation, but GSH content decreased.[25]

Kogure and his collaborators[21] incubated minced brain under oxygen or nitrogen gas without employing exogenous free radical initiators. Oxygenation of minced brain following decapitation ischemia yielded increased levels of TBA reactants and conjugated dienes, in contrast to anaerobically incubated preparations. Both aerobic and anaerobic incubation of brain minces facilitated a loss of alpha-tocopherol and GSH, but the level of GSSG was unchanged. Thus, lipid peroxidation can be induced by oxygenation of brain tissue *in vitro* without the use of exogenous prooxidants, although the magnitude of the rise in lipid peroxides is smaller than that reported by Rehncrona and his collaborators.[32] Moreover, the results of Kogure's experiments indicate that lipid peroxidation of a moderate degree is not accompanied by accumulation of GSSG. (The control level of GSSG reported by Kogure and his collaborators is several fold higher than the value presented by Rehncrona and his collaborators[25] and Cooper and his collaborators,[26] but is comparable to the value in another study by Rehncrona and his collaborators.[33] Thus, admitting the technical limits of analytical accuracy, a slight possibility is present that the relatively high basal level of GSSG in Kogure's study has masked the actual increase in GSSG content after reoxygenation.)

We studied the effect of postischemic reoxygenation on cerebral lipid peroxidation in relation to the dietary intake of vitamin E.[31] Homogenates prepared from vitamin E-deficient, -normal and -supplemented brains, which were previously rendered ischemic for 30 minutes by decapitation, were incubated under air or nitrogen gas for 60 minutes. The extent of peroxidation in brain tissue was estimated by a TBA test and by diene conjugation in total lipid extracts. The brain level of alpha-tocopherol and total and free fatty acids was also determined. Aerobic incubation increased TBA reactants in all dietary groups (FIG. 6): the effect was largest in the vitamin E-deficient group, intermediate in the vitamin E-normal group, and smallest in the vitamin E-supplemented group. By contrast, nitrogen incubation did not alter the basal level of TBA reactants except for a small rise associated with vitamin E deficiency. Conjugated dienes changed in parallel with TBA reactants (FIG. 7). Alpha-tocopherol decreased after aerobic incubation and also, to a lesser degree, after nitrogen incubation in each dietary-group (FIG. 8). Only in the reoxygenated samples of the vitamin E-deficient group was there a significant fall in total PUFA (TABLE 1). The levels of free fatty acids continuously increased throughout ischemia and subsequent incubation (TABLE 2). The level of free PUFA, however, was similar after aerobic and nitrogen incubation in each dietary group, and was not affected by vitamin E.

Our experiments demonstrate that two catabolic pathways of fatty acyl chains of cerebral phospholipids are operative during ischemia followed by reoxygenation *in vitro*. One is hydrolysis of ester bond, yielding free fatty acids; the other is direct peroxidation of polyunsaturated acyl chains. The former process continues throughout

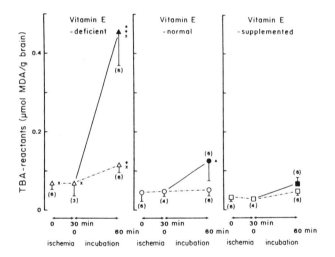

FIGURE 6. Cerebral thiobarbituric acid (TBA) reactants measured as malonyldialdehyde (MDA) after ischemia and subsequent incubation with synthetic air (closed symbols) or nitrogen gas (open symbols) in vitamin E-varied rats. The values are means ± standard deviation; if no bars are shown, the standard deviation falls within the symbol. Numbers of samples are in parentheses. The level of thiobarbituric acid reactants is always higher after aerobic incubation than in controls and after ischemia within each dietary group ($p < 0.01$), but no symbols are shown. *$p < 0.01$ vs. nitrogen incubation in the same dietary group; $^+p < 0.01$ vs. vitamin E-normal group; and $^xp < 0.05$ vs. vitamin E-supplemented group under the comparable experimental condition. (Yoshida *et al.*[31] With permission from the *Journal of Neurochemistry*.)

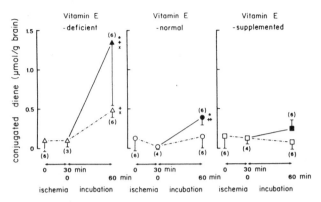

FIGURE 7. Cerebral conjugated dienes in total lipid extracts after ischemia and subsequent incubation with synthetic air (closed symbols) and nitrogen gas (open symbols) in vitamin E-varied rats. The values are the means ± standard deviation. The numbers of samples are in parentheses. $*p < 0.05$ vs. controls and ischemia; $^{++}p < 0.05$ versus nitrogen incubation within the same dietary group; $^{+}p < 0.05$ vs. vitamin E-normal group; and $^{x}p < 0.01$ vs. vitamin E-supplemented group under the comparable experimental condition. (Yoshida et al.[31] With permission from the *Journal of Neurochemistry.*)

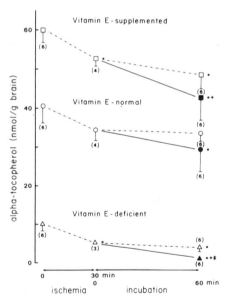

FIGURE 8. Cerebral alpha-tocopherol after ischemia and subsequent incubation under synthetic air (closed symbols) or nitrogen gas (open symbols) in vitamin E-varied rats. The values are the means ± standard deviation; if no bars are shown, the standard deviation falls within the symbol. The numbers of samples are in parentheses. $*p < 0.01$ vs. controls; $^{+}p < 0.01$ vs. ischemia; and $^{t}p < 0.01$ vs. nitrogen incubation within each dietary group. Significant differences ($p < 0.01$) always exist between the vitamin E-varied groups under the comparable experimental condition, but no symbols are shown. (Yoshida et al.[31] With permission from the *Journal of Neurochemistry.*)

TABLE 1. Cerebral Levels of Total Fatty Acids in Vitamin E (VE)-Varied Rats following Ischemia and Postischemic Incubation[31,a]

	Control	Ischemia (30 min)	Incubation (60 min) after ischemia	
			Nitrogen	Synthetic air
			VE-deficient	
	(6)	(3)	(6)	(6)
C 16:0	28.0 ± 1.8	28.3 ± 0.7	29.1 ± 1.9	28.0 ± 2.3
C 18:0	27.4 ± 2.5	24.2 ± 1.4	25.7 ± 2.2	27.1 ± 2.7
C 18:1	22.2 ± 2.4	22.4 ± 1.7	23.6 ± 2.2	20.5 ± 1.9
C 20:4	14.7 ± 1.1	14.1 ± 0.5	13.8 ± 0.7	11.7 ± 0.9[b,c,d,e]
C 22:6	9.4 ± 1.1	8.7 ± 0.4	8.1 ± 1.0	6.7 ± 0.5[b,c,e]
Sum	101.8 ± 7.6	97.7 ± 0.9	100.3 ± 6.5	94.1 ± 5.9
			VE-normal	
	(6)	(4)	(6)	(6)
C 16:0	29.5 ± 2.0	28.2 ± 2.2	29.4 ± 2.1	29.5 ± 2.6
C 18:0	26.5 ± 2.9	23.2 ± 1.2	24.0 ± 1.8	24.3 ± 2.4
C 18:1	24.0 ± 1.6	22.5 ± 2.6	24.4 ± 2.2	22.9 ± 2.7
C 20:4	14.1 ± 1.2	13.6 ± 1.4	13.9 ± 1.3	14.4 ± 1.4
C 22:6	10.0 ± 1.9	8.8 ± 0.7	8.5 ± 0.8	8.5 ± 0.9
Sum	104.2 ± 8.4	96.2 ± 5.9	100.2 ± 7.3	100.6 ± 8.3
			VE-supplemented	
	(6)	(4)	(6)	(6)
C 16:0	28.1 ± 2.0	27.7 ± 1.9	29.5 ± 3.6	28.5 ± 2.4
C 18:0	26.3 ± 4.9	24.2 ± 1.3	24.1 ± 2.3	25.2 ± 2.3
C 18:1	23.2 ± 2.2	21.0 ± 2.7	23.8 ± 1.8	21.4 ± 2.7
C 20:4	14.6 ± 1.4	13.4 ± 0.4	13.6 ± 1.1	14.2 ± 1.2
C 22:6	9.7 ± 1.2	8.2 ± 0.2	8.5 ± 1.1	8.8 ± 0.3
Sum	101.8 ± 8.9	94.6 ± 4.0	99.4 ± 9.2	98.2 ± 7.2

[a] Values are means ± SD in μmol/g of brain. The numbers in parentheses represent the number of samples.
[b] $p < 0.05$ vs. controls in the same row.
[c] $p < 0.01$ vs. ischemia in the same row.
[d] $p < 0.01$ vs. nitrogen incubation in the same row.
[e] $p < 0.01$ vs. VE-normal and -supplemented group after the same treatment.

ischemia and subsequent reoxygenation, and is not influenced by vitamin E. The latter is induced by postischemic reoxygenation and is modified by vitamin E. The modification by vitamin E of reoxygenation-induced peroxidation suggests free radical mediation. Although a selective decrease in total PUFA is an established index of lipid peroxidation, this method is far less sensitive than the TBA test or the conjugated diene assay; thus, a decrease was noted only in the vitamin E-deficient brains after reoxygenation. Oxygen is a prerequisite for oxidative degradation of biomembranes to proceed within unsaturated lipids. Our finding that sustained ischemic anoxia

TABLE 2. Cerebral Levels of Free Fatty Acids (FA) in Vitamin E (VE)-Varied Rats following Ischemia and Postischemic Incubation[31,a]

| | Control | Ischemia (30 min) | Incubation (60 min) after ischemia | |
			Nitrogen	Synthetic air
		VE-deficient		
	(6)	(3)	(6)	(6)
C 16:0	0.11 ± 0.01	0.39 ± 0.02[b]	0.77 ± 0.08[b,c]	0.85 ± 0.14[b,c]
C 18:0	0.14 ± 0.04	0.42 ± 0.08[b]	0.98 ± 0.09[b,c]	0.99 ± 0.16[b,c]
C 18:1	0.06 ± 0.01	0.33 ± 0.07[b]	0.60 ± 0.07[b,c]	0.61 ± 0.06[b,c]
C 20:4	0.10 ± 0.02	0.48 ± 0.04[b]	0.87 ± 0.08[b,c]	0.85 ± 0.14[b,c]
C 22:6	0.01 ± 0.01	0.04 ± 0.01	0.04 ± 0.02[b,c]	0.16 ± 0.04[b,c]
Sum	0.41 ± 0.06	1.65 ± 0.09[b]	3.38 ± 0.28[b,c]	3.46 ± 0.49[b,c]
		VE-normal		
	(6)	(4)	(6)	(6)
C 16:0	0.11 ± 0.02	0.37 ± 0.03[b]	0.83 ± 0.07[b,c]	0.87 ± 0.13[b,c]
C 18:0	0.12 ± 0.02	0.49 ± 0.05[b]	1.07 ± 0.13[b,c]	1.12 ± 0.14[b,c]
C 18:1	0.06 ± 0.01	0.20 ± 0.07	0.58 ± 0.07[b,c]	0.72 ± 0.14[b,c]
C 20:4	0.09 ± 0.01	0.45 ± 0.08[b]	0.88 ± 0.09[b,c]	1.03 ± 0.15[b,c]
C 22:6	0.02 ± 0.01	0.06 ± 0.01	0.16 ± 0.04[b,c]	0.18 ± 0.04[b,c]
Sum	0.40 ± 0.05	1.56 ± 0.16[b]	3.52 ± 0.31[b,c]	3.93 ± 0.52[b,c]
		VE-supplemented		
	(6)	(4)	(6)	(5)
C 16:0	0.12 ± 0.01	0.37 ± 0.09[c]	0.83 ± 0.17[b,c]	0.81 ± 0.08[b,c]
C 18:0	0.12 ± 0.03	0.56 ± 0.13[b]	1.02 ± 0.18[b,c]	1.02 ± 0.06[b,c]
C 18:1	0.07 ± 0.01	0.23 ± 0.07[b]	0.72 ± 0.10[b,c]	0.64 ± 0.04[b,c]
C 20:4	0.09 ± 0.02	0.53 ± 0.11[b]	0.96 ± 0.10[b,c]	0.86 ± 0.06[b,c]
C 22:6	0.02 ± 0.01	0.03 ± 0.01	0.17 ± 0.05[b,c]	0.15 ± 0.04[b,c]
Sum	0.42 ± 0.05	1.72 ± 0.34[b]	3.71 ± 0.57[b,c]	3.48 ± 0.18[b,c]

[a] Values are means ± SD in $\mu mol/g$ of brain. The levels of given free FA are not significantly different between nitrogen incubation and aerobic incubation within each dietary group, nor do they differ among dietary groups after the same treatment. The numbers in parentheses represent the number of samples.
[b] $p < 0.01$ vs. controls in the same row.
[c] $p < 0.01$ vs. ischemia in the same row.

induces lipid peroxidation in vitamin E-deficient brains contradicts the oxygen requirement. One possible explanation is that a trace of oxygen remaining in "anoxic" brain would allow the slow propagation of free radical-mediated reactions owing to the defective defense. The decrease in cerebral vitamin E after nitrogen incubation is also difficult to understand unless one assumes the presence of residual oxygen in an ischemic milieu. Because there is no evidence for peroxidation of liberated PUFA after reoxygenation, esterified PUFA are the main targets of free radicals.

Siesjö and his collaborators[34] studied the influence of acidosis on free radical formation and lipid peroxidation in brain homogenates. The homogenates fortified with ferrous ions, and in some experiments, with ascorbic acid, were equilibrated with 5-15% oxygen at pH values of 7.0, 6.5, 6.0, and 5.0 with subsequent measurements of TBA reactants, as well as of water- and lipid-soluble antioxidants, and total fatty acids. At pH 7.0, the contents of TBA reactants, GSSG, and oxidized ascorbate increased, and the content of alpha-tocopherol decreased, whereas the levels of total PUFA remained unchanged. Lowering pH to 6.5-6.0 grossly exaggerated the formation of TBA reactants and resulted in a decrease in total PUFA; alpha-tocopherol decreased further, but an additional increase in GSSG and oxidized ascorbate did not occur. Thus, in the condition of marked tissue acidosis, changes in alpha-tocopherol content mirrored those in TBA reactants (FIG. 9), and water-soluble antioxidants did not appear to quench free radicals.

In conclusion, those *in vitro* studies[21,25,31,32,34] have made it clear that nonenzymatic lipid peroxidation is potentiated by postischemic reoxygenation, impairment of vitamin E defense, and tissue lactic acidosis.

DO FREE RADICALS PRODUCE BRAIN DAMAGE IN ISCHEMIA?

Although the results of *in vitro* experiments are clear-cut, they merely illustrate the fact that brain tissue has a capacity to undergo nonenzymatic lipid peroxidation

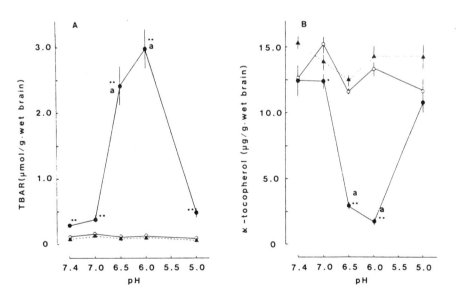

FIGURE 9. Production of thiobarbituric acid reactants (TBAR) (A) and alpha-tocopherol content (B) in brain cortical tissue homogenates exposed *in vitro* to 100% nitrogen gas (open circles) and 5% oxygen/95% nitrogen (filled circles) for 45 minutes at 37°C. Control samples (filled triangles) were taken prior to incubation. Values are means ± standard error of mean. **$p < 0.001$ vs. control values; $^{a}p < 0.001$ vs. pH 7.0 values. (Siesjö et al.[34] With permission from the *Journal of Cerebral Blood Flow and Metabolism*.)

as other tissues do. It should be emphasized that any conclusions must be tentative, owing to the difficulty of extrapolating results from brain homogenates or minces to an *in vivo* situation. The problem must be solved by analyses of the brain tissue subjected to regional ischemia and/or reperfusion following global ischemia. So far, we have considered TBA reactants and conjugated dienes to be the indices of free radical-mediated lipid peroxidation. It is known, however, that prostaglandin endo-peroxides are positive in a TBA test.[35] Similarly, lipoxygenase products contain conjugated diene structures. Furthermore, a selective loss of phospholipid-bound PUFA may be an index too insensitive to detect an early phase of lipid peroxidation. More specific and sensitive measures that can be applicable to *in vivo* situations need to be explored to prove unequivocally the existence of nonenzymatic lipid peroxidation in the future.

Yamamoto and his collaborators[22] examined if alpha-tocopherol would modify the sequelae of temporary forebrain ischemia. Pretreatment with alpha-tocopherol suppressed the rise in lipid peroxides both in the brain and serum, improved neurological outcome, and promoted resynthesis of tissue ATP during postischemic reperfusion. Their study implies that alpha-tocopherol plays a role in protecting cellular damage by scavenging free radicals and lipid peroxides formed by oxygen supply through blood reperfusion. There are no reports, to my knowledge, to study the effect of alpha-tocopherol administration on morphological outcome after ischemia, that is, a size of infarction and a density of neuronal necrosis. At present, though the evidence that free radical formation and subsequent lipid peroxidation contribute to ischemic brain

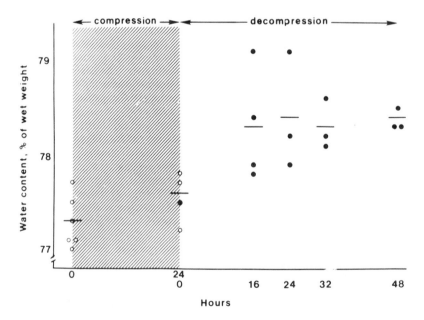

FIGURE 10. Brain water content during and after right brain compression in rats raised on regular rat pellets. Each circle represents right cerebral water content from one animal. Mean values are shown by horizontal lines. Open circles indicate no Evans blue staining, and closed circles indicate the presence of dye staining. (Yoshida *et al.*[36] With permission from *Neurology.*)

TABLE 3. Brain Water Content (Percent) and Swelling Percentage in Control and Brain-Compressed Rats Fed Vitamin E-Deficient, -Normal, and -Supplemented Diets. The Experimental Groups of Animals Underwent 24 Hours of Compression followed by 24-Hour Decompression.[36,a]

	Vitamin E-deficient	Vitamin E-normal	Vitamin E-supplemented
Controls	(n = 6)	(n = 6)	(n = 6)
Water content of right cerebrum	77.4 ± 0.3	77.3 ± 0.2	77.1 ± 0.3
Water content of left cerebrum	77.2 ± 0.5	77.3 ± 0.4	77.0 ± 0.4
Percent swelling of R/L	0.9 ± 2.2	0.3 ± 1.7	0.2 ± 1.9
Right brain compressed	(n = 6)	(n = 6)	(n = 6)
Water content of right cerebrum	79.1 ± 0.8	78.6 ± 0.6	78.5 ± 0.8
Water content of left cerebrum	77.0 ± 0.2	76.8 ± 0.3	77.4 ± 0.5
Percent swelling of R/L	10.4 ± 4.3[b]	8.5 ± 3.8[b]	5.5 ± 3.4[b,c]

[a] A one-way analysis of variance of water contents in left cerebrum demonstrated no population differences between the six groups. An analysis of swelling percentages revealed significant differences. Values are mean ± SD; n, number of animals.
[b] Different from corresponding controls with $p < 0.01$.
[c] Different from vitamin E-deficient experimental group with $p < 0.05$.

damage has been accumulating, it is still circumstantial and inconclusive, and much more information is required to settle the issue.

POSTTRAUMATIC BRAIN EDEMA AND EFFECTS OF VITAMIN E

We studied the degree of edema resulting from focal brain compression in rats raised on vitamin E-deficient, -normal, or -supplemented diets.[36] After release of 24 hours of epidural compression, edema developed ipsilaterally (FIG. 10) and was characterized by extravasation of serum protein, increased water and sodium content, and little change in potassium. The degree of swelling and increase of sodium in the previously compressed area were most pronounced in the vitamin E-deficient group and mildest in the vitamin E-supplemented group (TABLE 3). Degradative processes of biomembranes seem to participate in the pathogenesis of brain edema.

Then, cerebral content of total fatty acids and vitamin E was assayed at 24 hours postdecompression after a 24-hour period of compression.[37] Levels of all individual fatty acids in the previously compressed brain region were less by 20 to 25% in the vitamin E-deficient group than in noncompressed sides; by 6 to 10% in the vitamin E-normal group; and by 2 to 5% in the vitamin E-supplemented group (TABLE 4). The selective loss of total PUFA did not occur in this edema model, and brain levels

TABLE 4. Brain Total Fatty Acids in Right Brain-Compressed Rats Fed by Vitamin E-Varied Diets. The Animals Underwent 24 Hours of Compression followed by 24-Hour Decompression.[37,a]

	Vitamin E-deficient (n = 5)	Vitamin E-normal (n = 6)	Vitamin E-supplemented (n = 7)
Palmitic acid			
Right cerebrum	93 ± 10	112 ± 17	122 ± 16
Left cerebrum	122 ± 6	. 121 ± 10	124 ± 11
Right/left ratio	0.76 ± 0.06[b]	0.92 ± 0.10[c]	0.98 ± 0.12[c]
Stearic acid			
Right cerebrum	88 ± 10	109 ± 17	115 ± 15
Left cerebrum	117 ± 6	118 ± 10	119 ± 11
Right/left ratio	0.75 ± 0.08[b]	0.92 ± 0.9[c]	0.97 ± 0.12[c]
Oleic acid			
Right cerebrum	93 ± 13	117 ± 17	123 ± 14
Left cerebrum	125 ± 12	129 ± 10	127 ± 14
Right/left ratio	0.75 ± 0.11[b]	0.90 ± 0.09[c]	0.98 ± 0.14[c]
Arachidonic acid			
Right cerebrum	41 ± 6	50 ± 7	52 ± 6
Left cerebrum	52 ± 3	54 ± 4	56 ± 4
Right/left ratio	0.78 ± 0.11[b]	0.92 ± 0.08[c]	0.93 ± 0.10[c]
Docosahexanoic acid			
Right cerebrum	49 ± 5	58 ± 9	61 ± 6
Left cerebrum	61 ± 4	62 ± 6	65 ± 5
Right/left ratio	0.80 ± 0.07[b]	0.94 ± 0.09[c]	0.95 ± 0.10[c]

[a] Values are the mean ± SD in mmol/kg dry weight. Right/left ratio is calculated in individual brains. n, number of animals.
[b] $p < 0.05$, compared with the respective controls.
[c] $p < 0.05$, compared with the values of brain-compressed, vitamin E-deficient group.

of vitamin E were not altered by compression in any dietary group (TABLE 5). Thus, we found no evidence that vitamin E serves as a free radical scavenger after this type of brain injury.

Regional cerebral blood flow was studied autoradiographically in the same edema model.[38] Mean cortical blood flow was reduced to 0.48 ∼ 0.50 mL/g/min following 2 or 24 hours of compression. Early (2 hours) following subsequent decompression, a mixed pattern of hypoperfusion and hyperperfusion was observed. Twenty-four hours later, regional heterogeneities were less marked. Comparisons among animal groups raised on vitamin E-deficient, -normal, and -supplemented diets 2 hours after decompression revealed marked reductions in blood flow in the previously compressed cortex (dorsolateral cortex) of the first two groups and hyperemia of the underlying hippocampus (TABLE 6). The vitamin E-supplemented rats showed increased flow in the previously compressed cortex. In addition, vitamin E supplementation tended to eliminate regional blood flow gradients between subjacent zones (FIG. 11). The blood flow study suggests that the beneficial effects of vitamin E on posttraumatic brain edema may be mediated hemodynamically.

TABLE 5. Brain Alpha-Tocopherol in Controls and Right Brain-Compressed Rats Fed by Vitamin E-Varied Diets. The Animals Underwent 24 Hours of Compression followed by 24-Hour Decompression.[37,a]

	Vitamin E-deficient (n = 6)	Vitamin E-normal (n = 6)	Vitamin E-supplemented (n = 5)
Controls			
Right cerebrum	83 ± 8	162 ± 21	265 ± 17
Left cerebrum	81 ± 10	166 ± 18[b]	257 ± 25[b,c]
Right/left ratio	1.04 ± 0.16	0.99 ± 0.19	1.06 ± 0.16
	(n = 5)	(n = 6)	(n = 7)
Right brain-compressed			
Right cerebrum	91 ± 12	172 ± 19	273 ± 20
Left cerebrum	89 ± 9	163 ± 17[b]	260 ± 17[b,c]
Right/left ratio	1.02 ± 0.15	1.06 ± 0.08	1.06 ± 0.13

[a] Values are the mean ± SD in μmol/kg dry weight. Right/left ratio is calculated in individual brains. n, number of animals.

[b] $p < 0.05$, compared with vitamin E-deficient group.

[c] $p < 0.05$, compared with vitamin E-normal group. There is no significant difference between the control and brain-compressed animals in each dietary group.

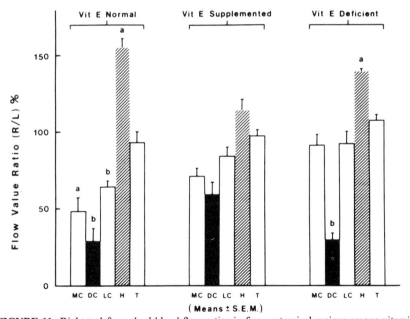

FIGURE 11. Right-to-left cerebral blood flow ratios in five anatomical regions among vitamin E-normal, -supplemented, and -deficient rats. Cerebral blood flow was determined 2 hours after decompression following 24-hour compression. MC: medial cortex; DC: dorsolateral cortex; LC: lateral cortex; H: hippocampus; T: thalamus. [a]$p < 0.01$, [b]$p < 0.05$ vs. corresponding regional cerebral blood flow in vitamin E-supplemented group. (Busto et al.[38] With permission from the Annals of Neurology.)

TABLE 6. Regional Cerebral Blood Flow in Right Brain-Compressed Rats Raised on Diets Varying in Vitamin E Content[38,a]

Group	Region				
	Medial Cortex	Dorsolateral Cortex[b]	Lateral Cortex	Hippocampus	Thalamus
VE-deficient (n = 4)					
Right cerebrum	1.14 ± 0.08	0.39 ± 0.06	1.27 ± 0.14	1.13 ± 0.14	1.18 ± 0.06
Left cerebrum	1.27 ± 0.11	1.30 ± 0.09	1.37 ± 0.09	0.81 ± 0.09	1.16 ± 0.05
R/L ratio[c]	0.91 ± 0.06	0.30 ± 0.04[e,f]	0.92 ± 0.02	1.39 ± 0.02[d,e]	1.01 ± 0.02
VE-normal (n = 4)					
Right cerebrum	0.55 ± 0.11	0.34 ± 0.09	0.99 ± 0.03	1.20 ± 0.02	1.03 ± 0.10
Left cerebrum	1.16 ± 0.09	1.20 ± 0.02	1.57 ± 0.09	0.78 ± 0.03	1.10 ± 0.06
R/L ratio[c]	0.48 ± 0.09[d,e]	0.29 ± 0.08[d,f]	0.64 ± 0.04[e,f]	1.56 ± 0.06[d,e]	0.93 ± 0.07
VE-supplemented (n = 6)					
Right cerebrum	0.80 ± 0.06	0.66 ± 0.11	1.12 ± 0.12	0.74 ± 0.08	1.00 ± 0.07
Left cerebrum	1.16 ± 0.11	1.10 ± 0.11	1.33 ± 0.14	0.65 ± 0.05	1.04 ± 0.07
R/L ratio[c]	0.71 ± 0.06[g]	0.59 ± 0.08[f]	0.84 ± 0.06	1.14 ± 0.07	0.96 ± 0.04

[a] All values are in milliliters per gram minute, expressed as means ± SEM. Cerebral blood flow was measured 2 hours after decompression following 24 hours of right brain compression. A two-way analysis of variance of rCBF values in each region in left hemisphere showed no significant differences among the six groups (three control groups and three groups of brain-compressed rats). Significant differences existed between medial cortex and lateral cortex of VE-deficient rats, and the corresponding regions of VE-normal rats ($p < 0.05$).
[b] This region of right cerebrum was the center of the previous compression site.
[c] Calculated in individual animals.
[d] $p < 0.01$ vs. VE-supplemented group by Dunn's test.
[e] $p < 0.05$ vs. VE-supplemented group by Dunn's test.
[f] $p < 0.01$ vs. control group by Student's t test.
[g] $p < 0.05$ vs. control group by Student's t test.

CONCLUSION

The hypothesis that free radicals produce brain damage after ischemia and trauma remains attractive. It may remain, however, an unproven hypothesis until free radicals are quantitatively measured in brain tissue that is subjected to various insults *in vivo*. Nonetheless, the contribution of the proposal of the hypothesis is apparent; it has directed our attention to changes occurring at the molecular level of biomembranes. Accordingly, metabolic cascades of membrane phospholipids and behaviors of endogenous antioxidants in cerebral ischemia and trauma are being unraveled. Vitamin E may act as a free radical scavenger and/or may exert its action by modulating blood rheology. It is obvious that the research task of clarifying mechanisms of neuronal death as well as of discovering strategies to protect brain is demanding.

REFERENCES

1. SIESJÖ, B. K. 1984. J. Neurosurg. **60:** 883-908.
2. DEMOPOULOS, H., E. FLAMM, M. SELIGMAN, R. POWER, D. PIETRONIGRO & J. RANSOHOFF. 1977. *In* Oxygen and Physiological Function. F. F. Jöbsis, Ed.: 491-508. Professional Information Library. Dallas, Texas.
3. FLAMM, E. S., H. B. DEMOPOULOS, M. L. SELIGMAN, R. G. POSER & J. RANSOHOFF. 1978. Stroke **9:** 445-447.
4. DEMOPOULOS, H. B., E. S. FLAMM, D. D. PIETRONIGRO & M. L. SELIGMAN. 1980. Acta Physiol. Scand. **492** (Suppl.): 91-119.
5. YOSHIDA, S., S. INOH, T. ASANO, K. SANO, M. KUBOTA, H. SHIMASAKI & N. UETA. 1980. J. Neurosurg. **53:** 323-331.
6. YOSHIDA, S., S. INOH, T. ASANO, K. SANO, M. KUBOTA, H. SHIMASAKI & N. UETA. 1982. *In* Cerebral Ischemia: Clinical and Experimental Approach. H. Handa, H. J. M. Barnett, M. Goldstein & Y. Yonekawa, Eds.: 7-18. Igakushoin. Tokyo, New York.
7. SIESJÖ, B. K. 1978. Brain Energy Metabolism. John Wiley & Sons. Chichester, New York, Brisbane, Toronto.
8. KOGURE, K., R. BUSTO, R. J. SCHWARTZMAN & P. SCHEINBERG. 1980. Ann. Neurol. **8:** 278-290.
9. DAWSON, R. M. C. & J. EICHBERG. 1965. Biochem. J. **96:** 634-643.
10. BAZÁN, JR., N. G. 1970. Biochim. Biophys. Acta **218:** 1-10.
11. AVELDAÑO, M. I. & N. G. BAZÁN. 1975. J. Neurochem. **25:** 919-920.
12. YOSHIDA, S., M. IKEDA, R. BUSTO, M. SANTOSO, E. MARTINEZ & M. D. GINSBERG. 1986. J. Neurochem. **47:** 744-757.
13. IKEDA, M., S. YOSHIDA, R. BUSTO, M. SANTISO & M. D. GINSBERG. 1986. J. Neurochem. **47:** 123-132.
14. MARION, J. & L. S. WOLFE. 1979. Biochim. Biophys. Acta **574:** 25-32.
15. SUN, G. Y. & L. L. FOUDIN. 1984. J. Neurochem. **43:** 1081-1086.
16. EDGAR, A. D., J. STROSZNAJDER & L. A. HORROCKS. 1982. J. Neurochem. **39:** 1111-1116.
17. GAUDET, R. J. & L. LEVINE. 1979. Biochem. Biophys. Res. Commun. **86:** 893-901.
18. GAUDET, R. J., I. ALAM & L. LEVINE. 1980. J. Neurochem. **35:** 653-658.
19. MOSKOWITZ, M. A., K. J. KIWAK, K. HEKIMIAN & L. LEVINE. 1984. Science **224:** 886-889.
20. WOLFE, L. S. 1982. J. Neurochem. **38:** 1-14.
21. KOGURE, K., B. D. WATSON, R. BUSTO & K. ABE. 1982. Neurochem. Res. **7:** 437-454.
22. YAMAMOTO, M., T. SHIMA, T. UOZUMI, T. SOGABE, K. YAMADA & T. KAWASAKI. 1983. Stroke **14:** 977-982.
23. WATSON, B. D., R. BUSTO, W. J. GOLDBERG, M. SANTISO, S. YOSHIDA & M. D. GINSBERG. 1984. J. Neurochem. **42:** 268-274.
24. MACMILLAN, V. 1982. J. Cereb. Blood Flow Metab. **2:** 457-465.

25. REHNCRONA, S., J. FOLBERGROVÁ, D. S. SMITH & B. K. SIESJÖ. 1980. J. Neurochem. **34:** 477-486.
26. COOPER, A. J. L., W. A. PULSINELLI & T. E. DUFFY. 1980. J. Neurochem. **35:** 1242-1245.
27. PULSINELLI, W. A. & T. E. DUFFY. 1983. J. Neurochem. **40:** 1500-1503.
28. SMITH, D. S., S. REHNCRONA & B. K. SIESJÖ. 1980. Anesthesiology **53:** 186-194.
29. YOSHIDA, S., K. ABE, R. BUSTO, B. D. WATSON, K. KOGURE & M. D. GINSBERG. 1982. Brain Res. **245:** 307-316.
30. ABE, K., S. YOSHIDA, B. D. WATSON, R. BUSTO, K. KOGURE & M. D. GINSBERG 1983. Brain Res. **273:** 166-169.
31. YOSHIDA, S., R. BUSTO, B. D. WATSON, M. SANTISO & M. D. GINSBERG. 1985. J. Neurochem. **44:** 1593-1601.
32. REHNCRONA, S., D. S. SMITH, B. ÅKESSON, E. WESTERBERG & B. K. SIESJÖ. 1980. J. Neurochem. **34:** 1630-1638.
33. REHNCRONA, S., B. K. SIESJÖ & D. S. SMITH. 1980. Acta Physiol. Scand. **492:** (Suppl.): 135-140.
34. SIESJÖ, B. K., G. BENDEK, T. KOIDE, E. WESTERBERG & T. WIELOCH. 1985. J. Cereb. Blood Flow Metab. **5:** 253-258.
35. SHIMIZU, T., K. KONDO & O. HAYAISHI. 1981. Arch. Biochem. Biophys. **206:** 271-276.
36. YOSHIDA, S., R. BUSTO, M. D. GINSBERG, K. ABE, E. MARTINEZ, B. D. WATSON & P. SCHEINBERG. 1983. Neurology **33:** 166-172.
37. YOSHIDA, S., R. BUSTO, K. ABE, M. SANTISO & M. D. GINSBERG. 1985. Neurology **35:** 126-130.
38. BUSTO, R., S. YOSHIDA, M. D. GINSBERG, O. ALONSO, D. W. SMITH & W. J. GOLDBERG. 1984. Ann. Neurol. **15:** 441-448.

Oxygen Free Radical-Mediated Heart Injury in Animal Models and during Bypass Surgery in Humans

Effects of α-Tocopherol[a]

R. FERRARI,[b,e] S. CURELLO,[b]
G. M. BOFFA,[b] E. CONDORELLI,[b] E. PASINI,[b]
G. GUARNIERI,[c] AND A. ALBERTINI[d]

[b] Cattedra di Cardiologia
Università di Brescia
25100 Brescia, Italy

[c] Cattedra di Biochimica
dell'Università di Bologna
Bologna, Italy

[d] Cattedra di Chimica
Università di Brescia
25100 Brescia, Italy

INTRODUCTION

The recognition that oxygen is essential for the metabolism and function of the myocardium must not blind us to the fact that it has several toxic effects. It is well-known that oxygen supplied at concentrations greater than those in normal air might damage plants, animals, and aerobic bacteria.[1] There is a considerable body of evidence that as much as 21% $O_2^{\cdot-}$ has slowly manifested damaging effects.[2,3] These effects vary considerably with the type of organism used, its age, and diet.

The inherent nature of the oxygen molecule makes it susceptible to univalent reduction reactions in the cell to form superoxide anions ($O_2^{\cdot-}$), a highly reactive free radical.[4,5] Other reactive products of oxygen metabolism can be formed from subsequent intracellular reduction of $O_2^{\cdot-}$, including oxygen peroxide (H_2O_2) and the hydroxyl radical ($\cdot OH$). These radical species are capable of various toxic effects: lipid peroxidation of membranes, inactivation of sulfhydryl enzymes, cross-linking of proteins, and DNA breakdown.[6-8]

[a] This work was supported by the Italian C.N.R. Grant 087432.

[e] Address for correspondence: R. Ferrari, Cattedra di Cardiologia, Università degli Studi, c/o Spedali Civili, P.le Spedali Civili, 1, 25100 Brescia, Italy.

In the myocardium, however, there is a series of defense mechanisms able to protect the cell against the cytotoxic oxygen metabolites. These include the enzymes superoxide dismutase (SOD) and glutathione peroxidase (GPD), plus other endogenous antioxidants like α-tocopherol, ascorbic acid, and cysteine.[6,9]

SOD exists in two isoenzymatic forms, the Cu-Zn SOD, localized in the mitochondrial matrix. This enzyme directly detoxifies $O_2^{\cdot -}$ radicals, forming H_2O_2 according to the equation: $O_2^{\cdot -} + O_2^{\cdot -} + 2H^+ \rightarrow H_2O_2 + O_2$. H_2O_2 is then removed by catalase and by GPD. GPD metabolized H_2O_2 and lipid peroxides, using reduced glutathione (GSH) as electron donor. GSH is then converted to oxidized glutathione (GSSG), which, in turn, is reduced to GSH by the NADPH-dependent enzyme glutathione reductase. The concerted action of this mechanism and the presence in relevant concentrations of the endogenous antioxidant is essential for the survival of aerobic organisms in an atmosphere of 20% oxygen.

FREE RADICALS AND MYOCARDIAL TISSUE INJURY

The possibility that oxygen-free radicals could be involved in myocardial tissue injury has recently been developed together with the recognition of the existence of a reperfusion-mediated myocardial damage. Undoubtedly the availability of techniques, such as surgical reperfusion, angioplasty, and thrombolysis, for the restoration of blood flow to the ischemic myocardium has revived interest in the reperfusion phenomenon.[10–13] It is clear that reperfusion occupies a central role in the protection of the ischemic myocardium, as, without it, no recovery is possible at all. Restoration of flow to the myocytes, however, is not necessarily beneficial, and it might result in numerous further negative consequences, thus directly favoring the occurrence of cell death.[13–16]

The causal factor determining cell death during reperfusion, however, is still unknown. Different possible mechanisms have been suggested as triggers for reperfusion damage, including depletion of high energy phosphates[17] and of catecholamines,[18] accumulation of calcium[19–21] and of lysophosphoglycerides, or activation of phospholipases.[22] Recently it has also been suggested that reperfusion induces a burst of oxygen free radicals which, in turn, can cause dysfunction of membrane permeability, leading to disturbance in ion transport and tissue calcium accumulation associated with cell necrosis.[15,16,23–26]

Several mechanisms appear to be responsible for the formation of oxygen free radicals during myocardial ischemia and reperfusion. The mitochondria are one of the most important sources of oxygen free radicals in the myocardium, and their production of $O_2^{\cdot -}$ and H_2O_2 is enhanced under ischemia and reperfusion, the electron transport chain being in the reduced state.[27,28]

The xanthine oxidase pathway is also an important site of free radical production, particularly during ischemia, when cytosolic calcium increases and adenosine triphosphate (ATP) is broken down to AMP, which is ultimately metabolized to hypoxanthine. The above-mentioned elevation of cytosolic calcium concentration enhances the conversion of xanthine dehydrogenase, an enzyme located in the endothelium of the capillaries of coronary arteries, to xanthine oxidase.[29,30] According to this concept, when molecular oxygen is reintroduced to cells containing high concentrations of hypoxanthine, this enzyme caused the release of $O_2^{\cdot -}$ and H_2O_2. The existence of this enzyme in several animal species, however, including humans, has been recently reassessed.[31] Endoperoxide intermediates, resulting from the conversion of arachidonic acid, also lead to the production of oxygen free radicals by leukocytes and other cell types in the heart.[32,33]

Another possible mechanism of free radical generation are the neutrophils. The neutrophils accumulate in the vascular space of reperfused ischemic myocardium, where they may adhere to the endothelium and release oxygen free radicals.[34] Although there are multiple stimuli for neutrophil migration, one chemoattractant may arise from the interaction of plasma lipids with oxygen free radicals derived from the activity of cycloxygenase or xanthine oxidase on their respective substrates. Engler *et al.*[35] have proposed that capillary plugging by leukocytes contributes to the occurrence of "no reflow" after reperfusion of ischemic myocardial tissue. Finally, the auto-oxidation of catecholamines could provide another source of free radicals.[36,37]

It is also important to note that the ischemic process alters the cellular defense mechanisms against oxygen toxicity. In particular, it has been shown that severe ischemia induces a marked and specific decline in the activity of mitochondrial SOD.[16,24] Furthermore, severe ischemia results in a decline of tissue levels of GSH. Under these conditions, the resumption of coronary flow on reperfusion causes a further reduction of tissue GSH and massive accumulation and release of GSSG, leading to a fall in the GSH/GSSG ratio to below ten. These findings are of particular importance because tissue accumulation of GSSG accompanied by release into the coronary effluent is a sensitive index of oxidative stress.[24]

Myocardial tissue injury induced by free radicals is usually thought to be due to the activation of lipid peroxidation in cellular and subcellular membranes. Various authors have reported tissue accumulation and release into the coronary effluent of malondialdehyde, a major by-product of lipid peroxidation,[22,38] which could be responsible for the loss of integrity of cell membranes during ischemia and reperfusion. This pathogenetic mechanism has been linked to the alterations of calcium homeostasis that ultimately mediate cell death. In this context, the importance of alterations to the cellular redox-potential during postischemic reperfusion should also be stressed. The described shift of the glutathione status towards oxidation, together with the loss of the total protein sulfhydryl groups, which occurs in reperfusion,[24] may exert detrimental effects on myocardial function by influencing many enzyme activities and regulatory processes even before the onset of peroxidative damage.

CLINICAL RELEVANCE OF OCCURRENCE OF OXIDATIVE STRESS IN HUMANS DURING POSTISCHEMIC REPERFUSION

Despite the large body of experimental evidence on the role of oxygen in ischemic and reperfusion-induced myocardial injury, the relevance of oxygen free radical-mediated damage in analogous clinical situations is still unknown. This is partly due to the inadequacy of reliable indexes able to detect, in humans, the occurrence of oxidative damage. Presently, and in other studies,[39–41] we are attempting to resolve this problem by measuring the arterial and coronary sinus difference of GSH and GSSG release in coronary artery disease (CAD) patients subjected to different periods of global ischemia followed by reperfusion during coronary artery bypass grafting. Because of the high rate of glutathione auto-oxidation and disappearance in the blood, we have determined plasma levels of GSH and GSSG with a method modified by us:[42] treating the blood, immediately after collection, with thiol reagents, 5,5'-dithio-

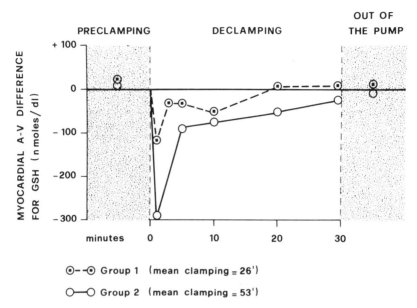

FIGURE 1. Myocardial arteriovenous difference for GSH of CAD patients subjected to open heart surgery.

bis(2-nitrobenzoic acid) (DTNB) for GSH, and *N*-ethylmaleimide (NEM) for GSSG determination, respectively.

In FIGURES 1 and 2 are reported the data regarding arterial-coronary sinus difference for GSH and GSSG in 16 patients. They have been divided into two groups, according to the duration of the cross-clamping period: less than 30 minutes (group 1, mean cross-clamping period 25.2 ± 1.3 min) or longer than 30 minutes (group 2, mean cross-clamping period: 55.2 ± 2.9 min). Before clamping in all patients there was a small positive arteriovenous difference for GSH and GSSG. During global ischemia there was no flow in the coronary sinus. During reperfusion after 25 min of clamping there was a transient release of GSH and GSSG into the coronary sinus, reaching a peak 5 min after the onset of reperfusion. During the following 15 min the GSH and the GSSG concentrations in the coronary sinus declined and fell below the arterial values. On the contrary, reperfusion after 55 min of clamping resulted in a pronounced and sustained release of GSH from the myocardium, and at the end of the procedure the concentration of GSH and GSSG in the coronary sinus greatly exceeded the arterial levels.

The results obtained in the two groups of patients reported here show that, as in animal studies, reperfusion results in an oxidative stress, depending on the duration of the ischemic period. When the period of clamping was reduced to 25 min, reperfusion resulted in a small and transient rise of GSH and GSSG in the coronary sinus. This, probably, represents a washout process.

Reperfusion reinstated after 55 min of ischemia led to an important release of GSH and GSSG, which was still continuing at the end of the procedure. This is similar to the effects of reperfusion after prolonged ischemia in the isolated heart and presumably implies oxidative stress. We suggest that these cases illustrate some aspects of pathophysiology of reperfusion of the human heart. They indicate that reperfusion may induce oxidative damage after a prolonged period of ischemia and suggest that oxygen free radicals may be involved in reperfusion damage. These findings are of importance, as they constitute the rationale for therapeutic interventions designed to improve the efficacy of myocardial reperfusion.

PROTECTION BY REDUCING CYTOTOXIC OXYGEN METABOLITES

Indirect evidence that cytotoxic oxygen metabolites play an important role in the genesis of myocardial ischemic and reperfusion damage comes from studies focused on the possibility of protecting heart muscle from ischemic and reperfusion injury with substances able to interfere with oxygen metabolism. Depletion of neutrophils by administration of hydrouria[43] or neutrophil antiserum[44] has been found to limit the extent of canine myocardial injury after temporary coronary occlusion. The extent to which neutrophil-mediated myocardial damage is due to leukotrienes and lysosomal enzymes, however, rather than oxygen radicals, remains uncertain.[45]

More direct evidence of oxygen radical-induced myocardial damage is derived from the observation that treatment with SOD[45,46] reduces the amount of myocardial damage in occlusion-reperfusion preparations of canine myocardial ischemic injury. Accordingly, the effect of allopurinol, an inhibitor of xanthine oxidase, has been evaluated by several laboratories. Animals pretreated with allopurinol 24 hours before

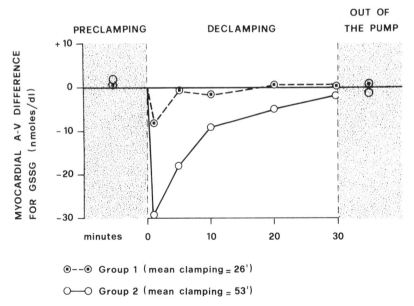

FIGURE 2. Myocardial arteriovenous difference for GSSG of CAD patients subjected to open heart surgery.

the induction of regional myocardial ischemia had significantly smaller infarcts than those that were not treated.[47] Similar experiments, undertaken by Chamber et al.[48] and Ambrosio et al.,[49] confirmed these results. Reimer and Jennings, however, recently reported that allopurinol did not limit infarct size in canine hearts when the extent of tissue injury was quantitated 4 days after 40 min of ischemia followed by reperfusion.[50]

Other antioxidants shown to be able to reduce reperfusion damage are ionol,[51] N-(2-mercaptopropionyl)glycine,[52] dimethylthiourea, and catalase.[53] We have recently investigated the role of N-acetyl-cysteine, a sulfhydryl group donor that is transported in the cell where it is deacetylated and thus increases the available thiol pool, including reduced glutathione.[54] The results have shown highly protective effects, but only when the compound is administered several minutes before the onset of ischemia. In the following discussion, we specifically consider the effects of α-tocopherol deficiency on myocardial oxidative damage and its protective effects against reoxygenation and reperfusion injury. Part of these results have been published before.[55-59]

EFFECT OF α-TOCOPHEROL DEFICIENCY ON MYOCARDIAL MITOCHONDRIAL METABOLISM

Little is known about the action of α-tocopherol at the mitochondrial level. Nason and Lehman[60] and Schwartz and Baumgartner[61] postulate that α-tocopherol plays a specific role in mitochondrial electron transport, functioning either as a cofactor or as a structural agent. Oliveira et al.[62] found appreciable levels of α-tocopherol present only in the inner mitochondrial membrane where the bulk of the enzymes of the electron transport system are located.

We have investigated the possible antioxidant role of α-tocopherol against toxic reactions mediated by oxygen metabolites in the rabbit heart mitochondria from control and α-tocopherol-deficient animals.[59] Experiments were performed using male albino rabbits maintained either on a standard diet (control) or fed for 1 month with a diet deficient of α-tocopherol[63] (deficient animals). A third group was selected from the α-tocopherol-deficient rabbits from the 28th to the 30th day and reswitched to control diet plus 25 mg/kg of α-tocopherol administered intraperitoneally twice daily (rehabilitated animals). FIGURE 3 shows some of the results obtained. Clearly the function (respiratory control ratio, RCR) of mitochondria isolated for α-tocopherol-deficient rabbits was depressed, and the formation of $O_2^{\cdot-}$ radicals was greatly enhanced. SOD activity, however, was only slightly reduced, suggesting that the impairment of mitochondrial function in α-tocopherol-deficient rabbits may be caused by increased formation of $O_2^{\cdot-}$ radicals beyond the neutralizing capacity of the SOD. Because α-tocopherol is an effective compound that may neutralize $O_2^{\cdot-}$ radicals,[64] it is possible that its deficiency, induced by the diet, accentuated the production and the toxicity of these radicals. In accordance with this hypothesis are the results reported in FIGURE 3, showing that the restoration of the control diet and the dose regimen of α-tocopherol administered to the deficient rabbits prevented the decline in mitochondrial function and the formation of $O_2^{\cdot-}$ radicals without modifying SOD activity. These data, therefore, indicate that in rabbit heart the presence of α-tocopherol may play an important role in the protection of mitochondrial membrane against the oxidative reactions mediated by $O_2^{\cdot-}$ radicals.

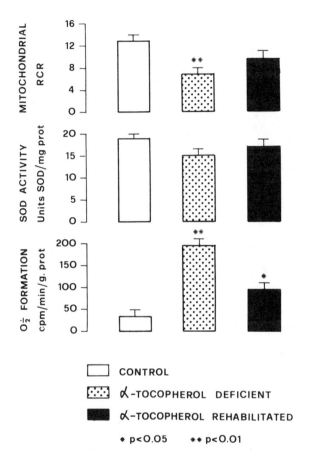

FIGURE 3. Oxidative phosphorylation capacity, superoxide dismutase (SOD) activity, and $O_2^{\cdot -}$ radical formation in cardiac mitochondria isolated from control, α-tocopherol-deficient, and rehabilitated, freshly excised, nonperfused rabbit hearts. The data represents the mean ± SE of six separate experiments; p relates to the significance of the difference for the control and the relative treated series of experiments. Mitochondrial function was measured in terms of respiratory control ratio (RCR), which is the ratio of oxygen consumed in the presence of ADP to that after phosphorylation of ADP. SOD activity was measured spectrophotometrically[59] and the formation of endogenous $O_2^{\cdot -}$ radicals by the chemiluminescence method previously described.[59]

EFFECTS OF α-TOCOPHEROL ADMINISTRATION DURING HYPOXIA AND REOXYGENATION

As already discussed, readmission of oxygen (reoxygenation) following a period of oxygen deprivation in the presence of normal coronary flow (hypoxia) may contribute to the exacerbation of the hypoxic damage, leading to a phenomenon called oxygen paradox.[14] In the series of experiments described in FIGURES 4 and 5, we have investigated whether α-tocopherol protects the myocardium when it is partially deprived of oxygen and then reoxygenated.

Isolated and perfused rabbit hearts were used, and the hypoxic and reoxygenation damage was determined in terms of mechanical function, enzyme release, tissue con-

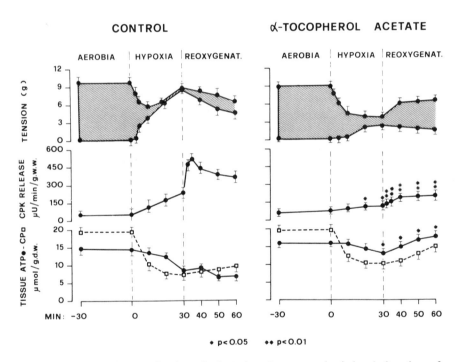

* p < 0.05　　** p < 0.01

FIGURE 4. Effect of α-tocopherol on the hypoxic and reoxygenation-induced alterations of mechanical function, CPK release, and tissue content of ATP and CP of the isolated Langendorff-perfused rabbit hearts. The hearts were perfused aerobically for 30 minutes and then with the hypoxic (PO$_2$ < 6 mm Hg) substrate-free buffer for 30 minutes, followed by reoxygenation with the normal aerobic medium. Coronary flow was maintained at 25 mL/min throughout. α-Tocopherol was infused into the aortic inflow cannula at a rate of 23.2 nM/min 20 minutes before the onset of hypoxia and for the entire period of hypoxia and reoxygenation. Results are mean ± SE of six separate experiments. CPK and tissue content of ATP and CP have been determined enzymatically as previously described.[58]

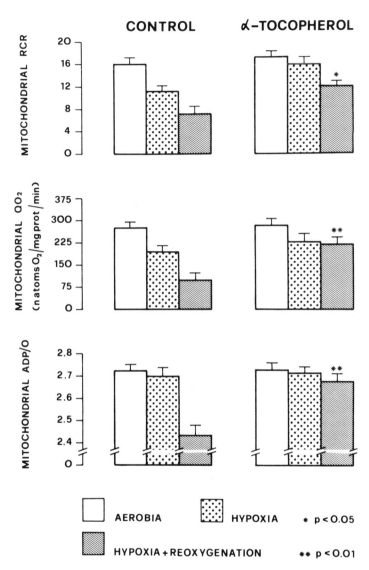

FIGURE 5. Effects of α-tocopherol on the hypoxic and reoxygenation-induced alterations of mitochondrial function of the isolated Langendorff-perfused rabbit hearts. Mitochondrial function was determined as previously described.[55,56] During the various perfusions, α-tocopherol was infused directly into the aortic cannula at a rate of 23.2 nM/min, as described in the text. P relates to the significance of the difference relative to the values obtained for mitochondria isolated from hearts that had been perfused under aerobic conditions.

tents of ATP and creatine phosphate (CP) (FIG. 4), and isolated mitochondrial function. α-Tocopherol acetate (1.1 mg) was infused into the aortic inflow cannula at a rate 1.0 mL/min 20 minutes before inducing hypoxia, and it was continued for the remainder of the perfusion. Hypoxia was induced by gassing the Krebs Henseleit solution with 95% $N_2 + 5\%$ CO_2 and by replacing glucose with mannitol.

FIGURE 4 shows that when hypoxic substrate-free perfusion was introduced (at 0 on the time scale), developed tension declined and resting tension increased. These changes in mechanical performance were only partially reversed during reoxygenation. In addition, reoxygenation induced a further release of creatine phosphokinase (CPK) in the coronary effluent and no recovery of tissue content of ATP and CP. The infusion of α-tocopherol at a rate of 23.2 nM/min modified the response to hypoxia and subsequent reoxygenation. When α-tocopherol was present, the hypoxic-induced increase of diastolic tension was reduced, and on reoxygenation there was a better recovery of tissue ATP and of developed tension.

Furthermore α-tocopherol almost completely abolished the exacerbation of CPK leakage caused by reintroduction of oxygen. FIGURE 5 refers to the data obtained for mitochondrial function. When α-tocopherol was present in the perfusion medium during hypoxia and reoxygenation, mitochondrial function was better maintained. These results show that α-tocopherol protects saline-perfused rabbit heart muscle against some of the deleterious consequences of hypoxic, substrate-free perfusion and reoxygenation. As α-tocopherol has no effect on spontaneous heart rate or peak developed tension, it is difficult to explain its protective effect in terms of a diminished rate of energy utilization consequent upon a reduction in cardiac work. Also, because coronary flow was constant, its beneficial effect is unlikely to have been due to an enhanced delivery of O_2. It is possible that the membrane stabilization exerted by α-tocopherol is important for its protective effects. α-Tocopherol associates with the sulfide-containing proteins and the polyunsaturated phospholipids in biological membranes,[64] thereby enhancing membrane stability. Conversely, vitamin E deficiency results in biological membranes becoming abnormally permeable.[65]

The ability of α-tocopherol to function as an antioxidant may also be of importance, particularly in preventing or reducing the exacerbation of damage that occurs during reoxygenation.[66] This exacerbation of tissue damage during reoxygenation has a complex etiology. When, after a period of hypoxia, the supply of oxygen is restored, cardiac contraction begins to increase at a time when relatively little energy is available and the mitochondria are functioning badly. Under these conditions it might be anticipated that the balance between energy supply and energy utilization would deteriorate further. Inasmuch as α-tocopherol protects mitochondrial function and maintains the high energy phosphate reserves, it should provide some degree of protection. Also, because of its antioxidant properties, it may prevent the occurrence of the O_2 toxicity phenomenon. This O_2 toxicity may be a consequence of the spontaneous formation of lipid peroxides.[67] Allison[68] has already shown how lipid peroxidation, induced by O_2, increases lysosomal permeability in heart muscle cells, thereby causing hydrolytic enzymes to be released into the cytosol and hence exacerbating the damage caused by the pre-existing period of inadequate oxygenation. By terminating the autocatalytic peroxidation sequences that may involve polyunsaturated fatty acids, lipids, and other easily oxidizable groups, such as the sulfhydryls,[69,70] α-tocopherol should provide some protection against the damage caused when O_2 is reintroduced after a period of hypoxia or anoxia. It must be pointed out, however, that in our acute *in vitro* experiments, α-tocopherol was used as α-tocopherol acetate, and we do not know if, or to what extent, α-tocopherol acetate, which is supposed to lack antioxidant properties, has been hydrolyzed, making "free" α-tocopherol available to act as an antioxidant.

EFFECTS OF α-TOCOPHEROL ADMINISTRATION DURING ISCHEMIA AND REPERFUSION

Previously reported experiments[56] and the data shown in FIGURE 6 demonstrate that when administered to hearts subjected to ischemia and reperfusion, α-tocopherol acetate failed to maintain normal sarcolemmal permeability and mechanical function. This is in contrast with the positive data obtained during hypoxia, and it seems to be related to the fact that under a condition of severe coronary flow reduction, like ischemia, α-tocopherol acetate is not hydrolyzed to free α-tocopherol, which is acting as an antioxidant.

FIGURE 6, in fact, also shows that when the same concentration of α-tocopherol (0.2 mM) was bound to 5% of bovine serum albumin, it partially modified the response of the hearts to ischemia and reperfusion, thus yielding some protection. When α-tocopherol albumin was present, the increase in diastolic pressure developed significantly more slowly, although it was of the same magnitude. During reperfusion, there was no further increase of diastolic pressure, and the developed pressure began to increase earlier and to a greater extent in the α-tocopherol bound to the albumin group than in control hearts. In addition, in these treated hearts there was less CPK release on reperfusion and better recovery of tissue contents of ATP and CP.

In an attempt to clarify the ability of free α-tocopherol to protect the ischemic myocardium by functioning as an antioxidant, we have also determined its effect on cellular content and release of GSH and GSSG. The data are shown in FIGURES 7 and 8, respectively. In these experiments, only α-tocopherol bound with albumin was used. In hearts perfused under aerobic conditions, there was a small release of GSH and almost no release of GSSG, independently from α-tocopherol infusion. Sixty minutes of ischemia did not significantly alter GSH and GSSG release (FIG. 8), while tissue content of GSH was significantly reduced in both control or α-tocopherol-infused hearts (FIG. 7). Tissue content of GSSG after ischemia was not significantly different from that obtained after aerobic perfusion. During reperfusion of the control hearts, there was a marked and sustained release of GSH and GSSG with a further reduction of cellular GSH. Furthermore, in this group, tissue content of GSSG was significantly increased after the readmission of coronary flow, despite the reperfusion-induced release of GSSG. Presence of α-tocopherol during ischemia and reperfusion was able to reduce the release of GSH and GSSG and attenuate the cellular accumulation of GSSG occurring on reperfusion.

These results indicate that α-tocopherol when bound with albumin protects saline-perfused rat heart muscle against some of the deleterious consequences of severe ischemia and reperfusion. The protection has been shown in several different ways, including altered rates of enzyme leakage, slowed rate of diastolic pressure development, improved recovery of developed pressure and of tissue ATP and CP, and preservation of the glutathione status during ischemia and reperfusion. We have previously pointed out that ischemia induces metabolic alterations capable of reducing the defense mechanisms against oxygen toxicity. The prime alteration seems to lie at the level of mitochondrial superoxide dismutase, its activity being reduced by 50% after severe ischemia.[16,40] The readmission of molecular oxygen is likely to stimulate the production of O_2 radicals above the neutralizing capacity of mitochondrial SOD. Under these conditions, the second line of defense against oxygen toxicity, GPD, is highly stimulated. A severe reduction of GSH/GSSG ratio, with enhanced GSSG content, was found after reperfusion in the control hearts, indicating that myocardial oxidative damage had occurred. All of these alterations are known to cause distur-

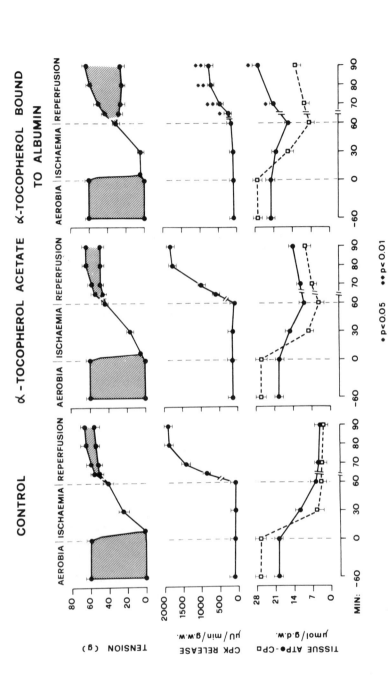

FIGURE 6. Effect of α-tocopherol acetate and of α-tocopherol bound to albumin on the ischemic- and reperfusion-induced alterations of mechanical function, CPK release, and tissue content of ATP and CP of the isolated and perfused rabbit hearts. The hearts were perfused aerobically for 60 minutes and made ischemic for 60 minutes by reducing coronary flow from 25 mL/min to 1 mL/min. After ischemia the hearts were reperfused for another 30 minutes. α-Tocopherol acetate or bound with albumin was infused into the aortic inflow cannula 60 minutes before the onset of ischemia, and the infusion was continued during ischemia and reperfusion. 0.2 mM of α-tocopherol was bound to 5% bovine serum albumin. The solution was stirred, sonicated, and filtered. α-Tocopherol concentration in the final perfusate was 1.4×10^{-5} M. Results are the mean ± SE of at least six separate experiments. CPK and tissue content of ATP and CP were determined as previously described.[57]

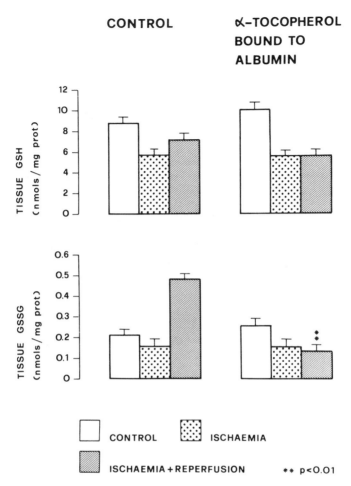

FIGURE 7. Effects of α-tocopherol bound with albumin on the ischemic- and reperfusion-induced alterations of glutathione status. All the determinations were performed in the homogenate, as previously described.[57] Under aerobic and reperfusion conditions the hearts were perfused at a mean coronary flow of 25 mL/min. Ischemia was induced by reducing coronary flow 1 mL/min. Results are given as mean ± SE of six experiments. Test of significance relates to the significance of the difference caused by the presence of α-tocopherol.

bances in calcium transport,[44] alterations of membrane permeability,[45] and impairment of muscle contraction, which can account for the poor recovery of metabolic and mechanical function observed in this group during reperfusion. The exogenous administration of α-tocopherol, acting as a natural antioxidant, could have reduced the occurrence of the oxidative stress occurring during reperfusion, and it could also have terminated the autocatalytic peroxidation sequence likely to occur in cellular and subcellular membranes under our experimental conditions. The finding that the reperfusion-induced release and the tissue accumulation of GSSG was significantly reduced in the series of hearts treated with α-tocopherol support this hypothesis. Finally, it is worthwhile recalling here that, at least in the isolated and perfused rabbit hearts, free α-tocopherol has a stronger protective effect than α-tocopherol acetate.[56] This finding indirectly suggests that the mechanism of action of α-tocopherol might be connected with its antioxidant effects, as α-tocopherol acetate is supposed to lack antioxidant properties. Our results also indicate that in *in vitro* experiments α-tocopherol acetate probably is not completely hydrolyzed and that binding of α-tocopherol with albumin is advantageous, particularly in an asanguineous medium, as we used.

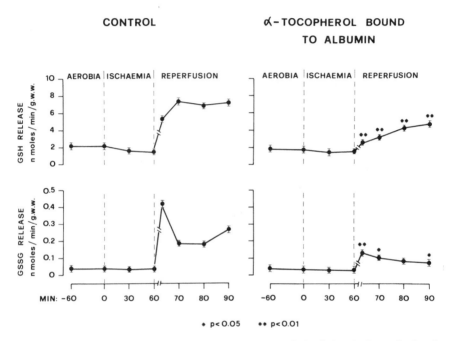

FIGURE 8. Effect of α-tocopherol on the ischemic- and reperfusion-induced release of reduced (GSH) and oxidized (GSSG) glutathione from isolated, Langendorff-perfused rabbit hearts. When α-tocopherol was present, it was infused continuously (see text) through the entire perfusion. Results are mean ± SE of six separate experiments. Test of significance relates to the significance of the difference caused by the presence of α-tocopherol.

SUMMARY

There is evidence that oxygen free radicals play a role in myocardial ischemic and reperfusion injury. We investigated the effect of ischemia and reperfusion on glutathione status. Reperfusion after prolonged ischemia (60 min) induced an important release of reduced (GSH) and oxidized (GSSG) glutathione, concomitant with an increase of tissue GSSG and no recovery of mechanical function, indicating that reperfusion results in oxidative stress. These alterations are associated with tissue and mitochondrial calcium accumulation, loss of mitochondrial function, and membrane damage. We also determined the arteriocoronary sinus difference for GSH and GSSG of 16 CAD patients undergoing coronary artery bypass. Patients were divided in two groups according to the length of clamping period: 25 ± 2 min (group 1), and 55 ± 6 min (group 2). In group 1, reperfusion resulted in a transient release of GSH, GSSG, CPK, and lactate, with return to preclamping values in 10 minutes. In group 2, reperfusion determined a sustained and pronounced release of GSH, GSSG, CPK, and lactate during declamping, suggesting the occurrence of an oxidative stress. Using an *in vitro* model, administration of α-tocopherol bound with albumin showed protection of mitochondrial function, improved recovery of contraction, and reduced oxidative stress during reperfusion.

ACKNOWLEDGMENTS

We thank Miss Afra Benini for secretarial assistance in preparing the manuscript and Miss Michela Palmieri and Miss Cristina Capelli for their technical assistance.

REFERENCES

1. MORRIS, J. G. 1976. J. Appl. Bacteriol. **40:** 220-229.
2. HALLIWELL, B. & M. C. GUTTERIDGE. 1984. Biochem. J. **219:** 1-14.
3. McINTYRE, T. M. & N. P. CURTHOYS. 1980. Int. J. Biochem. **12:** 545-551.
4. BULKLEY, G. B. 1983. Surgery **94:** 407-414.
5. FRIDOVICH, I. 1978. Science **201:** 875-880.
6. FREEMAN, B. A. & M. D. CRAPO. 1982. Lab. Invest. **47:** 412-426.
7. HOCHSTEIN, P. & S. K. JAIN. 1981. Fed. Proc. Fed. Am. Soc. Exp. Biol. **40:** 183-188.
8. TAPPEL, A. L. 1973. Fed. Proc. Fed. Am. Soc. Exp. Biol. **32:** 1870-1874.
9. CHANCE, B., H. SIES & A. BOVERIS. 1979. Physiol. Rev. **59:** 527-605.
10. G.I.S.S.I. (Gruppo Italiano per lo studio della Streptochinasi nell'infarto miocardico). 1986. Lancet **1:** 397-400.
11. GRUNTZIG, A. R., A. SENNING & W. E. SIEGENTHALER. 1979. N. Engl. J. Med. **301:** 61-68.
12. GANZ, W., N. BUCHBINDER, H. MARCUS, A. MONDKAR, J. MADDAHI, Y. CHARUZI, L. O'CONNOR, W. SHELL, M. C. FISHBEIN, R. KASS, A. MIYAMOTO & H. J. C. SWAN. 1981. Am. Heart J. **104:** 4-13.
13. FERRARI, R., C. CECONI, S. CURELLO, A. CARGNONI, E. CONDORELLI, S. BELLOLI, A. ALBERTINI & O. VISIOLI. 1988. J. Mol. Cell. Cardiol. **20** (Suppl. 2): 119-133.
14. HEARSE, D. J. 1977. J. Mol. Cell. Cardiol. **9:** 607-616.
15. FERRARI, R., A. ALBERTINI, S. CURELLO, C. CECONI, F. DI LISA, R. RADDINO & O. VISIOLI. 1986. J. Mol. Cell. Cardiol. **18:** 487-498.
16. FERRARI, R., C. CECONI, S. CURELLO, A. CARGNONI, C. AGNOLETTI, G. M. BOFFA & O. VISIOLI. 1986. Eur. Heart J. **7:** 3-12.
17. JENNINGS, R. B., H. K. HAWKINS, J. E. LOWE, M. C. HILL, S. KLOTTMAN & K. REIMER. 1978. Am. J. Pathol. **92:** 187-214.
18. GAUDEL, Y., H. S. KARAGUEUZIAN & J. DE LEIRIS. 1979. J. Mol. Cell. Cardiol. **11:** 717-731.
19. SHEN, A. C. & R. B. JENNINGS. 1972. Am. J. Pathol. **67:** 441-452.
20. KATZ, A. M. & F. C. MESSINEO. 1983. Circ. Res. **48:** 1-20.
21. FERRARI, R., A. ALBERTINI, S. CURELLO, C. CECONI, F. DI LISA, R. RADDINO & O. VISIOLI. 1986. J. Mol. Cell. Cardiol. **18:** 487-498.

22. WEGLICKI, W. B., B. M. WAITE & A. C. STAM. 1972. J. Mol. Cell. Cardiol. **4:** 195-201.
23. MEERSON, F. Z., V. E. KAGAN, YU P. KOZLOV, L. M. BELKINA & YU V. ARKHIPENKO. 1982. Basic Res. Cardiol. **77:** 465-485.
24. FERRARI, R., C. CECONI, S. CURELLO, C. GUARNIERI, C. M. CALDARERA, A. ALBERTINI & O. VISIOLI. 1985. J. Mol. Cell. Cardiol. **17:** 937-945.
25. FREEMAN, B. A. & M. D. CRAPO. 1982. Lab. Invest. **47:** 412-416.
26. MCCORD, J. 1985. N. Engl. J. Med. **312:** 159-163.
27. FERRARI, R., S. BONGRANI, F. CUCCHINI, F. DI LISA, C. GUARNIERI & O. VISIOLI. 1982. Effects of molecular oxygen and calcium on heart metabolism during reperfusion. *In* Coronary Arterial Spasm. M. E. Bertrand, Ed.: 46-59.
28. TURNER, J. F. & A. BOVERIS. 1980. Biochem. J. **191:** 421-430.
29. BRAUNWALD, E. & R. A. KLONER. 1985. J. Clin. Invest. **76:** 1713-1719.
30. MCCORD, J. 1985. N. Engl. J. Med. **312:** 159-163.
31. DOWNEY, J. M., D. J. HEARSE & D. M. YELLON. 1988. J. Mol. Cell. Cardiol. **20** (Suppl. II): 55-63.
32. KUEHL, F. A., J. L. HUMES & M. L. TORCHIANA. 1979. Adv. Inflamm. Res. **I:** 419-430.
33. HALLIWELL, B. & J. M. C. GUTTERIDGE. 1984. Biochem. J. **219:** 1-14.
34. KORTHUIS, R. J., D. N. GRANGER, M. I. TOWNSLEY & A. E. TAYLOR. 1982. Circ. Res. **57:** 599-611.
35. ENGLER, R. L., G. W. SCHMID-SCHONBEIN & R. S. PAVELEC. 1983. Am. J. Pathol. **111:** 98-111.
36. BURTON, K. P., M. J. MCCORD & G. GHAI. 1984. Am. J. Physiol. **246:** H776-H783.
37. SINGAL, P. K., N. KAPUR, K. S. DHILLON, R. E. BEANISH & N. S. DHALLA. 1982. Can. J. Physiol. Pharmacol. **60:** 1390-1397.
38. JOLLY, S. R., N. J. KANE, M. B. BAILIE, G. D. ABRAMS & B. R. LUCCHESI. 1984. Circ. Res. **54:** 277-285.
39. FERRARI, R., C. CECONI, S. CURELLO, A. CARGNONI, A. ALBERTINI & O. VISIOLI. 1986. Oxygen utilization and toxicity at myocardial level. *In* Biochemical Aspects of Physical Exercise. G. Benzi, L. Packer & N. Siliprandi. Eds.: 145-156. Elsevier. Amsterdam.
40. FERRARI, R., C. CECONI, S. CURELLO, A. CARGNONI & D. MEDICI. 1986. J. Mol. Cell. Cardiol. **18:** 67-69.
41. CURELLO, S., C. CECONI, D. MEDICI, R. FERRARI. 1986. J. Appl. Cardiol. **1:** 311-327.
42. CURELLO, S., C. CECONI, A. CARGNONI, R. FERRARI & A. ALBERTINI. 1987. Clin. Chem. **33/8:** 1448-1449.
43. MULLANE, K. M., N. READ, J. A. SALMON & S. MONCADA. 1984. J. Pharmacol. Exp. Ther. **228:** 510-515.
44. ROMSON, J. L., B. G. HOOK, S. L. KUNKEL, G. D. ABRAMS, M. A. SCHORK & B. R. LUCCHESI. 1983. Circulation **67:** 1016-1027.
45. WERNS, S. W., M. Y. SHEA & B. R. LUCCHESI. 1986. Circulation **74:** 1-5.
46. WERNS, S. W., M. Y. SHEA, B. R. LUCCHESI, C. COHEN, G. D. ABRAMS, B. PITT & B. R. LUCCHESI. 1986. Circ. Res. **56:** 895-912.
47. WERNS, S. W., M. J. SHEA, J. E. MITSOS, R. C. DYSKO, J. C. FANTONE, M. A. SCHORK, G. D. ABRAMS, B. PITT & B. R. LUCCHESI. 1986. Circulation **73:** 518-602.
48. CHAMBERS, D. E., D. A. PARKS, G. PATTERSON, R. ROY, J. M. MCCORD, S. YOSCHIDA, L. F. PARMLEY & J. M. DOWNEY. 1985. J. Mol. Cell. Cardiol. **17:** 145-153.
49. AMBROSIO, G., L. C. BECHER, G. M. HUTCHINS, H. F. WEISMAN & M. L. WEISFELDT. 1986. Circulation **74:** 1424-1433.
50. REIMER, K. A. & R. B. JENNINGS. 1985. Circulation **71:** 1069-1073.
51. MEERSON, F. Z., V. E. KAGAN, YU P. KOZLOV, L. M. BELKINA & YU V. ARKHIPENKO. 1982. Basic Res. Cardiol. **77:** 465-485.
52. MITSOS, S. E., T. E. ASKEW & J. C. FANTONE. 1983. Circulation **73:** 1077-1086.
53. ZHU, W. X., R. BOLLI, M. L. MYERS, C. J. HARTLEY & R. ROBERTS. 1985. Circulation **72** (III): 74 (Abstr.).
54. CECONI, C., S. CURELLO, A. CARGNONI, R. FERRARI, A. ALBERTINI & O. VISIOLI. 1988. J. Mol. Cell. Cardiol. **20:** 5-13.
55. FERRARI, R., O. VISIOLI, C. GUARNIERI & C. M. CALDARERA. 1982. Acta Vitaminol. Enzymol. **5:** 11-22.

56. FERRARI, R., C. CECONI, S. CURELLO, A. CARGNONI, C. CONDORELLI & R. RADDINO. 1985. Acta Vitaminol. Enzymol. **7:** 61-70.
57. FERRARI, R., A. CARGNONI, C. CECONI, S. CURELLO, A. ALBERTINI & O. VISIOLI. 1987. Role of oxygen in the myocardial ischaemic and reperfusion damage: Protective effects of vitamin E. *In* Clinical and Natriuretic Aspects of Vitamin E. O. Hayaishi & M. Mino. Eds.: 209-226. Elsevier. Amsterdam.
58. GUARNIERI, C. R. FERRARI, O. VISIOLI, C. M. CALDARERA & W. G. NAYLER. 1978. J. Mol. Cell. Cardiol. **10:** 893-906.
59. GUARNIERI, C., F. FLAMIGNI, C. ROSSONI-CALDARERA & R. FERRARI. 1982. Adv. Myocardiol. **3:** 621-627.
60. NASON, A. & I. R. LEHMAN. 1965. J. Biol. Chem. **22:** 511-529.
61. SCHWARZ, K. & W. BAUMGARTNER. 1970. Kinetic studies in mitochondrial enzymes during respiratory decline relating to the mode of action of tocopherol. *In* The Fat Soluble Vitamins. H. F. Deluca & J. W. Suttie, Eds.: 317. Univ. of Wisconsin Press. Madison, WI.
62. OLIVEIRA, M. M., W. B. WEGLICKI, A. NASON & P.P. NAIR. 1969. Biochim. Biophys. Acta **180:** 98-113.
63. YOUNG, J. M. & J. S. DINNING. 1951. J. Biol. Chem. **193:** 743-747.
64. NISHIKIMI, M., H. YAMADA & K. YAGI. 1980. Biochim. Biophys. Acta **627:** 100-108.
65. ORNE-JOHNSON, W. H. & H. BEYNERT. 1969. Biochem. Biophys. Res. Commun. **36:** 905-911.
66. HEARSE, D. J., S. M. HUMPHREY, W. G. NAYLER, A. SLADE & D. BORDER. 1975. J. Mol. Cell. Cardiol. **8:** 205-215.
67. BAIRD, M. B., H. R. MASSIE & M. J. PIEKIELNYAK. 1977. Chem. Biol. Interact. **16:** 145-153.
68. ALLISON, A. C. 1965. Nature **205:** 141-143.
69. DRAPER, H. H. & A. S. CSALLANY. 1969. Fed. Proc. **28:** 1960-1965.
70. TAPPEL, A. L. 1962. Vitamins **20:** 493-510.

The Role of Vitamin E and Carotenoids in Preventing Oxidation of Low Density Lipoproteins[a]

HERMANN ESTERBAUER,[b] GEORG STRIEGL,
HERBERT PUHL, SABINE OBERREITHER, MARTINA
ROTHENEDER, MOHAMMED EL-SAADANI, AND
GÜNTHER JÜRGENS

*Institute of Biochemistry and
Institute of Medical Biochemistry
University of Graz
A-8010 Graz, Austria*

INTRODUCTION

It is well-established that an increased plasma cholesterol content is mainly due to increased levels of the low density lipoprotein (LDL), that cholesterol deposits in fatty streaks and atherosclerotic plaques stem primarily from LDL, and that high levels of plasma LDL are closely associated with an increased risk of atherosclerosis.[1-4]

Early atherosclerotic lesions are characterized by a massive accumulation of cells filled with lipid droplets rich in cholesterylesters and cholesterol. Such cells are called foam cells because of their foamy appearance. Most of these arterial foam cells in atherosclerotic lesions have developed from resident tissue macrophages or from blood monocytes that entered the arterial intima in response to chemotactic factors (for review see ref. 5 and 6). Recently it has been shown by several groups[7-17] that oxidatively modified LDL (o-LDL) possesses a number of functional properties that could explain the formation of foam cells and several other aspects of atherogenesis.

In vitro, LDL can be oxidized by incubating it in cultures of endothelial cells,[7,9] smooth muscle cells,[9,11] monocytes, or macrophages.[10,16] Also, incubation of LDL in cell-free medium results in oxidation, and in both systems, that is, cell-free medium or cells, the rate and extent of oxidation is strongly enhanced by micromolar amounts of iron or copper ions, whereas EDTA, BHT, vitamin E, and other antioxidants prevent or retard the oxidative modification. It is assumed that the structural and functional properties of cell-oxidized LDL are very similar if not identical to LDL oxidized in a cell-free medium.[17] Strong evidence exists that oxidation of LDL is a

[a] This work was supported by the Association for International Cancer Research (U.K.) and by the Austrian Science Foundation, project no. P 6176 B.

[b] Correspondence should be addressed to Prof. Dr. H. Esterbauer, Institute of Biochemistry, University of Graz, Schubertstr. 1, A-8010 Graz, Austria.

free radical process by which the LDL particle is depleted of its antioxidants, and the polyunsaturated fatty acids 18:2 and 20:4 are degraded in a lipid peroxidation process.[12,18–21] In this process a number of highly reactive products such as malonaldehyde, 4-hydroxynonenal, various other aldehydes, lipid peroxides, lysophosphatides, and other products rapidly accumulate in the LDL particle. Indirect evidence suggests that these products then interact with the amino acid side chains of the apo-B and modify it in such a way that new epitopes are formed that are no longer recognized by the apo-B/E receptor but by the scavenger receptor.[17,22–26] It has been shown that native LDL treated with increasing concentration of malonaldehyde[22,23,25] or 4-hydroxynonenal[24,26]progressively loses its affinity for the LDL receptor, and if more than 16% of the lysines are blocked by one of these aldehydes, the LDL particle is then internalized by way of the scavenger receptor.

In support of the hypothesis that lipid peroxidation plays a crucial role in the progression of atherosclerosis is also that atherosclerotic lesions of human aorta contain lipid peroxides,[27] that normal LDL contains a subfraction with some properties of o-LDL,[28] and that in atheroma of Watanabe rabbits, malonaldehyde-modified apolipoprotein (apo-B) occurs.[29] Moreover, it has been shown that the antiatherogenic effect of probucol, a drug used for the treatment of hypercholesterolemia, is partly related to its antioxidant effects.[30] Probucol is basically a dimer of the well-known chain-breaking antioxidant BHT (FIG. 1).

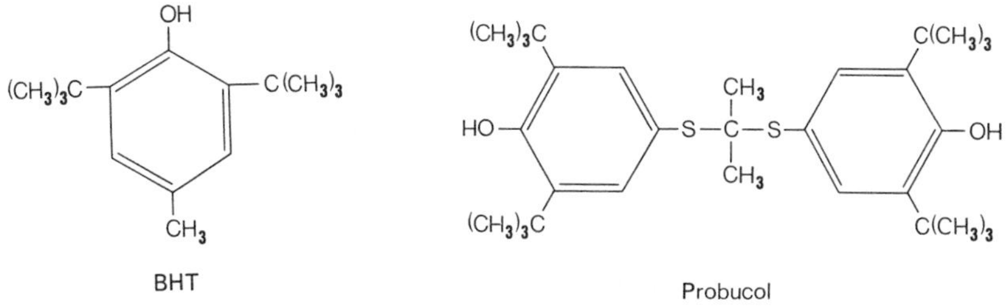

FIGURE 1. Formula of probucol and BHT.

The various results briefly summarized above strongly suggest, but of course do not definitely prove, a causal relationship between modification of LDL by lipid peroxidation and atherosclerosis. If it is so, antioxidants, in particular those contained in LDL, should play a central role at the biochemical level by preventing or retarding oxidative modification of LDL.

POLYUNSATURATED FATTY ACIDS AND ANTIOXIDANTS IN LDL

When we first began our work on oxidation of LDL, we tried to find exact data on the composition of LDL with regard to fatty acids and antioxidants in the literature. Much to our surprise, such data were not available. It seems that LDL research of recent years had mainly concentrated on apo-B and its function and on the biological and physical primary properties of LDL.

Inasmuch as a good knowledge of the polyunsaturated fatty acid (PUFA) and antioxidant content in LDL is a basic requirement for lipid peroxidation studies, we have determined these values in a number of LDL preparations from different donors (TABLE 1, for experimental details see ref. 12 and 21). It is known that in LDL these fatty acids are mainly bound to phospholipids and cholesterol and to a lesser extent to triglycerides.

The major PUFA that can undergo lipid peroxidation are 18:2 and 20:4; they mainly amount to one-half of all fatty acids in LDL. The molecular weight of LDL is about 2.5 million, expressed on a molar base; one LDL molecule therefore, on average, contains about 1000 molecules 18:2 and 130 molecules 20:4. There are, however, great variations between the LDL from different donors, as can be seen by the range given in TABLE 1. The LDL with the lowest arachidonic acid content contained only 48 molecules 20:4 per LDL particle, whereas the highest content was 250 molecules 20:4 per LDL molecule. The high variability in the PUFA content may be associated with the individual dietary conditions of the donors. The same is likely valid for the variability of the antioxidants (TABLE 1; for experimental details see ref. 21). The major antioxidant in LDL is alpha-tocopherol, followed by retinyl-stearate, gamma-tocopherol, beta-carotene, and lycopene. It should be noted here that the donor that had the highest vitamin E content in the LDL (3.96 nmole/mg) had taken 150 mg vitamin E/day for 1 month prior to blood donation. It is plausible that the high variability of PUFA and antioxidants influences the susceptibility of LDL towards oxidation and the quantity of the individual products that can be formed by the oxidative degradation of the PUFA. This is consistent with our experimental

TABLE 1. Mean Values of Fatty Acids and Antioxidants in Human LDL; n Gives the Number of LDL Preparations (see TABLE 2) Investigated. All Values Are Given in nmole/mg LDL.[a]

	Mean ± SD	Range
Fatty acids (n = 11)		
14:0	28 ± 11	14 ± 46
16:0	278 ± 36	221 − 333
16:1	20 ± 7	15 − 33
18:0	49 ± 10	39 − 67
18:1	161 ± 36	123 − 229
18:2	413 ± 88	272 − 543
20:4	57 ± 30	19 − 100
Total FA	930 ± 152	770 − 1164
Total PUFA	422 ± 95	300 − 574
Antioxidants		
Alpha-tocopherol (n = 18)	2.57 ± 0.66	1.26 − 3.96
Gamma-tocopherol (n = 19)	0.20 ± 0.06	0.11 − 0.32
Beta-carotene (n = 16)	0.15 ± 0.09	0.05 − 0.36
Lycopine (n = 16)	0.08 ± 0.04	0.02 − 0.16
Retinylstearate (n = 5)[b]	0.57 ± 0.26	0.20 − 0.72

[a] Antioxidants/PUFA (mole/mole) 1 : 110.
[b] See Note Added in Proof.

findings[12,14,21] that each LDL preparation shows its own characteristic behavior in the oxidation experiments, as reflected by the duration of the lag phase, the rate of oxidation, and the amount of lipid peroxidation products formed.

In our work, we find that, in general, a positive correlation exists between the amount of vitamin E and carotenoids and the resistance of an LDL preparation against oxidation, as measured by the amount of malondialdehyde (MDA) formed after the incubation with 10 μM Cu^{2+} for certain periods of time. There were also strong exceptions, however, and we therefore had the suspicion that antioxidants other than vitamin E and carotenoids might play a significant role, too. (See Note Added in Proof.)

The total amount of the individual antioxidants in LDL varied widely from donor to donor, and obviously no intercorrelation existed between the content of vitamin E, carotenoids, and retinoids (TABLE 2). Thus we have found LDL with high vitamin E and high beta-carotene (LDL-10), high vitamin E and low beta-carotene (LDL-6), and low vitamin E and low beta-carotene (LDL-2).

In our opinion, much more data are needed, in particular for retinylesters, to make a statistical evaluation regarding classes of LDL defined according to antioxidant status, in a systematic way, as done by F. Gey[4] for plasma antioxidants. In this evaluation, it would also be good to know whether in plasma a free exchange of all or some of the antioxidants exists between different classes of lipoproteins or chylomicrons. Knowledge of this subject is very limited. For example, some studies say that LDL is the main carrier of vitamin E, whereas others claim that the plasma tocopherol content correlates with the HDL level. A recent *in vivo* study[31] with deuterated alpha-tocopherol (oral administration of 15 mg) shows that vitamin E is secreted by the intestine into chylomicrons; the chylomicron remnants are then taken up by the liver, from which the vitamin E is secreted in VLDL and is finally more or less equally distributed between LDL and HDL.

According to epidemiological studies (479 healthy persons, 40-49 years of age), the plasma vitamin E content varies from 20.07 to 28.3 μM.[4] With an average concentration of 3 mg LDL/mL plasma and our vitamin E measurements in isolated LDL, only about 30-40% of the total plasma vitamin E is contained in LDL.

RELATIONSHIP BETWEEN THE ONSET OF LIPID PEROXIDATION IN LDL AND THE CONSUMPTION OF ANTIOXIDANTS

It has been shown[8] that the addition of vitamin E to the cell culture medium prevented its oxidation by cells, as measured by the increase of MDA; even more importantly, the LDL reisolated from the vitamin E-supplemented culture was not taken up by the macrophage scavenger receptor. Later, it was shown by us that *in vitro* oxidation of LDL only occurs if the particle is depleted of its endogeneous content of alpha-tocopherol, gamma-tocopherol, and beta-carotene.[12,20,21,32] To follow exactly the time curves of the decrease of the various antioxidants of LDL and to follow the onset of lipid peroxidation appeared rather difficult. The problems we faced in this attempt were briefly as follows. Each LDL preparation differed from the others by its oxidizability in response to the addition of Cu^{2+} ions as prooxidant (our standard condition of stimulation LDL oxidation is 16 mole Cu^{2+} ions per mole LDL); the experimental observation of the progress of oxidation in a particular experiment

TABLE 2. Individual Values of Alpha-Tocopherol, Gamma-Tocopherol, Beta-Carotene, Lycopine, Retinylstearate,[a] and PUFA 18:2 and 20:4 in Human LDL. The Values Given Are in nmole/mg LDL.

LDL Number	LDL Prepared from Blood of	α-Tocopherol	γ-Tocopherol	β-Carotene	Lycopine	Retinylstearate[a]	18:2	20:4
1	1 female	n.e.[b]	0.11	0.17	0.02	n.e.	313	19
2	1 female	1.61	0.11	0.10	0.07	n.e.	272	25
3	1 female + 1 male	2.25	0.16	n.e.	n.e.	n.e.	373	30
4	1 female + 1 male	2.35	0.21	0.14	0.07	n.e.	419	28
5	2 females	2.94	0.22	0.13	0.04	n.e.	n.e.	n.e.
6	1 male	3.96	0.09	0.05	0.09	n.e.	n.e.	n.e.
7	2 females + 3 males	2.61	0.24	0.22	0.14	n.e.	n.e.	n.e.
8	1 female + 1 male	2.98	0.28	0.36	0.15	n.e.	n.e.	n.e.
9	2 females + 1 male	2.93	0.28	0.35	0.16	n.e.	n.e.	n.e.
10	2 females	3.49	0.25	0.11	0.10	n.e.	n.e.	43
11	1 female + 3 males	2.48	0.17	0.11	0.08	n.e.	386	n.e.
12	2 females + 1 male	2.91	0.11	0.18	0.02	n.e.	327	20
13	1 male	1.76	0.18	0.12	0.06	n.e.	474	48
14	2 females + 1 male	2.24	0.17	0.10	0.14	n.e.	n.e.	n.e.
15	3 females + 2 males	2.18	0.19	0.14	0.09	n.e.	498	69
16	2 females + 2 males	2.43	0.32	n.e.	n.e.	n.e.	432	100
17	1 male	2.3	0.16	0.05	0.04	0.28	509	83
18 (P113)	1 female + 3 males	1.26	0.21	0.05	0.04	0.77	543	93
19 (P114)	4 males	2.32	0.23	0.07	0.06	0.20	n.e.	n.e.
20 (P111)	2 females + 1 male	n.e.	n.e.	n.e.	n.e.	0.72	n.e.	n.e.
21 (P112)	2 males	n.e.	n.e.	n.e.	n.e.	0.62	n.e.	n.e.
	mean ± SD	2.51 ±0.66	0.20 ±0.06	0.15 ±0.09	0.08 ±0.04	0.57 ±0.26	413 ±88	51 ±30

[a] See Note Added in Proof.
[b] Not estimated.

afforded the measurement of many samples in short time intervals, which in turn means large quantities of precious LDL. Nevertheless, in some experiments the exact time of the onset of lipid peroxidation was missed, and in others, again, the time when the LDL was depleted of its antioxidants could not be accurately determined by the discontinuous measurements. When we tried to repeat the oxidation experiments with the same batch of the LDL preparation (dialyzed and therefore free from EDTA and BHT), stored overnight at 4°C, we repeatedly observed (although not always) that it was easier to oxidize than the fresh preparation, although the antioxidants did not measurably change during this short storage.

FIGURE 2 shows one of these kinetic experiments.[32] Here, the decrease of alpha- and gamma-tocopherol, lycopine, and beta-carotene was measured in 10-minute in- tervals, and the decrease of linoleic acid and arachidonic acid was measured in 30- minute intervals. It is evident that massive lipid peroxidation only occurred after the consumption of the antioxidants. The exact time when the LDL had lost all its antioxidants and entered into the lipid peroxidation propagation phase, however, could not be deduced from this experiment. At the time when the experiment, shown in FIGURE 2, was performed, we did not yet know that retinylstearate (see Note Added in Proof) was an important additional endogenous antioxidant in LDL (see TABLE 1 and 2). The result of another LDL oxidation experiment where retinylstearate (see Note Added in Proof) was also measured is shown in TABLE 3. Here we measured

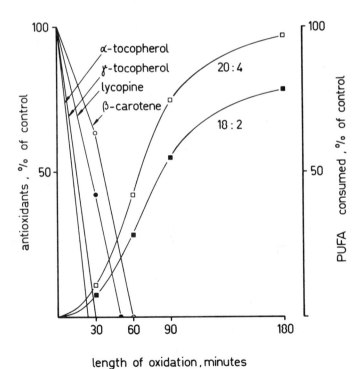

FIGURE 2. Kinetics of the consumption of antioxidants and PUFA during oxidation of LDL. (Esterbauer *et al.*[32] With permission from Elsevier.)

TABLE 3. Relationship between the Decrease of Lipophilic Antioxidants in LDL and the Increase of Peroxides.[a]

Time	Peroxides	α-Tocopherol	γ-Tocopherol	β-Carotene	Lycopine	Retinylstarate[b]
0	5	1.26	0.21	0.049	0.040	0.77
10	5	0	0	0.049	0.030	0.48
20	5	0	0	0.025	0.011	0.27
30	5	0	0	0.015	0.004	0.15
60	10	0	0	0	0	0
90	40	0	0	0	0	0
120	83	0	0	0	0	0

[a] The incubation mixture contained 0.25 mg LDL/mL, 0.01 M phosphate buffer, pH 7.4, and 0.16 M NaCl. Oxidation was initiated by addition of 1.66 μM CuCl$_2$. The values given are nmole/mg LDL.
[b] See Note Added in Proof.

as index of lipid peroxidation, instead of the loss of PUFA, the increase of lipid peroxides by a rapid iodometric assay specifically developed by us for analysis of lipoproteins.[33] The data of this experiment clearly show that the antioxidants are consumed in the sequence alpha-tocopherol, gamma-tocopherol, lycopine, retinylstear-ate (see Note Added in Proof), beta-carotene, and that peroxides in LDL do not increase to a measurable extent as long as the LDL contains antioxidants. This means that even if the LDL has lost its vitamin E (already 10 minutes after the initiation of the oxidation), it is not oxidized, indicating that it is still sufficiently protected by the remaining retenoids and carotenoids. The experiment in TABLE 3 shows finally that the onset of lipid peroxidation was somewhere between 30 and 60 minutes after the initiation of the oxidation. Again the exact time cannot be determined from this experiment. To overcome this problem, we have recently developed a procedure that allows us to follow the oxidation of LDL continuously.

CONTINUOUS MONITORING OF *IN VITRO* OXIDATION OF LDL

The primary products of lipid peroxidation are lipid hydroperoxides of the general structure $-CH=CH-CH=CH-CHOOH-$ with an absorption maximum around 235 nm. Inasmuch as o-LDL is, like native LDL, fully soluble in buffer, the generation of such conjugated lipid hydroperoxides can directly be measured by recording the ultraviolet (UV) spectrum of the aqueous LDL solution. This is different from all other biological systems (microsomes, mitochondria cells, tissue homogenate), where lipid peroxidation was studied. In such cases the conjugated dienes can only be obtained by analyzing the lipid extracts.

FIGURE 3 shows the UV spectrum of an LDL solution measured at different times after the addition of Cu^{2+} as a prooxidant. Native LDL showed a maximum at 222 nm, which is probably due to the absorption of the apo-B. With increasing oxidation time, the absorbance in the 220-230 nm region increased due to the formation of conjugated lipid hydroperoxides. To prove that the increase of the absorption is caused by the lipid part of the LDL and not by changes in the apo-B, native and oxidized

LDL were delipidated, and the UV spectra of the apo-B (in 0.15% aqueous SDS) and lipids (in hexane) were measured and compared. No difference existed between the spectra of the apo-B from native and oxidized LDL, whereas the spectrum of the lipids extracted from the oxidized LDL showed a strong absorption maximum at 234 nanometers. Furthermore, an excellent correlation (r = 0.99) exists between the amount of conjugated lipid hydroperoxides as measured by the change of the absorbance at 234 nm (ΔA, ϵ = 29500) and the amount of malonaldehyde measured by the thiobarbituric acid (TBA) assay or peroxides (measured by the iodometric method,[33] see FIGURE 4).

The fact that the formation of conjugated dienes in the LDL particle can be measured directly, that is, without prior extraction of the lipids, offers the possibility to continuously monitor the time course of their formation, that is, the time course of oxidation. For that, an aliquot of the LDL solution to be investigated is placed in a 1 cm quartz cuvette; the initial absorption at 234 nm is set to zero, and the increase of the absorption is continuously recorded. Another aliquot of the same LDL solution is used for measuring (discontinuously) the decrease of the antioxidants.

FIGURES 5 and 6 show two such experiments. In the one (FIG. 5), LDL (0.25 mg/mL) dissolved in oxygen saturated 0.01 M phosphate buffer, pH 7.4, 0.16 M NaCl was supplemented with 1.6 μM CuCl$_2$, and the oxidation was continuously monitored by measuring the increase of the 234 nm absorption. It can be seen that

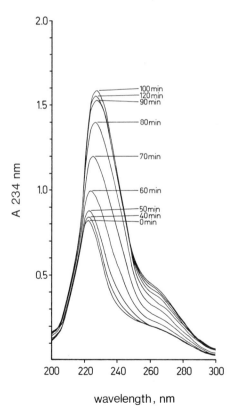

FIGURE 3. Change of the UV spectrum of LDL during oxidation. LDL (0.25 mg/mL) in oxygen-saturated 0.01 M phosphate buffer, pH 7.4, and 0.16 M NaCl; oxidation was initiated by addition of 1.66 μM CuCl$_2$. Spectra measured against a reference solution without LDL.

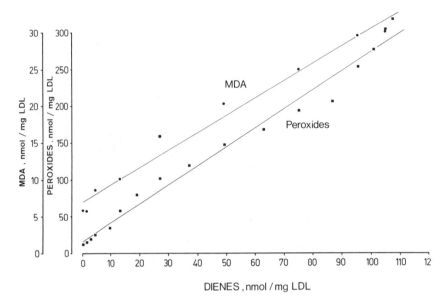

FIGURE 4. Relationship between the amount of conjugated dienes, peroxides, and MDA in o-LDL. Experimental conditions as in FIGURE 3. The amount of dienes was calculated from the increase of the absorbance at 234 nm. $\epsilon = 29500$; MDA was determined by the TBA assay, and peroxides by the iodometric method are described in reference 33.

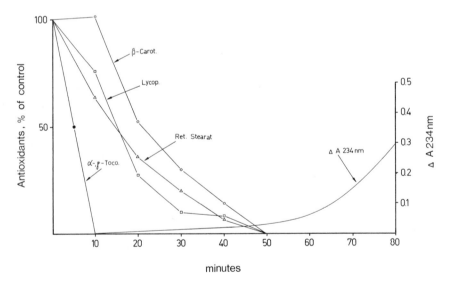

FIGURE 5. Kinetics of the consumption of antioxidants and formation of conjugated dienes during oxidation of LDL. Experimental conditions as in FIGURE 3. The diene increase was measured by continuously monitoring the increase of the 234 nm absorption. Retinylstearate, see also Note Added in Proof.

the oxidation process can be clearly divided into a lag phase and a propagation phase. During the lag phase, which lasted in this particular experiment 60 minutes, the antioxidants are progressively consumed in the sequence vitamin E, lycopine, retinylstearate (see Note Added in Proof), and beta-carotene. During the lag phase there is only a small and linear increase of the diene absorption. Such a small increase can, in fact, be expected, because the scavenging of lipid peroxyradicals by vitamin E, and likely also by the other antioxidants, leads to lipid hydroperoxides according to ($LOO \cdot$ + vit E → $LOOH$ + vit E $\cdot$). When the LDL is depleted of its antioxidants, the rate of the diene formation progressively increases, indicating that the lipid peroxidation process has entered into its propagation phase. In this particular experiment, the absorption increased up to 160 min to a maximum ΔA of 0.6 and then slowly decreased again. In the other experiment (FIG. 6), all experimental conditions were identical to the experiment shown in FIGURE 5, except that the LDL solution was

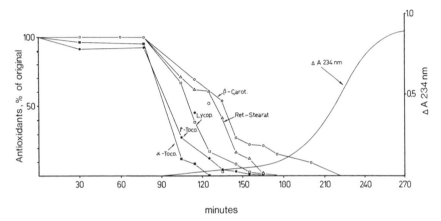

FIGURE 6. Effect of ascorbate on the consumption of antioxidants and formation of conjugated dienes during oxidation of LDL. The experimental conditions were as in FIGURE 5, except that the LDL solution was supplemented with 10 μM ascorbate prior to addition of $CuCl_2$. Retinylstearate, see also Note Added in Proof.

supplemented with 10 μM ascorbic acid immediately prior to starting the experiment by the addition of 1.6 μM Cu^{2+} as prooxidant. It can be seen that this water-soluble antioxidant increases the duration of the lag phase from about 60 min (without ascorbate) to 180 minutes. The endogenous antioxidants present in the LDL are completely protected by ascorbate for about 80 minutes. Thereafter, their consumption proceeds in the same sequence as in the ascorbate free medium.

The continuous monitoring of the LDL oxidation by the measurement of the 234 nm diene absorption is a very convenient and accurate method for determining the oxidizability of LDL and the effect of antioxidants. FIGURES 7 and 8 show such measurements for 2.5 and 5 μM ascorbate and 0.41 and 0.83 μM urate. Both compounds retard LDL oxidation in a concentration-dependent manner, but have no marked effect on the rate of the LDL oxidation during the propagation phase; that is, the slope of the curves is not affected by these antioxidants. The concentration of ascorbate or urate used in these experiments (FIGURES 7 and 8) is in the range as

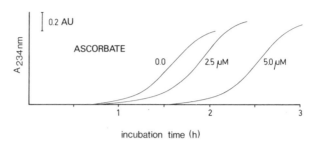

FIGURE 7. Effect of ascorbate on the lag phase of LDL oxidation as measured by the increase of the diene absorption. The LDL solution was supplemented with 0, 2.5, and 5.0 μM ascorbate prior to addition of $CuCl_2$. Other conditions are as in FIGURE 5.

found in plasma. This indicates that the water-soluble antioxidants are of equal importance as the endogenous lipophilic antioxidants of LDL itself for its protection against oxidation in the plasma.

More difficult to study is the effect of externally added lipophilic antioxidants. First we tried to enrich LDL with alpha-tocopherol. For that study, alpha-tocopherol (0 to 60 μg/mg LDL) dissolved in ethanol was equally distributed on the wall of a small round bottom flask by evaporating the ethanol on a rotary evaporator. The LDL solution was added and the flask was rotated for 3 hours. The LDL was then recovered and reisolated by ultracentrifugation, and the alpha-tocopherol content was determined. In all LDL samples prepared in this way, the alpha-tocopherol content was lower than in the original LDL. The original LDL had 0.78 nmole alpha-tocopherol/mg LDL, with a lag phase of 38 min; the "enriched" LDL had 0.0, 0.17, 0.52, 0.82, and 1.03 nmole alpha-tocopherol/mg LDL, with lag phases of 9, 13, 13, 13, 18, and 17 minutes. Thus it appears that the enrichment procedure was not successful and led in fact to a depletion of the endogeneous antioxidants, most likely through oxidation.

In a second experiment, alpha-tocopherol was added directly as an ethanolic solution (TABLE 4). Here we found an increase of the lag phase from 47 min (control LDL with 2.32 nmole alpha-tocopherol/mg LDL) to 76 min in the system supple-

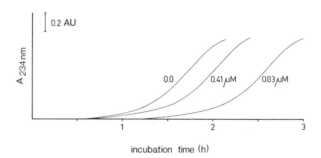

FIGURE 8. Effect of urate on the lag phase of LDL oxidation as measured by the increase of the diene absorption. The LDL solution was supplemented with 0, 0.41, and 0.83 μM urate prior to addition of $CuCl_2$.

TABLE 4. Effect of Antioxidants on the Lag Phase of LDL Oxidation

System	Lag Phase (min)
Ascorbate	
control LDL, no. 18 (TABLE 2)	72
+ 5 μM ascorbate (= 20 nmole/mg LDL)	129
+ 10 μM ascorbate (= 40 nmole/mg LDL)	200
Urate	
control LDL, no. 18 (TABLE 2)	76
+ 0.83 μM urate (= 3.32 nmole/mg LDL)	129
+ 1.66 μM urate (= 6.64 nmole/mg LDL)	200
Alpha-tocopherol	
control LDL, no. 19 (TABLE 2), + 10 μl EtOH	47
+ 0.58 μM tocopherol (2.3 nmole/mg LDL)	51
+ 1.16 μM tocopherol (4.6 nmole/mg LDL)	50
+ 2.32 μM tocopherol (9.2 nmole/mg LDL)	56
+ 4.64 μM tocopherol (18.4 nmole/mg LDL)	76
Retinylstearate	
control LDL, no. 19 (TABLE 2), + 10 μl DMSO	20
+ 0.26 μM retinylstearate (1.04 nmole/mg)	26
+ 0.52 μM retinylstearate (2.08 nmole/mg)	33
+ 1.04 μM retinylstearate (4.16 nmole/mg)	61

[a] The incubation mixtures (1 mL) contained 0.25 mg LDL/mL, 0.01 M phosphate buffer, pH 7.4, and 0.16 M NaCl. Oxidation was initiated by addition of 1.66 μM $CuCl_2$. Alpha-tocopherol was added in 10 μL ethanol; synthetic retinylstearate was added in 10 μL dimethylsulfoxide.

mented with an additional 18.4 nmole alpha-tocopherol/mg LDL. The question, however, remains, How much of the added vitamin E was, in fact, incorporated into the LDL? The same is true for the experiment with synthetic retinylstearate supplementation. In the particular experiment shown in TABLE 4, the lag phase of the control LDL decreased from 47 min to 20 min, due to the addition of 10 μL DMSO; with synthetic retinylstearate dissolved in the same volume of DMSO, the lag phase could be increased from 20 min to 61 minutes.

[NOTE ADDED IN PROOF: During the conference and when the manuscript was prepared, we thought that the additional antioxidant was retinylstearate. The substance in question showed the same retention time in reversed phase HPLC and the same fluorescence behavior as synthetic retinylstearate. Recently, however, we obtained evidence that the HPLC peak contains a further fluorescent substance that also decreases during LDL oxidation as shown in FIGURES 5 and 6 for retinylstearate. A similar observation was also made by F. Hoffmann-La Roche, Basel (personal communication with F. Gey). The structure of this substance is presently being investigated.]

REFERENCES

1. GOLDSTEIN, J. L. & M. S. BROWN. 1978. Low-density lipoprotein pathways and its relation to atherosclerosis. Annu. Rev. Biochem. **46:** 897-930.

2. BROWN, M. S. & J. L. GOLDSTEIN. 1986. A receptor-mediated pathway for cholesterol homeostasis. Science 232: 34-47.
3. GOTTO, A. M. 1987. Plasma lipoproteins. New Comprehensive Biochemistry, Vol. 14. A. Neuberger & L. L. M. van Deenen, Eds. Elsevier. Amsterdam.
4. GEY, K. F. 1986. On the antioxidant hypothesis with regard to arteriosclerosis. Bibl. Nutr. Dieta 37: 53-91.
5. SOUTAR, A. K. & B. L. KNIGHT. 1985. Regulation of macrophage functions by lipoproteins. In Mononuclear Phagocytes: Physiology and Pathology. (R. Dean & W. Jessup, Eds.) Elsevier. Amsterdam.
6. BROWN, M. S. & J. L. GOLDSTEIN. 1983. Lipoprotein metabolism in the macrophage: Implications for cholesterol deposition in atherosclerosis. Annu. Rev. Biochem. 52: 223-261.
7. HENRIKSEN, T., E. M. MAHONEY & D. STEINBERG. 1981. Enhanced macrophage degradation of low density lipoprotein previously incubated with cultured endothelial cells: Recognition by receptors for acetylated low density lipoproteins. Proc. Natl. Acad. Sci. USA 78: 6499-6503.
8. STEINBRECHER, U. P., S. PARTHASARATHY, D. S. LEAKE, J. L. WITZTUM & D. STEINBERG. 1984. Modification of low density lipoprotein by endothelial cells involves lipid peroxidation and degradation of low density lipoprotein phospholipids. Proc. Natl. Acad. Sci. USA 81: 3883-3887.
9. MOREL, D. W., P. E. DiCORLETO & G. M. CHISOLM. 1984. Endothelial and smooth muscle cells alter low density lipoprotein in vitro by free radical oxidation. Arteriosclerosis 4: 357-364.
10. CATHCART, M. K., D. W. MOREL & G. M. CHISOLM. 1985. Monocytes and neutrophils oxidize low density lipoprotein making it cytotoxic. J. Leukocyte Biol. 38: 341-350.
11. HEINECKE, J. W., L. BAKER, H. ROSEN & A. CHAIT. 1986. Superoxide-mediated modification of low density lipoprotein by arterial smooth muscle cells. J. Clin. Invest. 77: 757-761.
12. ESTERBAUER, H., G. JÜRGENS, O. QUENHENBERGER & E. KOLLER. 1987. Autoxidation of human low density lipoprotein: Loss of polyunsaturated fatty acids and vitamin E and generation of aldehydes. J. Lipid Res. 28: 495-509.
13. HEINECKE, J. W. 1987. Free radical modification of low-density lipoprotein: Mechanisms and biological consequences. Free Radical Biol. Med. 3: 65-73.
14. JÜRGENS, G., H. F. HOFF, G. M. CHISOLM, III & H. ESTERBAUER. 1987. Modification of human serum low density lipoprotein by oxidation—characterization and pathophysiological implications. Chem. Phys. Lipids 45: 315-336.
15. QUINN, M. T., S. PARTHASARATHY, L. G. FONG & D. STEINBERG. 1987. Oxidatively modified low density lipoproteins: A potential role in recruitment and retention of monocytes/macrophages during atherogenesis. Proc. Natl. Acad. Sci. USA 84: 2995-2998.
16. RAYMOND, T. L., S. A. REYNOLDS & J. A. SWANSON. 1987. In vitro incubation of low-density lipoproteins with inflammatory cells causes enhanced degradation by macrophages in culture. Inflammation 11: 335-344.
17. STEINBRECHER, U. P., J. L. WITZTUM, S. PARTHASARATHY & D. STEINBERG. 1987. Decrease in reactive amino groups during oxidation or endothelial cell modification of LDL. Arteriosclerosis 7: 135-143.
18. JÜRGENS, G., M. EL-SAADANI, G. STRIEGL & H. ESTERBAUER. 1988. LDL modified by endogeneous lipid peroxidation products. In Modified Lipoproteins. Proceedings of the Eighth International Symposium on Atherosclerosis, Venice, October 7-8. 13-20. CIC Edizioni Internazionali s.r.l., Roma.
19. STEINBRECHER, U. P. 1987. Oxidation of human low density lipoprotein results in derivatization of lysine residues of apolipoprotein B by lipid peroxide decomposition products. J. Biol. Chem. 262: 3603-3608.
20. ESTERBAUER, H., G. JÜRGENS & O. QUEHENBERGER. 1988. Modification of human low density lipoprotein by lipid peroxidation. In Oxygen Radicals in Biology and Medicine. M. Simic, Ed. 369-373. Plenum. New York, NY.
21. ESTERBAUER, H., O. QUEHENBERGER & G. JÜRGENS. 1988. Oxidation of human low density lipoprotein with special attention to aldehydic lipid peroxidation products. In

Free Radicals: Methodology and Concepts. C. Rice-Evans & B. Halliwell, Eds.: 243-368. Richelieu Press. London.

22. FOGELMAN, A. M., I. SHECHTER, J. SAEGER, M. HOKOM, J. S. CHILD & P. A. EDWARDS. 1980. Malondialdehyde alteration of low density lipoproteins leads to cholesteryl ester accumulation in human monocyte-macrophages. Proc. Natl. Acad. Sci. USA **77:** 2214-2218.

23. HABERLAND, M. E., A. M. FOGELMAN & P. A. EDWARDS. 1982. Specificity of receptor-mediated recognition of malondialdehyde-modified low density lipoprotein. Proc. Natl. Acad. Sci. USA **79:** 1712-1716.

24. JÜRGENS, G., J. LANG & H. ESTERBAUER. 1986. Modification of human low density lipoprotein by the lipid peroxidation product 4-hydroxynonenal. Biochim. Biophys. Acta **875:** 103-114.

25. HABERLAND, M. E. & A. M. FOGELMAN. 1987. The role of altered lipoproteins in the pathogenesis of atherosclerosis. Am. Heart J. **113:** 573-577.

26. HOFF, H. F., G. M. CHISOLM, III, D. W. MOREL, G. JÜRGENS & H. ESTERBAUER. 1988. Chemical and functional changes in LDL following modification by 4-hydroxynonenal. *In* Oxy-Radicals in Molecular Biology and Pathology. P. A. Cerutti, J. M. McCord & I. Fridovich, Eds.: 459-472. Alan R. Liss, Inc. New York.

27. GLAVIND, J., S. HARTMANN, J. CLEMMESEN, K. E. JESSEN & H. DAM. 1952. Studies on the role of lipoperoxides in human pathology. Acta. Pathol. Microbiol. Scand. **30:** 1-6.

28. AVOGARO, P., G. BITTOLO BON & G. CAZZOLATO. 1988. Presence of a modified low density lipoprotein in humans. Arteriosclerosis **8:** 79-87.

29. HABERLAND, M. E., D. FONG & L. CHENG. 1988. Malondialdehyde-altered protein occurs in atheroma of Watanabe heritable hyperlipidemic rabbits. Science **241:** 215-218.

30. KITA, T., Y. NAGANO, M. YOKODE, K. ISHI, N. KUME, A. OOSHIMA, H. YOSHIDA & C. KAWAI. 1987. Probucol prevents the progression of atherosclerosis in Watanabe heritable hyperlipidemic rabbit, an animal model for familial hypercholesterolemia. Proc. Natl. Acad. Sci. USA **84:** 5928-5931.

31. TRABER, M. G., K. U. INGOLD, G. W. BURTON & H. J. KAYDEN. 1987. Absorption and transport of deuterium-substituted 2R,4′R,8′R-α-tocopherol in human lipoproteins. Lipids **23:** 791-797.

32. ESTERBAUER, H., G. JÜRGENS, H. PUHL & O. QUEHENBERGER. 1989. Role of oxidatively modified LDL in atherogenesis. *In* Medical, Biochemical and Chemical Aspects of Free Radicals. O. Hayaishi, E. Niki, M. Kondo & T. Yoshikawa, Eds.: 1203-1209. Elsevier. Amsterdam.

33. EL-SAADANI, M., H. ESTERBAUER, M. EL-SAYED, M. GOHER, A. Y. NASSAR & G. JÜRGENS. 1989. A spectrophotometric assay for lipid peroxides in serum lipoproteins using a commercially available reagent. J. Lipid Res. **30:** 627-630.

Plasma Vitamins E and A Inversely Correlated to Mortality from Ischemic Heart Disease in Cross-Cultural Epidemiology

K. FRED GEY[a]

Vitamin Research Department
F. Hoffmann-La Roche & Co., Ltd.
Basel, Switzerland

PEKKA PUSKA[a]

Public Health Institute
Helsinki, Finland

INTRODUCTION

An elevated plasma level of total cholesterol, of LDL (low density lipoprotein) cholesterol, or of the LDL/HDL (high density lipoprotein) ratio predicts, even if combined with other classical risk factors (such as hypertension and smoking), the increased risk of ischemic heart disease (IHD) to at most 50 percent. The remaining risk may, at least in part, be related to dietary factors. Thus, various diets are associated with a lower morbidity and mortality from IHD, for example, the vegetarian diet or the Mediterranean diet (literature cited in ref. 1). Potential benefits may mainly be expected from essential polyunsaturated fatty acids (PUFA), as well as from essential

[a] On behalf of principal investigators and collaborators of the International Collaborative Study on the Fatty Acid-Antioxidant Hypothesis of Arteriosclerosis and of the Optional Study on Antioxidant Vitamins and PUFAs, WHO/MONICA Project: Georg Alfthan, Helsinki, Finland; Florence Bernasconi, Basel, Switzerland; Daniel Brunner, Tel Aviv, Israel; Ernst Bühler, Basel, Switzerland; I. M. Eckstein, Schleiz, GDR; Alun Evans, Belfast, Northern Ireland; Flaminio Fidanza, Perugia, Italy; Horst Georgi, Basel, Switzerland; Horst Heine, Berlin, GDR; Lothar Heinemann, Berlin, GDR; Paul Jordan, Basel, Switzerland; Kim Klarlund, Copenhagen, Denmark; Mario Mancini, Naples, Italy; Ulrich K. Moser, Basel, Switzerland; Reto Muggli, Basel, Switzerland; J. Müller, Schwedt, GDR; Tapio Nikkari, Tampere, Finland; Michael F. Oliver, Edinburgh, Scotland; Pekka Puska, Helsinki, Finland; Rudolph A. Riemersma, Edinburgh, Scotland; Günther Ritzel, Basel, Switzerland; Paolo Rubba, Naples, Italy; Matti Salo, Tampere, Finland; Marianne Schroll, Roskilde, Denmark; Willy Schüep, Basel, Switzerland; H. Schüler, Cottbus, GDR; Erkki Vartiainen, Helsinki, Finland; Jean-Pual Vuilleumier, Basel, Switzerland; Claus Wagenknecht, Berlin, GDR; and David A. Wood, Edinburgh, Scotland.

antioxidants, such as the vitamins A, C, and E, carotenoids, and selenium. The important role of antioxidant vitamins is suggested by several findings (literature cited in ref. 1): (1) Chronic marginal deficiency of vitamin C or E causes arteriosclerosis-like lesions in rodents, piglets, and primates.[2,3] Supplements of vitamins A and/or E counteract the spontaneous arteriosclerosis of the middle-aged hen in the egg-laying period.[4] (2) Exogenous peroxidized PUFA damage the endothelium and heart muscle cells and provoke proliferation of smooth muscle cells. This cytotoxicity can be prevented by vitamins C and E. (3) Hypoxia with subsequent reoxygenation (as conceivable for a transitory impairment of coronary flow) produces a sudden burst of oxygen radicals that can overcharge protective enzymes such as superoxide dismutase. Oxygen radicals will seriously damage arteries in animal models as soon as the physiological radical scavengers, such as the vitamins E, C, and glutathione, are exhausted.[5-8] (4) Oxygen radicals cause peroxidative breakdown of the PUFA of LDL when the lipid-soluble radical scavengers of LDL are consumed. Thereby α- and γ-tocopherol disappear first, whereas carotenoids and retinyl esters form some last barrier against the modification of apolipoprotein-B (apo-B), which may be mediated to a great extent by hydroxyalkenals, that is, by fragments of peroxidized PUFA.[9,10] Correspondingly, LDL can be modified by incubation with cells (endothelial cells, smooth muscle cells, monocytes, and neutrophils), and this modification, as well as cytotoxicity, can again be counteracted by vitamin E.[11-14] Peroxide- or alkenal-modified LDL, in contrast to normal LDL, is taken up by monocytes/macrophages that can thereby be transformed into arteriosclerotic lipid-laden foam cells. This transformation has been assumed to be an early, if not even initial step, in the formation of the arteriosclerotic plaque.[9-18] In the arteriosclerotic aorta of the Watanabe heritable hyperlipemic rabbit, malondialdehyde-modified apo-B has been demonstrated,[19] and fresh surgical specimens of human atherosclerotic plaques contain modified LDL that is bound/degraded by monocytes/macrophages.[20] (5) Probucol, a drug with a radical scavenging phenol structure, reduces (in part presumably independent of its hypocholesterolemic potential) LDL modification and lipid storage in macrophages, as well as the progression of arteriosclerosis in the Watanabe heritable hyperlipemic rabbit.[21-24] (6) Modified LDL occurs regularly in small amounts in human plasma,[25] which can be significantly diminished by oral supplements of vitamin E.[26] (7) Patients with IHD have increased plasma levels of thiobarbituric acid-reactive material (an indicator of increased susceptibility of LDL towards lipid peroxidation), which can be decreased by vitamin C and/or E. (8) A low plasma level of lipid-standardized vitamin E is a risk factor in early angina pectoris.[27]

All this suggestive evidence leads to the crucial question of whether in the human a poor status of antioxidant vitamins is linked to a high mortality from IHD. This question can hardly be answered by dietary surveys, because they have too many inherent weaknesses. For instance, the present food tables are incomplete for carotenoids. They often do not differentiate between preformed vitamin A and its provitamin β-carotene, and worst of all, the dietary vitamin E cannot be properly calculated at all in the products of the modern food industry. Clearly, the vitamin status is more properly defined by the measurement of plasma levels. This has actually been done in the current cross-cultural investigation known as the *Optional Study on Antioxidant Vitamins and PUFAs of the WHO/MONICA Project* (initiated as the International Collaborative Study on the Fatty Acid-Antioxidant Hypothesis of Arteriosclerosis). Up to now, all essential antioxidants of plasma have been compared in 12 European populations, with up to 4-fold differences of age-specific mortality from IHD. The presently available data show, in confirmation of earlier data,[1,28-30] that vitamin E has the strongest inverse correlation to IHD mortality, and that vitamin A is also inversely related to IHD mortality.

SUBJECTS AND METHODS

In the current cross-sectional surveys, groups of about 100 apparently healthy males, of 40-49 years of age, from regions with different rates of mortality from IHD, were compared during the standard period of January through April with regard to the plasma status of the principal essential antioxidants, that is, vitamins A, C, and E, β-carotene, and selenium. The study populations were, in accordance with the well-known North-South gradient of IHD in the northern hemisphere, representative for regions with different incidences of death: (1) highest incidence, that is, yearly > 300 deaths from IHD [International Classification of Diseases, 9th Ed. WHO, No. 410-414] per 100,000 males, 40-59 years of age: North Karelia, Finland (481 deaths/ 100,000 for 1983 and 469/100,000 for 1987; $n = 92$ in 1983; $n = 161$ in 1987) > Southwest Finland (359/100,000; $n = 82$) and Edinburgh, Scotland (293/100,000; $n = 108$); (2) medium incidence, that is, approximately 150-250/100,000: peripheral Belfast, Northern Ireland (254/100,000; $n = 124$) > Glostrup-Copenhagen, Denmark (208/100,000; $n = 114$) = Schleiz, GDR (208/100,000; $n = 106$) > Cottbus, GDR (182/100,000; $n = 44$) = Schwedt, GDR (186/100,000; $n = 102$) > Tel Aviv, Israel (154/100,000; $n = 103$); (3) low incidence, that is, approximately 110/ 100,000: Thun, foothills of the Alps in Switzerland (112/100,000; $n = 220$) and Sapri, Southern Italy (107/100,00, $n = 77$). All subjects were selected at random, except for the large cohort of Swiss industrial employees in Thun. The latter, however, were in every respect representative for this age group of the working population of German-speaking Switzerland. Most details and analytical methods have been described elsewhere.[1,28-30]

In individuals ($n = 1176$ or 1336) biologically substantial, Spearman's rank correlation coefficients ($r_s > 0.3$) occurred between absolute plasma vitamin A (retinol) and absolute vitamine E (α-tocopherol; $r_s = 0.33$), as well as between these lipid-soluble vitamins and cholesterol ($r_s = 0.23$ and 0.55, respectively), triglycerides ($r_s = 0.38$ and 0.49), and the sum of cholesterol and triglycerides ($r_s = 0.39$ and 0.63, respectively). Therefore, in the present report, plasma vitamins E and A were standardized by nonlinear adjustment to 220 mg cholesterol plus 110 mg triglycerides/ dL (FIG. 1), that is, to a rather common plasma lipid level for European populations. Thereby, both vitamins became independent of the combination of cholesterol and triglycerides ($r_s < 0.005$), and lipid-standardized vitamins A and E varied practically independently ($r_s = 0.12$). The α-tocopherol: cholesterol plus triglyceride ratio is known to identify the plasma status of vitamin E almost as powerfully as the previously suggested α-tocopherol: total lipid ratio and slightly better than the α-tocopherol: cholesterol ratio.[1,31]

RESULTS AND DISCUSSION

The hitherto available populations do not reveal a consistent correlation of IHD mortality with the median of selenium ($r^2 = 0.02$), β-carotene ($r^2 = 0.01$), and vitamin C ($r^2 = 0.00$). This does not, however, exclude indirect, and in some populations even important correlations, for example, in those with a particularly low vitamine C status.[1,28] Thus, in the hitherto available individuals ($n = 1176$), the plasma level of lipid-standardized vitamin E tends to parallel the vitamin C level

(Spearman's rank correlation coefficeint $r_s = 0.28$), but a particularly strong correlation exists in populations with low vitamin C medians (*e.g.* in Edinburgh with 20.2 μM vitamin C, $r_s = 0.53$, or Glostrup with 28.4 μM vitamin C, $r_s = 0.52$), in contrast to populations with high vitamin C values (*e.g.* Tel Aviv with 57.4 μM, $r_s = 0.15$ or Sapri with 35.2 M, $r_s = 0.16$). This may suggest that a critical vitamin C level limits the regeneration of vitamine E,[1,32,33] and will thus deteriorate the vitamin E status. Correspondingly, *in vitro* vitamin E delays the disappearance of vitamin E during peroxidative LDL damage.[10]

The absolute plasma level of vitamin E (α-tocopherol), the quantitatively most important lipid-soluble antioxidant, varies in individuals (FIG. 1, top) on the one hand

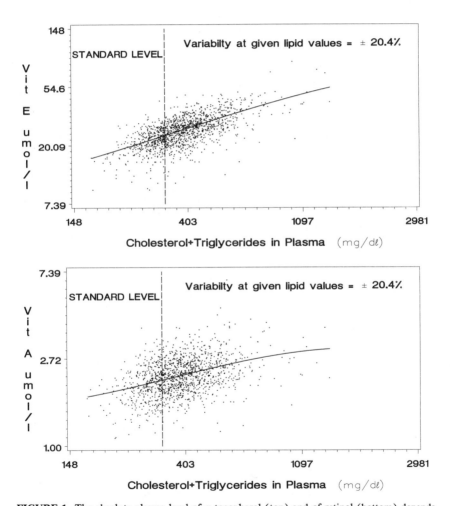

FIGURE 1. The absolute plasma level of α-tocopherol (top) and of retinol (bottom) depends on one hand on the level of lipoproteins (represented by the sum of cholesterol and triglycerides) and on the other hand on the vitamin concentration within the lipoproteins. The latter is indicated by the vertical variability (coefficient of variation).

with the level of cholesterol and triglycerides, which represent practically the sum of LDL and VLDL (very low density lipoproteins), but on the other hand with the vitamin concentration within the lipids and lipoproteins, respectively. The about 7-fold increase of lipids from hypo- to hyperlipidemia may raise the absolute vitamin E level to roughly 3-fold, but at any given lipoprotein level, its vitamin concentration can also vary up to 4-fold, with a coefficient of variation as great as 20 percent. Because of these variations, any judgements on vitamin E status of plasma is restricted to two conditions: (a) The absolute level of vitamin E may only be considered as long as plasma lipids are almost identical. We actually compared absolute α-tocopherol levels (FIG. 2) in 8 (out of 12) study populations, inasmuch as their plasma cholesterol was of the common European order (220-240 mg/dL), and did not differ significantly ($p > 0.05$). (b) If, by contrast, the lipid levels show the common wide variation, the vitamin E level requires lipid-standardization, for example, to mean values. This precaution was needed for the evaluation of the complete series of our populations that includes hypo- and hypercholesterolemic study sites (Italy, Israel, and North Karelia, respectively). Actually, the vitamin E level of all individuals was adjusted to a normal level, that is, 220 mg cholesterol plus 110 mg triglycerides per deciliter (FIG. 3). The lipid-adjusted vitamin E value thus becomes an indicator of the vitamin E concentration within the lipoproteins related to vitamin E variations, that is, within VLDL and LDL.

Retinol, which accounts for approximately 90-95% of total vitamin A in plasma, is actually carried by a specific lipoprotein, the retinol-binding protein.[34] Nevertheless, as already observed in many studies, the absolute retinol level also varies positively with the combination of plasma cholesterol and triglycerides, and in the individuals of the present study the variability of retinol (FIG. 1, bottom) was practically identical with that of vitamin E. This fact could be due to a coupling of the hepatic secretion of both retinol-binding protein and VLDL. The latter is known to be the exclusive vehicle by which both alpha-tocopherol and retinyl esters enter the blood plasma. Normally, an average (but with great variations between individuals) of about 2-8% of the vitamin A activity in plasma occurs as esterified retinol in the fractions of VLDL and finally of LDL.[34-38] In any case, retinol levels may only be interpreted with the same precautions (FIGURES 2 and 3) as for vitamin E in spite of the fact that lipid standardization of retinol has, to our knowledge, never been done before.

In the eight study populations, which lack a significant difference in the median of plasma cholesterol ($p > 0.05$), the latter is obviously not directly related ($r^2 = 0.05$) to the IHD mortality (FIG. 2, bottom). By contrast, the medians of the absolute plasma level of both tocopherol and retinol show an inverse association, with up to 3-fold difference in IHD mortality (FIG. 2, top). In these eight populations with a common European cholesterol level, the $r^2 = 0.55$ ($p = 0.003$) and $r^2 = 0.51$ ($p = 0.046$) for absolute vitamin A and E, respectively, indicate in a one-variable model that 55% and 51%, respectively, of the IHD risk can be attributed to the absolute amounts of vitamin E and A, respectively.

Of course, after inclusion of populations with particularly low and high medians of plasma cholesterol, the latter becomes directly and significantly ($p < 0.01$) related to the IHD risk in our 12 populations with an $r^2 = 0.51$ (FIG. 3, bottom). Nevertheless, when vitamins E and A are lipid-standardized they remain inversely related to the IHD mortality. The $r^2 = 0.49$ ($p = 0.01$) for lipid-standardized vitamin E is of the same order as that of absolute vitamin E in the eight populations of common cholesterol, whereas the $r^2 = 0.33$ ($p = 0.07$) for lipid-standardized retinol is somewhat lower (FIG. 3, top). In conclusion, the inverse association of both lipid-soluble vitamins with the IHD mortality may in any case be independent from the concurrent lipoprotein level. This is, in principle, confirmed by partial regression analysis (which

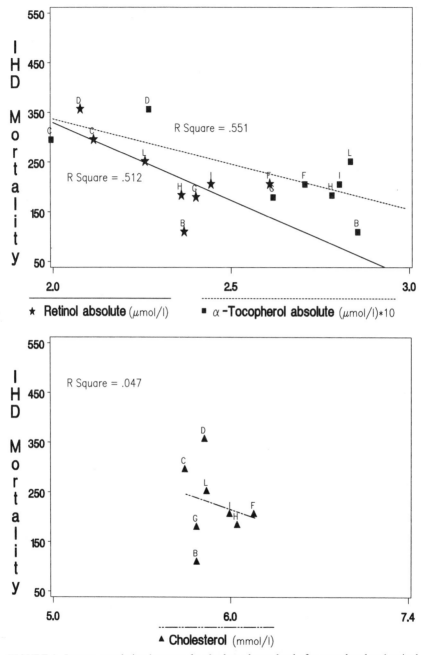

FIGURE 2. Inverse correlation between the absolute plasma level of α-tocopherol and retinol, respectively, and the age-specific IHD mortality (per 100,000) in eight populations with similar total plasma cholesterol, which lacks significant differences ($p > 0.05$) and has no direct correlation to the IHD mortality (bottom). The points represent the medians.

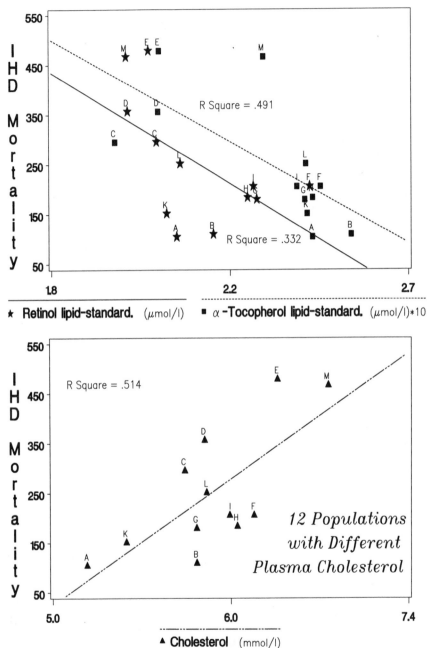

FIGURE 3. Inverse correlation between lipid-standardized plasma α-tocopherol and retinol, respectively, to the age-specific IHD mortality (per 100,000) in the complete series of study populations (12 populations with different plasma cholesterol, top) the cholesterol of which reveals a direct correlation to the IHD mortality (bottom). A represents the median of the study sample of Sapri, Southern Italy; B, Thun, Switzerland; C, Edinburgh, Scotland; D, Southwest Finland; E, North Karelia, Finland, 1982; F, Glostrup-Copenhagen, Denmark; G, Cottbus, GDR; H, Schwedt, GDR; I, Schleiz, GDR; K, Tel Aviv, Israel; L, Belfast, Northern Ireland; and M, North Karelia, Finland, 1987.

corrects on one hand the linear correlation between the median of cholesterol and IHD mortality, and on the other hand the residual correlation between the medians of lipid-standardized vitamins and cholesterol), because it yields $r^2 = 0.69$ ($p <$ 0.001) for the medians of lipid-standardized vitamin E to IHD mortality, and $r^2 =$ 0.74 ($p < 0.001$) for lipid-standardized retinol, respectively. The lipid-standardized vitamins E and A vary almost independently in individuals ($r_s = 0.12$) and may thus be separate risk factors of IHD.

If the medians of individually lipid-standardized vitamins E and A are combined in a two-variable model, the actual IHD mortality is predicted with $r^2 = 0.53$ ($p <$ 0.01). In consequence, the remaining half of IHD risk must be due to other factors, among which cholesterolemia may be most important in the present populations.

If the correlation between the medians of cholesterol and IHD is excluded by partial regression analysis, the combination of lipid-standardized vitamins E and A predicts the actual IHD mortality with $r^2 = 0.89$ ($p < 0.001$) (FIG. 4). Corresponding results are obtained when the medians of cholesterol and of vitamins E and A are combined in a three-variable model. In the eight populations with similar cholesterol level, the three-variable model (which uses cholesterol with absolute levels of vitamins E and A) predicts the actual IHD mortality, with an $r^2 = 0.81$ ($p = 0.06$) (FIG 5, top). In all 12 populations (considering cholesterol together with lipid-standardized vitamins E and A), the prediction formula fits the actual IHD mortality almost perfectly, that is, with $r^2 = 0.94$ ($p < 0.001$) (FIG. 5, bottom). In conclusion, in the hitherto available study propulations, 81-94% of the IHD risk can be statistically predicted by these three independent risk factors, that is, by the combination of cholesterol and vitamins E and A.

In the initial phase of the current cross-sectional study, the PUFA status was measured in the adipose tissue of four populations.[39] Low IHD in Italy was associated with a higher ratio of polyunsaturated/saturated fatty acids (P/S ratio) and a higher level of linoleic acid than in IHD-prone populations (Finland and Scotland). A corresponding moderate trend might also exist in the subsequent populations, the PUFA status of which has been measured in the membrane phospholipids of the erythroctye and buccal mucosae. In individuals of subsequent populations, however, the Spearman's rank correlation coefficient of α-tocopherol and PUFA has been very low and inconsistent (mostly around $r_s = 0.1$, with the exception of $r_s = 0.2$ for linoleic acid and α-tocopherol in erythrocytes only and of $r_s = 0.3$ for the P/S ratio and α-tocopherol in buccal mucosa). In consequence, it is unlikely that vitamin E and PUFA just behave similarly, at least not in the individuals of the more recent populations. This assumption is consistent with a well-known high variation of vitamin E content of vegetable oils,[40] the consumption of which cannot simply improve vitamin E status.[41,42]

The present cross-sectional data from European populations seem substantially to complement experimental data that suggest physiological functions of α-tocopherol as protectors of lipoproteins against peroxidation and apo-B modification, respectively (see INTRODUCTION). The same may be true for retinyl esters of LDL. Although retinyl esters might be weaker radical scavengers than α-tocopherol, their molar concentration in LDL is still about one-fourth that of α-tocopherol and markedly above γ-tocopherol and carotenoids. But most important, retinyl esters form a sort of last barrier against PUFA peroxidation and apo-B modification, respectively.[10] Retinyl esters parallel free retinol (as actually measured in the present study) in human plasma to some extent.[34-38] In vitro, as well as epidemiologically, vitamins E and A appear to act as synergists, although they can vary almost independently in isolated LDL[10] and in plasma lipids (see METHODS). In consequnce, the present epidemiological data may extend the oxidative modification hypothesis to the mortality

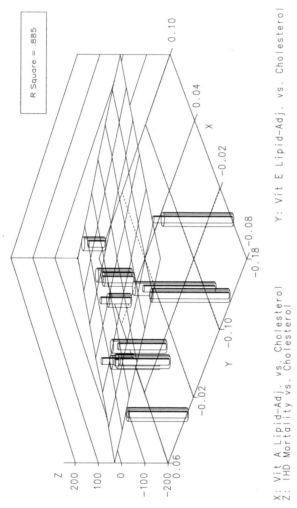

R Square = .885

X: Vit A Lipid-Adj. vs. Cholesterol   Y: Vit E Lipid-Adj. vs. Cholesterol
Z: IHD Mortality vs. Cholesterol

FIGURE 4. Multiple partial regression analysis (residual analysis) of age-specific IHD mortality. The x and y axes indicate the residuals (of medians of the logarithms) of lipid-adjusted vitamins after regressing them on cholesterol; the z axis indicates the IHD mortality after regressing it by cholesterol as well. In consequence, the new variables, x, y, and z, represent those portions of the corresponding original medians that have no dependence on cholesterol. The subsequent regression of such residuals results in the plane above the figure, where the outer columns represent actual values and the inner pillars the corresponding predicted values. Thus, r^2 means that 89% of the actual IHD mortality can be predicted by the combination of both lipid-standardized vitamins after exclusion of cholesterol.

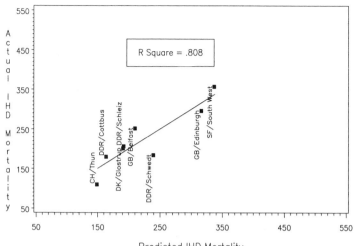

Predicted IHD Mortality
based on log median of plasma vitamins E & A absolute and cholesterol

12 Populations with Different Levels of Plasma Cholesterol

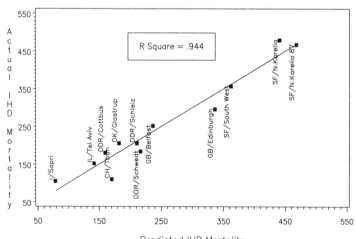

Predicted IHD Mortality
based on log median of plasma cholesterol and lipid—standardized vit A & E

FIGURE 5. Optional MONICA Study on Antioxidant Vitamins and PUFA. Multiple regression analysis of age-specific IHD mortality (per 100,000) with three variables, that is, the logarithms of the medians of plasma cholesterol, of α-tocopherol, and of retinol. For the 8 populations with similar cholesterol levels (top), the absolute vitamin values were used, whereas for the complete series of 12 populations with different cholesterol (bottom), the corresponding lipid-standardized values were used. The plot shows the strong correlation between actual and predicted IHD mortality.

from IHD in the human. This hypothesis postulates that antioxidants that block the modification of LDL *in vivo* might slow the progress of atherosclerosis, at least in the early steps leading to the fatty streak lesion, in which macrophage-derived foam cells contain most of the stored lipid.[9-26] Aside from the above-mentioned antioxidative protection of LDL, further effects of vitamins E and A, respectively, on the cellular and subcellular level may be considered as well. Tissue uptake of α-tocopherol is carried out by the specific LDL receptors, as well as by an unspecific uptake, together with lipids when they are liberated by lipoprotein lipase or even by thermodynamic partitioning. Correspondingly, vitamin A can be taken up specifically by cell receptors of the retinol-binding protein, as well as unspecifically, for example, after action of lipoprotein lipase on retinyl ester-carrying lipoproteins. The uptake of either antioxidant vitamin by cells may increase their antioxidant potential, and in consequence perhaps helps to overcome critical phases of plaque formation, such as the degradation of modified LDL taken up by monocytes/macrophages. Vitamin E may also be able to specifically exert some well-known antiarteriosclerotic functions, for example, by alteration of eicosanoid formation,[43-46] immunoresponses,[47,48] platelet behavior,[49] and stabilization of membrane structures.[45] Vitamin A, as an extremely potent morphogen, is known to regulate cell differentiation, as well as the expression of several proteins, and particularly arterial glycoproteins and immunoresponses as well.[50]

The current cross-sectional study reveals lipid-soluble vitamins E and A as important hitherto underrated risk factors of IHD, which substantially complement the previously known classical risk factors, particularly hypercholesterolemia. Thus the present data suggest that one considers the risk of hyperlipemia no longer only quantitatively, but from now on, also qualitatively, that is, with regard to the concentration of the antioxidant vitamins E and A within atherogenic lipoproteins. A potentially protective plasma status of both vitamins, as presumably needed for "optimum health" (as defined by WHO), may be achieved relatively easy by dietary measures, although at least for vitamin E, the present RDA presumably needs to be multiplied.[29,51] The optimization of the status of antioxidant vitamins for IHD prevention becomes particularly intriguing because population-based intervention trials on the reduction of classical risk factors (cholesterolemia, blood pressure, and smoking) have shown only weak and debatable overall benefits.[52] Of course, the IHD-preventive potentials of lipid-soluble vitamins A and E require reconfirmation by a continuation of the present cross-cultural comparisons and by pertinent prospective studies in individuals. Two prospective studies of the blood-bank type have not yet indicated a dependence of subsequent IHD mortality on vitamin E status,[53,54] but these data demand reservation because of several methodological problems, for example, the considerable loss of α-tocopherol on prolonged storage of serum in freezing temperatures, lack of both standardization for cholesterol plus triglycerides, and simultaneous consideration of lipid-standardized vitamin A. Clearly, preventive potentials of vitamins E and A regarding the morbidity and mortality from IHD can conclusively be proven only by population-based controlled intervention trials with specific supplements of these vitamins.

SUMMARY

In eight study populations in which the medians of total plasma cholesterol did not differ significantly (mean 5.8 mM, $p > 0.05$) and therefore did not correlate with the IHD mortality ($r^2 = 0.05$), the median of absolute plasma level of vitamin E (α-

tocopherol) was inversely related to the IHD mortality ($r^2 = 0.55$; $p = 0.003$). Vitamin A behaved similarly ($r^2 = 0.51$; $p = 0.046$). The absolute levels of vitamins E and A together with cholesterol predicted (by multiple regression analysis) the IHD mortality of these eight populations fairly well ($r^2 = 0.81$; $p = 0.06$). Considering all 12 study populations analyzed thus far, total plasma cholesterol correlated with the IHD mortality directly as expected ($r^2 = 0.51$; $p < 0.01$), but the median of the plasma α-tocopherol individually standardized for cholesterol and triglycerides (220 mg/dL + 110 mg/dL, respectively) maintained a strong inverse association with the IHD mortality ($r^2 = 0.49$; $p = 0.01$). In the partial regression analysis, lipid-standardized vitamin E exhibited an even stronger inverse correlation with IHD mortality ($r^2 = 0.69$; $p < 0.001$). Again, vitamin A behaved similarly to vitamin E, that is, after lipid-standardization of individuals ($r^2 = 0.33$; $p = 0.07$), as well as in the cholesterol-independent partial regression analysis ($r^2 = 0.74$; $p < 0.001$). Both vitamins may act singularly, for after lipid-standardization they vary *de facto* independently ($r_s = 0.012$) in individuals. The combination of vitamins E and A as obtained by multiple partial regression predicted the actual IHD mortality to a large extent ($r^2 = 0.89$; $p < 0.001$), whereas the three-variable prediction model, with the median of total cholesterol and of individually lipid-standardized vitamins E and A, fit the actual IHD mortality of these 12 populations almost completely ($r^2 = 0.94$; $p < 0.001$). In conclusion, the plasma status of vitamins E and A are important, hitherto underrated risk factors of IHD, which may act independently, but can, if combined, predict at least 53% of the cross-cultural differences of IHD mortality. After inclusion of total cholesterol into a multivariate model, up to 94% of the IHD mortality can be predicted. The present epidemiological data are in agreement with the hypothesis that these vitamins have physiological functions in the protection of lipoproteins against peroxidation and atherogenic apo-B modifications, respectively, but that does not exclude additional beneficial effects of vitamin E and A in the arterial wall.

REFERENCES

1. GEY, K. F. 1986. On the antioxidant hypothesis with regard to arteriosclerosis. Bibl. Nutr. Dieta **37:** 53-91.
2. NELSON, J. S. 1980. Pathology of vitamin E deficiency. *In* Vitamin E, A Comprehensive Treatise. L. J. Machlin. Ed.: 397-428. Dekker. New York, NY.
3. LIU, S.-K., E. P. DOLENSEK & J. P. TAPPE. 1984. Cardiomyopathy associated with vitamin E deficiency in seven gelada baboons. J. Am. Vet. Med. Assoc. **185:** 1347-1350.
4. WEITZEL, G., H. SCHOEN, K. F. GEY & E. BUDDECKE. 1956. Lipid-soluble vitamins and atherosclerosis. Hoppe-Seyler's Zeitschr. Physiol. Chem. **304:** 247-272.
5. FERRARI, R., C. CECONI, S. CURELLO, A. CARGNONI, E. CONDORELLI & R. RADDINO. 1985. Role of oxygen in myocardial ischemic and reperfusion damage: Effect of tocopherol. Acta Vitiminol. Enzymol. **7** (Suppl.): 61-70.
6. FERRARI, R., S. CURELLO, G. M. BOFFA, E. CONDORELLI, E. PASINI, G. GUARNIERI & A. ALBERTINI. 1989. Oxygen free radical-mediated heart injury in animal models and during bypass surgery in humans. This volume.
7. MARUBAYASHI, S., K. DOHI, K. SUGINO & T. KAWASAKI. 1989. The protective effect of administered α-tocopherol against hepatic damage caused by ischemia-reperfusion or endotoxemia. This volume.
8. YOSHIDA, S. 1989. Brain injury after ischemia and trauma: The role of vitamin E. This volume.
9. ESTERBAUER, H., G. JÜRGENS, O. QUEHENBERGER & E. KOLLER. 1987. Antioxidation

of human low density lipoprotein; loss of polyunsaturated fatty acids and vitamin E and generation of aldehydes. J. Lipid Res. **28:** 495-509.

10. ESTERBAUER, H., G. STRIEGEL, H. PUHL, S. OBERREITHER, M. ROTHENEDER, M. EL-SAADANI & G. JÜRGENS. 1989. The role of vitamin E and carotenoids in preventing oxidation of low density lipoproteins. This volume.

11. MOREL, D. W., J. R. HESSLER & G. M. CHISOLM. 1983. Low density lipoprotein cytotoxicity induced by free radical peroxidation of lipid. J. Lipid Res. **24:** 1070-1076.

12. STEINBRECHER, U. P., S. PARTHASARATHY, D. S. LEAKE, J. L. WITZTUM & D. STEINBERG. 1984. Modification of low density lipoprotein by endothelial cells involves lipid peroxidation and degradation of low density lipoprotein phospholipids. Proc. Natl. Acad. Sci. USA **81:** 3883-3887.

13. VAN HINSBERGH, V. W. M., M. SCHEFFER, L. HAVEKES & H. J. M. KEMPEN. 1986. Role of endothelial cells and their products in the modification of low-density lipoproteins. Biochim. Biophys. Acta **878:** 49-64.

14. STEINBRECHER, U. P., J. L. WITZTUM, S. PARTHASARATHY & D. STEINBERG. 1987. Decrease in reactive amino groups during oxidation or endothelial cell modification of LDL. Arteriosclerosis **7:** 135-143.

15. BROWN, M. S. & J. L. GOLDSTEIN. 1983. Lipoprotein metabolism in the macrophage: Implications for cholesterol deposition in artherosclerosis. Annu. Rev. Biochem. **52:** 223-261.

16. PARTHASARATHY, S., D. J. PRINTZ, D. BOYD, L. JOY & D. STEINBERG. 1986. Macrophage oxidation of low density lipoprotein generates a modified form recognized by the scavenger receptor. Arteriosclerosis **6:** 505-510.

17. HOFF, H. F., J. O'NEIL, G. M. CHISOLM III, T. B. COLE, O. QUEHENBERGER, H. ESTERBAUER & G. JÜRGENS. 1989. Modification of low density lipoprotein with 4-hydroxynonenal induces uptake by macrophages. Arteriosclerosis **9:** 538-549.

18. HABERLAND, M. E. & A. M. FOGELMAN. 1987. The role of altered lipoproteins in the pathogenesis of atherosclerosis. Am. Heart J. **113:** 573-577.

19. HABERLAND, M. E., D. FONG & L. CHENG. 1988. Malondialdehyde-altered protein occurs in atheroma of Watanabe heritable hyperlipemic rabbits. Science **241:** 215-218.

20. SHAIK, M., S. MARTINI, J. R. QUINEY, P. BASKERVILLE, A. E. LA VILLE, N. L. BROWSE, R. DUFFIELD, P. R. TURNER & B. LEWIS. 1988. Modified plasma-derived lipoproteins in human atherosclerotic plaques. Atherosclerosis **69:** 165-172.

21. PARTHASARATHY, S., S. G. YOUNG, J. L. WITZTUM, R. C. PITTMANN & D. STEINBERG. 1986. Probucol inhibits oxidative modification of low density lipoprotein. J. Clin. Invest. **77:** 641-644.

22. YAMOMOTO, A., S. TAKAICHI, H. HARA, O. NISHIKAWA, S. YOKOYAMA, T. YAMAMURA & T. YAMAGUCHI. 1986. Probucol prevents lipid storage in macrophages. Atherosclerosis **62:** 209-217.

23. KITA, T., Y. NAGANO, M. YOKODE, K. ISHII, N. KUME, A. OOSHIMA, H. YOSHIDA & C. KAWAI. 1987. Probucol prevents the progression of atherosclerosis in Watanabe heritable hyperlipemic rabbit, an animal model for familial hypercholesterolemia. Proc. Natl. Acad. Sci. USA **84:** 5928-5931.

24. CAREW, T. E., D. C. SCHWENKE & D. STEINBERG. 1987. Antiatherogenic effect of probucol unrelated to its hypocholesterolemic effect: Evidence that antioxidants *in vivo* can selectively inhibit low density lipoprotein degradation in macrophage-rich fatty streaks and slow the progression of atherosclerosis in the Watanabe heritable hyperlipemic rabbit. Proc. Natl. Acad. Sci. USA **84:** 7725-7729.

25. AVOGARO, P., G. BITTOLO-BON & G. CAZZOLATO. 1988. Presence of a modified low density lipoprotein in humans. Arteriosclerosis **8:** 79-87.

26. BITTOLO-BON, G., G. CAZZOLATO, M. SACCARDI & P. AVOGARO. 1987. Presence of a modified LDL in humans: Effect of vitamin E. *In* Clinical and Nutritional Aspects of Vitamin E. O. Mayaishi & M. Mino, Eds.: 109-120. Elsevier. Amsterdam.

27. RIEMERSMA, R. A., D. A. WOOD, C. C. A. MACINTYRE, R. ELTON, K. F. GEY & M. F. OLIVER. 1989. Low plasma vitamin E and C: Increased risk of angina in Scottish men. This volume.

28. GEY, K. F., H. B. STÄHELIN, P. PUSKA & A. EVANS. 1987. Relationship of plasma vitamin C to mortality from ischemic heart disease. Ann. N.Y. Acad. Sci. **498:** 110-123.
29. GEY, K. F., G. B. BRUBACHER & H. B. STÄHELIN. 1987. Plasma levels of antioxidant vitamins in relation to ischemic heart disease and cancer. Am. J. Clin. Nutr. **45:** 1368-1377.
30. GEY, K. F. 1989. Inverse correlation of vitamin E and ischemic heart disease. Int. J. Vit. Nutr. Res. Suppl. **30:** 224-237.
31. THURNHAM, D. I., J. A. DAVIES, B. J. CRUMP, R. D. SITUNAYAKE & M. DAVIS. 1986. The use of different lipids to express serum tocopherol: Lipid ratios for the measurement of vitamin E status. Ann. Clin. Biochem. **23:** 514-520.
32. NIKI, E. 1987. Interation of ascorbate and α-tocopherol. Ann. N.Y. Acad. Sci. **498:** 186-199.
33. NIKI, E., Y. YAMAMOTO, M. TAKAHASHI, E. KOMURO & Y. MIYAMA. 1989. Inhibition of oxidation of biomembranes by tocopherol. This volume.
34. OLSON, J. A. 1984. Serum levels of vitamin A and carotenoids as reflectors of nutritional status. J. Natl. Cancer Inst. **73:** 1439-1444.
35. SMITH, F. R. & D. W. S. GOODMAN. 1976. Vitamin A transport in human vitamin A toxicity. N. Engl. J. Med. **294:** 805-808.
36. WILSON, D., I.-F. CHAN, K. N. BUCHI & S. C. HORTON. 1985. Postchallenge plasma lipoprotein retinoids: Chylomicron remnants in endogenous hypertriglyceridemia. Metabolism **34:** 551-558.
37. BANKSON, D. D., R. M. RUSSELL & J. SADOWSKI. 1986. Determination of retinyl esters and retinol in serum or plasma by normal-phase liquid chromatography: Method and applications. Clin. Chem. **32:** 35-40.
38. SCHINDLER, R. & A. KLOPP. 1986. Transport of esterified retinol in fasting human blood. Int. J. Vit. Nutr. Res. **56:** 21-27.
39. RIEMERSMA, R. A., D. A. WOOD, S. BUTLER, R. A. ELTON, M. OLIVER, M. SALO, T. NIKKARI, E. VARTIAINEN, P. PUSKA, K. F. GEY, P. RUBBA, M. MANCINI & F. FIDANZA. 1986. Linoleic acid content of adipose tissue and coronary heart disease. Br. Med. J. **292:** 1423-1427.
40. MCLAUGHIN, P. J. & J. L. WEIHRAUCH. 1979. Vitamin E content of foods. J. Am. Diet. Assoc. **75:** 647-665.
41. LEHMANN, J., M. W. MARSHALL, H. T. SLOVER & J. M. IACONO. 1977. Influence of dietary fat level and dietary tocopherols on plasma tocopherols of human subjects. J. Nutr. **197:** 1006-1015.
42. LEHMANN, J., H. L. MARTIN, E. L. LASHLEY, M. W. MARSHALL & J. T. JUDD. 1986. Vitamin E in foods from high and low linoleic acid diets. J. Am. Diet. Assoc. **86:** 1208-1216.
43. DOUGLAS, C. E., A. C. CHAN & P. C. CHOY. 1986. Vitamin E inhibits platelet phospholipase A_2. Biochim. Biophys. Acta **876:** 639-645.
44. CHAN, A. C. & M. K. LEITH. 1981. Decreased prostacyclin synthesis in vitamin E-deficient rabbit aorta. Am. J. Clin. Nutr. **34:** 2341-2347.
45. DIPLOCK, A. T., G.-L. XU, C.-L. YEOW & M. OKIKIOLA. 1989. Relationship of tocopherol structure to biological activity, tissue uptake, and prostaglandin biosynthesis. This volume.
46. REDDANNA, P., J. WHELAN, J. R. BURGESS, M. L. ESKEW, G. HILDENBRANDT, A. ZARKOWER, R. W. SCHOLZ & C. C. REDDY. 1989. The role of vitamin E and selenium on arachidonic acid oxidation by way of the 5-lipoxygenase pathway. This volume.
47. MEYDANI, S. N., M. MEYDANI, P. M. BARKLUND, S. LIU, R. A. MILLER, J. G. CANNON, R. ROCKLIN & J. B. BLUMBERG. 1989. Effect of vitamin E supplementation on immune responsiveness of the aged. This volume.
48. TENGERDY, R. P. 1989. Vitamin E, immune response, and disease resistance. This volume.
49. JANDAK, J., M. STEINER & P. D. RICHARDSON. 1988. Reduction of platelet adhesiveness by vitamin E supplementation in humans. Thromb. Res. **49:** 393-404.
50. OLSON, J. A. 1984. Vitamin A. In Handbook of Vitamins. L. J. Machlin, Ed.: 1-43. Dekker. New York, NY.
51. DIPLOCK, A. T. 1987. Dietary supplementation with antioxidants. Is there a case for exceeding the recommended dietary allowance? Free Radical Biol. & Med. **3:** 199-201.
52. MCCORMICK, J. & P. SKRABANEK. 1988. Coronary heart disease is not preventable by population interventions. Lancet **ii:** 839-841.

53. SALONEN, J. T., R. SALONEN, I. PENTTILAE, J. HERRANEN, M. JAUHIAINEN, M. KAN-
    TOLA, R. LAPPETELAEINEN, P. H. MAEENPAEAE, G. ALFTHAN & P. PUSKA. 1985.
    Serum fatty acids, apolipoproteins, selenium and vitamin antioxidants and the risk of
    death from coronary artery disease. Am. J. Cardiol. 56: 226-231.
54. KOK, F., A. M. DE BRUIJN, R. VERMEEREN, A. HOFMAN, A. VAN LAAR, D. DE BRUIN,
    R. J. J. HERMUS & H. A. VALKENBURG. 1987. Serum selenium, vitamin antioxidants
    and cardiovascular mortality: A 9-year follow-up study in the Netherlands. Am. J. Clin.
    Nutr. 45: 462-468.

Effect of Vitamin E Supplementation on Immune Responsiveness of the Aged[a]

SIMIN NIKBIN MEYDANI,[b,e] MOHSEN MEYDANI,[b]
PATRICE M. BARKLUND,[b] SANDRA LIU,[b]
RICHARD A. MILLER,[c] JOSEPH G. CANNON,[b]
ROSS ROCKLIN,[d] AND JEFFREY B. BLUMBERG [b]

[b] *USDA Human Nutrition Research Center on Aging*
Tufts University
Boston, Massachusetts 02111

[c] *Department of Biochemistry*
Boston University School of Medicine
Boston, Massachusetts 02118

[d] *Fisons Corporation*
Bedford, Massachusetts 01730

INTRODUCTION

Considerable evidence indicates that aging is associated with altered regulation of the immune system.[1] Well-documented, age-related functional changes have been defined for both humoral and cell-mediated responses.[2-4] Although all four major cell types of the immune system, that is, stem cells, macrophages, T cells, and B cells show age-related changes, the major alterations occur in the T cells.[5] *In vivo*, T-cell dependent cell-mediated functions such as primary delayed-type hypersensitivity (DTH),[6,7] graft versus host reaction,[2] and resistance to challenge with syngeneic and allogeneic tumors and parasites[5] are depressed with age. *In vitro*, the proliferative response of human and rodent lymphocytes to phytohemagglutinin (PHA) and concanavalin A (Con A) as well as natural killer cell (NK) activity in mice becomes depressed with age.[2]

Cooperation between monocytes and lymphocytes is essential in antigen recognition, lymphocyte differentiation and eventual antibody production, and development of the effector state of cellular immunity or the DTH phase.[8] In addition to presenting antigen, macrophages synthesize interleukin-1 (IL-1), which induces the production

[a]This study was supported in part by USDA Contract #53-3K06-5-10, NIA Grant #IR23AG05791-02, and a Grant from Hoffmann-La Roche Inc., Nutley, NJ.

[e]Address correspondence to Simin Nikbin Meydani, USDA Human Nutrition Research Center on Aging, Tufts University, 711 Washington Street, Boston, MA 02111.

of interleukin-2 (IL-2) by the activated T cells. Macrophages have high levels of arachidonic acid (AA) in their membrane phospholipids. Upon stimulation, mouse peritoneal macrophages release up to 50% of their AA content in the form of oxygenated metabolites, that is, prostaglandins (PG), hydroxyeicosatetraenoic acid (HETE), and leukotrienes (LT).[9,10] These compounds, in addition to their effect on the biological activities of macrophages, suppress lymphocyte proliferation and lymphokine synthesis.[11–13] Other oxidative metabolites of activated macrophages such as H_2O_2 have also been shown to suppress lymphocyte proliferation.[14,15]

Increased PGE_2 production by macrophages from aged rats[16] and mice[17] has been reported. Furthermore, Rosenstein and Strauser[18] were able to achieve substantial enhancement of aged spleen cell responsiveness *in vitro* and *in vivo* with indomethacin, a cyclooxygenase inhibitor. One of the biological changes associated with aging is an increase in free radical formation with subsequent damage to cellular processes. Several studies have investigated the free radical theory of aging and the role of antioxidants, including vitamin E, on the life expectancy of rodents.[19]

It has been suggested by Harman[20] that vitamin E and other antioxidants may increase longevity by influencing the immune system and reducing age-related diseases. An immunological basis for many age-associated diseases such as amyloidosis, atherosclerosis, and cancer has been proposed by Walford *et al.*[21] Antioxidant supplementation has been shown to be protective against some of these diseases in animals including cancer[22] and amyloidosis.[23] Oxygen metabolites, such as H_2O_2 and eicosanoids, especially PGE_2 are produced by activated macrophages and depress lymphocyte proliferation. Thus, free radical formation associated with aging may be an underlying factor in the depressed immune response observed in senescent rodents, and improved antioxidant status might be effective in stimulating the immune response during aging.

ANIMAL STUDIES

The immunostimulatory effect of vitamin E has been reported in several animal species.[24–27] These studies indicate that the dietary α-tocopherol requirement for maintenance of optimal immune responsiveness may be higher than the levels necessary for normal growth and reproduction. An increase in average life span of short-lived autoimmune-prone NZB/NZW mice receiving vitamin E supplements was reported by Harman.[28] Such observations prompted us to evaluate the effect of vitamin E supplementation on the cell-mediated immune response of aged mice. We found that 500 ppm dietary vitamin E supplementation of 24-month-old C57BL/6J mice for 6 weeks significantly increased splenocyte proliferation in response to the mitogens Con A and lipopolysaccharide (LPS), but not to PHA, relative to control animals fed 30 ppm of the vitamin (TABLE 1).[29] In addition, vitamin E supplementation significantly increased DTH to 2,4-dinitro-7-fluorobenzene. This immunostimulatory effect of vitamin E was associated with an increased production of IL-2 and a decreased synthesis of PGE_2 (TABLE 1). No stimulatory effect of vitamin E was noted on NK-mediated cytotoxicity; however, when the mice were immunized with sheep red blood cells (SRBC), a condition associated with increased oxidative stress prior to assessment, the supplemented mice had a greater NK-mediated cytotoxicity.[30]

Similar results were obtained in our laboratory when comparing the effect of an *in vitro* addition of d-α-tocopherol (4 μg/mL in autologous serum) on the mitogen-induced proliferative response of splenocytes from young and old mice fed corn oil

TABLE 1. Effect of Vitamin E on Immune Response of Aged Mice

Age (Months)	Dietary Vitamin E (ppm)	Serum α-Tocopherol (μg/dL)	DTH[a] (percent)	Con A[b] Lymphocyte Proliferation (ccpm)	LPS[c] Lymphocyte Proliferation (ccpm)	PGE$_2$[d] (μg/g)	IL-2[e] (units/mL)
3	30	236 ± 39	59.9 ± 13.8	119,661 ± 35,491	25,074 ± 5,149	2.60 + 0.08	27 + 4
24	30	168 ± 50	21.0 ± 6.1[f]	5,578 ± 1,844[f]	5,940 ± 2,369[f]	3.20 ± 0.07[f]	12 ± 3[f]
24	500	457 ± 54[f]	45.1 ± 7.0	45,665 ± 17,098	21,260 ± 4,474	2.30 ± 0.10	23 ± 6

[a] Delayed-type hypersensitivity skin test response to 2,4-dinitrofluorobenzene assessed by percent ear swelling.
[b] Blastogenic response of lymphocytes to T-cell mitogen Con A (5μg/mL) expressed as corrected counts per minute (average cpm of mitogen-stimulated cultures minus average cpm of cultures without mitogen) of [³H]thymidine incorporation.
[c] As in footnote b, but with B-cell mitogen E. coli lipopolysaccharide W (100 μg/mL).
[d] Ex-vivo synthesis by incubated spleen homogenates at 37°C for 10 min determined by RIA.
[e] Interleukin-2 activity from supernatants harvested from Con A-stimulated cultured spleen cells with 1 unit = amount of recombinant IL-2 (standard), which causes half maximal incorporation of [³H]thymidine in 5×10^3 cytotoxic T cell lines (CTLL) in culture.
[f] Significantly different from the other two groups at $p < 0.05$. All values are mean ± SEM.

or fish oil diets (unpublished data). Whereas α-tocopherol alone was not mitogenic, it significantly enhanced the mitogenic response of splenocytes to PHA and Con A. Vitamin E produced a greater response in young mice than in old mice maintained on either diet. This effect might be due to a greater utilization and/or incorporation of α-tocopherol in the cells from young mice. Furthermore, a higher percent increase in mitogen-induced proliferation was observed in mice fed corn oil than those fed fish oil. This difference may be due to a higher tocopherol requirement associated with fish oil consumption.[31] These studies indicate that vitamin E supplementation improves the impaired immune response of aged mice. Further studies are required to determine the optimal level of vitamin E as well as the effect of longer term supplementation on the immune response of aged rodents.

HUMAN STUDIES

Very few studies have examined the effect of vitamin E supplementation in humans. Goodwin and Garry[32] in their survey of elderly subjects consuming megadoses of vitamin supplements did not see any correlation between vitamin E intake and tests of lymphocyte proliferation and DTH. Interpretation of this survey is complicated by the fact that several vitamin supplements were used by each subject, and the interaction between different nutrients present confounding variables. Harman and Miller[33] supplemented 103 patients from a chronic care facility with 200 or 400 mg α-tocopheryl acetate/day but did not see any beneficial effect on antibody development against influenza virus vaccine. Unfortunately, data on the health status, medication use, antibody-titers, and other relevant parameters were not reported. Chavance et al.[34] conducted an epidemiological survey on the relationship between nutritional and immunological status in healthy French subjects over 60 years of age. They reported that plasma vitamin E levels were positively correlated with positive DTH responses to diphtheria toxoid, candida, and Trichophyton antigens. In men only, positive correlations were also observed between vitamin E levels and the number of positive DTH responses. Subjects with α-tocopherol levels greater than 135 mg/L were found to have higher helper-inducer/cytotoxic-suppressor ratios. Blood vitamin E concentrations were negatively correlated with the number of infectious disease episodes in the three preceding years.

Therefore, we designed a study to investigate the effect of vitamin E supplementation on the immune response of healthy elderly subjects living in a metabolic research unit where environmental factors and intake of other nutrients were carefully controlled.

Thirty-two men and women from the Boston, MA area, 60 years of age and older with no known medical illness and no prescription medication (other than an occasional laxative and/or analgesic) were recruited. Potential volunteers using vitamin supplements and nonsteroidal antiinflammatory drugs (including aspirin and indomethacin) were excluded. The study was approved by the Tufts University Human Investigation Review Committee (HIRC). All volunteers signed an HIRC-approved written consent form. Volunteers were randomly assigned to a placebo or vitamin E-supplemented group. Subjects resided and consumed all their meals at the Metabolic Research Unit of the USDA Human Nutrition Research Center on Aging at Tufts University. A three-day cycle menu, consisting of foods typical to the American diet and adequate in all nutrients, was served throughout the study. The amount of food provided to each subject was calculated based on his or her caloric requirement to maintain constant weight. Subjects were weighed weekly and their vital signs monitored daily. During the first seven days of the study, all subjects received a placebo capsule with breakfast and with dinner, at which time 3 fasting blood samples and 24-hour urinary collection (every other day) were obtained for different analyses as baseline or presupplementation values. Subjects were then administered a DTH skin test. After the 48-hour evaluation of the skin test was completed, the placebo group continued consuming two placebo capsules containing soybean oil, while the vitamin E group consumed two vitamin E capsules containing 400 IU *dl*-α-tocopheryl acetate in soybean oil (Hoffmann-La Roche, Inc. Nutley, NJ) daily until completion of the study. After 30 days of supplementation, three fasting blood and 24-hour urine samples were collected for different analyses as postsupplementation values.

DTH was assessed using multitest CMI (Merieux Institute, Inc. Miami, FL) containing the following recall antigens: tetanus toxoid, diphtheria toxoid, streptococcus, mycobacterium tuberculosis, candida, Trichophyton, and Proteus. The diameter of positive reaction was measured 24 and 48 hours following the administration of the test. The antigen score was calculated as total number of positive antigens, and the cumulative score was calculated as total diameter of induration of all the positive reactions.

Mitogenic response of Ficoll Hypaque-separated peripheral blood mononuclear cells (PBMC) to T-cell mitogens Con A and PHA were assessed as described before.[29] Con A and PHA-stimulated IL-2 formation was measured according to the methods of Gillis *et al.*[35]

Endotoxin-stimulated IL-1 production was measured by the method of Mizel *et al.*[36] Precursor frequencies for helper T cells (PHTL) were measured using the limited dilution assay described by Miller *et al.*[37] PGE_2 production by PBMC was measured using RIA.[38] Blood and urine samples were used for a complete nutritional status evaluation. Plasma and white blood cell α and γ-tocopherol levels were measured by HPLC.[39] Plasma lipid peroxides were measured as thiobarbituric reactive substances according to the method of Yagi *et al.*[40] Data was analyzed using a two-tailed paired Student's *t* test or paired Wilcoxon Ranked Signed test, depending on the distribution of the parameter.

The plasma α-tocopherol levels in the supplemented group increased from 1104 ± 62 to 3055 ± 272 μg/dL ($p < 0.001$), whereas no change was observed in the placebo group (1127 ± 75 before vs. 1028 ± 61 μg/dL after supplementation). No significant changes were observed in either the placebo or the vitamin E-treated group in plasma vitamin A, vitamin C, total carotenoids, hemoglobin, hematocrit, platelet count, total white blood cell count, or the percentages of lymphocytes and neutrophils.

Although there was no significant change in DTH as measured by the cumulative score and the total number of positive antigens (antigen score) in the placebo group, both cumulative scores and antigen scores were significantly increased in the vitamin E-treated group ($p < 0.05$). Furthermore, the percent change in the cumulative score in the vitamin E group was significantly higher than that of the placebo group ($p < 0.05$).

The mitogenic response of lymphocytes to Con A (but not to PHA) was significantly improved in the vitamin E-treated group ($p < 0.05$), whereas no significant change was noted in the placebo group.

Con A-stimulated IL-2 formation was significantly increased in the vitamin E-treated group ($p < 0.05$), whereas no significant change was observed in the placebo group. The percent change in the IL-2 level of the vitamin E-treated group was also higher than that of the placebo group ($p < 0.005$).

TABLE 2. Effect of Vitamin E Supplementation on Immune Responsiveness of Healthy Elderly Subjects

Test	Placebo	Vitamin E
Delayed-type Hypersensitivity		
Cumulative Score	NE[a]	+[b]
Antigen Score	NE	+
Lymphocyte Proliferation		
to Con A	NE	+
to PHA	NE	NE
IL-2 Production		
to Con A	NE	+
to PHA	NE	+
IL-1 Production	NE	NE
PHTL	NE	NE
PGE$_2$ Production	NE	−[c]
Plasma Lipid Peroxide	NE	−

[a] NE = No statistically significant effect.
[b] + = Statistically significant increase.
[c] − = Statistically significant decrease.

No significant effect of vitamin E supplementation on the PHTL, endotoxin-stimulated IL-1 production, or serum immunoglobulin levels was observed. Plasma lipid peroxides were significantly reduced in the vitamin E-treated group ($p < 0.001$), whereas no change in the placebo group was observed. PGE$_2$ production by PBMC was significantly reduced in the vitamin E-treated group only. The percent reduction in PGE$_2$ production was significantly higher in the vitamin E-treated group compared to the placebo treated group ($p < 0.005$). The results are summarized in TABLE 2.

In conclusion, our animal and clinical studies indicate that vitamin E supplementation improves T-cell mediated immune responses in aged mice and healthy elderly subjects. The degree of improvement in immune status varied depending on the individual, with some showing no improvement at all.

This immunostimulatory effect of vitamin E appears to be mediated by a decrease in PGE$_2$ production and plasma lipid peroxides. Further clinical trials are necessary to establish the required level of vitamin E needed to achieve optimal immune responsiveness. It will also be necessary to determine the duration of this efficacy before an increased intake of α-tocopherol can be recommended for the elderly.

REFERENCES

1. SISKIND, G. W. 1980. Immunological aspects of aging: an overview. *In* Biological Mechanism in Aging. R. T. Schimke, Ed.: 455-467. U. S. Department of Agriculture, National Institutes of Health, Bethesda, MD.
2. KAY, M. M. B. 1979. An overview of immune aging. Mech. Ageing Dev. **9:** 39-59.
3. HALLGREN, H. M., C. E. BUCKLEY, V. A. GILBERSTEN & E. J. YUNIS. 1973. Lymphocyte phytohemagglutinin responsiveness, immunoglobulins and autoantibodies in aging humans. J. Immunol. **4:** 1101-1111.

4. BUCKLEY, C. G., E. G. BUCKLEY & F. C. DORSEY. 1974. Longitudinal changes in serum immunoglobulin levels in older humans. Fed. Proc. **33:** 2036-2039.

5. MAKINODAN, T. 1981. Cellular basis of immunologic aging. *In* Biological Mechanisms in Aging. R. T. Shimke, Ed.: 488-500. U. S. Department of Agriculture, National Institutes of Health, Bethesda, MD.

6. ROBERTS-THOMPSON, I. C., V. YVONSCHAIYUD & S. WHITTINGHAM. 1974. Aging, immune response and mortality. Lancet **II:** 368-370.

7. GOODWIN, J. S., R. P. SEARLES & K. S. K. TUNG. 1982. Immunological responses of a healthy elderly population. Clin. Exp. Immunol. **48:** 403-410.

8. UNANUE, E. R. 1980. Cooperation between mononuclear phagocytes and lymphocytes in immunity. N. Engl. J. Med. **303:** 977-985.

9. HUMES, J. L., R. J. BONNEY, L. PEBES *et al.* 1977. Macrophage synthesize and release prostaglandins in response to inflammatory response. Nature **269:** 149-150.

10. BONNEY, R. J., E. E. OPAS & J. L. HUMES. 1985. Lipoxygenase pathway of macrophages. Fed. Proc. **44:** 2933-2936.

11. GOODWIN, J. S., R. P. MESSNER & G. T. PEAKE. 1974. Prostaglandin suppression of mitogen stimulated leukocytes in culture. J. Clin. Invest. **54:** 368-378.

12. WEBB, D. R., T. J. ROGERS & I. NOWOWIEJSKI. 1980. Endogenous prostaglandin synthesis and the control of lymphocyte function. Ann. N.Y. Acad. Sci. **332:** 260-270.

13. ROLA-PLESZCZYNSKI, M. 1985. Immunoregulation by leukotrienes and other lipoxygenase metabolites. Immunology Today **6:** 302-307.

14. METZGER, Z., J. T. HOFFELD & J. J. OPPENHEIM. 1980. Macrophage mediated suppression. I. Evidence of participation of both hydrogen peroxide and prostaglandins in suppression of murine lymphocyte proliferation. J. Immunol. **124:** 983-988.

15. ZOSCHKE, D. C. & R. P. MESSNER. 1984. Suppression of human lymphocyte mitogenesis mediated by phagocyte-released reactive oxygen species: Comparative activities in normal and in chronic granulomatous disease. Clin. Immunol. Immunopathol. **32:** 29-40.

16. BASH, J. A. 1983. Cellular immunosenescence in F344 rats: Decline in responsiveness to phytohemagglutinin involves changes in both T cells and macrophages. Mech. Ageing Dev. **21:** 323-333.

17. BARTOCCI, A., F. M. MAGGI, R. D. WELKER & F. VERONESE. 1982. Age-related immunosuppression: Putative role of prostaglandins. *In* Prostaglandins and Cancer. T. J. Powles, R. S. Backman, K. V. Honn & P. Ramwell, Eds.: 725-730. Alan R. Liss. New York, NY.

18. ROSENSTEIN, M. M. & H. R. STRAUSER. 1980. Macrophage induced T-cell mitogen suppression with age. J. Reticuloendothelial Soc. Med. **27:** 159-166.

19. BLUMBERG, J. B. & S. N. MEYDANI. 1986. Role of dietary antioxidants in aging. *In* Nutrition and Aging. H. Munro & M. Hutchinson, Eds. Vol. **5:** 85-97. Academic Press. New York, NY.

20. HARMAN, D. 1982. The free-radical theory of aging. *In* Free Radicals in Biology. W. A. Pryor, Ed. Vol. **5:** 255-273. Academic Press. New York, NY.

21. WALFORD, R. L., S. R. S. GOTTESMAN & R. H. WEINDRUCH. 1981. Immunopathology of aging. Annu. Rev. Gerontol. Geriatr. **2:** 3-15.

22. HORVARTH, P. M. & C. IP. 1983. Synergistic effect of vitamin E and selenium in the chemoprevention of mammary carcinogenesis in rats. Cancer Res. **43:** 5335-5341.

23. MEYDANI, S. N., E. S. CATHCART, R. E. HOPKINS, M. MEYDANI, K. C. HAYES & J. B. BLUMBERG. 1986. Antioxidants in experimental amyloidosis of young and old mice. *In* Fourth International Symposium of Amyloidosis. G. G. Glenner, E. P. Asserman, E. Benditt, E. Calkins, A. S. Cohen & D. ZUCKER-FRANKLIN, EDS.: 683-692. PLENUM. NEW YORK, NY.

24. TENGERDY, R. & J. C. BROWN. 1977. Effect of vitamins E and A on humoral immunity and phagocytosis in *E. coli* infected chickens. Poultry Sci. **56:** 957-963.

25. CORWIN, L. M. & J. SHLOSS. 1980. Role of antioxidants on the stimulation of the mitogenic response. J. Nutr. **110:** 916-923.

26. LARSEN, H. J. & S. TOLLERSRUD. 1981. Effect of dietary vitamin E and selenium on the phytohaemagglutinin response of pig lymphocytes. Am. J. Vet. Sci. **31:** 301-305.

27. BENDICH, A. & E. GABRIEL. 1986. Dietary vitamin E requirement for optimum immune response in the rat. J. Nutr. **116:** 675-681.

28. HARMAN, D. 1980. Free radical theory of aging: Beneficial effect of antioxidants on the lifespan of male NZB mice: Role of free radical reactions in the deterioration of the immune system with age and in the pathogenesis of systemic lupus erythematosus. Age **3:** 64-73.

29. MEYDANI, S. N., M. MEYDANI, C. P. VERDON, A. C. SHAPIRO, J. B. BLUMBERG & K. C. HAYES. 1986. Vitamin E supplementation suppresses prostaglandin E_2 synthesis and enhances the immune response in aged mice. Mech. Aging Dev. **34:** 191-201.

30. MEYDANI, S. N., G YOGEESWARAN, S. LIU, S. BASKAR & M. MEYDANI. 1988. Fish oil and tocopherol induced changes in natural killer cell mediated cytotoxicity and PGE_2 synthesis in young and old mice. J. Nutr. **118:** 1245-1252.

31. MEYDANI, S. N., A. C. SHAPIRO, M. MEYDANI, J. McCAULEY & J. B. BLUMBERG. 1987. Effect of age and dietary fat (fish oil, corn oil, and coconut oil) on tocopherol status of C57BL/6Nia mice. Lipids **22:** 345-350.

32. GOODWIN, J. S. & T. J. GARRY. 1983. Relationship between megadose vitamin supplementation and immunological function in a healthy elderly population. Clin. Exp. Immunol. **51:** 647-653.

33. HARMAN, D. & R. W. MILLER 1986. Effect of vitamin E on the immune response to influenza virus vaccine and incidence of infectious disease in man. Age **9:** 21-23.

34. CHAVANCE, M., G. BRUBACHER, B. HERBERTH, G. VERNES, T. MISTACKI, F. DETI, C. FOURNIER & C. JANOT. 1985. Immunological and nutritional status among the elderly. *In* Nutrition, Immunity, and Illness in the Elderly. R. K. Chandra, Ed.: 137-142. Pergamon Press. New York, NY.

35. GILLIS, S., M. M. FERN, W. OU & K. A. SMITH. 1978. T-cell growth factor: Parameters of production and a quantitative micro-assay for activity. J. Immunol. **120:** 2027-2032.

36. MIZEL, S., J. OOPENHEIM & D. ROSENSTREICH. 1978. Characterization of lymphocyte-activating factor (LAF) produced by macrophage cell line, P388D. J. Immunol. **120:** 1497-1503.

37. MILLER, R. 1984. Age associated decline in precursor frequency for different T cell mediated reactions with preservation of helper or cytotoxic effect per precursor cell. J. Immunol. **132:** 63-68.

38. MEYDANI, S. N. & J. DUPONT. 1982. Effect of zinc deficiency on prostaglandin levels in different organs of the rat. J. Nutr. **112:** 1098-1104.

39. BIERI, J. G., T. J. TOLLINERY & G. L. CATIGANI. 1979. Simultaneous determination of alpha-tocopherol and retinol in plasma or red cells by high pressure liquid chromatography. Am. J. Clin. Nutr. **32:** 2143-2149.

40. YAGI, K. 1982. Assay for serum lipid peroxide level and its clinical significance. *In* Lipid Peroxides in Biology and Medicine. K. Yagi, Ed.: 223-242. Academic Press. New York, NY.

Low Plasma Vitamins E and C

Increased Risk of Angina in Scottish Men[a]

RUDOLPH A. RIEMERSMA, DAVID A. WOOD,
CECILIA C.A. MACINTYRE, ROB ELTON,
K. FRED GEY,[b] AND MICHAEL F. OLIVER

Cardiovascular Research Unit
University of Edinburgh
Edinburgh EH8 9XF, Scotland

[b] *Vitamin Research Department*
F. Hoffman-La Roche Co. Ltd.
CH-4002 Basel, Switzerland

INTRODUCTION

Classical risk factors, such as raised serum cholesterol or LDL cholesterol, blood pressure, and smoking status do not fully explain an individual's risk for coronary heart disease.[1] We[2-5] and others[6,7] have identified that low levels of the essential fatty acid linoleic acid in adipose tissue and plasma phospholipids, reflecting a long-term low intake of dietary linoleate,[8] are new risk factors for coronary heart disease, independent of classical risk factors.[5,6]

There is a close association between the content of the natural antioxidant vitamin E and the linoleic acid content of plant oils. Previous studies suggested that the antioxidant status was low in apparently healthy men in Scotland.[9]

We wished to test the hypothesis that those with a low antioxidant status are at enhanced risk for coronary heart disease, and that the enhanced risk is independent of classical risk factors. This short paper, represents a preliminary report of a case-control study of occult angina pectoris in Edinburgh men, aged 35-54.

POPULATION AND METHODS

The basic design of this case-control study has been published.[5] Briefly, 125 patients with previously unknown angina pectoris were detected from a systematic sample of 6000 Edinburgh men, aged 35-54 registered with the Lothian Health Board central

[a] This study was supported by a Grant from the British Heart Foundation.

register using the World Health Organization (WHO) chest pain questionnaire.[10] A stratified sample (n = 430) of control subjects (no reported history of coronary heart disease (CHD) and negative to the WHO chest pain questionnaire) was taken.

All men were invited to a clinic and had a full medical examination, including family history, anthropometric measurements, blood pressure, and nonfasting blood samples for serum lipids (cholesterol, HDL cholesterol, and triglycerides) and plasma antioxidant vitamins C and E.[11] Fatty acid composition of adipose tissue and platelets was used as an index of linoleate intake.[5] The response rate for the patients was 83% and 76% for the controls. For the sake of clarity, the published anthropometric and serum lipid results[5] of the apparently healthy men and those with angina pectoris are presented in TABLE 1.

STATISTICS

Statistical comparisons between patients with angina and controls were made by a nonparametric Wilcoxon rank sum test. Contingency tables were analyzed by chi-square. Logistic regression was used to investigate the relationship between factors and the risk of angina (PLR program, BMDP Statistical Software 1983, University of California Press).

RESULTS

Plasma vitamin C levels were lower in patients with a positive WHO chest pain questionnaire than in comparable controls (TABLE 2). Plasma vitamin E levels were not different between patients and controls. When the results are expressed as vitamin E/cholesterol molar ratio, however, to allow for the well-known association between these factors, patients with CHD had a significantly lower vitamin E status also (TABLE 2).

TABLE 1. Risk Factors in Healthy Controls and Patients with New Angina

	Controls[a] (n = 430)	Angina[a] (n = 125)
Age (years)	47.8 (0.3)	46.8 (0.6)
Percent cigarette smokers	29	46[b]
Blood pressure (S/D)	137/84	140/86
Cholesterol (mM)	6.27 (0.06)	6.19 (0.11)
HDL cholesterol (mM)	1.18 (0.02)	1.13 (0.03)
Weight/height^2 (kg/m^2 × 10^{-1})	2.52 (0.02)	2.59 (0.05)
Adipose linoleate (percent)	9.81 (0.14)	8.77 (0.18)[a]

[a] Mean (SEM)
[b] $p < 0.01$. Data from reference 5.

TABLE 2. Plasma Antioxidant Vitamins C and E in Healthy Controls and Patients with New Angina

	Controls (n = 396)	Angina (n = 111)
Vitamin C (μM)	30.5 (1.1)	23.6 (1.7)[a]
Vitamin E (μM)	10.3 (0.1)	9.8 (0.3)
Vitamin E/Cholesterol ratio (μM/mM)	1.66 (0.02)	1.58 (0.03)[b]

[a] $p < 0.001$.
[b] $p < 0.01$.

There were significantly more patients in the lowest quintile of the plasma vitamin C and E distribution of the apparently healthy men than might have been expected (both $p < 0.01$). The relative risk for angina pectoris for men in the lowest quintile of vitamin C was 2.6 to 1 (vs. highest quintile of vitamin C). The confidence interval was 1.3-5.2 ($p < 0.01$).

The enhanced risk for angina by low plasma vitamin C was independent of classical risk factors (blood pressure, total and HDL cholesterol) (not shown), but smoking status removed the association between low vitamin C levels and angina.

The relative risk for angina for men in the lowest quintile of the cholesterol-adjusted vitamin E distribution was 2.2 to 1 (vs. highest quintile), with a confidence interval from 1.0-4.5 ($p < 0.01$). The enhanced risk remained after adjustment for classical risk factors for CHD, including smoking status ($p < 0.01$). When the new CHD risk factor, adipose tissue linoleate, was introduced, however, the relative risk decreased and was no longer significant ($p < 0.07$).

DISCUSSION

This case-control study of middle-aged Edinburgh men shows that those whose plasma vitamin C and E levels fall in the lowest quintile of the normal plasma concentrations have an increased risk of angina. The strength of these relations to the disease are as strong as that of serum cholesterol.[12] For plasma vitamin E, this is independent of classical risk factors for CHD, including smoking status. When adipose linoleate was introduced into the logistic model, however, the relation between low vitamin E levels and angina disappeared.

The association between low plasma vitamin C levels and angina is confounded by cigarette smoking. This does not mean that low plasma vitamin C levels are not important in the etiology of CHD, but it could point to a possible mechanism whereby smoking predisposes to CHD.

An important aspect of our study is that patients with angina were detected by a self-administered WHO chest pain questionnaire and were, like their general practitioner, unaware of the nature of their chest pain. They are therefore unlikely to have changed their dietary habits.[3] Also, the design of our study (studying cases and control simultaneously) excluded the possibility of a confounding influence of seasonal variations in these antioxidant vitamins.[13]

Prospective studies suggested no major role for vitamin E in the development of CHD in Finland,[14] the Netherlands,[15] and Switzerland[9] and also not for vitamin C in Switzerland.[9] The very low levels of plasma vitamin E in the first study may be attributed to deterioration during prolonged storage (7 years) at −20 C. It is difficult to reconcile this, however, with apparently no sample deterioration under similar laboratory conditions in the Dutch study.

The high Swiss levels were measured without delay, and the lack of relation was attributed to the optimal level of vitamin E and C in Basel.[9] For vitamin C, an alternative explanation may be that matching for smoking status removed the association between low plasma vitamin C and CHD, as it did in our study.

In summary, in Scotland where plasma antioxidant status is low,[9] low plasma antioxidants predispose to angina, and this association is not explained by the confounding influence of classical risk factors (relative weight, cholesterol, and blood pressure). For vitamin C, the association is closely linked to a smoking habit. When adjusted for adipose linoleate, a new independent risk factor for CHD, the association between low plasma vitamin E and angina was no longer significant. Thus a diet low in this essential fatty acid and/or vitamin E predisposes to angina.

SUMMARY

Cross-cultural studies suggest that low plasma antioxidant levels contribute to the high incidence of coronary heart disease (CHD) in Scotland. One hundred twenty-five cases of angina *without* reported history were identified by a postal WHO chest pain questionnaire from a systemic population sample of 6000 Edinburgh men (35-54 years). Classical CHD risk factors (lipids, blood pressure, smoking, and relative weight), plasma vitamins, and a new independent CHD risk factor, adipose tissue linoleate, were measured in angina (n = 125) and healthy controls (n = 430). Cigarette smoking was common in angina (46% vs. 29%, p <0.01), and adipose tissue linoleate was lower (8.77 ± 0.18% vs. 9.81 ± 0.14% (p <0.01). Classical CHD risk factors were not different. Vitamin E/cholesterol molar ratio (μm/mM) was lower in angina than in controls: 1.58 ± 0.03 vs. 1.66 ± 0.02 (p <0.01). Plasma vitamin C was also lower in angina than in controls: 23.6 ± 1.7 vs. 30.5 ± 1.1 μM (p <0.001). The relative risk of angina for those in the lowest versus those in the highest quintile of the vitamin E/cholesterol ratio distribution was 2.2:1, irrespective of other risk factors (p <0.009). Adipose tissue linoleate removed the association between vitamin E and angina. The relative risk of angina for those in the lowest versus those in the highest quintile of plasma vitamin C was 2.6 :1 (p <0.01), and the increased risk was also independent of classical risk factors, but closely related to a smoking habit. Low plasma vitamin E or adipose linoleate predisposes to angina, and smoking may increase the risk of angina by lowering plasma vitamin C levels in Scottish men.

REFERENCES

1. HELLER, R. F., S. CHINN, H. TUNSTALL PEDOE & G. ROSE. 1984. How well can we predict coronary heart disease? Findings in the United Kingdom Heart Disease Prevention Project. Br. Med. J. **288:** 1409-1411.

2. LOGAN, R. L., M. THOMSON, R. A. RIEMERSMA *et al.* 1978. Risk factors for ischaemic heart disease in normal men aged 40. Lancet **1:** 949-955.
3. WOOD, D. A., S. BUTLER, R. A. RIEMERSMA, M. THOMSON & M. F. OLIVER. 1984. Adipose tissue and platelet fatty acids and coronary heart disease in Scottish men. Lancet **2:** 117-121.
4. RIEMERSMA, R. A., D. A. WOOD, S. BUTLER *et al.* 1986. Linoleic acid content in adipose tissue and coronary heart disease. Br. Med. J. **292:** 1423-1427.
5. WOOD, D. A, R. A. RIEMERSMA, S. BUTLER *et al.* 1987. Linoleic and eicosapentaenoic acids in adipose tissue and platelets and the risk of coronary heart disease. Lancet **1:** 177-183.
6. MIETTINEN, T. A., V. NAUKKARIENEN, J. K. HUTTUNEN, S. MATTILA & T. KUMLIN. 1982. Fatty acid composition of serum lipids predicts myocardial infarction. Br. Med. J. **285:** 933-936.
7. NIKKARI, T., M. SALO, J. MAATELA & A. AROMAA. 1983. Serum fatty acids in Finnish men. Atherosclerosis **49:** 139-148.
8. VAN STAVEREN, W. A., P. DEURENBERG, M. B. KATAN *et al.* 1986. Validity of the fatty acid composition of subcutaneous fat tissue of the diet of separate individuals. Am. J. Epidemiol. **123:** 455-463.
9. GEY, K. F., H. B. STÄHELIN, P. PUSKA & A. EVANS. 1987. Relationship of plasma level of vitamin C to mortality from ischemic heart disease. Ann. N.Y. Acad. Sci. **498:** 110-120.
10. ROSE, G. A., H. BLACKBURN, R. F. GILLUM & R. J. PRINCAS. 1982. *In* Cardiovascular survey methods. 2nd Ed. World Health Organization. Geneva.
11. VUILLEUMIER, J. P., H. E. KELLER, D. GYSEL & F. HUNZIKER. 1983. Clinical chemical methods for the routine assessment of the vitamin status in human populations. Part I: The fat-soluble vitamins A and E, and beta-carotene. Int. J. Vit. Nutr. Res. **53:** 265-272.
12. The Pooling Project Research Group. 1978. Relationship of blood pressure, serum cholesterol, smoking habit, relative weight, and ECG abnormalities to incidence of major coronary events. J. Chronic Dis. **31:** 201-305.
13. RIEMERSMA, R. A. 1989. Unpublished observations.
14. SALONEN, J. T., R. SALONEN, I. PENTILLA *et al.* 1985. Serum fatty acids, apolipoproteins, selenium and vitamin antioxidants and the risk of death from coronary artery disease. Am. J. Cardiol. **56:** 226-231.
15. KOK, F. J., A. M. DE BRUIJN, R. VERMEEREN *et al.* 1987. Serum selenium, vitamin antioxidants, and cardiovascular mortality: a 9-year follow-up study in the Netherlands. Am. J. Clin. Nutr. **45:** 462-468.

Nutritional Assessment of Vitamin E in Oxidative Stress[a]

MAKOTO MINO, MASAYUKI MIKI,
MUNENORI MIYAKE, AND TORU OGIHARA

Department of Pediatrics
Osaka Medical College
2-7 Daigakucho
Taskatsuki, Japan

INTRODUCTION

As the assessment of human vitamin E status from a clinical standpoint has generally relied on serum or plasma tocopherol concentrations, it has been previously supposed that newborn infants are in a marginally vitamin E-deficient state due to their low plasma tocopherol concentrations and increased hydrogen peroxide hemolysis.[1-3] Estimates of nutritional vitamin E status based only on plasma levels, however, are now recognized as being subject to error because these levels tend to fluctuate in relation to plasma lipids.[4-6] Horwitt[4] thus proposed plasma tocopherol expressed in terms of total lipids (tocopherol/lipid ratio) as a very reliable index of vitamin E status, and several clinical studies of the nutritional status of vitamin E have been undertaken based on this index.[4-6] Martinez[7] and Desai[8] reported that this ratio in newborn infants appeared to be within an acceptable range (more than 0.8),[4] indicating that newborn infants may be in no vitamin E-deficient status. On the basis of our findings with respect to red blood cell (RBC) tocopherol, which is also thought to be an expression of vitamin E status,[9-11] the majority of newborn infants displayed a normal vitamin E status,[12] in spite of increased susceptibility of RBC to oxidant stress. Tocopherol acts as a chain-breaking antioxidant in biomembranes, whereas its transport to biomembranes occurs by way of lipoproteins in plasma. Both biomembranes and plasma lipids may be exposed to oxygen radicals that are produced by a variety of mechanisms. This includes a case of recurrent hypoxic and hyperoxic states, mimicking ischemic and reperfusion systems, which are induced by respiratory distress states in premature infants with mechanical ventilations; a case of excited polymorphonuclear cell (PMN) functions and platelet aggregations induced by inflammation, that were induced by infections; or a case of hemorrhages, where active oxygen may be generated around the focuses. In this study, nutritional assessment of vitamin E

[a]This work was supported by a Grant-in-Aid (61480225) for Scientific Research from the Ministry of Education, Science, and Culture, Japan, and by a Grant for Maternal and Child Health Research from the Ministry of Health and Welfare of Japan. We are also grateful to the Eisai Co. Ltd. for financial assistance and the provision of an assay reagent for tocopherol determination.

AAPH: 2,2'-azobis(2-aminidopropane) dihydrochloride

$$HCL \cdot HN = C - \underset{\underset{NH_2}{|}}{\overset{\overset{CH_3}{|}}{C}} - N = N - \underset{\underset{CH_3}{|}}{\overset{\overset{CH_3}{|}}{C}} - C = NH \cdot HCl$$

$$\xrightarrow[O_2]{} HCl \cdot HN = C - \underset{\underset{NH_2}{|}}{\overset{\overset{CH_3}{|}}{C}} - O_2 \cdot + N_2$$

(Radical initiator)

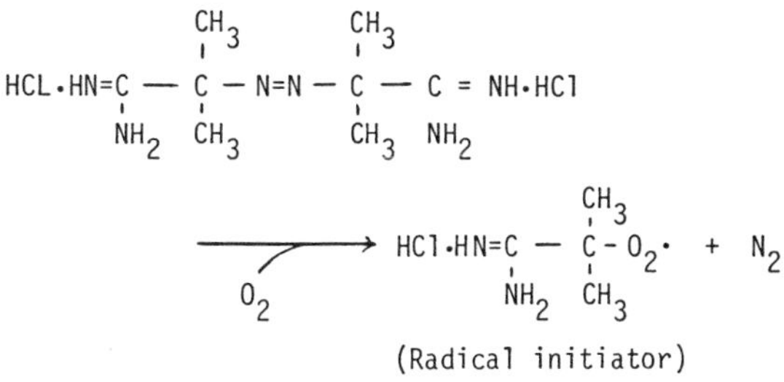

FIGURE 1. Peroxyl radical formation in AAPH reaction.

was investigated on the basis of peroxidizability of RBC ghosts and lipoprotein fractions exposed to oxidant stress. As an oxidant stress agent, an azocompound, AAPH [2,2'-azobis(2-aminido-propane) dihydrochloride] was used, inasmuch as it is known that AAPH initiates free radicals at a constant rate by unimolecular thermal decomposition, and the rate of generation of free radicals can be easily controlled and measured by adjusting the concentration of the initiator (FIG. 1).

MATERIAL AND METHODS

Subjects

1. Premature Infants

All the infants ranging from 1,750 to 2,500 g birth weight from our neonatal nursery were examined during the period from birth to 7 days of life. No infants had either delivery complications or evidence of intrauterine malnutrition, and all had an Apgar score of 7 or more during both the first minute and five minutes of life.

2. Pregnant Women

All the women investigated had no complications during gestation, and blood was drawn immediately before delivery.

3. Healthy Adults

Laboratory personnel were enrolled in this study. A health check was performed before examination.

4. Cord Blood Was Obtained Immediately after Birth from Women with a Normal Pregnancy and Normal Delivery.

The study protocol was approved by the ethics committee of the college, and the studies were performed after informed concent was obtained from either the individuals or the parents.

Laboratory Analysis

Heparinized blood was drawn after 4 hours and after overnight fasting in the infants and adults, respectively, and immediately before delivery in the pregnant women. The heparinized blood was first provided to obtain platelet-rich plasma from which platelet pellets were separated. After removal of the platelet-rich plasma, the RBC were washed three times with saline to form a packed cell layer. The RBC ghosts were prepared from the packed cells using Burton's method,[13] the procedure being described in previous reports.[12,14] PMN were isolated by dextran sedimentation and hypotonic lysis of RBC and suspended in 2 mL of Hanks' balanced solution at a concentration of 1×10^9 cells/mL to provide samples for tocopherol assay.[15] Buccal mucous cells were collected by a previously described method.[16] Lipoproteins were fractionated by ultracentrifugation in accordance with the method of Hatch and Lees.[17]

Reaction

In order to induce oxidative stress we used an azocompound, AAPH, at final concentrations of 8.7 mM and 20 mM for RBC ghosts and lipoprotein lipids, respectively, in accordance with a slight modification of Yamamoto's method.[18] Reaction was carried out at 37°C either with RBC ghosts adjusted on the basis of 2 mg of the protein content, or with lipoprotein fractions on the basis of 1 mg of lipid in phosphate buffer (pH 7.4).

Assay Systems

All the assay systems used in the present study have been described in previous reports.[12,14,16]

TABLE 1. Tocopherol Concentrations in Biological Samples[a]

	Neonates	Adults
Plasma (μg/dL)	401.9 ± 154.9 (81)	808.7 ± 23.5 (19)
Tocopherol/lipid ratio	1.43 ± 0.34 (67)	1.75 ± 0.28 (19)
RBC (μg/dL packed cells)	178.8 ± 57.0 (81)	201.5 ± 58.1 (19)
Platelet (μg/mg protein)	0.20 ± 0.09 (6)	0.22 ± 0.07 (22)
PMN (μg/10^9 cells)	2.66 ± 0.61 (11)	5.54 ± 1.53 (20)
Buccal mucous cell (μg/mg protein)	23.8 ± 12.6 (17)	49.3 ± 17.8 (18)

[a] The given values represent the mean ± SD. Numbers of cases are indicated in parentheses.

RESULTS

Tocopherol Concentrations in the Samples Obtained from Premature Infants

Tocopherol concentrations in plasma, RBC, platelets, PMN, and buccal mucous cells of premature infants and healthy adults were compared, as shown in TABLE 1. No deficiency was demonstrated in the RBC and platelets of premature infants, as compared with adults, whereas the concentrations in PMN and buccal mucous cells were approximately one half of the adult levels. In addition, the plasma tocopherol/lipid ratios, as a proposed index of available vitamin E status,[4] was within an acceptable level (more than 0.8) in premature infants, indicating no deficiency. On the basis of the above tocopherol concentrations, it is not clear whether or not premature infants are deficient in vitamin E.

First, we used RBC in which the tocopherol concentrations were similar for premature infants and adults, although RBC in premature infants were highly susceptible to oxidant stress with hydrogen peroxide. When RBC were oxidized with AAPH to produce hemolytic stress, it was observed that RBC in human cord blood were more susceptible than those of adults, as shown in TABLE 2, in spite of very similar tocopherol concentrations in both RBC. An increased susceptibility of RBC in cord blood to AAPH is generally thought to be consistent with that shown in the hydrogen peroxide hemolysis tests.

TABLE 2. Time Course of Hemolysis in Adult and Cord Blood RBC Reacted with AAPH, at a Final Concentration of 8.7 mM[a]

	Reaction time (min)				
	0	30	60	90	120
Cord blood	1.6 ± 0.2	1.8 ± 0.2	34.1 ± 11.5	84.3 ± 28.5	89.9 ± 23.1
Adult blood	0.2 ± 0.2	0.5 ± 0.2	11.9 ± 3.8	36.7 ± 25.4	49.3 ± 28.8

[a] Mean ± SD; n = 5.

*Oxygen Uptake in RBC Ghosts and Lipoprotein Lipids
in Reaction with AAPH*

When the RBC ghosts and lipoproteins reacted with AAPH solutions, the oxygen uptake pattern in cord and adult ghosts was similar, occurring at a slow rate in the first phase and a faster rate during the second phase. Analysis of this oxygen uptake pattern suggests that the tocopherol in the ghosts was consumed at a constant rate during the first phase, and that, after tocopherol content decreased to the lowest levels, phase 2, characterized by an increased oxygen consumption, commenced as shown in FIGURE 2. These finding are consistent with those of a previous study concerning RBC ghosts by Yamamoto *et al.*[18] The rapid uptake of oxygen in phase 2, occurring immediately after the tocopherol became totally depleted in the ghosts and LDL, suggested an extensive propagation of the chain oxidative reactions in the membrane lipids and lipoprotein lipids, whereas the slow oxygen uptake in phase 1 suggests that the chain propagation is constantly inhibited by tocopherol remaining in the lipids.

In these patterns, the oxygen consumption rate in phase 1 was denoted by R-1 and that in phase 2 by R-2, and both of these were expressed in mole oxygen consumption per second. The length of R-1 was referred to T-inhibition (T_{inh}), expressed in seconds.

*Kinetic Study of Oxygen Consumption in RBC Ghosts
of Cord and Adult Blood*

Tocopherol Content in Ghosts and Oxygen Consumption in Phase 1

A comparison of cord, mother, and adult RBC ghost tocopherol content showed that total tocopherol concentrations, including alpha and gamma forms, were very

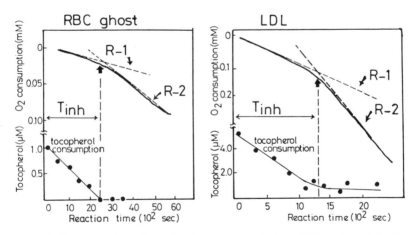

FIGURE 2. Oxygen uptake and tocopherol consumption during oxidation of RBC ghosts and LDL reacted with AAPH. T_{inh} = length of phase 1; R = rate of oxygen consumption (decrease of O_2, moles/s).

TABLE 3. Peroxidizability of Cord, Mother, and Adult RBC Ghosts Reacted with AAPH

	Cord (n = 11)	Mother (n = 7)	Adult (n = 10)
Total tocopherol (μM)	1.67 ± 0.47	1.37 ± 0.26	1.67 ± 0.18
Alpha-tocopherol	1.54 ± 0.47	1.25 ± 0.23	1.49 ± 0.17
Gamma-tocopherol	0.13 ± 0.13	0.12 ± 0.04	0.18 ± 0.04
Active H (μM)[a]	7246 ± 1527[d]	5602 ± 2754	3460 ± 788
Active H (No.)[b]	1.94 ± 0.23	1.79 ± 0.26	1.63 ± 0.25
T_{inh} (s)	2021 ± 542	1927 ± 386	2089 ± 492
R-1 (10^{-9}M/s)	27.7 ± 7.1	24.6 ± 6.6	24.7 ± 4.4
R-2 (10^{-9}M/s)	56.6 ± 7.1[d]	49.9 ± 8.9	46.9 ± 7.1
KCL in R-1[c]	13.5 ± 2.4	11.2 ± 3.2	12.1 ± 2.1
KCL in R-2	27.5 ± 3.5[d]	24.2 ± 4.3	22.7 ± 3.7

[a] Total active H/2 mg of ghost proteins.
[b] Average numbers of active H in one molecule of fatty acid calculated from fatty acid composition in membrane lipids.
[c] The KCL (kinetic chain length) is defined as the ratio of oxygen uptake rate to radical formation rate. KCL (in R-1 or R-2) = R-1 or R-2/R-initiation. R-initiation was calculated from the rate of tocopherol consumption (2 × Δtocopherol) in the ghosts reacted with AAPH.
[d] Mean ± SD; $p < 0.05$ (vs. adult).

similar (TABLE 3). The three types of ghosts were exposed to AAPH reaction, and then T_{inh} as well as R-1 were similar in the three types. As shown in FIGURE 3, T_{inh} was found to be closely correlated with ghost tocopherol content, whereas there was no correlation between oxygen consumption rate in R-1 and the tocopherol content. Thus, during the periods in which tocopherol was consumed at a constant rate by reaction with AAPH, oxygen uptake occurred at only a low rate, as long as any tocopherol remained in the ghosts; the chain propagation was constantly inhibited by this tocopherol, regardless of its amount in the initial phase. Therefore, there may be no essential differences in T_{inh} and R-1 among the three types of ghosts (TABLE 3).

Fatty Acid Composition of Ghosts and Quantity of Active Bisallylic Hydrogen (active H)

Since the rapid uptake of oxygen in R-2 following total tocopherol depletion in the ghosts suggests an extensive propagation of the chain reaction in the membrane lipids, the peroxidizability of the membranes was subsequently investigated with respect to fatty acid compositions.

Fatty acid content and composition are shown in terms of both lipids and membrane proteins in TABLE 4. The amounts of fatty acids in terms of membrane proteins were larger in the ghosts from cord RBC than in those from the RBC of healthy adults, whereas the corresponding amounts in mothers were variable. The cord ghosts were rich in polyunsaturated fatty acids (PUFA), particularly arachidonic acid and eicos-

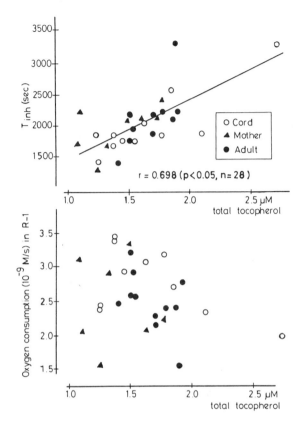

FIGURE 3. Relationships between T_{inh}, R-1, and tocopherol content in RBC ghosts.

atrienoic acid, as compared with the other ghosts. From the PUFA compositions and the amounts in the three types of ghosts the quantities of active bisallylic hydrogen (active H) were calculated. This probably constitutes another index for peroxidizability of the ghost membranes. As shown in TABLE 4, the amounts of the active H numbers in the cord ghosts were also larger than in the adult RBC ghosts on the basis of both membrane lipids and proteins.

Relationship between Oxygen Uptake and Active H

FIGURE 4 shows the relationships between the amounts of active H numbers and either the values of R-1 or R-2. The amounts of active H numbers in the ghosts were closely correlated with R-2, but poorly correlated with R-1. This also indicates that the rate of suppression of chain propagation by the remaining tocopherol was not greatly affected by the amount of active H, whereas the propagation rate is proportional to the amount of active H in the tocopherol-depleted membranes. As shown in TABLE 3, R-2 in cord ghosts was significantly greater than in adult RBC ghosts, suggesting high peroxidizability of cord RBC membranes, as compared with adult RBC membranes.

From these data, kinetic chain length was calculated for the three types of ghosts, as also shown in TABLE 3. The kinetic chain length is defined as the ratio of oxygen uptake rate to radical formation rate,[18] and is determined by the conventional inhibitor method with tocopherol, as shown in data in FIGURE 2. The kinetic chain length number (KCL) indicates that when one radical is generated from AAPH solution, the given numbers of molecules of fatty acids are oxidized in R-1 or in R-2, respectively. TABLE 5 shows the kinetic chain lengths in R-1 and R-2 for the three types of ghosts. With respect to the oxygen uptake in R-1, the kinetic chain length did not differ significantly among all three types of ghosts and was shorter than that calculated in R-2 for all the ghosts. This confirmed again that chain propagation proceeded actively in the latter phase, but was effectively suppressed in the initial phase, because of the tocopherol remaining in the ghosts. Moreover, with respect to the second phase of oxygen uptake, the kinetic chain length was longer in the cord ghosts as compared with the adult ghosts, indicating that cord ghosts are far more susceptible to oxidant stress.

TABLE 4. Membrane Fatty Acid Constituents in Ghosts from Cord, Mother, and Adult RBC

	Cord (n = 11)	Mother (n = 7)	Adult (n = 10)
Fatty acids (FA)			
(μmol/2 mg protein)	3742 ± 683^a	3171 ± 1491	2235 ± 413
FA composition (mole-percent)			
14:0	0.7 ± 0.2	0.7 ± 0.2	0.6 ± 0.2
16:0	37.5 ± 2.9	34.9 ± 3.7	35.5 ± 9.3
16:1	0.7 ± 0.3	0.5 ± 0.2	0.2 ± 0.2
18:0	15.9 ± 2.4	13.2 ± 2.0	16.9 ± 0.6
18:1	10.2 ± 1.2	13.2 ± 1.3	13.9 ± 0.8
18:2	4.7 ± 0.8^a	12.7 ± 5.0	10.6 ± 0.9
20:3	2.4 ± 0.3^a	0.8 ± 0.4	0.8 ± 0.3
20:4	16.4 ± 2.1^a	11.1 ± 1.5	11.9 ± 1.7
22:0	0.5 ± 0.2	0.7 ± 0.4	0.5 ± 0.1
22:4	1.5 ± 0.5	1.1 ± 0.3	1.5 ± 0.2
22:6	6.9 ± 1.3	7.7 ± 1.3	5.9 ± 1.5
unknown	1.4 ± 0.5	2.5 ± 0.9	3.3 ± 1.1
Active H			
(No.)[b]	1.94 ± 0.23^a	1.79 ± 0.26	1.63 ± 0.25
(μM)[c]	7246 ± 1528^a	5602 ± 2754	3640 ± 788

[a] $p < 0.05$.
[b] Average numbers of active hydrogen in one molecule of fatty acid calculated from fatty acid composition.
[c] Total numbers of active hydrogen in 2 mg ghost protein.

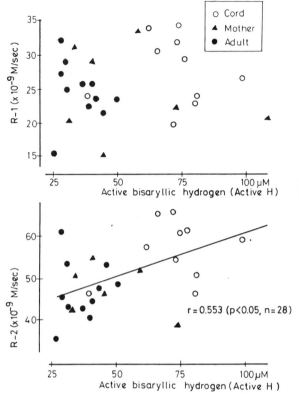

FIGURE 4. Relationships between R-1, R-2, and active H numbers.

TABLE 5. Peroxidizability of Cord and Adult Lipoproteins Reacted with AAPH

	LDL		HDL	
	Cord	Adult	Cord	Adult
Total tocopherol[a]	1.47 ± 0.37^c	1.96 ± 0.42	1.45 ± 0.13^c	2.02 ± 0.18
Alpha-tocopherol	1.31 ± 0.35^c	1.82 ± 0.40	1.38 ± 0.15^c	1.86 ± 0.20
Gamma-tocopherol	0.07 ± 0.02^c	0.22 ± 0.02	0.12 ± 0.01^c	0.29 ± 0.02
Active H (No.)[b]	1.27 ± 0.29^c	1.62 ± 0.16	1.36 ± 0.20^c	1.61 ± 0.25
Active H/tocopherol	87 ± 17^c	75 ± 11	96 ± 13^c	69 ± 12
T_{inh} (s)	595 ± 140^c	854 ± 271	402 ± 89^c	924 ± 384
R-1 (10^{-9}M)	50 ± 5^c	45 ± 3	57 ± 5^c	50 ± 4
R-2 (10^{-9}M)	95 ± 12^c	122 ± 15	129 ± 15^c	138 ± 5

[a] μg/mg lipids.
[b] Average numbers of active H in one molecule of fatty acid calculated from fatty acid composition of lipoproteins.
[c] Mean $\pm$ SD; $p < 0.05$ (sample numbers were 10 each).

Kinetic Study of Oxygen Consumption in Lipoproteins of Cord and Adult Blood Reacted with AAPH

Oxygen Consumption Patterns in Cord and Adult Lipoproteins Reacted with AAPH

In this study, oxygen consumption patterns were investigated with respect to the two major types of lipoproteins, LDL and HDL. FIGURE 5 shows the oxygen consumption patterns in cord and adult HDL fractions reacted with AAPH. Patterns of R-1 and R-2 similar to those observed in RBC ghosts were noted in both HDL. A marked difference occurred in T_{inh}, which was much shorter for cord HDL than for adult HDL.

Fatty Acid Composition in Cord and Adult Lipoproteins

TABLE 6 shows the fatty acid composition of LDL and HDL. The proportion of linoleic acid in cord LDL and HDL was lower than in the adult case, whereas the arachidonic acid in cord lipoproteins was higher. The calculated amount of active H, however, was ultimately smaller in cord than in adult lipoproteins.

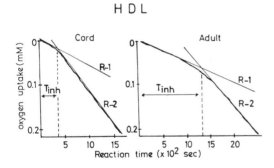

FIGURE 5. Oxygen consumption patterns in cord and adult lipoproteins reacted with AAPH.

Peroxidizability in Lipoproteins of Cord and Adult Blood

As shown in TABLE 5, tocopherol content in LDL and HDL lipids was lower in cord blood than in adult blood, and thus the active H/tocopherol ratio in cord blood was larger. This may indicate a greater susceptibility to peroxidation in cord lipoproteins, even though average numbers of active H were smaller in cord than in adult lipoproteins. T_{inh} in reaction with AAPH was also closely correlated with tocopherol content in both lipoproteins (FIG. 5). Therefore, the T_{inh} was actually shorter in cord

TABLE 6. Fatty Acid Composition of LDL and HDL in Cord and Adult Blood

	LDL		HDL	
Fatty acids	Cord (n = 20)	Adult (n = 16)	Cord (n = 20)	Adult (n = 16)
14:0	1.6 ± 0.2	1.2 ± 0.3	0.9 ± 0.2	0.8 ± 0.3
16:0	39.1 ± 3.1	24.5 ± 2.3	42.5 ± 2.6	30.1 ± 2.2
18:0	5.4 ± 0.9	3.2 ± 0.4	10.3 ± 1.9	7.2 ± 1.5
18:1	22.7 ± 3.6	14.0 ± 1.5	15.2 ± 2.1	11.8 ± 1.4
18:2	14.7 ± 3.3	46.1 ± 4.4	11.5 ± 2.1	35.3 ± 7.0
18:3	0.4 ± 0.4	0.5 ± 0.2	0.2 ± 0.1	0.3 ± 0.1
20:3	1.5 ± 0.2	0.5 ± 0.1	2.5 ± 0.3	0.8 ± 0.1
20:4	8.2 ± 1.9	5.0 ± 0.7	11.1 ± 1.7	6.5 ± 1.4
20:5	0.5 ± 0.2	1.5 ± 0.7	0.4 ± 0.2	2.0 ± 1.5
22:4	0.2 ± 0.1	0.2 ± 0.1	0.4 ± 0.1	0.2 ± 0.1
22:5	0.2 ± 0.1	0.2 ± 0.1	0.2 ± 0.1	0.3 ± 0.2
22:6	3.3 ± 1.1	1.9 ± 0.6	2.9 ± 0.7	2.6 ± 0.9
Active H[a]	1.27 ± 0.29	1.62 ± 0.16	1.36 ± 0.20	1.61 ± 0.25

[a] Average numbers of active hydrogen in one molecule of fatty acids.

than in adult lipoproteins (TABLE 6). In addition, the finding that the R-1 was greater in cord than in adult lipoproteins suggests that peroxidation in the lipoprotein lipids reacting with AAPH may develop faster for cord than for adult lipoproteins even during the periods in which tocopherol remained in the lipoproteins. Thus, R-1 was correlated with the ratio of active H to tocopherol content (FIGURES 7 and 8). On

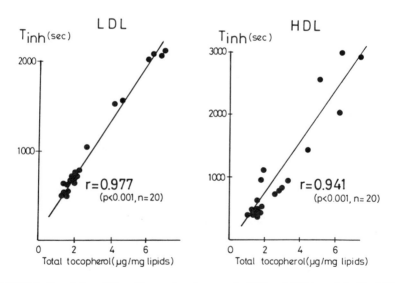

FIGURE 6. Correlation of T_{inh} with tocopherol content in LDL and HDL reacted with AAPH.

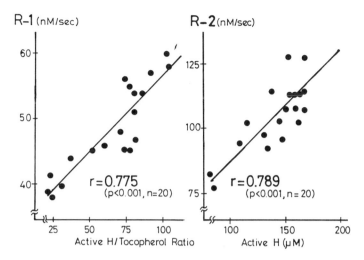

FIGURE 7. Correlation of active H with oxygen consumption rates in phase-1 (R-1) and phase-2 (R-2) of LDL reacted with AAPH.

the other hand, oxygen uptake in R-2 during reaction with AAPH became faster in adult than in cord lipoproteins after tocopherol was exhausted, because greater R-2 was observed in adult lipoproteins as compared with cord lipoproteins (TABLE 6). The R-2 was closely correlated with active H in lipoprotein lipids, as in the case of RBC ghosts (FIGURES 7 and 8).

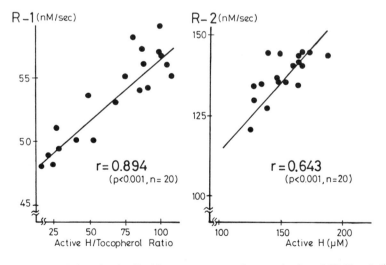

FIGURE 8. Correlation of active H with oxygen consumption rates in phase-1 (R-1) and phase-2 (R-2) of HDL reacted with AAPH.

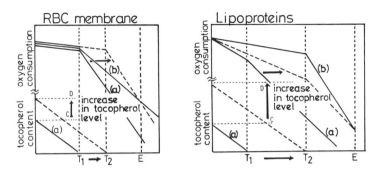

FIGURE 9. Changes in peroxidizability of neonatal membranes and lipoproteins lipids with increase in tocopherol levels (from C to D). (a): neonate; (b): adult; E: end point of oxidation.

DISCUSSION AND CONCLUSIONS

We propose the following ideas with regard to membrane and lipoprotein tocopherol and their peroxidizability. First, RBC membranes in cord blood and adult blood have a similar content of tocopherol, and cord RBC membranes can thus be protected from peroxidation to an extent similar to the adult RBC membranes during the periods while tocopherol still remains in the membranes. After the tocopherol has been consumed, however, peroxidizability in cord ghosts may increase to a greater extent than that in adult RBC ghosts, as demonstrated by the greater quantities of active H, as well as the R-2 and KCL in R-2 (TABLE 3). Therefore, neonatal membranes may be highly susceptible to oxidant stress. If, in neonatal membranes that are exposed to oxygen radicals under highly oxidative conditions, including hyperoxia induced by mechanical ventilation, or inflammation induced by infections,[19] the vitamin E content increases from C to D, as shown in FIGURE 9, then T_{inh} should be prolonged from T_1 to T_2, and then at the end point of propagation (E) the peroxidizability of neonatal membranes would be expected to be comparable to that of adult membranes. Thus, even though tocopherol content of neonatal and adult membranes is similar, more tocopherol content is required for protection of neonatal membranes under oxidative conditions. If tocopherol content in tissue cells is lower than that of adult cells, such as buccal cells and PMN, then far greater tocopherol concentration may be required.

As regards the kinetic study of lipoproteins, peroxidizability in R-1 was greater in cord, contrary to the case of cord RBC ghosts. This high peroxidizability of plasma lipids, including tocopherols, may confirm and explain the previous finding of Yoshioka[20] that levels of thiobarbituric acid reactive substances (as an index of lipid peroxides) are higher in neonatal blood, as compared with adult blood. As shown in FIGURE 9 (right), tocopherol requirements in lipoprotein lipids may also be expected to increase with respect to protection of lipoproteins from oxidative stress under highly oxidative conditions. The susceptibility of biomembranes to oxidative stress cannot be decided *in situ*, however, and remains obscure at present.

ACKNOWLEDGEMENTS

The authors wish to thank Dr. H. Niki and Dr. Y. Yamamoto for their kind assistance and discussion.

REFERENCES

1. Lo, S. S. & W. H. HITZIG. 1973. Vitamin E and hemolytic anemia in premature infants. Arch. Dis. Child. **48**: 360-365.
2. FARRELL, P. M. 1979. Vitamin E deficiency in premature infants. J. Pediatr. **95**: 869-872.
3. GROSS, S. J. & E. GABRIEL. 1985. Vitamin E status in premature infants fed human milk or infant formula. J. Pediatr. **106**: 635-639.
4. HORWITT, M. K., C. C. HARVEY, C. C. DAHM, JR. & M. T. SEARY. 1972. Relationship between tocopherol and serum lipid levels for determination of nutritional adequacy. Ann. N.Y. Acad. Sci. **203**: 223-236.
5. RUBINSTEIN, H. M., A. A. DIETZ & R. SRINAVASAN. 1969. Relation of vitamin E and serum lipids. Clin. Chim. Acta **23**: 1-6.
6. GONTZEA, I. & N. NICOLAU. 1972. Relationship between serum tocopherol level and dyslipemia. Nutr. Rep. Int. **5**: 225-231.
7. MARTINEZ, P. E., AL. L. CONCALVES, S. M. JORGE & I. D. DESAI. 1981. Vitamin E, placental blood and its relationship to maternal and newborn level of vitamin E. J. Pediatr. **99**: 298-300.
8. DESAI, I. D., M. A. SWANN, M. L. GARCIA TRAVERES, B. S. DURA DE OLIVERIA, B. PHARM & J. E. DURA DE OLIVERIA. 1980. Vitamin E status of agricultural migrant workers in South Brazil. Am. J. Clin. Nutr. **33**: 2669-2673.
9. KITAGAWA, M., S. NZAGAGAWA & M. MINO. 1983. Influence of plasma lipids and adiposity on red blood cell tocopherol level. Eur. J. Pediatr. **140**: 238-243.
10. MINO, M., S. NAKAGAWA, H. TAMAI & M. MIKI. 1983. Clinical evaluation of red blood cell tocopherol. Ann. N.Y. Acad. Sci. **393**: 175-178.
11. MINO, M., M. KITAGAWA & S. NAKAGAWA. 1985. Red blood cell tocopherol concentrations in a population of Japanese children and premature infants in relation to the assessment of vitamin E status. Am J. Clin. Nutr. **41**: 631-638.
12. TANAKA, H., M. MINO & T. TAKEUCHI. 1988. A nutritional evaluation of vitamin E status in very low birth weight infants with respect to changes in plasma and red blood cell tocopherol levels. J. Nutr. Sci. Vitaminol. **34**: 293-307.
13. BURTON, K. U., K. U. INGOLD & K. E. THOMPSON. 1981. An improved procedure for the isolation of ghost membranes from human red blood cells. Lipids **16**: 946.
14. MIKI, M., H. TAMAI, M. MINO, Y. YAMAMOTO & E. NIKI. 1987. Free-radical chain oxidation of red blood cells by molecular oxygen and its inhibition by alpha-tocopherol. Arch. Biochem. Biophys. **258**: 373-380.
15. ROSEN, H. & S. J. KLEBANOFF. 1976. Chemiluminescence and superoxide production by myeloperoxidase-deficient leukocytes. J. Clin. Invest. **58**: 50-60.
16. TAMAI, H., M. MANAGO, K. YOKOTA, M. KITAGAWA & M. MINO. 1988. Determination of alpha-tocopherol in buccal mucosal cells using an electrochemical detector. Int. J. Vit. Nutr. Res. **58**: 202-207.
17. OGIHARA, T., M. MIKI, M. KITAGAWA & M. MINO. 1988. Distribution of tocopherol among human plasma lipoproteins. Clin. Chim. Acta **174**: 299-306.
18. YAMAMOTO, Y., E. NIKI, J. EGUCHI, K. KAMIYA & H. SHIMAZAKI. 1985. Oxidation of biological membranes and its inhibition. Free radical chain oxidation of erythrocyte ghost membranes by oxygen. Biochim. Biophys. Acta **819**: 29-36.

19. FLOHE, L., R. BECKMANN, H. GIERTZ & G. LOSCHEN. 1985. Oxygen-centered free radicals as mediators of inflammation. *In* Oxidative Stress. H. Sies, Ed.: 403-436. Academic Press. London.
20. YOSHIOKA, T., Y. TAKEHARA, M. SHIMATANI, K. ABE & K. UTSUMI. 1982. Lipid peroxidation and antioxidants in rat liver during development. Tohoku J. Exp. Med. **137:** 391-400.

Modulation of Tissue Vitamin E Levels by Physical Exercise[a]

L. PACKER, A. L. ALMADA, L. M. ROTHFUSS, AND
D. S. WILSON

Department of Physiology-Anatomy
University of California
Berkeley, California 94720

INTRODUCTION

Increased metabolism can lead to an increase in free radicals produced by the electron transport system, which in turn leads to a response by cellular antioxidant systems. These systems include antioxygenic scavenging enzymes, and water- and lipid-soluble antioxidants. In particular, alpha-tocopherol (vitamin E) is the major chain-breaking lipid-soluble antioxidant that serves to interrupt lipid peroxidation. Hence, the vitamin E status in selective tissues may reflect the degree to which free radical generating reactions have transpired. We have employed different regimens of endurance exercise training on a treadmill, hypothesizing that exercise at a given intensity and duration can modulate cellular antioxidant systems through elevations in active oxygen species generation. Here we report studies using exercising and sedentary animals that have been placed on diets considered sufficient (32 IU/kg) and deficient (0 IU/kg) in vitamin E. The impact of exercise upon blood and tissue antioxidant status has been evaluated.

Other studies on human exercise have also been carried out with antioxidant supplementation. In this case we have investigated the effects of vitamin E and other antioxidants by measuring changes in blood vitamin E, glutathione status, and enzyme activity, that is, a noninvasive strategy. These studies are reported elsewhere.[1,24]

METHODS

Animals on Vitamin E-Sufficient Diets

Female Wistar rats, 9 weeks old, were housed in a room with 12 hour light/dark cycles in groups of 3 per cage. Animals had access to normal rat chow (Purina) and

[a]This work was supported by the NIH (CA479597), National Foundation for Cancer Research, Bethesda, MD, and Roche Vitamins and Fine Chemicals, Nutley, New Jersey.

311

water ad libitum. During the first week, all rats were exercised on a treadmill (Stanhope Scientific, Davis, California) at a 15% gradient at an average speed of 10 meters/minute. The aim of this procedure was to select rats that would run with minimal or no electrical stimulation. At the end of the first week, 12 rats were selected for the endurance study. Six rats were randomly assigned to the sedentary group and were exercised for 5 minutes on the treadmill at about 20 m/min, 3 days a week, for 12 weeks. The remaining six rats were trained for endurance for 12 weeks, 3 days per week with progressive increases in duration and intensity, so that for the final 2 weeks of the study the rats ran at an average speed of 30 m/min for 2 hours.

During the week following the last week of training, 4 rats (2 sedentary and 2 trained) were sacrificed on alternate days, and the various tissues and blood were removed for biochemical analysis as described in reference 2. White adipose tissue was dissected from the abdominal wall. All tissue samples were stored at −70°C until analysis. Activity of succinate cytochrome C reductase in tissue homogenates was measured as described in reference 2. Vitamin E, ubiquinone, and ubiquinol contents of the tissues were analyzed by HPLC as described in reference 3. The statistical significance of differences between sedentary and endurance-trained groups was analyzed by Student's t test.

Animals on Vitamin E-Deficient Diets

Weanling female Sprague-Dawley rats were randomized into equal-sized sedentary and exercise groups. Animals within the trained group exercised 4 days per week. Each training session commenced with a 5 minute warm-up run at an intensity of 9-11 m/min, followed by a gradual progression until the desired exercise intensity was reached. After 7 weeks animals were running approximately 65 minutes per day at an intensity of 20-21 meters per minute. Thereafter, an increase in the duration and intensity to 120 m/day at 25-27 m/min was instituted and maintained until the eleventh week. After week 11 the animals in the exercise group were confined to their cages and remained sedentary for 4 weeks. Two almost identical studies with vitamin E-deficient rats were conducted in succession, hereafter referred to as study I and study II.

For preparation of vitamin E-deficient diets, tocopherol-stripped corn oil was used as the source of dietary lipid. After diets were prepared, they remained under refrigeration.

Tissue sampling, HPLC analysis of vitamin E, ubiquinones, and ubiqunols, and statistical analysis were performed as described above.[3,4]

RESULTS AND DISCUSSION

Rationale

We have previously proposed that physically active individuals will have higher dietary requirements for the antioxidant vitamins E and C.[5] But this hypothesis has not received careful experimental scrutiny. With the recent development of sensitive and accurate methods for the measurement of vitamin E and other lipid-soluble antioxidants, such as ubiquinols,[3] such studies became feasible. In addition to allowing the simultaneous detection of vitamin E and ubiquinones 9 and 10, this technique also makes it possible to quantitate reduced and oxidized species of the ubiquinones. Because ubiquinones are likely to be major sites for free radical generation by mito-chondrial electron transport activity[6] and inasmuch as vitamin E is the major lipid-soluble, chain-breaking antioxidant[7] present in mitochondrial membranes,[8] it was of interest to follow the changes in both of these parameters simultaneously in a variety of tissues from sedentary and endurance-trained animals.

In a previous series of studies from this laboratory, Davies *et al.* found that severe vitamin E deficiency in rats led to decreased maximal exercise endurance capacity in untrained animals.[9] This was paralleled by an increase in stable-free radical electron spin resonance (ESR) signals, increased lipid peroxidation (malondialdehyde), a loss of mitochondrial respiratory control efficiency, and a decreased latency of lysosomal enzymes, collectively indicative of oxidative damage to tissues. Similar alterations were observed in vitamin E-sufficient animals following a single session of maximal en-durance exercise. Taken together, these findings suggest that the cellular damage produced by exhaustive exercise resembles the damage seen in vitamin E deficiency.

In another study we reported that vitamin E deficiency in rats leads to a decrease in endurance capacity for endurance exercise-trained animals.[10] This was attended by a significant fall in tissue (skeletal muscle and liver) vitamin E content.

The present studies further address these issues by following tissue changes in vitamin E concentration as they are affected by exercise under two conditions: animals receiving a diet sufficient in vitamin E level and, animals receiving a diet devoid of vitamin E.

Vitamin E-Sufficiency Experiments

The tissues of sedentary and endurance-trained rats fed a normal diet were analyzed for the levels of ubiquinones, vitamin E, and mitochondrial succinate cytochrome C reductase. The results indicate that the increases in mitochondrial markers (succinate cytochrome C reductase and ubiquinones) observed in endurance-trained animals[11] are not paralleled by increases in vitamin E levels (TABLE 1 and ref. 4).

Succinate cytochrome C reductase activities in various rat tissues expressed per gram of tissue wet weight ranged from 0.6 to 11.8 μmol/min (TABLE 1). The highest activity was found in heart, the lowest in white quadriceps. Activities in skeletal muscles were in the order: red quadriceps > soleus > plantaris > white quadriceps. Liver and brown adipose tissue (BAT) showed similar activities. As has been described by a number of previous studies (see ref. 11 for review), endurance training shows tissue-specific increases in the mitochondrial content. We found that endurance training produced large increases in the succinate cytochrome C reductase activity of red quadriceps (96%) and plantaris muscles (146%) and a smaller but significant increase of 56% in soleus. No significant change occurred in white quadriceps, cardiac muscle, and liver. Succinate cytochrome C reductase activity in BAT also increased in response to the stimulus of 12 weeks of endurance training.

Vitamin E levels of the various tissues in sedentary and endurance-trained rats compare well with a previous report.[12] Among the various skeletal muscle subtypes, white quadriceps showed the lowest values for vitamin E and ubiquinones 9 and 10,

TABLE 1. Tissue Vitamin E and Cytochrome C Reductase in Animals Maintained on a Diet Containing 32 IU dl-Alpha Tocopheryl Acetate/kg Diet

	Cytochrome C Reductase[a]		Vitamin E[b]	
	Sedentary	Trained	Sedentary	Trained
White quadriceps	0.6 ± 0.1	0.7 ± 0.1	19.6 ± 2.3	16.4 ± 1.5
Red quadriceps	3.6 ± 0.4	7.1 ± 0.6[d]	29.3 ± 3.4	29.0 ± 2.3
Plantaris	1.3 ± 0.1	3.2 ± 0.2[e]	26.6 ± 3.0	24.3 ± 1.4
Soleus	2.5 ± 0.4	3.9 ± 0.1[e]	27.7 ± 1.8	24.0 ± 1.9
Heart	11.8 ± 0.8	10.8 ± 0.8	63.6 ± 5.4	53.6 ± 1.3
Brown adipose tissue	8.1 ± 1.1	13.6 ± 1.9[c]	330.1 ± 32.3	348.7 ± 41.3
Liver	7.9 ± 0.8	6.9 ± 1.1	64.0 ± 7.3	49.8 ± 2.7
White adipose tissue	—	—	63.8 ± 5.0	75.6 ± 1.3
Lung	—	—	64.5 ± 4.7	59.2 ± 2.2

[a] Values are means ± SE in μmol/min^{-1}/g wet wt^{-1}; n = 6.
[b] Values are means ± SE in nmol/g wet wt^{-1}; n = 6.
[c] $p < 0.05$; significantly different from sedentary group.
[d] $p < 0.01$.
[e] $p < 0.001$.

whereas the highest values for these parameters were found in red quadriceps. Vitamin E content of cardiac muscle, white adipose tissue, liver, and lung was similar in the sedentary group of rats. Ubiquinone contents, however, were very different. The highest vitamin E and ubiquinone levels were seen in brown adipose tissue. Endurance training showed no statistically significant effect on the vitamin E content of any of the tissues that were examined. The concentrations of ubiquinones were significantly ($p < 0.01$) increased in red quadriceps and soleus, however, as well as in white and brown adipose tissue. This unexpected discrepancy between responses of ubiquinones and vitamin E to endurance exercise training indicates that vitamin E/total ubiquinone 9 ratios significantly decrease in tissues with a positive adaptation in succinate cytochrome C reductase activity and ubiquinone 9 and 10 content, in response to endurance training, but remain constant in other tissues.

Reduced ubiquinones (ubiquinols) prevail in white adipose tissue, BAT, and liver, whereas in all other tissues, the oxidized form is predominant. Endurance training did not have any significant effect on this parameter. The ratio of total ubiquinone 9 (sum of oxidized plus reduced ubiquinones) to total ubiquinone 10 shows remarkable differences for the various tissues but was not significantly influenced by endurance training. (Data elsewhere.[4])

One of the most notable changes that accompanies the adaptation of animals to endurance exercise is an increased biogenesis of mitochondria in skeletal muscles. In this study, the mitochondrial content increased in response to endurance training, as has been demonstrated before.[11,13] Red quadriceps, soleus, and plantaris muscle showed a large increase in succinate cytochrome C reductase activity, whereas liver, cardiac, and white skeletal muscle did not show this positive adaptation in mitochondrial activity to endurance training. The significantly increased ubiquinone content of adipose tissue can be attributed to an increase in adipocyte number per gram of tissue, resulting from a decrease in the triglyceride content per adipocyte in endurance-trained rats.[14] There is no concomitant increase in vitamin E levels, however, as would be expected from a relative increase in the number of adipocytes per gram tissue due to lipolysis. This discordance between ubiquinone and vitamin E adipocyte content may underscore a rudimentary difference between the two: ubiquinone status reflects both endogenous (*de novo* biosynthesis) and exogenous (dietary) contributions, only the latter source being operative with respect to vitamin E. Ultimately this implies that the maintenance of a protective vitamin E/cellular component ratio requires additional intake of the vitamin. The lower vitamin E levels in trained rats could render the tissue more susceptible to lipid peroxidation. This could be related to our previous finding that some of the mitochondrial oxidative pathways in BAT are inactivated with acute exercise.[2]

Ubiquinones, like succinate cytochrome C reductase, are predominantly located in the inner membranes of mitochondria, and hence ubiquinones can also be taken as markers of mitochondrial biogenesis. We found a positive association between the activity of succinate cytochrome C reductase and total ubiquinone content in red quadriceps and soleus muscle of sedentary and trained rats. Exercise-induced increases in the total ubiquinones of skeletal muscles have been described before.[15] Interestingly, ubiquinones in plantaris muscle did not increase significantly with endurance training, although succinate cytochrome C reductase showed a highly significant increase of 146 percent. At this moment we do not have a satisfactory explanation for this finding. We have also examined the distribution of ubiquinones 9 and 10 in the various tissues. Most remarkable is the striking difference in the relative contents of ubiquinone 9 and 10 in white and red quadriceps muscle (FIG. 1). Ubiquinones are also the major site for the generation of superoxide radicals.[6] Because the flux of reducing equivalents through the mitochondrial electron transport chain is increased by exercise, it was important to evaluate the effect of changes in this component of the inner mitochondrial membrane on the lipid-soluble antioxidant, vitamin E.

Factors that influence the vitamin E content of tissues are poorly defined. If fat solubility was the major factor dictating the tissue vitamin E content, then white and brown adipose tissues would be expected to have similar concentrations of this lipid-soluble vitamin. We found, however, that the vitamin E content of brown adipose tissue is at least fivefold higher than that of white adipose tissue. Inasmuch as there is nearly a 100-fold difference in the mitochondrial content between the two tissues, at least part of the difference in vitamin E content may be attributed to the mito-chondrial compartment. Draper and Alaupovic[8] have shown that a major portion of tissue vitamin E is concentrated in the mitochondrial membrane where the respiratory electron transport system is located. Because the muscle mitochondrial content and its electron transport activity increase with exercise, we also expected a parallel increase in muscle vitamin E content. This was not observed, however. There is no correlation between the mitochondrial content of skeletal muscle and its major lipid-soluble antioxidant, vitamin E. It is clear from FIGURE 1 that mitochondria from trained rats have lower vitamin E content per unit oxidative capacity as defined by the total ubiquinone 9 content.

Vitamin E-Deficiency Experiments

Although the above studies provided information regarding static indices of vitamin E status as affected by exercise, prospective data from a wider variety of tissues, which might reveal changes in tissue vitamin E kinetics, was lacking. Our experiments were designed to test how moderate and increased levels of exercise training modulate such kinetics. Two different exercise protocols of varying impact upon adaptive increases in mitochondrial content were used. As shown in FIGURE 2, moderate exercise during

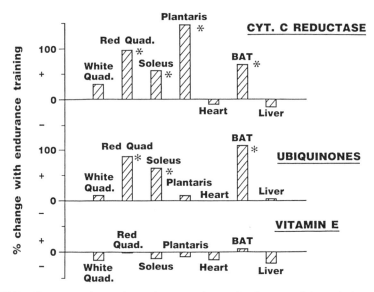

FIGURE 1. Percentage changes in succinate cytochrome C reductase activity, ubiquinone, and vitamin E content with endurance training. Asterisk indicated significantly different from sedentary group.

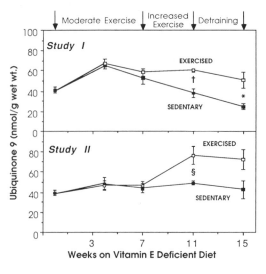

FIGURE 2. Effect of exercise on the profile of red quadricep ubiquinone levels in vitamin E-deficient rats. Significantly more ubiquinone 9 in exercised animals: $*p < 0.05$; $\S p < 0.02$; $\dagger p < 0.001$.

the first seven weeks did not lead to such an increase based on ubiquinone concentration as being a marker of mitochondrial content. During the period between weeks seven and eleven, however, when the exercise intensity and duration were increased, proliferation of mitochondria was indicated. In study I, exercised animals displayed a relative increase (or absolute maintenance) of ubiquinone 9 content relative to the sedentary group; during the 7-11 week period, an absolute increase in ubiquinone content was seen in study II-exercised animals. In study I, mitochondrial ubiquinone content was slightly maintained in the exercised animals relative to the sedentary group. During the detraining period, ubiquinone content was maintained at higher levels in the exercised as compared to the sedentary animals. Nevertheless, during this latter period, red quadricep vitamin E content fell significantly more in the exercised group than in the sedentary controls (FIG. 3). In both studies, red quadricep vitamin E analysis gave similar results with respect to exercise and detraining.

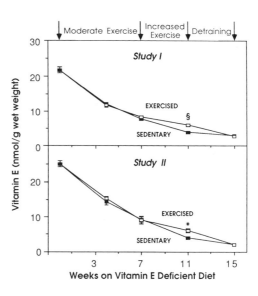

FIGURE 3. Kinetics of vitamin E depletion in red quadricep. Significantly more vitamin E in exercised animals: $*p < 0.05$; $\S p < 0.01$.

The vitamin E depletion kinetic profiles of six tissues investigated are shown in FIGURE 4. As expected, initial levels of vitamin E in tissues differed markedly, with adrenal and brown adipose tissue having the highest initial levels. Liver and white adipose tissue began at levels almost a magnitude lower, with red and white quadriceps displaying even lower initial levels. These values are in general agreement with initial vitamin E levels in rat tissues reported by Bieri *et al.*[16]

The vitamin E depletion in red and white quadriceps, white adipose tissue, and adrenal gland showed that significantly higher vitamin E levels were maintained in the exercised animals as compared to the sedentary controls after 11 weeks of exercise.

These differences disappear after four weeks of detraining (week 15). Levels of vitamin E are reported per gram wet weight of the tissue; thus we cannot evaluate the contribution of tissue volume changes to tissue vitamin E content. Indeed, shrinkage of adipose tissue with exercise has been reported,[14] and the larger values for vitamin

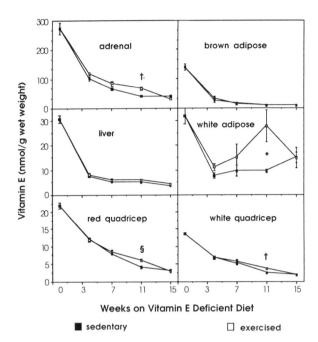

FIGURE 4. Effect of exercise training on vitamin E depletion kinetics in rat tissues. Significantly more vitamin E in exercised animals: *$p < 0.02$; §$p < 0.01$; †$p < 0.001$.

E per gram wet weight may therefore reflect such changes rather than a net exercise-induced increase of this vitamin. After week 7, a marked abdominal hyperadiposity among sedentary animals was observed, suggesting a dilution of vitamin E concentration per adipocyte in members of this group.[17] An additional factor is that of the rapid growth displayed by weanling animals. It is of interest that 15 weeks of maintenance on vitamin E-deficient diet did not completely deplete this vitamin in any tissue studied.

The changes in vitamin E levels observed in the various tissues with increased exercise training intensity suggest that several mechanisms may be operative. The most obvious is that exercise may induce a redistribution of vitamin E among the various tissues by way of blood transport systems, thus exhibiting an apparent tissue-specific retention of vitamin E. It has been reported that white adipose tissue is unlikely to be a labile exchange site for vitamin E.[16,17] Alternately, it is known from both *in vitro*[18] and *in vivo*[19] studies that vitamin E may be regenerated by vitamin C, and perhaps by free radical reductases (L. Packer, unpublished results). Exercise may alter levels of the hydrophilic antioxidants vitamin C[20] and glutathione,[21] and other water- and lipid-soluble antioxidants, resulting in a modified vitamin E regenerative capacity, or in an increased scavenging of the free radicals that otherwise could oxidize vitamin E. The adrenal gland, harboring very high levels of both vitamins C and E, may serve as an ideal organ in which to further investigate this interaction. Indeed, the observation that the majority of vitamin E within adrenal tissue exists as the free vitamin (alpha-tocopherol), whereas other tissues also contain significant levels of an irreversible oxidation product of alpha-tocopherol, alpha-tocopherylquinone,[22] suggests that this organ possesses a regulatory role in intertissue vitamin E distribution. Hence, regeneration, sparing, and/or redistribution of vitamin E may account for the apparent retention of vitamin E in tissues of exercised as compared to sedentary animals (during weeks 7-11). This effect is reversible, as shown (FIG. 5) by the detraining-induced disappearance of statistically significant differences in vitamin E content between the two animal groups (by week 15); this indicates that chronic exercise mitigates vitamin E depletion.

Values for the vitamin E/ubiquinone ratios in red quadriceps at week 11 were 5.83 and 5.08 for sedentary and exercised groups, respectively. After 4 weeks of detraining, the ratios were 5.90 and 3.03 for sedentary and exercised, respectively. The greater fall in vitamin E relative to ubiquinone possibly reflects retention of ubiquinone in the exercised group, or a prolonged stimulation of *de novo* ubiquinone biosynthesis following the cessation of exercise. Perhaps retention of ubiquinone is partially governed by mitochondrial vitamin E concentrations. Additionally, elevated levels of ubiquinones may appreciably alter intracellular vitamin E depletion kinetics. Furthermore, a biphasic depletion of whole tissue vitamin E levels has been observed, consisting of a fast, and a slower, more stable component, based upon studies with animals maintained on vitamin E-deficient[16] and supplemented[12] diets. This may be a manifestation of intracellular compartmental shifts in vitamin E content.

These observations have important implications for the possible role of antioxidants and free radicals in physical exercise and training. We have shown that the vitamin E content of muscle and liver from endurance-trained rats is lower than that of tissues from sedentary counterparts when the animals are fed a vitamin E-deficient diet.[10] In this study we have examined the quantitative relationship between the components of free radical formation in the electron transport chain and the antioxidant vitamin E, which are specifically located in the membrane compartment. The increased electron transport activity brought about by endurance exercise training would be expected to generate, through ubiquinone electron transport reactions, superoxide ions[6] and activate a subsequent cascade of reactions involved in the removal of superoxide (by superoxide dismutase) and organic and inorganic hydroperoxides by peroxidase and catalase.[23] Our results demonstrate that the adaptive increase in the mitochondrial

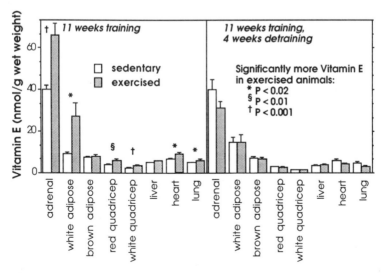

FIGURE 5. Effect of training and detraining on tissue vitamin E levels in vitamin E-deficient rats.

content of muscle is not paralleled by an increase in muscle vitamin E content among animals consuming vitamin E-sufficient diets. Conversely, in exercised animals provided vitamin E-deficient diets, we have described elevations of muscle mitochondrial content that were paralleled by higher levels of vitamin E, relative to sedentary controls.

CONCLUDING REMARKS

Evidence of oxidative damage accompanying exercise has been reported, but free radical production, which is thought to be responsible, cannot be quantitated. Changes in endogenous antioxidants (concentration and redox status), however, reflect free radical generation. Tissues of endurance-trained rats maintained on a normal diet showed positive and adaptive increases over sedentary animals in mitochondrial content and activity (e.g. increased ubiquinones).

It was shown that levels of vitamin E per unit of mitochondrial activity decreased with exercise training. This may be indicative of a higher degree of lipid peroxidation susceptibility in tissues of exercising animals. The fact that this is displayed by animals receiving "sufficient" amounts of dietary vitamin E suggests that higher amounts of vitamin E may be needed in the diet of exercising animals in order to maintain optimal tissue levels of this essential antioxidant. This may be of special importance, because our earlier studies[2] showed that the damaging effects of vitamin E deficiency in tissues are very similar to the damaging effects accompanying acute exercise to exhaustion.

From our study on the effects of chronic exercise training on induced tissue vitamin E depletion, it was found that an exercise protocol equivalent to endurance training results in a positive increase in mitochondrial markers, as it did with vitamin E-sufficient animals. When tissue vitamin E fell to very low levels in certain tissues, however, as seen in red and white quadriceps and adrenal, increased vitamin E levels were associated with the training. Detraining mediated an additional decline of vitamin E in these tissues.

Endurance training modulates the biokinetics of vitamin E depletion in tissues, which may reflect the induction of vitamin E redistributional, sparing, and/or regenerative systems that come into play in different degrees and in different tissues, depending upon the initial tissue vitamin E content and the exercise training protocols.

REFERENCES

1. VIGUIE, C. A., L. PACKER & G. A. BROOKS. 1988. Muscle trauma does not change blood antioxidant status. Med. Sci. Sports 20(2): S10.
2. GOHIL, K., S. HENDERSON, S. E. TERBLANCHE, G. A. BROOKS & L. PACKER. 1984. Effects of training and exhaustive exercise on the mitochondrial oxidative capacity of brown adipose tissue. Biosci. Rep. 4: 987-993.
3. LANG, J., K. GOHIL & L. PACKER. 1986. Simultaneous determination of tocopherols, ubiquinols, and ubiquinones in blood, plasma, tissue homogenates, and subcellular fractions. Anal. Biochem. 157: 106-116.
4. GOHIL, K., L. M. ROTHFUSS, J. LANG & L. PACKER. 1987. Effect of exercise training on tissue vitamin E and ubiquinone content. J. Appl. Physiol. 63: 1338-1341.
5. PACKER, L. 1986. Oxygen radicals and antioxidants in endurance exercise. In Biochemical

Aspects of Physical Exercise. G. Benzi, L. Packer & N. Siliprandi, Eds.: 73-92. Elsevier. New York, NY.
6. BOVERIS, A., E. CADENAS & A. O. M. SHOPPANI. 1976. Role of ubiquinone in the mitochondrial generation of hydrogen peroxide. Biochem. J. **156:** 435-444.
7. BURTON, G. W., K. H. CHEESEMAN, T. DOBA, K. V. INGOLD & T. F. SLATER. 1983. Vitamin E as an antioxidant *in vitro* and *in vivo. In* Biology of Vitamin E. Ciba Foundation Symposium **101:** 4-18. London. Pitman.
8. DRAPER, H. H. & P. ALAUPOVIC. 1959. Intracellular distribution of radioactive vitamin E and its metabolites in rat liver. Fed. Proc. **18:** 218.
9. DAVIES, K. J. A., A. T. QUINTANILHA, G. A. BROOKS & L. PACKER. 1982. Free radical and tissue damage produced by exercise. Biochem. Biophys. Res. Commun. **107:** 1178-1205.
10. AIKAWA, K. M., A. T. QUINTANILHA, B. O. DE LUMEN, G. A. BROOKS & L. PACKER. 1984. Exercise endurance training alters vitamin E tissue levels and red cell hemolysis in rodents. Biosci. Rep. **4:** 253-257.
11. HOLLOSZY, J. O. & F. W. BOOTH. 1976. Biochemical adaptation to endurance exercise in muscle. Annu. Rev. Physiol. **38:** 237-291.
12. MACHLIN, L. J. & E. GABRIEL. 1982. Kinetics of tissue alpha-tocopherol uptake and depletion following administration of high levels of vitamin E. Ann. N.Y. Acad. Sci. **393:** 48-59.
13. DAVIES, K. J. A., L. PACKER & G. A. BROOKS. 1981. Biochemical adaptations of mito-chondria, muscle, and whole animal respiration to endurance training. Arch. Biochem. Biophys. **209:** 538-553.
14. BUKOWIECKI, L., J. LUPIEN, N. FOLLEA, A. PARADIS, D. RICHARD & J. LEBLANC. 1980. Mechanism of enhanced lipolysis in adipose tissue of exercise-trained rats. Am. J. Physiol. **239:** E422-E429.
15. BEYER, R., P. MORALES-CORRAL, B. RAMP, K. KREITMAN, M. FALZON, S. RHEE, T. KUHN, M. STEIN, M. ROSENWASSER & K. CARTWRIGHT. 1984. Elevation of tissue coenzyme Q (ubiquinone) and cytochrome C concentrations by endurance exercise in the rat. Arch. Biochem. Biophys. **234:** 323-329.
16. BIERI, J. G. 1972. Kinetics of alpha-tocopherol depletion and repletion. Ann. N.Y. Acad. Sci. **203:** 181-191.
17. GALLO-TORRES, H. E. 1980. Transport and metabolism. *In* Vitamin E: A Comprehensive Treatise. L. J. Machlin, Ed.: 226. Dekker. New York, NY.
18. BENDICH, A., L. J. MACHLIN, Q. SCANDURRA, G. W. BURTON & D. M. WAYNER. 1986. The antioxidant role of vitamin C. Adv. Free Radical Biol. Med. **2:** 419-444.
19. BENDICH, A., P. DIAPOLITO, E. GABRIEL & L. J. MACHLIN. 1984. Interaction of dietary vitamin C and vitamin E in guinea pig immune response to mitogens. J. Nutr. **114:** 1588-1593.
20. GLEESON, M., J. D. ROBERTSON & R. J. MANGHAN. 1987. Influence of exercise on ascorbic acid status in man. Clin. Sci. **73:** 501-515.
21. LEW, H., S. PYKE & A. QUINTANILHA. 1985. Changes in the glutathione status of plasma, liver and muscle following exhaustive exercise in rats. FEBS Lett. **185:** 262-266.
22. MELLORS, A. & M. M. BARNES. 1966. The distribution and metabolism of alpha-tocopherol in the rat. Br. J. Nutr. **20:** 69-77.
23. HALLIWELL, B. & J. M. C. GUTTERIDGE. 1985. Free Radicals in Biology and Medicine. Oxford University Press. New York, NY.
24. GOHIL, K., L. PACKER, B. DE LUMEN, G. A. BROOKS & S. E. TERBLANCHE. 1986. Vitamin E deficiency and vitamin C supplements: Exercise and mitochondrial oxidation. J. Appl. Physiol. **60(6):** 1986-1991.

The Antioxidant Abnormality in the Stress-Susceptible Pig

Effect of Vitamin E Supplementation[a]

GARRY G. DUTHIE AND JOHN R. ARTHUR

Rowett Research Institute
Aberdeen AB2 9SB
Scotland, United Kingdom

BACKGROUND

In many herds of swine, a large proportion of the animals have inherited the porcine stress (PS) syndrome. When these pigs are subjected to relatively minor stresses, such as transportation, exercise, mating, and parturition, they develop a tachycardia and hyperventilate. Areas of localized cyanosis appear on the skin surface, and a characteristic limb rigidity occurs. A rapid and fatal increase in body temperature of 1°C every 5 minutes ensues and is referred to as malignant hyperthermia (MH). At postmortem, muscle is found to be oedematous and severely disrupted.[1] The porcine stress/malignant hyperthermia syndrome (PS/MH) is a major loss of revenue to the pig industry both through increased mortality and reduced meat quality. In West Germany and Belgium, the incidence of PS syndrome can be up to 80-90 percent.[2] Even in the United States, where the incidence is relatively low, lost revenue due to PS syndrome in 1972 was $250 million,[3] although improved management procedures have reduced losses.[4] MH also occurs in dogs,[5] cats,[6] horses,[7] and deer[8] and can be triggered by exposure to halothane anesthesia.[2] This has led to the identification of an analagous syndrome in humans[9] with an incidence in anesthetized patients of between 1:4,500[10] and 1:40,000.[11] The inheritance of PS syndrome is through a recessive gene so that the heterozygote does not develop the fulminant MH response.[12] In humans, inheritance may be by dominant mode,[11] and in addition to halothane, environmental stressors similar to those that trigger the response in pigs may initiate MH in humans.[13]

The similarities of the MH response in pigs and humans indicate that the pig is an appropriate model for studying the human syndrome.[9] The biochemical lesion responsible for PS/MH syndrome is unknown, although there is general agreement that the fulminant response involves a cell membrane disorder that leads to uncontrolled increases in myoplasmic calcium levels.[14] In this paper, we suggest that this

[a] We thank Dr. Peter Hoppe for his support of this work which was funded by BASF, West Germany.

322

membrane disorder reflects an antioxidant abnormality that increases susceptibility of cell membranes to damage by free radicals. In addition, we present data that indicate that increasing the dietary intake of vitamin E ameliorates, at the biochemical level, the PS/MH syndrome.

METHODS

The following references give the methods used to obtain the results described in this paper and are listed according to analyte: vitamin E,[15] vitamin C,[16] malonaldehyde,[17] conjugated dienes,[18] glutathione peroxidase,[19] glucose-6-phosphate dehydrogenase,[20] catalase,[21] superoxide dismutase,[22] hydrocarbon production,[23] erythrocyte lipid peroxidation,[23] erythrocyte deformability,[24] pyruvate kinase,[20] creatine kinase,[20] reduced and oxidized glutathione,[25] fatty acid profiles,[26] and tissue vitamin C production.[27]

SIMILARITIES BETWEEN PS/MH SYNDROME AND VITAMIN E DEFICIENCY

Polyunsaturated fatty acids in cell membranes of vitamin E-deficient animals are more susceptible to free radical-mediated peroxidation than are those of vitamin E-sufficient individuals. As a result, vitamin E-deficient animals have increased plasma concentrations of products of lipid peroxidation such as conjugated dienes and malonaldehyde.[28] A loss of cell membrane integrity leads to the enhanced leakage of enzymes such as pyruvate kinase and creatine kinase from cells into plasma.[28] Compared with material from vitamin E-sufficient animals, homogenates of tissue from vitamin E-deficient animals produce increased quantities of hydrocarbons such as ethane and pentane,[28] and erythrocytes also show increased malonaldehyde production[29] and decreased deformability[30] when incubated with hydrogen peroxide. Similar differences were found between British Landrace homozygous stress-susceptible and stress-resistant pigs of the same breeding stock and age (TABLE 1). The pigs had consumed an identical diet with a recommended vitamin E content of 10 IU/kg.[31] Nevertheless the stress-susceptible pigs showed all the signs for a reduced capacity to cope with oxidant stress that are typical of an animal deficient in vitamin E.

Despite these differences, the PS/MH pigs were not deficient in vitamin E, insofar as tissue concentrations of tocopherol were identical in the stress-susceptible and stress-resistant animals (TABLE 2). Moreover, in contrast to a previous report,[32] there was no significant decrease in the activity of selenium-dependent glutathione peroxidase (GSHPx) in blood or organs of PS/MH pigs compared with normal pigs. GSHPx activity was, in fact, higher in longissimus dorsi muscle of the PS/MH pigs (TABLE 3). The activities of other antioxidant enzymes such as superoxide dismutase, catalase, and glucose-6-phosphate dehydrogenase were also similar in PS/MH and normal pigs (TABLE 4). Concentrations of reduced glutathione, however, were increased in erythrocytes and muscle of PS/MH pigs (TABLE 5), which may indicate an adaptive response to a sustained oxidant stress.[33,34]

TABLE 1. Indices of Cell Membrane Damage and Indicators of Free Radical-Mediated Lipid Peroxidation in Stress-Susceptible (SS) and Stress-Resistant (SR) Pigs Consuming Diet Containing 10 IU Vitamin E/kg[a]

Parameter	SS	SR	p
Pyruvate kinase (mU/mL plasma)	1028 ± 182	256 ± 51	<0.001
Creatine kinase (mU/mL plasma)	1431 ± 296	563 ± 156	<0.001
Malonaldehyde (nmoles/mL plasma)	2.0 ± 0.3	1.2 ± 0.1	<0.025
Conjugated dienes (U/mL plasma)	157 ± 9	130 ± 7	<0.050
Erythrocyte peroxidation (1.5% H_2O_2 absorbance units at 535 nM)	0.24 ± 0.02	0.10 ± 0.02	<0.001
Erythrocyte deformability (30 min incubation with 0.3% H_2O_2, msec)	2.31 ± 0.61	0.67 ± 0.09	<0.060
Pentane production by longissimus dorsi homogenates (pmoles/mg protein/h)	15.3 ± 5.2	7.01 ± 1.2	<0.020

[a] Data as mean ± SE; ten animals per group. Comparisons made with Student's t test.

TABLE 2. Vitamin E Concentrations in Blood and Tissues of Stress-Susceptible (SS) and Stress-Resistant (SR) Pigs Consuming Diet Containing 10 IU Vitamin E/kg[a]

Vitamin E	SS	SR	p
Plasma (μg/mL)	0.9 ± 0.1	1.0 ± 0.1	NS
Erythrocyte (μg/g Hb)	1.4 ± 0.3	1.0 ± 0.3	NS
Liver (μg/g)	2.7 ± 0.5	2.0 ± 0.4	NS
Heart (μg/g)	3.5 ± 0.3	3.1 ± 0.4	NS
Semitendinous (μg/g)	2.5 ± 0.3	2.5 ± 1.1	NS
Longissimus dorsi (μg/g)	2.7 ± 0.8	1.7 ± 0.2	NS
Serratus (μg/g)	2.3 ± 0.4	2.1 ± 0.4	NS

[a] Data as mean ± SE. NS denotes not significantly different.

TABLE 3. Glutathione Peroxidase Activities in Blood and Tissues of Stress-Susceptible (SS) and Stress-Resistant (SR) Pigs[a]

Glutathione peroxidase	SS	SR	p
Whole blood (U/mL)	19.2 ± 2.34	21.1 ± 0.4	NS
Liver (U/mg protein)	0.275 ± 0.043	0.287 ± 0.015	NS
Heart (U/mg protein)	0.061 ± 0.011	0.077 ± 0.011	NS
Semitendinous (U/mg protein)	0.027 ± 0.003	0.025 ± 0.004	NS
Longissimus dorsi (U/mg protein)	0.023 ± 0.002	0.017 ± 0.003	<0.01

[a] Diet contained 10 IU vitamin E/kg and 0.15 mg selenium/kg.

TABLE 4. Activities of Antioxidant-Related Enzymes in Erythrocytes of Stress-Susceptible (SS) and Stress-Resistant (SR) Pigs

Enzyme	SS	SR	p
Superoxide dismutase (μg/g Hb)	639 ± 55	620 ± 14	NS
Catalase (K/g Hb)	160 ± 8	162 ± 14	NS
Glucose-6-phosphate dehydrogenase (U/g Hb)	11.5 ± 0.9	12.3 ± 0.8	NS

The increased indices of lipid peroxidation in PS/MH pigs do not reflect an obvious deficiency in vitamin E or in the major antioxidant enzymes that were measured (TABLES 2 and 4). Thus we examined the possibility that the increased pentane production by muscle homogenates of PS/MH pigs was due to an increase in ω-6 fatty acid content. However, there were no differences in fatty acid profiles of longissimus dorsi muscle between stress-susceptible and stress-resistant pigs (FIG. 1), suggesting that the cell membranes of PS/MH pigs do not have an increase in peroxidizable substrate, but that substrate that is present is more susceptible to free radical-mediated peroxidation.

EFFECTS OF VITAMIN E SUPPLEMENTATION ON INDICES OF LIPID PEROXIDATION IN PS/MH PIGS

Although the stress-susceptible and stress-resistant pigs appeared to be of similar vitamin E status, there were some differences in their response to supplementation with large amounts of vitamin E (235 IU/kg) (TABLE 6). Concentrations of vitamin

TABLE 5. Concentrations of Reduced (GSH) and Oxidized (GSSG) Glutathione in Erythrocytes and Tissues of Stress-Susceptible (SS) and Stress-Resistant (SR) Pigs[a]

	GSH		
	SS	SR	p
Erythrocyte (mg/g Hb)	99.2 ± 13.8	49.3 ± 13.5	$p < 0.025$
Longissimus dorsi (μg/mg protein)	2.08 ± 0.22	1.23 ± 0.24	$p < 0.05$
Liver (μg/mg protein)	2.83 ± 0.49	2.30 ± 0.17	NS
	GSSG		
	SS	SR	p
Erythrocyte (mg/g Hb)	ND	ND	—
Longissimus dorsi (μg/mg protein)	ND	ND	—
Liver (μg/mg protein)	0.59 ± 0.20	0.53 ± 0.21	NS

[a] ND denotes not detectable.

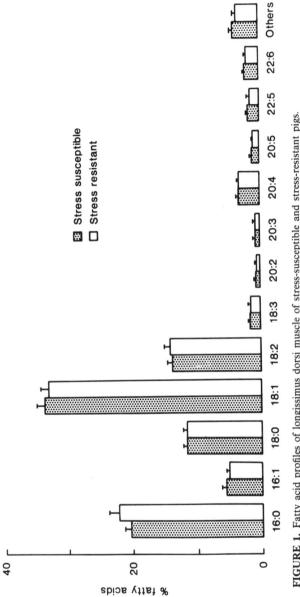

FIGURE 1. Fatty acid profiles of longissimus dorsi muscle of stress-susceptible and stress-resistant pigs.

TABLE 6. Effects of Supplementation with Vitamin E (+E) on Plasma and Tissue Vitamin E Contents, Indices of Cell Membrane Damage and Indicators of Free Radical-Mediated Lipid Peroxidation in Stress-Susceptible (SS) and Stress-Resistant (SR) Pigs[a]

Parameter	Group				RSD	Pig type effect (p)	Vitamin E effect (p)	Interaction (p)
	SS+E	SS	SR+E	SR				
Vitamin E, plasma (µg/mL)	2.2	1.2	2.5	1.0	0.4	NS	<0.001	NS
Vitamin E, longissimus dorsi (µg/g)	3.8	2.7	4.8	1.7	0.6	NS	<0.001	NS
Vitamin E, semitendinous (µg/g)	6.3	2.5	7.3	2.6	0.8	NS	<0.001	NS
Pyruvate kinase (mU/mL)	574	1029	255	256	269	<0.001	<0.05	<0.05
Creatine kinase (mU/mL)	790	1431	294	563	456	<0.001	<0.01	NS
Malonaldehyde (nmoles/mL)	2.72	4.24	2.59	3.06	0.69	<0.02	<0.005	<0.05
Erythrocyte peroxidation (absorbance at 535 nm)	0.06	0.33	0.04	0.07	0.10	<0.001	<0.001	<0.001
Pentane production by longissimus dorsi (pmoles/mg protein/h)	2.3	15.5	1.7	7.0	4.9	<0.02	<0.01	NS
Pentane production by semitendinous (pmoles/mg protein/h)	2.3	15.3	1.7	7.0	4.9	<0.02	<0.01	NS

[a] At 10 weeks of age British Landrace stress-susceptible and stress-resistant pigs were offered, ad libitum, rations containing either 10 IU vitamin E/kg or an increased amount of 235 IU vitamin E/kg (as α-tocopherol acetate). Five weeks later, 6 mL of blood was removed from the jugular vein of each pig. After another week, pigs were sacrificed, and tissue samples were frozen in liquid nitrogen. Residual standard deviations (RSD) were obtained using analysis of variance.

E in plasma and in longissimus dorsi and semitendinous muscles increased to a similar extent in both groups of pigs, but only the PS/MH pigs showed a reduction in plasma pyruvate kinase and creatine kinase activities. In addition, plasma malonaldehyde concentration, erythrocyte peroxidation, and pentane production by muscle homogenates of PS/MH pigs were markedly reduced by the vitamin E supplementation. These results are consistent with decreased free radical-mediated lipid peroxidation and improved cell membrane integrity of vitamin E-supplemented stress-susceptible pigs. Vitamin E supplementation did not affect the stress-resistant pigs to the same extent.

EFFECTS OF TRANSPORTATION AND VITAMIN E SUPPLEMENTATION ON PS/MH PIGS

Further evidence of a beneficial effect of vitamin E supplements in stress-susceptible pigs was obtained in a trial where the animals were transported for 30 minutes prior to measurement of indices of cell membrane integrity and of lipid peroxidation (FIG. 2). Plasma creatine kinase and malonaldehyde increased after transport of the PS/MH pigs, but these changes were partially prevented by supplementation with vitamin E. No effects of transport or vitamin E were noted in the stress-resistant animals.

EFFECTS OF VITAMIN E AND VITAMIN C SUPPLEMENTATION

As stress-susceptible pigs have reduced plasma vitamin C concentrations,[35] it is possible that their apparent antioxidant abnormality reflects a reduction in endogenous vitamin C production, with resultant impaired regeneration of vitamin E. Production of vitamin C, however, by liver homogenate using sodium glucuronate as substrate was not inhibited in PS/MH pigs (FIG. 3). Nevertheless, as lipid hydroperoxides can inhibit vitamin C synthesis in vitro,[27] the possibility still exists that endogenous vitamin C production in PS/MH pigs is reduced. Supplementation of the diet with large amounts of vitamin C (1000 mg/kg) had some effect on the PS/MH pigs. It further reduced plasma pyruvate kinase activities and muscle glutathione concentrations in pigs given a diet with added vitamin E (FIG. 4). It did not amplify, however, the effect of vitamin E in reducing plasma malonaldehyde levels.

Dietary supplementation with vitamins C and E also had significant effects of PS/MH pigs exposed to halothane (TABLE 7). Eight hours after halothane exposure, there was a marked increase in plasma pyruvate kinase and creatine kinase activities in both unsupplemented (10 IU vitamin E/kg) and supplemented pigs. A highly significant effect of the antioxidant supplementation was apparent, however, indicating that the vitamins had limited effects of halothane treatment on cell membrane integrity. Plasma malonaldehyde was significantly lower in supplemented pigs compared with unsupplemented pigs and remained unchanged between 0 and 8 hours. In unsupplemented pigs, however, there was a decrease in plasma malonaldehyde subsequent to halothane exposure.

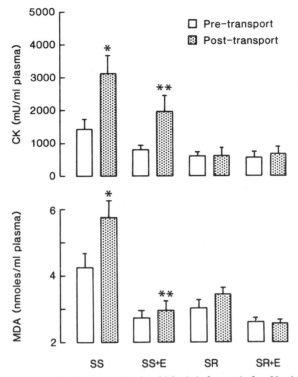

FIGURE 2. Plasma creatine kinase and malonaldehyde before and after 30 min transportation. Stress-susceptible (SS) and stress-resistant (SR) pigs consumed diets containing either 10 or 235 IU vitamin E/kg (+E). *Denotes significant difference between pre- and posttransportation ($p < 0.05$). **Denotes significant difference between supplemented and unsupplemented stress-susceptible pigs posttransport ($p < 0.05$ and $p < 0.001$ for creatine kinase and malonaldehyde, respectively).

FIGURE 3. *In vitro* ascorbate production by liver homogenates of stress-susceptible and stress-resistant pigs, using sodium glucuronate as substrate.

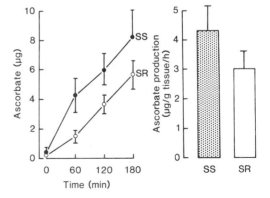

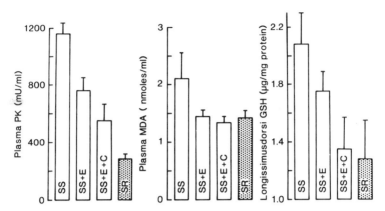

FIGURE 4. Effects of vitamin E or vitamin E + C supplementation on plasma pyruvate kinase activity (PK), plasma malonaldehyde concentration (MDA), and longissimus dorsi muscle glutathione (GSH) concentrations. SS denotes stress-susceptible pigs. Because there were no significant effects of vitamin supplementation on stress resistant pigs, the data are pooled.

DISCUSSION

PS/MH pigs resemble animals that are vitamin E-deficient insofar as they exhibit signs of free radical-mediated damage to cell membranes. This is illustrated by the increased leakage of pyruvate kinase and creatine kinase from muscle to plasma and the increased plasma malonaldehyde and conjugated diene concentrations. The latter changes are indicative of increased peroxidation of membrane polyunsaturated fatty acids. The indices of free radical-mediated damage are further increased by the stress of transport and halothane exposure; the latter stress is a potent producer of free radicals.[36] This indicates a reduced ability of PS/MH pigs to accommodate a sudden increase in free radical load. Susceptibility to free radicals is further emphasized by enhanced *in vitro* peroxidation of red blood cells and muscle homogenates: this is also characteristic of vitamin E-deficient animals. The stress-susceptible pig, therefore, appears to have a defect in its antioxidant defense mechanisms. This can be partially corrected at the biochemical level by increasing the dietary intake of vitamin E. Such supplementation lowers the indices of lipid peroxidation in plasma, even when the pig is stressed and confers protection to erythrocytes and muscle tissue when they are exposed to free radicals *in vitro*.

The PS/MH pigs are not, however, vitamin E-deficient. Furthermore, although increased peroxidation of cell membranes can arise from deficiencies in antioxidant enzymes or increases in polyunsaturated fatty acid content of cell membranes, we did not find any deficiency in the major antioxidant enzymes or increased proportions of ω-3 and ω-6 fatty acids in PS/MH pigs. Moreover, there is less total fat and therefore potentially less substrate for peroxidation in such pigs.[37] This does not exclude the possibility that the PS/MH pig is deficient in other putative antioxidants such as the muscle peptides carnosine, homocarnosine, and anserine.[38] The increase in reduced glutathione in tissues of stress-susceptible pigs possibly reflects an adaptive response to a sustained oxidant stress. Increased dietary intake of antioxidants may as a con-

TABLE 7. Plasma Pyruvate Kinase, Creatine Kinase, and Malonaldehyde of Stress-Susceptible Pigs Immediately following Halothane Inhalation and 8 Hours Later[a]

Parameter	Unsupplemented		Supplemented		Coefficient of variation	Supplementation effect (p)	Time effect (p)	Interaction (p)
	0 h	8 h	0 h	8 h				
Pyruvate kinase (mU/mL)	499	1966	487	1184	0.547[b] 0.679[c]	<0.01	<0.001	<0.01
Creatine kinase (mU/mL)	635	5983	526	3308	0.696[b] 0.878[c]	<0.01	<0.001	<0.06
Malonaldehyde (nmoles/mL)	2.65	2.35	1.86	1.86	0.112[b] 0.140[c]	<0.001	<0.05	<0.05

[a] Eighty-four German Landrace x Pietrain Cross stress-susceptible pigs were fed rations containing either 10 IU vitamin E/kg or supplemented with 250 IU α-tocopherol acetate and 500 mg vitamin C/kg (as L-ascorbic acid) from weaning. At 30 kg live weight, pigs were exposed to halothane until muscle rigidity developed. Immediately, halothane was withdrawn, and 8 h later, a 5 mL blood sample was removed from the vena cava. Data have been subjected to split plot analysis of variance.

[b] Denotes within animal error.

[c] Denotes between animal error.

sequence decrease the requirement for endogenous glutathione and result in a decrease in its synthesis. Activities of the enzymes involved in glutathione synthesis in PS/MH pigs, however, have yet to be determined.

We also considered that the decreased plasma vitamin C concentrations in the PS/MH pigs reflect a lower endogenous vitamin C production, with resultant impaired efficiency of regeneration of vitamin E and increased peroxidation of cell membranes. Although *in vitro* production of vitamin C is not affected in the PS/MH pig, endogenous production *in vivo* could still be inhibited by increased tissue hydroperoxide concentrations. Addition of vitamin C to a vitamin E-supplemented diet has some effect on cell membrane integrity of PS/MH pigs. Nevertheless this does not necessarily imply a functionally dependant relationship between these vitamins, but may merely reflect an additive but independent effect of a membrane and cytoplasmic antioxidant.

Another possibility is that the PS/MH pig has a metabolic defect leading to sudden increased production and/or increased leakage of free radicals from mitochondrial oxidative phosphorylation that exceeds the capacity of the available supply of antioxidants. Also, increased phospholipase A_2 activity[39] in muscle of PS/MH pigs may lead to a rapid release of peroxidizable substrates such as arachidonic acid and lipid hydroperoxides from cell membranes that could overwhelm cytoplasmic antioxidants such as glutathione peroxidase. The protection conferred by vitamin E may thus reflect its inhibitory effect on phospholipase A_2 activity;[40] effects of phospholipase A_2 inhibitors on PS/MH pigs may be worthy of further investigation.

In conclusion, the stress response in PS/MH pigs may be triggered by a sudden free radical load that overwhelms antioxidant defense mechanisms by as yet undefined mechanisms. The free radical load can arise from halothane inhalation or through increased oxidative phosphorylation during stress. Subsequent rapid peroxidation of cell membranes would cause a release of calcium from sarcoplasmic reticulum, with resultant development of characteristic limb rigidity and also uncoupling of metabolic processes. This could divert production of chemical energy as ATP to that of heat, thus causing the observed rise in body temperature.

Whether analogous increases in indices of lipid peroxidation are present in MH-susceptible humans has yet to be ascertained. Our preliminary experiments indicate, however, that antioxidant supplementation reduces the incidence of stress-related mortalities in pigs during transportation procedures. The possible beneficial effect of vitamin E supplementation with MH-susceptible humans may be worthy of investigation.

ACKNOWLEDGMENTS

We are grateful to Dr. Ian Bremner for his suggestions during revisions of the manuscript.

REFERENCES

1. MITCHELL, G. & J. J. A. HEFFRON. 1982. Porcine stress syndromes. Adv. Food Res. **28:** 167-230.

2. WEBB, A. J. 1980. The halothane test: A practical method of eliminating porcine stress syndrome. Vet. Rec. **106:** 410-412.

3. HALL, J. T. 1972. Economic importance of pork. *In* Proceedings of Pork Quality Symposium. R. G. Cassens, F. Giesler & Q. Kolb, Eds. IX-XII. Univ. of Wisconsin Extension. Madison, WI.

4. GRANDIN, T. 1980. The effect of stress on livestock and meat quality prior to and during slaughter. Int. J. Stud. Anim. Prod. **1:** 313-337.

5. SHORT, C. E. & R. R. PADDLEFORD. 1973. Malignant hyperthermia in the dog. Anestheisology **39:** 462-463.

6. DE JONG, R. H., H. E. HEAVNER & D. W. AMORY. 1974. Malignant hyperpyrexia in the cat. Anesthesiology **41:** 608-609.

7. KLEIN, L. V. 1975. Case report: A hot horse. Vet. Anesth. **2:** 41-42.

8. PERTZ, L. & D. P. SUNBERG. 1978. Malignant hyperthermia induced by atropine and xylazine in a fallow deer. J. Am. Vet. Med. Assoc. **173:** 124.

9. GRONERT, G. A. 1980. Malignant hyperthermia. Anesthesiology **53:** 395-423.

10. LIEDING, K. G. & M. D. GRAHAM. 1981. Malignant hyperthermia. Cause and treatment. Arch. Otolaryngology **107:** 758-760.

11. ELLIS, F. R. & J. J. A. HEFFRON. 1985. Clinical and biochemical aspects of malignant hyperpyrexia. Rec. Adv. Anaesthesia **15:** 173-207.

12. REIK, T. R., W. E. REMPEL, L. J. McGARTH & P. B. ADDIS. 1983. Further evidence on the inheritance of the halothane reaction in pigs. J. Anim. Sci. **57:** 826-831.

13. WINCARD, D. W. 1974. Malignant hyperthermia: A human stress syndrome. Lancet **2:** 1450-1451.

14. O'BRIEN, P. J. 1987. Etiopathogenetic defect of malignant hyperthermia: Hypersensitive calcium-release channel of skeletal muscle sarcoplasmic reticulum. Vet. Res. Commun. **11:** 527-559.

15. TAYLOR, S. L., M. P. LAMDEN & A. L. TAPPEL. 1976. Sensitive fluorometric method for tissue tocopherol analysis. Lipids **11:** 530-538.

16. GLEESON, M., J. D. ROBERTSON & R. J. MAUGHAN. 1987. Influence of exercise on ascorbic acid status in man. Clin. Sci. **73:** 501-505.

17. SATOH, K. 1978. Serum lipid peroxides in cerebrovascular disorders detected by new colorimetric method. Clin. Chim. Acta **90:** 37-43.

18. HUNTER, M. I. S. & J. B. MOHAMED. 1986. Plasma antioxidants and lipid peroxidation products in Duchene muscular dystrophy. Clin. Chim. Acta **155:** 123-132.

19. PAGLIA, D. E. & W. N. VALENTINE. 1967. Studies on the quantitative and qualitative characterisation of erythrocyte glutathione peroxidase. J. Lab. Clin. Med. **70:** 158-169.

20. DUTHIE, G. G. & J. R. ARTHUR. 1987. Blood antioxidant status and plasma pyruvate kinase activity of halothane reacting pigs. Am. J. Vet. Res. **48:** 309-310.

21. AEBI, H. 1985. Catalase *in vitro.* Methods Enzymol. **105:** 121-126.

22. ARTHUR, J. R. & R. BOYNE. 1985. Superoxide dismutase and glutathione peroxidase activities in neutrophils from selenium deficient and copper deficient cattle. Life Sci. **36:** 1569-1575.

23. DUTHIE, G. G., J. R. ARTHUR, F. NICOL & M. WALKER. 1989. Increased indices of lipid peroxidation in stress susceptible pigs and effects of vitamin E. Res. Vet. Sci. **46:** 226-230.

24. KIKUCHI, Y., T. ARAI & T. KOYAMA. 1983. Improved filtration method for red cell deformability measurement. Med. Biol. Eng. Comput. **21:** 270-276.

25. ALLEN, K. G. D. & J. R. ARTHUR. 1987. Inhibition by 5-sulphosalicylic acid of the glutathione reductase recycling assay for glutathione. Clin. Chim. Acta **162:** 237-239.

26. ARTHUR, J. R. 1988. Effects of selenium and vitamin E status on plasma creatine kinase activity in calves. J. Nutr. **118:** 747-755.

27. CHATTERJEE, I. B. 1970. Biosynthesis of L-ascorbate in animals. Methods Enzymol. **18:** 28-34.

28. DUTHIE, G. G., J. R. ARTHUR & C. F. MILLS. 1987. Tissue damage in vitamin E deficient rats is not detected by expired ethane and pentane. Free Rad. Res. Comm. **4:** 21-25.

29. CYNAMON, H. A., J. N. ISENBERG & C. H. NGUYEN. 1985. Erythrocyte malondialdehyde release *in vitro:* A functional measure of vitamin E status. Clin. Chim. Acta **151:** 169-176.

30. HALLIWELL, B. & J. M. C. GUTTERIDGE. 1985. Free Radicals in Biology and Medicine. Clarendon Press. Oxford.
31. DUTHIE, G. G., J. R. ARTHUR, S. P. SIMPSON & F. NICOL. 1988. Plasma pyruvate kinase activity vs. creatine kinase activity as an indicator of the porcine stress syndrome. Am. J. Vet. Res. 49: 508-510.
32. SCHANUS, E. G., F. SCHENDEL, R. E. LOVRIEN, W. E. REMPEL & C. McGRATH. 1981. Malignant hyperthermia (MH): Porcine erythrocyte damage from oxidation and glutathione peroxidase deficiency. The Red Cell, Fifth Ann Arbor Conf. S. J. Brewer, Ed. 323-336. Alan R. Liss. New York, NY.
33. MEISTER, A. 1983. Selective modification of glutathione metabolism. Science 220: 472-477.
34. ALLEN, K. G. D., J. R. ARTHUR, P. C. MORRICE, F. NICOL & C. F. MILLS. 1988. Copper deficiency and tissue glutathione concentration in the rat. Proc. Soc. Exp. Biol. Med. 187: 38-43.
35. DUTHIE, G. G., J. R. ARTHUR & P. HOPPE. 1988. Porcine stress syndrome, free radicals and vitamin E. In Oxygen Radicals in Biology and Medicine. Fourth ICOR Conference, San Diego. 605-609. Plenum. New York.
36. MONIG, J. & K. D. ASMUS. 1984. One-electron reduction of halothane (2-Bromo-2-chloro-1,1,1-trifluorethane) by free radicals. Radiation chemical model system for reductive metabolism. J. Chem. Soc. Perkin Trans. 2: 2057-2063.
37. DUTHIE, G. G., J. R. ARTHUR, C. F. MILLS, P. MORRICE & F. NICOL. 1987. Anomalous tissue vitamin E distribution in stress-susceptible pigs after dietary vitamin E supplementation and effects on plasma pyruvate kinase and creatine kinase activities. Livestock Prod. Sci. 17: 169-178.
38. KOHEN, R., Y. YAMAMOTO, K. C. CUNDY & B. N. AMES. 1988. Antioxidant activity of carnosine, homocarnosine, and anserine present in muscle and brain. Proc. Natl. Acad. Sci. 85: 3175-3179.
39. CHEAH, K. S. 1984. Skeletal-muscle mitochondria and phospholipase A_2 in malignant hyperthermia. Biochem. Soc. Trans. 12: 358-360.
40. VANKUIJK, F. J. G. M., A. SEVANIAN, G. J. HANDELMAN & E. A. DRATZ. 1987. A new role for phospholipase A_2: Protection of membranes from lipid peroxidation damage. Trends Biochem. Sci. 12: 31-34.

Vitamin E, Immune Response, and Disease Resistance[a]

ROBERT P. TENGERDY

Department of Microbiology
Colorado State University
Fort Collins, Colorado 80523

INTRODUCTION

It is now well-established that vitamin E stimulates body defenses against infectious disease. The subject has been covered in previous reviews.[1-5] Vitamin E enhances humoral and cellular immune responses and increases phagocytic functions. Its effect is most pronounced in infectious diseases where immune phagocytosis is the main defensive mechanism. It is least effective where cell-mediated immunity is the main defense. Vitamin E is effective as a dietary supplement or as an injection, especially in adjuvant vaccines. The effective dietary dose for optimal immune protection is about 4-6 times higher than vitamin E levels found in normal diets. Inasmuch as vitamin E deficiency predictably leads to impaired immune function and disease resistance, this review is restricted to the effect of vitamin E supplementation on immunity and disease resistance. The review is focused on the comparison of dietary supplementation and injection of vitamin E in the form of adjuvant vaccines.

DIETARY SUPPLEMENTATION OF VITAMIN E

Dietary supplementation of vitamin E increased the resistance of laboratory animals,[6-9] farm animals,[4,10-15] and humans[6-20] against infectious diseases. Dietary supplementation of vitamin E is now recommended in modern farm animal production practice for poultry, swine, sheep, and cattle to maintain a high level of immune protection in the face of a high level of feeding required by an increasing demand for higher meat, egg, and milk production.[21] Vitamin E supplementation is most effective for farm animals under stress. Vitamin E supplementation appears to be beneficial in elderly persons to reduce the incidence or severity of infectious diseases.[16,22,23] It has been used in the treatment of diabetes mellitus,[18] autoimmune diseases,[17,20] and genetic disorders.[24] Vitamin E may reduce corticosteroid levels induced by stress.[25] Vitamin E, together with vitamins A and C, may participate in cancer prevention, by potentiating immunosurveillance against tumors.[26]

[a] This work was supported by a Grant from Hoffmann-La Roche Inc.

335

The disease protective effect of vitamin E may be attributed principally to the antioxidant function of this vitamin. Antioxidants protect cells from peroxidation damage, protect the lipids in cell membranes, and modulate the biosynthesis of important cell regulators, prostaglandins, thromboxane, and leukotrienes.

The immunoenhancing effect of vitamin E compared with a synthetic antioxidant was demonstrated in an early experiment in our laboratory in 1973 (TABLE 1).[6] Both the synthetic antioxidant DPPD and vitamin E stimulated cell proliferation in immunopoietic organs, such as the spleen, increased the number of antibody-producing plasma cells, and caused a shift from IgM to IgG antibody production. The effect of vitamin E, however, was clearly superior.

The direct effect of vitamin E on immune-competent lymphocytes was demonstrated in *in vitro* mouse spleen cell cultures (TABLE 2).[27] A detailed explanation of this observation was provided later by *in vitro* experiments of Tanaka *et al.*[28] and Corwin and co-workers.[29] Vitamin E apparently stimulated primarily T-helper cells, amplifying or even bypassing the cooperative effect of macrophages. Synthetic antioxidants, such as 2-mercaptoethanol have a similar, albeit lesser, effect.[27] In the complex cell-cell interactions triggering and regulating immune responses, cell membrane-bound vitamin E probably plays an important role. A possible clue is the observation that vitamin E decreases membrane fluidity in platelets.[5] The close association of vitamin E with arachidonic acid in the membrane and the presence of a

TABLE 1. Antioxidant Effect on Humoral Immunity in Mice Immunized with Sheep Red Blood Cells (SRBC)[a]

Treatment of mice	Body weight g	Spleen weight g	PFC[d] per 10^6 cells	HA[e] $\log_2$ titer	
				Without IgM	With IgG
WLB[b] chow	28.0 ±2.1	0.016 ±0.021	1,225 ±85	7.3 ±0.2	< 1
WLB chow + 222 mg DPPD[c]/kg	27.0 ±2.3	0.123 ±0.032	5,461 ±292	7.5 ±0.9	3.5 ±0.2
WLB + 2,035 mg vitamin E/kg	25.6 ±2.4	0.114 ±0.024	7,863 ±295	7.9 ±0.4	4.1 ±0.9
Vitamin E-deficient diet	18.5 ±1.5	0.059 ±0.007	419 ±25	6.8 ±1.2	< 1
Vitamin E-deficient diet + 222 mg DPPD/kg	18.3 ±2.4	0.073 ±0.010	562 ±32	6.5 ±1.2	< 1
Vitamin E-deficient diet + 2.0 g vitamin E/kg	26.3 ±1.9	0.120 ±0.021	6,520 ±300	7.5 ±0.5	3.5 ±0.2

[a] Each value represents the average of 10 mice. The values given are means ±SD; p <0.01 between controls and treatment groups.
[b] WLB: Wayne laboratory blocks.
[c] DPPD: N_1N_1 diphenyl-*p*-phenylenediamine.
[d] PFC: plaque-forming cells.
[e] HA: hemagglutination.

TABLE 2. Effect of Vitamin E on PFC Count of SRBC-Stimulated Spleen Cells in Single-Cell Suspension Culture[27]

μg dl-alpha-tocopheryl acetate added per culture[a]	PFC per culture[b]	
	normal spleen cells	nonadherent cells
	18,360	471
1.8	36,990	3,109
5.0	34,471	2,875
50.0	25,786	209

[a] Solubilized in Emulphor®.
[b] 10^6 normal or column-separated spleen cells were cultured for 5 days before counting.

newly discovered membrane-bound Se containing glutathione peroxidase[30] may hint at the role of vitamin E in these cell-cell interactions.

Vitamin E has enhanced mitogenic stimulation of lymphocytes and granulocytes in vitro.[8,9,29,31] This in vitro stimulation does not always correspond to increased immune functions and protection in vivo.[3,4] Vitamin E and other antioxidants enhance the proliferation, chemotaxis, and bactericidal killing power of polymorphonuclear leukocytes (PMN).[19,32] Vitamin E as an antioxidant protects PMN from peroxidative damage, but an excessive dose may reduce the intracellular killing power of PMN that depends on peroxidative damage to the engulfed bacteria by the H_2O_2 generated. In an infant with congenital deficiency of glutathione synthetase and abnormal PMN function, vitamin E treatment corrected the overproduction of H_2O_2 and the decreased ability to iodinate protein and kill bacteria.[24] In diabetic patients, vitamin E restored monocyte chemotaxis and motility.[18] Vitamin E also may counteract drug toxicity to PMN and other cells of the immune response.[33]

The modulation of prostaglandin, thromboxane, and leukotriene biosynthesis by vitamin E is well-documented and most likely plays an important role in immunoregulation.[5,34-37] In general, a suppression of lipoxygenation of arachidonic acid by vitamin E may lead to immunoenhancement,[38] but the data reported in the literature are not unequivocal, perhaps due to the apparent bidirectional nature of the response. Lower doses of vitamin E stimulated, and higher doses suppressed, lipoxygenation in leukocytes.[36]

The involvement of possible prostaglandin (PG) modulation by vitamin E in disease protection was first demonstrated in our laboratory by comparing a known PG inhibitor, aspirin, with vitamin E in suppressing PG levels in immunopoietic organs and reducing mortality of E. coli infected chickens (TABLE 3).[39] The PG modulation and consequent immune protection by vitamin E also depends on nutritional interactions. For example, vitamin A, which is also a prostaglandin and immunomodulator, counteracted the effect of vitamin E on PGE_1 and PGE_2 levels, mortality, and antibody titer, but enhanced the phagocytic clearance of bacteria from the blood (TABLE 4).[40]

Dietary lipids also interact with vitamin E in regulating prostaglandin levels and immune responses. A saturated fat enhanced PGE_2 suppression by vitamin E with a corresponding increase in antibody titer; an unsaturated fat acted opposite, perhaps by reducing the effective concentration of vitamin E available for PG modulation (TABLE 5).

In assessing the expected benefit of vitamin E supplementation for disease protection, nutritional interactions with minerals (Se, Zn), other vitamins, lipids, and

TABLE 3. Correlation between Prostaglandin (PG) Levels and Mortality in *E. coli*-Infected Chickens[39]

Treatment[a]	PGF$_2$	PGE$_2$	PGE$_1$	Percent[c] mortality
	PG in bursa, μg/g wet tissue[b]			
Control	71.9 ± 8	22.5 ± 1.9	94.0 ± 14.8	80
Vitamin E	36.2 ± 3.8	21.2 ± 2.7	32.5 ± 6.4	36
Aspirin	39.7 ± 4.6	12.2 ± 1.0	70.0 ± 5.9	42
Vitamin E + Aspirin	12.4 ± 3.6	2.9 ± 1.0	23.3 ± 7.7	0
Noninfected	44.2	27.4	46.6	0

[a] All chickens except noninfected controls were injected with 1×10^9 *E. coli*. Vitamin E dietary supplement: 300 mg/kg diet; aspirin 50 mg/kg body weight, injected intraperitoneally on the day before infection and daily thereafter.
[b] n = 8. PG radioimmunoassays from bursa taken from sacrificed birds 5 min after infection.
[c] Counted 2 days postinfection.

TABLE 4. Interaction of Vitamins A and E in Disease Protection[40]

Diet[a]	Percent mortality	Blood clearance[b] *E. coli* cells × 10^4/mL	Hemagglutination log 2 titer	PGE$_1$ μg/g[c]	PGE$_2$ μg/g
Control	53	7.9 ± 0.7a	9.0 ± 1.0a	1.9	3.2
Vitamin E	25	6.4 ± 0.9b	11.0 ± 0.8b	1.3	1.8
Vitamin A	22	6.3 ± 0.7b	11.1 ± 0.7b	2.5	3.4
Vitamin E+A	39	6.0 ± 1.6b	8.6 ± 0.7b	1.5	3.6

[a] Vitamin E, 300 mg/kg; vitamin A, 60,000 IU/kg.
[b] 20 immunized chicks per group were challenged with 3.0×10^8 *E. coli* cells on day 21. The average number of *E. coli* cells remaining in the blood one hour after challenge is shown. Means followed by different letters indicate significant differences ($p < 0.01$).
[c] Measured by radioimmunoassay in the bursa.

TABLE 5. Interaction of Dietary Lipids and Vitamin E on Prostaglandin (PGE$_2$) Level and Antibody Titer to SRBC in Chickens[a]

Diet	PGE$_2$ (pg/mg) in bursa	Antibody log$_2$ titer
Control	33.1	2.7
Control + E	21.0	2.9
3% safflower oil	32.6	2.7
3% safflower oil + E	22.6	2.3
3% beef tallow	30.3	2.8
3% beef tallow + E	15.5	3.0

[a] Source: C.F. Nockels, unpublished data.

protein-calorie nutrition should be considered.[41] Bendich *et al.*[9] and Watson and Leonard[26] reported positive interaction between vitamins E and C. We found interaction between vitamins E and A.[40] Selenium is a known potentiator of vitamin E activity, and other minerals may also interact with vitamin E.[41] Lipids, especially unsaturated fats, increase the demand for vitamin E and interfere with immunoenhancement.[34] High protein-calorie nutrition, common in modern farm animal management, increases the demand for vitamin E and may alter susceptibility to infections.[21]

Environmental stress is another modifier of vitamin E action. Stress, such as nutritional imbalance, heat and cold, crowding, noise, and transportation may predispose to infectious diseases by lowering the defensive mechanisms of the body. The chemical modulators of stress, such as corticosteroids, have a pronounced immunosuppressive effect, associated with increased prostaglandin levels, and also affect the bioavailability of nutrients.[25] A stress-induced infection may cause diarrhea and decreasing feed utilization, thus further increasing disease susceptibility. Perhaps the reason for the reported effectiveness of vitamin E administration to stressed animals, lactating cows, and cattle in transit or feedlots is the early interference with this interlocking chain of events that eventually leads to disease.[42]

THE ADJUVANT ACTION OF VITAMIN E

Vitamin E has a particularly strong effect on immune responses when *dl*-alphatocopheryl acetate, the oily form, is incorporated into water-in-oil adjuvants. A striking observation was made in comparing the effect of dietary supplementation of vitamin E and adjuvant administration of vitamin E on the vaccination of sheep with *Clostridium perfringens* type D toxin against enterotoxemia. While the dietary treatment gave enhanced humoral immunity and increased protection upon challenge with virulent *C. perfringens,* the adjuvant vaccine, although containing only a fraction of the vitamin E that was used in dietary treatment, was far more effective (TABLE 6).[43]

TABLE 6. Comparison of *Clostridium perfringens* Antitoxin D Titers in Vitamin E Adjuvant and Conventionally Immunized Lambs[43]

Group	Mean antibody titer[a]	
	before vaccination	after vaccination (7 days)
Vaccinated, control diet	0.312 ± 09 (n=12)	0.513 ± 0.22 (n=12)
Vaccinated, vitamin E diet	0.332 ± 0.10 (n=12)	0.725 ± 0.14 (n=12)
Vitamin E adjuvant, control diet	0.446 ± 0.14 (n=3)	1.64 ± 0.25 (n=3)
Vitamin E adjuvant, vitamin E diet	0.354 ± 0.12 (n=3)	1.046 ± 0.24 (n=3)

[a] Measured in an ELISA test. Titer expressed in absorbance units at 405 nm and 1:200 serum dilution. The pelleted diet was supplemented with 300 mg/kg vitamin E and fed for 5 weeks.

TABLE 7. Correlation of Humoral Immunity and Infection in Rams Vaccinated with *B. ovis* against Epididymitis[45]

Group	No. in Group	No. Infected	Overall Infectivity	Peak ELISA[a] Titer ± SD
Bacterin[b]	9	4	44.4	0.27 ± 0.15
B. ovis-vitamin E	9	2	22.2	0.42 ± 0.25
B. ovis-FIA[c]	9	4	44.4	0.35 ± 0.16
Vitamin E placebo	8	3	37.5	0.14 ± 0.08
FIA placebo	8	5	62.5	0.15 ± 0.09
Aluminum Hydroxide control	9	6	66.7	0.26 ± 0.18

[a] Enzyme-linked immunosorbent assay: titer is expressed in OD units at 485 nm and 1:200 serum dilution.

[b] Killed *B. ovis* cells in Al (OH)$_3$.

[c] Freund's incomplete adjuvant.

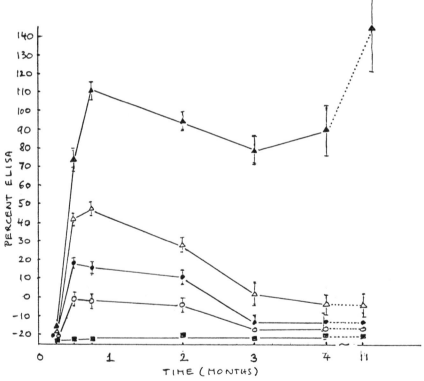

FIGURE 1. ELISA antibody titers of rams immunized with *Brucella* vaccines. ▲, *B. ovis* vitamin E adjuvant vaccine; △, Al(OH)$_3$ precipitated *B. ovis* bacterin; ●, Rev 1 (*B. melitensis*) in vitamin E adjuvant; ○, Rev 1; ■, Control; n = 10-20. Titers are expressed as optical density in percentage of reference standards.

Adjuvants are most effective with antigens that are not very immunogenic by themselves, such as many protein antigens.[44] In comparing the immune response of guinea pig against bovine serum albumin (BSA), the vitamin E adjuvant gave significantly better response than a Freund's incomplete adjuvant formulation or the aqueous solution of BSA. The vitamin E adjuvant vaccination also proved superior with whole cell bacterial vaccines, such as a *Brucella ovis* vaccine against ram epididymitis (TABLE 7).[45] In a current field trial in Peru, this vaccine competed successfully against the best commercially available vaccines (FIG. 1).

Water-in-oil adjuvants partially serve as a stable depot for the gradual slow release of an antigen, stimulating the cells of the immune response for a long time. The ordered orientation of antigen molecules in the oil-water boundary, hydrophobic regions in the oil, hydrophilic regions in the water, may provide the necessary cross-linking for effective presentation to macrophages and lymphocytes. At this point it may be hypothesized that when vitamin E is the oil phase in an adjuvant, the attraction of chemotactic cells, PMN, dendritic cells, macrophages, and lymphocytes to the adjuvanted antigen elicits a local inflammatory and immune response, which is amplified by vitamin E. All the vitamin E administered in the adjuvant is targeted to the cells contacting the adjuvant; thus the effective concentration of vitamin E is much higher than in dietary supplementation.

A number of water-in-oil adjuvants, such as Freund's adjuvant, vitamin A, saponin, and retinol are surface-active agents that may alter cell membrane behavior and cell-cell interactions.[46] These adjuvants activate phospholipase A to form surface-active lysophosphatidylcholine (lysolecithin).[47] Lysolecithin inhibits prostaglandin synthesis.[48]

The vitamin E adjuvant produces the same indicators of immunoenhancement and disease protection as dietarily administered vitamin E, except at an elevated level: increased humoral immunity, increased mitogenic stimulation of T and B cells, increased phagocytosis by PMN, increased delayed-type hypersensitivity, and a moderate inflammatory reaction. Interestingly, in contrast to Freund's adjuvant, which causes a strong inflammatory reaction that prohibits its use in human or veterinary medicine, the vitamin E adjuvant has a mild inflammatory response, due to the antiinflammatory property of vitamin E. Vitamin E adjuvant vaccines may be particularly beneficial to immunocompromised populations, such as the elderly.

SUMMARY

Vitamin E as a dietary supplement or as part of an adjuvant vaccine formulation increases humoral and cell-mediated immunity and disease resistance in laboratory animals, farm animals, and humans. Adjuvant administration has far greater effect than dietary supplementation. Vitamin E as an antioxidant protects the cells of the immune response from peroxidative damage; possibly through a modulation of lipoxygenation of arachidonic acid, vitamin E alters cell membrane functions and cell-cell interactions. The most pronounced effect of vitamin E is on immune phagocytosis. Dietary supplementation is beneficial to animals, especially under stress, in decreasing susceptibility to infections. Vitamin E adjuvant vaccines have provided greater immunoprotection against enterotoxemia and epididymitis in sheep than conventional vaccines.

REFERENCES

1. TENGERDY, R. P. 1980. Effect of vitamin E on immune responses. *In* Vitamin E, a Comprehensive Treatise. L. J. Machlin, Ed.: 429-443. Dekker. New York, NY.
2. TENGERDY, R. P., M. M. MATHIAS & C. F. NOCKELS. 1981. Vitamin E, immunity and disease resistance. *In* Diet and Resistance to Disease. M. Phillips & A. Baetz, Eds.: 27-42. Plenum. New York, N.Y.
3. TENGERDY, R. P., M. M. MATHIAS & C. F. NOCKELS. 1984. Effect of vitamin E on immunity and disease resistance. *In* Vitamins, Nutrition and Cancer. K. N. Prasad, Ed.: 118-122. Karger. Basel.
4. TENGERDY, R. P. 1986. Nutrition, immunity and disease resistance. *In* Proceedings of the Sixth International Conference on Production Disease in Farm Animals, Belfast, N. Ireland, pp. 175-182.
5. CARPENTER, M. P. 1986. Effects of vitamin E on the immune system. *In* Vitamins and Cancer. F. L. Meyskens & K. N. Prasad, Eds.: 199-211.
6. TENGERDY, R. P., R. H. HEINZERLING, G. L. BROWN & M. M. MATHIAS. 1973. Enhancement of the humoral immune response by vitamin E. Int. Arch. Allergy Appl. Immunol. **44:** 221-227.
7. HEINZERLING, R. H., R. P. TENGERDY, L. L. WICK & D. C. LUEKER. 1974. Vitamin E protects mice against *Diplococcus pneumoniae* type I infection. Infect. Immun. **10:** 1292-1295.
8. BENDICH, A., E. GABRIEL & L. J. MACHLIN. 1986. Dietary vitamin E requirement for optimum immune responses in the rat. J. Nutr. **116:** 675-681.
9. BENDICH, A., P. D'APOLITO, E. GABRIEL & L. J. MACHLIN. 1984. Interaction of dietary vitamin C and vitamin E on guinea pig immune responses to mitogens. J. Nutr. **114:** 1588-1593.
10. SMITH, L. K. & H. R. CONRAD. 1987. Vitamin E and selenium supplementation for dairy cows. Roche Technical Symposium. March 11. Daytona, FL. 47-66.
11. MORRILL, J. L. & P. G. REDDY. 1987. Effect of vitamin E on immune responses and performance of dairy calves. Roche Technical Symposium. March 11. Daytona, FL. 34-46.
12. CIPRIANO, J. E., J. L. MORRILL & N. V. ANDERSON. 1982. Effect of dietary vitamin E on immune responses of calves. J. Dairy Sci. **65:** 2357-2361.
13. ELLIS, R. P. & M. W. VORTIES. 1976. Effect of supplemental dietary vitamin E on the serologic response of swine to *E. coli* bacteria. J. Am. Vet. Med. Assoc. **168:** 231-232.
14. TEIGE, J., S. TOLLERSRUD, A. LUND & H. J. LARSEN. 1982. Swine dysentery: The influence of dietary vitamin E and selenium on the clinical and pathological effects of *Treponema hyodysenteriae* infection in pigs. Res. Vet. Sci. **32:** 95-100.
15. LARSEN, H. J. & S. TOLLERSRUD. 1981. Effect of dietary vitamin E and selenium on the phytohemagglutinin responses of pig lymphocytes. Res. Vet. Sci. **31:** 301-305.
16. MEYDANI, S. N., J. B. BLUMBERG, G. YOGEESWARAN & M. MEYDANI. 1989. Antioxidants and the aging immune system. *In* Antioxidant Nutrients and the Immune Response. A. Bendich, M. Phillips & R. Tengerdy, Eds. Plenum. New York, NY. In press.
17. FERNANDES, G. 1989. Effect of omega-3-fatty acids and vitamin E supplements on autoimmune diseases. *In* Antioxidant Nutrients and the Immune Response. A. Bendich, M. Phillips & R. Tengerdy, Eds. Plenum. New York, NY. In press.
18. HILL, H. R., N. H. AUGUSTINE, M. L. RALLISON & J. I. SANTOS. 1983. Defective monocyte chemotactic responses in diabetes mellitus. J. Clin. Immunol. **3:** 70-77.
19. BOXER, L. A. 1989. Functional effects of leukocyte antioxidants on polymorphonuclear leukocyte behavior. *In* Antioxidant Nutrients and the Immune Response. A. Bendich, M. Phillips & R. Tengerdy, Eds. Plenum. New York, NY. In press.
20. AYRES, S., JR. & R. MIHAN. 1978. Is vitamin E involved in the autoimmune mechanism? Cutis **21:** 321-325.
21. STUART, R. L. 1987. Factors affecting vitamin E status of beef cattle. Roche Technical Symposium. March 11. Daytona, FL. 67-80.
22. CHAVANCE, M., G. BRUBACHER, B. HERBETH, G. VERNHES, T. MIKSTACKI, F. DETE,

C. FOURNIER & C. JANOT. 1984. Immunological and nutritional status among the elderly. *In* Topics of Aging Research in Europe. A. L. deWitz, Ed.: 231-237. Europe. Amsterdam.

23. BENDICH, A. 1989. Effect of antioxidant vitamins on cellular immune functions. *In* Antioxidant Nutrients and the Immune Response. A. Bendich, M. PHillips & R. Tengerdy, Eds. Plenum. New York, NY. In press.

24. BOXER, J. A., J. M. OLIVER, S. O. SPIELBERG, J. M. ALLEN & J. D. SHULMAN. 1979. Protection of granulocytes by vitamin E in glutathione synthetase deficiency. N. Engl. J. Med. **301:** 901-905.

25. WATSON, R. R. & T. M. PETRO. 1982. Cellular immune response, corticosteroid levels and resistance to *Listeria monocytogenes* and murine leukemia in mice fed a high vitamin E diet. Ann. N.Y. Acad. Sci. **393:** 205-210.

26. WATSON, R. R. & T. K. LEONARD. 1986. Selenium and vitamins A, E and C: Nutrients with cancer prevention properties. J. Am. Diabetic Assoc. **85:** 505-510.

27. CAMPBELL, P. A., H. R. COOPER, R. H. HEINZERLING & R. P. TENGERDY. 1974. Vitamin E enhances *in vitro* immune response by normal and non-adherent spleen cells. Proc. Soc. Exp. Biol. Med. **146:** 465-469.

28. TANAKA, T., H. FUJIWARA & M. TORISU. 1979. Vitamin E and immunity. I. Enhancement of helper T-cell activity. Immunology **38:** 727.

29. CORWIN, L. M. & R. K. GORDON. 1982. Vitamin E, biochemical, hematological and clinical aspects. Ann. N.Y. Acad. Sci. **393:** 437-451.

30. URSINI, F. & A. BINDOLI. 1987. The role of selenium peroxidases in the protection against oxidative damage of membranes. Chem. Phys. of Lipids **44:** 255-276.

31. BENDICH, A., E. GABRIEL & L. J. MACHLIN. 1983. Effect of dietary level of vitamin E on the immune system of the spontaneously hypertensive (SHR) and normotensive Wistar Kyoto (WKY) rat. J. Nutr. **113:** 1920-1926.

32. BOXER, L. A. 1986. Regulation of phagocyte function by alpha-tocopherol. Proc. Nutr. Soc. **45:** 333-338.

33. PICKERING, L. K., T. G. CLEARY, M. KLETZEL, Y.-M. WANG & M. M. PARRA. 1983. Modulation of polymorphonuclear leukocyte function by doxorubicin (adriamycin ®) and alpha tocopherol (vitamin E). J. Clin. Lab. Immunol. **11:** 95-100.

34. AFZAL, M., R. P. TENGERDY, S. J. BRODIE, J. C. DeMARTINI, R. P. ELLIS, R. L. JONES, & C. V. KIMBERLING. 1986. The immune response in rams experimentally infected with *Brucella ovis.* Res. Vet. Sci. **41:** 85-89.

35. MACHLIN, L. 1978. Vitamin E and prostaglandins. *In* Tocopherol, oxygen and biomembranes. C. deDuve & O. Hayashi, Eds.: 179-189. Elsevier. New York, NY.

36. GOETZL, E. J. 1980. Vitamin E modulates the lypoxygenation of arachidonic acid in leukocytes. Nature **288:** 183-185.

37. CHAN, A. C., C. E. ALLEN & P. V. J. HEGARTY. 1980. The effects of vitamin E depletion and repletion on PG synthesis in semitendinosus muscle of young rabbits. J. Nutr. **110:** 66-81.

38. LAWRENCE, L. M., M. M. MATHIAS, C. F. NOCKELS & R. P. TENGERDY. 1985. The effect of vitamin E on prostaglandin levels in the immune organs of chicks during the course of an *E. coli* infection. Nutr. Res. **5:** 497-509.

39. LIKOFF, R. O., D. R. GUPTILL, L. M. LAWRENCE, C. C. McKAY, M. M. MATHIAS, C. F. NOCKELS & R. P. TENGERDY. 1981. Vitamin E and aspirin depresses prostaglandins in protection of chickens against *E. coli* infection. Am. J. Clin. Nutr. **34:** 245-299.

40. TENGERDY, R. P. & J. C. BROWN. Effect of vitamin E and A on humoral immunity and phagocytosis in *E. coli*-infected chicken. Poult. Sci. **56:** 957-962.

41. BODWELL, C. E. & J. W. ERDMAN, JR. 1988. Nutrient Interactions. Dekker. New York, NY.

42. TENGERDY, R. P. 1989. Immunity and disease resistance in farm animals fed vitamin E supplement. *In* Antioxidant Nutrients and the Immune Response. A. Bendich, M. Phillips & R. Tengerdy, Eds. Plenum. New York, NY. In press.

43. TENGERDY, R. P., D. L. MEYER, L. H. LAUERMAN, D. C. LUEKER & C. F. NOCKELS. 1983. Vitamin E enhances humoral antibody response to *Clostridium perfringens,* type D, in sheep. Br. Vet. J. **139:** 147-152.

44. NERVIG, R. M., P. M. GOUGH, M. L. KAEBERLE & C. A. WHETSTONE, EDS. 1986.

Advances in Carriers and Adjuvants for Veterinary Biologics. Iowa State Univ. Press. Ames, IA.

45. AFZAL, M., R. P. TENGERDY, R. P. ELLIS, C. V. KIMBERLING & C. J. MORRIS. 1984. Protection of rams against epididymitis by a *B. ovis*-vitamin E adjuvant vaccine. Vet. Immunol. Immunopathol. **7**: 293-304.
46. ALLISON, A. C. 1979. Mode of action of immunological adjuvants. Reticuloendothel. Soc. **26**(Suppl.): 619-630.
47. MUNDER, P. G., M. MODOLELL, R. ANDREESEN, H. U. WELTZIEN & O. WESTPHAL. 1979. Lysophosphatidylcholine (lysolecithin) and its synthetic analogues. Immunomodulating and other biologic effects. Springer Sem. Immunopathol. **2**: 187-203.
48. SHIER, W. T. 1977. Inhibition of prostaglandin synthesis by lysolecithin. Biochem. Biophys. Res. Commun. **78**: 1168-1174.

Pharmacokinetics of Intravenous Vitamin E in Preterm Infants

SORAYA ABBASI, BRADFORD K. JENSEN,[a]
JEFFREY S. GERDES, VINOD K. BHUTANI,
AND LOIS JOHNSON

Department of Pediatrics
University of Pennsylvania School of Medicine
Section on Newborn Pediatrics
Pennsylvania Hospital
Philadelphia, Pennsylvania 19107
and
[a] Hoffmann-La Roche Inc.
Department of Drug Metabolism
Nutley, New Jersey 07110

INTRODUCTION

Vitamin E is a lipid antioxidant that protects unsaturated fatty acids from peroxidation and is an essential structural element of all biologic membranes. It is present in foods in proportion to the content of unsaturated fatty acids. Vitamin E deficiency is rare in adults in the absence of severe malabsorption[1-5] because of extensive tissue stores and readily available sources in the diet.

Premature infants are at risk for vitamin E deficiency because of low vitamin E stores,[6] immature intestinal function, and increased demands resulting from rapid growth rate and increased oxidative stress. Very low birthweight infants receive most nutrients by the intravenous route inasmuch as they do not tolerate enteral feeds and have limited muscle mass, which precludes intramuscular injection. The purpose of this study was to develop a pharmacokinetic profile for vitamin E following intravenous administration of variable doses to preterm infants.

METHODS

Study Population

Preterm infants with respiratory distress syndrome (RDS) were studied during the first 3 days of life in the intensive care nursery. These infants had mild to moderate respiratory distress and were treated with mechanical ventilation. They were not fed

345

TABLE 1. Vitamin E Infusion over 8 Hours[a]

	5 mg/kg	10 mg/kg	15 mg/kg	20 mg/kg	30 mg/kg
No. of infants	4	5	7	6	5
Birth weight (kg)	1.22 ±0.2	1.14 ±0.2	1.08 ±0.3	0.94 ±0.1	1.04 ±0.2
Gestational age (wk)	29.5 ±2.6	28.5 ±1.2	29.4 ±2.5	27.5 ±1.2	30.8 ±3.7
Sex (F/M)	2/2	1/4	3/4	2/4	5/0

[a] Data are means ± SD values.

and were receiving parenteral alimentation without vitamin supplementation during the first two days of life. After age 48 hours, multivitamins (1 unit vitamin E/kg) were added to the parenteral alimentation. Twenty-seven infants were given variable doses (5-30 mg/kg) of the Hoffmann-La Roche preparation of parenteral *dl*-alpha-tocopherol (vitamin E alcohol) by intravenous infusion over an 8 hour period. This preparation was used on an investigator's investigational new drug permit. An additional 19 infants were given vitamin E parenterally (5 and 10 mg/kg) over one hour. The patient characteristics and dosing information are presented in TABLES 1 and 2.

Methodology

Blood samples were obtained through indwelling umbilical artery catheters that had been placed for routine clinical management. Vitamin E concentrations were measured by the microcolorimetric method of Hashim[7] on 0.05 mL of serum, and/or high-pressure liquid chromatography after the method of Bieri.[8]

Informed Consent

The protocol was approved by the Research Review Committee of Pennsylvania Hospital. Informed consent was obtained from parents prior to the study.

TABLE 2. Vitamin E Infusion over 1 Hour[a]

	5 mg/kg	10 mg/kg
No. of infants	6	13
Birth weight (kg)	1.26 ± 0.20	1.13 ± 0.26
Gestational age (wk)	30.5 ± 1.6	29.2 ± 1.7
Sex (F/M)	3/3	8/5

[a] Data are means ± SD values.

Pharmacokinetic Analysis

The pharmacokinetic parameters were determined by model-independent analysis of the corrected vitamin E serum concentration time data up to 48 hours after intravenous infusion of drug. Vitamin E serum concentrations were corrected for baseline concentrations that were obtained immediately prior to the intravenous infusion of vitamin E. The terminal elimination rate constant (β) was determined by nonlinear regression of the terminal serum concentration time data up to 48 hours after initiation of the infusion. The area under the serum concentration time curves from time zero to infinity (AUC 0-∞) was calculated by summation of AUC 0-48 and AUC 48-∞. The AUC 0-48 AUC 48-∞ values were calculated by linear trapezoidal summation and by dividing the corrected serum concentration at 48 hours by β, respectively. The serum clearance (Cl_s) of vitamin E was determined by dividing the intravenous dose by AUC 0-∞. The postdistributive volume of distribution ($Vd\beta$) was determined by dividing the Cl_s by β.

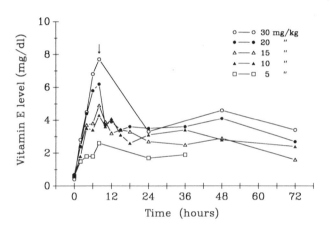

FIGURE 1. Serum vitamin E time profile for neonates that receive iv infusion over 8 hours. ↓ : end of infusion.

RESULTS

The mean uncorrected vitamin E serum concentration time profiles for neonates that received vitamin E by intravenous infusion over eight hours are shown in FIGURE 1. The mean uncorrected vitamin E serum concentration time profiles for neonates that received 5 mg/kg of vitamin E intravenously over one and eight hours are shown in FIGURE 2. FIGURE 3 shows the same data for infants who received 10 mg/kg of vitamin E over one and eight hours. The pharmacokinetic parameters obtained from model independent analysis of the individual corrected data are shown in TABLES 3 and 4. The parameters reflect the intravenously administered vitamin E pharmacokinetics because baseline vitamin E was assumed to remain constant.

Considerable variability in the terminal elimination rate constant (β) was observed in all groups as reflected by the percent coefficient of variation (SD ÷ x), which ranged from 56 to 106 percent. The mean harmonic half-life for the 5 mg/kg infused

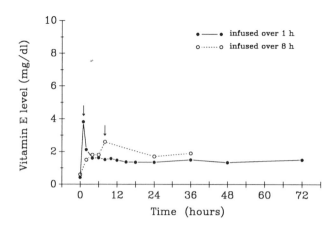

FIGURE 2. Serum vitamin E time profile of 5 mg/kg iv over 1 and 8 hours. ↓ : end of infusion.

over 8 hours (173 hours) and 30 mg/kg infused over 8 hours (139 hours) was quite long relative to the other doses. A small volume of distribution (0.31-0.72 L/kg) and serum clearance (1.41-5.67 mL/h/kg for 8 hour infusion and 5.75-8.36 mL/h/kg for 1 hour infusion) was also seen. The relatively long half-lives seen in this study are a reflection of the low serum clearance.

DISCUSSION

Vitamin E has recently received attention as a potential therapeutic agent to prevent or reduce clinical conditions thought to be associated with excessive production of oxidant radicals.[9-15] These clinical trials in human infants using the im, iv, and po routes have relied on serial vitamin E levels and the information from Colburn and Ehrenkranz' study of the clinical pharmacology of intramuscular injection of 20 mg/kg of

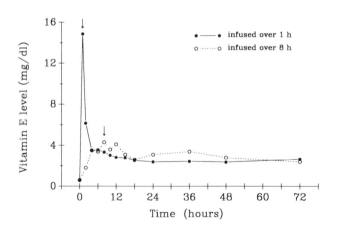

FIGURE 3. Serum vitamin E time profile of 10 mg/kg iv over 1 and 8 hours. ↓ : end of infusion.

TABLE 3. Pharmacokinetic Parameters of Vitamin E Infused over 8 Hours[a]

	5 mg/kg	10 mg/kg	15 mg/kg	20 mg/kg	30 mg/kg
Beta	0.004	0.010	0.013	0.016	0.005
(h^{-1})	±0.003	±0.006	±0.013	±0.009	±0.004
$T \frac{1}{2}^{b}$	173	69	53	43	139
(h)					
Vd Beta	0.42	0.31	0.54	0.50	0.72
(L/kg)	±0.25	±0.09	±0.26	±0.38	±0.20
Cls	1.41	2.84	4.50	5.67	2.99
(mL/h/kg)	±0.17	±0.91	±0.86	±2.72	±1.41

[a] Data are means ± SD values.
[b] Harmonic mean.

vitamin E in premature neonates to monitor dosage.[16] Extensive data on the use of oral E is available in both the human and animal literature. Parenteral preparations of the vitamin, however, are of recent origin and have not been studied extensively, except at very high dosage levels used for exploration of toxicity and tissue deposition in relation to elevated serum levels.[17–19]

There is an increasing need for the use of vitamin E by the intravenous route because of the improving survival of very low birth weight infants (< 1000 g) who have limited muscle mass and variable absorption. The present study was conducted to develop a pharmacokinetic profile of variable doses of vitamin E administered with rapid (in one hour) or slow infusion (over a period of 8 hours). In our study, rapid infusion of vitamin E, both with 5 and 10 mg/kg dose, resulted in high peak E levels at 1 hour and a sharp decrease to a steady level by 6 hours following infusion. Following slow infusion of α-tocopherol, serum concentrations increased significantly within 2 hours. Maximum serum concentrations occurred at the end of infusion. Serum vitamin E concentrations decreased rapidly in the first 24 hours and then remained stable over the next 48 hours. Increasing doses from 5 to 30 mg/kg resulted in higher peak serum E levels of 2.6 to 7.7 mg/dL.

TABLE 4. Pharmacokinetic Parameters of Vitamin E Infused over 1 Hour[a]

	5 mg/kg	10 mg/kg
Beta	0.025 ± 0.009	0.020 ± 0.012
(h^{-1})		
$T \frac{1}{2}^{b}$	34	52
(h)		
Vd Beta	0.34 ± 0.09	0.32 ± 0.09
(L/kg)		
Cls	8.36 ± 4.27	5.75 ± 2.75
(mL/h/kg)		

[a] Data are mean ± SD values.
[b] Harmonic mean.

Assessing the pharmacokinetic behavior of vitamin E is complicated by the fact that endogenous levels may interfere with rigorous analysis of the data. This difficulty is intensified when the study is conducted in neonates that may not be in optimal physiological condition and need hyperalimentation therapy that contains a dietary source of vitamin E. This aspect is well-demonstrated by the large variation in the elimination half-life of vitamin E.

In general, the pharmacokinetic parameters generated from slow intravenous infusion of vitamin E agree with a previous study[16] using composite profiles of neonates after a single 20 mg/kg intramuscular dose.

The small volume of distribution (0.31-0.72 L/kg) seen for vitamin E after intravenous infusion is puzzling because it should readily distribute throughout the body. Colburn and Ehrenkranz[16] suggest that the term better reflects the known physiochemical characteristics of vitamins, and that the body may clear an exogenous pharmacological dose more rapidly than dietary physiological doses. In addition, assumptions of constant baseline values of vitamin E during the study may have contributed to the small volume of distribution inasmuch as AUC 0-∞ was indirectly used in determining this parameter.

For the neonates receiving 5 mg/kg, the mean half-life of vitamin E was very long, approximately 173 hours. This long half-life is probably a consequence of this dose, which barely increased vitamin E serum concentrations over the baseline concentration of 0.6 mg/dL. Therefore, fluctuations of baseline values after this low dose would have a greater effect on pharmacokinetic parameters such as half-life.

Neonates in both the 5 mg/kg and 30 mg/kg were enrolled at a later age than others, and therefore received hyperalimentation with multivitamins during part of the study. Therefore, the long half-life seen for these two groups is more a reflection of the dietary source of vitamin E rather than decreased elimination of administered drug. Under both of these conditions, the assumption that baseline concentrations of vitamin E remain constant can lead to erroneous results and conclusions.

The results of this study indicate that the pharmacokinetics of vitamin E is independent of dose when given to neonates by intravenous infusion over a dose range of 5-30 mg/kg. Although the date is quite variable, the half-life, volume of distribution, and serum clearance of vitamin E did not appear to significantly increase or decrease with dose or rate of infusion. The peak vitamin E level, which occurred at the end of infusion, increased with increasing dose. This is an important aspect that should be useful in determination of dosage recommendations.

REFERENCES

1. FARRELL, P. M. 1980. Deficiency states, pharmacological effects, and nutrient requirements. In L. A. Machlin, Ed.: 520-622. Vitamin E: A Comprehensive Treatise. Part IIa. Dekker, New York, NY.
2. LEONARD, P. J. & M. S. LOSOWSKY. 1971. Effect of alpha-tocopherol administration on red cell survival in vitamin E-deficient human subjects. Am. J. Clin. Nutr. 24: 388-393.
3. SOKOL, R. J., M. GUGGENHEIM, S. T. IANNACCONE, P. E. BARKHAUS, C. MILLER, A. SILVERMAN, W. T. BALISTRERI & J. E. HEUBI. 1985. Improved neurologic function after long-term correction of vitamin E deficiency in children with chronic cholestasis. N. Engl. J. Med. 313: 1580-1586.
4. KAYDEN, H. J. 1972. Abetalipoproteinemia. Annu. Rev. Med. 23: 285-296.
5. MALLOY, M. J., J. P. KANE, D. A. HARDMAN, R. L. HAMILTON & K. B. DALAL. 1981.

Normotriglyceridemic abetalipoproteinemia. Absence of the B-100 apolipoprotein. J. Clin. Invest. **67:** 1441-1450.

6. DJU, M. Y., K. E. MASON & L. J. FILER, JR. 1952. Vitamin E (tocopherol) in human fetuses and placentae. Etud. Neo-Natales **1:** 49-61.

7. HASHIM, S. A. 1966. Rapid determination of tocopherol in macro and micro quantities of plasma. Am. J. Clin. Nutr. **19:** 136-145.

8. BIERI, J. G., T. J. TOLLIVER & G. L. CATIGNANI. 1979. Simultaneous determination of α-tocopherol and retinol in plasma or red blood cells by high pressure liquid chromatography. Am. J. Clin. Nutr. **32:** 2143-2149.

9. JOHNSON, L., D. SCHAFFER, G. QUINN *et al.* 1982. Vitamin E supplementation and the retinopathy of prematurity. Ann. N.Y. Acad. Sci. **393:** 473-495.

10. JOHNSON, L., G. E. QUINN, S. ABBASI *et al.* 1989. The effect of sustained pharmacologic vitamin E levels on the incidence and severity of retinopathy of prematurity (ROP): A controlled clinical trial. J. Pediatr. **114:** 827-838.

11. HITTNER, H. M., L. B. GODIO, A. J. RUDOLPH *et al.* 1981. Retrolental fibroplasia: Efficacy of vitamin E in a double-blind clinical study of preterm infants. N. Engl. J. Med. **305:** 1365-1371.

12. EHRENKRANZ, R. A., B. W. BONTA, R. C. ABLOW & J. B. WARSHAW. 1978. Amelioration of bronchopulmonary dysplasia after vitamin E administration. N. Engl. J. Med. **299:** 564-566.

13. EHRENKRANZ, R. A., R. C. ABLOW & J. B. WARSHAW. 1978. THe complication of oxygen use in the newborn infant. Clin. Perinatol. **5:** 437-450.

14. CHESWICK, M. L., M. JOHNSON *et al.* 1983. Protective effect of vitamin E (DL-alpha-tocopherol) against intraventricular haemorrhage in premature babies. Br. Med. J. **287:** 81-84.

15. KNIGHT, M. E. & R. R. ROBERTS. 1986. Disposition of intravenously administered pharmacologic doses of vitamin E in newborn rabbits. Pediatr. Pharmacol. Ther. **108:** 145-150.

16. COLBURN, W. A. & R. A. EHRENKRANZ. 1983. Pharmacokinetics of a single intramuscular injection of vitamin E to premature neonates. Pediatr. Pharmacol. **3:** 7-14.

17. PHELPS, D. L. & A. L. ROSENBAUM. 1977. The role of tocopherol in oxygen-induced retinopathy: Kitten model. Pediatrics **59:** 998-1005.

18. PHELPS, D. L. 1981. Local and systemic reactions to the parenteral administration of vitamin E. Dev. Pharmacol. Ther. **2:** 156-171.

19. PHELPS, D. L., A. L. ROSENBAUM, S. J. ISENBERG *et al.* 1987. Tocopherol efficacy and safety for preventing retinopathy of prematurity: A randomized, controlled, double-masked trial. Pediatrics **79:** 489-500.

Continuous Parenteral Infusion of Vitamin E Pharmacokinetics and Bilirubin Production in Premature Neonates[a]

DAVID K. STEVENSON, HENDRIK J. VREMAN,
JAMES E. FERGUSON II, LESLIE A. LENERT,
MARY B. LEONARD, AND RENA GALE

Department of Pediatrics
Stanford University School of Medicine
Stanford, California 94305

INTRODUCTION

Premature neonates produce more bilirubin on a per body weight basis than full-term infants.[1] Because the life span of red blood cells (RBC) in preterm infants is shorter than that in term infants,[1,2] hemolysis represents a major cause of jaundice of prematurity. Low serum levels and body stores of vitamin E have been implicated in the etiology of jaundice of prematurity,[3,4] by making premature infants more vulnerable to oxidant stresses.[5-8] Thus, it has been hypothesized that supplementation with vitamin E may protect the premature infant against hemolysis.[9] We have not been able, however, to prove this hypothesis in two randomized, controlled, double-blind studies, using a regimen of oral vitamin E supplementation during the first several days of life.[10,11] The purpose of the present study was to test the possible protective effect of injectable vitamin E (*dl*-alpha tocopherol) against increased bilirubin production in the premature infant, when administered by a continuous intra-arterial (umbilical artery) infusion over an 8-hour period, initiated within the first 24 hours of life. Furthermore, the study design allowed us to examine the blood levels of vitamin E simultaneously with heme degradation and subsequent bilirubin production.

[a]This work was supported by Grant RR-81 from the General Clinical Research Centers Program, Division of Research Resources, National Institutes of Health; by Grant HD-14426 from the National Institutes of Health; by the Christopher Taylor Harrison Fund; and by Hoffmann-La Roche, Inc. Pharmacokinetic analysis was assisted by Charles J. Hamori, Division of Neonatology, Stanford University School of Medicine.

METHODS

The first enzymatic step in heme degradation, catalyzed by heme oxygenase (HO), results in equimolar production of carbon monoxide (CO) and biliverdin. The latter is rapidly converted to bilirubin.[12-14] The CO is firmly bound to hemoglobin to form carboxyhemoglobin (HbCO). HbCO concentrations, when corrected for ambient air CO concentration (HbCOc), correlate with total body CO production, and therefore may be used as an index of total bilirubin production.[15]

Prior to enrollment in the study, written informed consent was obtained from the parents of each participant. The study included 38 premature infants of birth weight under 2,000 g, prospectively randomized in a double-blind manner for vitamin E (Viprimol™, Hoffmann-La Roche, Inc., 5 mg/kg body weight) or placebo (saline) administration, delivered by continuous intra-arterial infusion over an 8-hour period, and initiated within the first 24 hours of life. We recruited only infants without any major anomalies, free of clinical or laboratory signs of congenital infection, and whose mothers had not been treated with phenobarbital. Many of the infants were ventilated during the course of the study. Three infants in the study group and two in the control group received phototherapy. Prior to infusion of vitamin E (t = 0 h), blood was withdrawn for determination of baseline vitamin E, Hb, and HbCO levels. Subsequent vitamin E levels were obtained at 2, 4, 8, 24, and 48 hours after the initiation of the infusion. Hb and HbCO levels were also measured 48 hours after the infusion was started. Ambient air samples were collected at the time of blood sampling for HbCO. Total serum bilirubin levels were measured when clinically indicated, and the peak value within each 24-hour time period was used for statistical analysis. Serum vitamin E was determined by the modified fluorimetric assay of Hansen and Warwick.[16] The positive relationship of vitamin E levels and total lipid levels has been previously confirmed by our laboratory (unpublished data) and was judged not likely to contribute to the interpretation of the results in this study. HbCO concentrations were determined using a gas chromatographic method and were corrected for the CO content of ambient air.[17] The serum total bilirubin concentrations were measured using a UB Analyzer, UA-1 (Labo Science USA, Briarcliff Manor, NJ).

Before pharmacokinetic analysis, serum vitamin E concentrations were first corrected for baseline values (t = 0 h). Pharmacological parameters were determined using the "drugfun" program of the Prophet package (Division of Research Resources, National Institutes of Health). Each patient's results were fitted using a constant infusion, one compartment model with a weight of $1/y$. Elimination rate constant, half life, distribution volume, and clearance are reported as means ± SD.

RESULTS

The vitamin E-treated group of infants had a mean birth weight of 1,272 ± 379 g (mean ± SD), with a mean gestational age of 29 ± 2.7 weeks and a male (M):female (F) ratio of 12:7. The placebo group had a mean birth weight of 1,214 ± 318 g, with a mean gestational age of 29 ± 2.0 weeks and a M:F ratio of 11:8. There was no significant difference between the two groups for any of these parameters.

The baseline vitamin E, Hb, and HbCOc levels were comparable between the two groups, and no significant differences in the Hb and HbCOc levels were observed between day 1 and day 3, despite significant elevations in vitamin E level in the treated group (TABLE 1). No significant increase in serum vitamin E levels was noted between day 1 and day 3 in the placebo group. There was a significant difference in vitamin E levels on day 3 between the vitamin E- and placebo-treated groups. The serum bilirubin levels on days 2, 3, and 4 in the vitamin E-treated and placebo-treated groups were also not different. Only four infants in the vitamin E-treated group, and four in the placebo group were initially vitamin E-deficient (< 0.5 mg/dL). The mean uncorrected serum vitamin E levels during and after the 8-hour continuous intra-arterial infusion of 5 mg/kg of vitamin E, relative to the placebo group, are shown in FIGURE 1.

The elimination rate constant was $0.046 \pm 0.014 \text{ h}^{-1}$, with a half life of 16.7 ± 5.8 hours. Clearance of vitamin E was $8.9 \pm 9.1 \text{ mL/h/kg}$, and the distribution volume was $0.19 \pm 0.15 \text{ 1/kg}$.

DISCUSSION

The early intra-arterial administration of vitamin E by way of an 8-hour continuous infusion of 5 mg/kg resulted in significant elevation of vitamin E levels in the vitamin E-treated versus placebo-treated group within hours after birth. No significant differences, however, were found in the levels of Hb, HbCOc, or serum bilirubin over the first several days of life. The peak serum concentrations of vitamin E (which did not typically exceed 3.5 mg/dL) were reached near the end of the infusion; the concentrations decreased rapidly after 24 hours and then remained near the same average concentration when measured at 48 hours. Because this study was primarily designed to determine the effect of vitamin E on bilirubin production rates, and not to examine the pharmacokinetics of this drug, sampling was performed in a manner that prevented meaningful application of a two-compartment pharmacokinetic model,

TABLE 1. Concentration Data for Vitamin E–treated (n = 19) and Placebo-treated (n = 19) Groups of Premature Infants

	Day	Placebo		Vitamin E	
Hb^a (g/dL)	1	15.6 ± 1.7	(n = 19)	15.2 ± 1.3	(n = 17)
	3	15.2 ± 1.3	(n = 19)	14.6 ± 1.3	(n = 17)
HbCOc^a (% Hb)	1	1.0 ± 0.4	(n = 19)	0.9 ± 0.3	(n = 17)
	3	1.0 ± 0.5	(n = 19)	1.0 ± 0.4	(n = 17)
Bilirubin (mg/dL)	2	5.3 ± 1.2	(n = 18)	5.8 ± 1.7	(n = 15)
	3	7.1 ± 2.1	(n = 19)	7.9 ± 1.7	(n = 17)
	4	7.3 ± 2.5	(n = 16)	8.0 ± 1.9	(n = 11)
Vitamin E (mg/dL)	1	0.7 ± 0.3	(n = 19)	0.8 ± 0.5	(n = 19)
	3	0.9 ± 0.7	(n = 19)	$1.9 \pm 0.8^{b,c}$	(n = 15)

^{a} HbCO corrected for ambient CO.
^{b} $p < 0.0001$ compared with day 1.
^{c} $p < 0.001$ compared with placebo group.

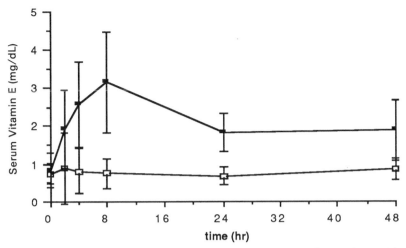

FIGURE 1 Serum vitamin E levels of premature infants during and after continuous 8-hour administration of either 5 mg/kg vitamin E (■) or a placebo solution (□).

which might be desirable for physiologic reasons (the high lipid solubility of the compound). Given the limitations of the data, a one-compartment model was applied for the analysis. Estimates of the parameters obtained, particularly the half-life, may vary substantially from the true population values. Additional factors, such as endogenous levels and uncontrolled exogenous sources of vitamin E, further confound the pharmacokinetic analysis and might be responsible for the great variability in plasma vitamin E levels seen in this study.

Our observations are similar to those reported by Smith *et al.*[10] and Fischer *et al.*[11] Both these studies, however, used an oral preparation of *d*-alpha-tocopheryl, polyethylene glycol-1,000-succinate, 50 mg/day for 3 days. In the study by Smith *et al.*, there were 30 premature infants with a mean birth weight of approximately 1,800 grams. All the infants in the study by Fischer *et al.*, had birth weights under 1,500 grams. In all three of the studies conducted at this institution, the majority of premature infants had initial vitamin E levels $\geq$ 0.5 mg/dL.

Premature neonates have relatively increased bilirubin production for their body weight,[1,15] related in large part to the fact that the RBC life span of premature infants is shorter than that of full-term infants, children, or adults.[2,18] One of the possible mechanisms for the increased hemolysis in premature infants is their greater susceptibility to oxidative injury of RBC membranes due to low serum vitamin E levels in serum and tissues.[6-9,19] Because vitamin E can react with free radicals and possibly other oxidizing compounds, the suggestion that vitamin E might have a beneficial effect on RBC membrane stability is reasonable.[20,21] In fact, other investigators have reported observations consistent with such an effect. Gross *et al.*[9,19] used daily intramuscular injections of 125 mg/kg/day for 5 days. Ten preterm infants with HbCO levels that were elevated at 3 days of age were compared to term infants. Five days of treatment with vitamin E resulted in a significant fall in the HbCO levels. Gross *et al.*[19] further showed that in a group of infants with birth weights less than 1,500 g, vitamin E supplementation during the first 3 days of life significantly increased vitamin E levels and decreased peak serum bilirubin levels on days 3 and 8. It is likely, however, that the initial vitamin E levels in the majority of infants studied by Gross *et al.*[9,19] were lower than those of the preterm infants studied by us.[10,11]

SUMMARY

We conclude that 5 mg/kg of vitamin E, administered intra-arterially as an 8-hour continuous infusion, significantly and predictably raises serum vitamin E levels into the supraphysiologic range with no apparent side effects. In a group of premature infants whose initial serum vitamin E levels were generally greater than or equal to 0.5 mg/dL, no decrease in bilirubin production was observed. Thus, vitamin E deficiency probably does not play a prominent role in jaundice of prematurity.

REFERENCES

1. COHEN, R. S., C. R. OSTRANDER, B. E. COWAN, G. B. STEVENS, A. O. HOPPER & D. K. STEVENSON. 1982. Pulmonary excretion rate of carbon monoxide: Differences between premature and full term infants. Biol. Neonate **41:** 289-93.
2. O'BRIEN, R. T. & H. A. PEARSON. 1971. Physiologic anemia of the newborn infant. J. Pediatr. **79:** 132-138.
3. WRIGHT, S. W., L. J. FILER, JR. & K. E. MASON. 1951. Vitamin E blood levels in premature and full term infants. Pediatrics **7:** 386-393.
4. DJU, M. Y., K. E. MASON & L. J. FILER, JR. 1952. Vitamin E (tocopherol) in human fetuses and placentae. Etudes Neonatales **1:** 49.
5. HASSAN, H., S. A. HASHIM, T. B. VAN ITALLIE & W. H. SEBRELL. 1966. Syndrome in premature infants associated with low plasma vitamin E levels and high polyunsaturated fatty acid diet. Am. J. Clin. Nutr. **19:** 147-157.
6. OSKI, F. A. & L. A. BARNESS. 1967. Vitamin E deficiency: A previously unrecognized cause of hemolytic anemia in the premature infant. J. Pediatr. **70:** 211-220.
7. RITCHIE, J. H., M. B. FISH, V. MCMASTERS & M. GROSSMAN. 1968. Edema and hemolytic anemia in premature infants: A vitamin E deficiency syndrome. N. Engl. J. Med. **279:** 1185-1190.
8. LOW, S. S., D. FRANK & W. H. HITZIG. 1973. Vitamin E and haemolytic anemia in premature infants. Arch. Dis. Child. **48:** 360-365.
9. GROSS, S. J., S. A. LANDAW & F. A. OSKI. 1977. Vitamin E and neonatal hemolysis. Pediatrics **59:** 995-997.
10. SMITH, D. W., R. S. COHEN, H. J. VREMAN, A. YEH, S. SHARRON & D. K. STEVENSON. 1985. Bilirubin production after supplemental oral vitamin E therapy in preterm infants. J. Pediatr. Gastroenterol. Nutr. **4:** 38-44.
11. FISCHER, A. F., D. INGUILLO, D. M. MARTIN, C. G. OCHIKUBO, H. J. VREMAN & D. K. STEVENSON. 1987. Carboxyhemoglobin concentration as an index of bilirubin production in neonates with birth weights less than 1,500 grams: A randomized double-blind comparison of supplemental oral vitamin E and placebo. J. Pediatr. Gastroenterol. Nutr. **6:** 748-751.
12. TENHUNEN, R., H. S. MARVER & R. SCHMID. 1969. Microsomal heme oxygenase. Characterization of the enzyme. J. Biol. Chem. **244:** 6388-6394.
13. BERK, P. D., F. L. RODKEY, T. F. BLASCHKE, H. A. COLLISON & J. G. WAGGONER. 1974. Comparison of plasma bilirubin turnover and carbon monoxide production in man. J. Lab. Clin. Med. **83:** 29-37.
14. LANDAW, S. A., E. W. CALLAHAN, JR. & R. SCHMID. 1970. Catabolism of heme *in vivo:*

Comparison of the simultaneous production of bilirubin and carbon monoxide. J. Clin. Invest. **49:** 914-925.

15. OSTRANDER, C. R., R. S. COHEN, A. O. HOPPER, B. E. COWAN, G. B. STEVENS & D. K. STEVENSON. 1982. Paired determinations of blood carboxyhemoglobin concentration and carbon monoxide excretion rate in term and preterm infants. J. Lab. Clin. Med. **100:** 745-755.

16. HANSEN, L. G. & W. J. WARWICK. 1978. An improved assay method for serum vitamin A and E using fluorometry. Am. J. Clin. Pathol. **70:** 922-925.

17. VREMAN, H. J., L. K. KWONG & D. K. STEVENSON. 1984. Carbon monoxide in blood: An improved microliter blood-sample collection system, with rapid analysis by gas chromatography. Clin. Chem. **30:** 382-386.

18. PEARSON, H. A. 1967. Lifespan of the fetal red blood cell. J. Pediatr. **70:** 166-71.

19. GROSS, S. J. 1979. Vitamin E and neonatal bilirubinemia. Pediatrics **64:** 321-323.

20. MOLENAAR, I., C. E. HULSTAERT & M. J. HARDONK. 1980. Role in function and ultrastructure of cellular membranes. *In* Vitamin E: A Comprehensive Treatise. L. J. Machlin, Ed.: 372-389. Dekker. New York, NY.

21. FRAGATA, M. & F. BELLEMARE. 1980. Model of singlet oxygen scavenging by α-tocopherol in biomembranes. Chem. Phys. Lipids **27:** 93-99.

Modeling Cortical Cataractogenesis: IX

Activity of Vitamin E and Esters in Preventing Cataracts and γ-Crystallin Leakage from Lenses in Diabetic Rats

J. R. TREVITHICK, H. A. LINKLATER,
K. P. MITTON, T. DZIALOSZYNSKI, AND
S. E. SANFORD[a]

Department of Biochemistry
University of Western Ontario
London, Ontario, Canada, N6A 5C1
and
[a] *Veterinary Services Laboratory*
Ontario Ministry of Agriculture and Food
Huron Park, Ontario, Canada, N0M 1Y0

INTRODUCTION

Several studies have demonstrated the efficacy of vitamin E in prevention or reduction of cataractogenesis. In 1982, Varma, Beachy, and Richards[1] reported that, *in vitro,* α-tocopherol (10^{-3} to 10^{-7} M) prevented the increase in rat lens malonaldehyde resulting from exposure of the lens to light of visible wavelengths. Also *in vitro* all rac-α-tocopherol (2.32 mM) has been found to reduce, by 44%, rabbit lens malondialdehyde produced by the presence of xanthine-XOD-FeCl$_3$ in the culture medium.

In a study using rabbits, Bhuyan, Bhuyan, and Podos[2] reported that α-tocopherol, 50 mg/kg body weight given intramuscularly daily, abolished the increase in aqueous and vitreous humor H_2O_2 induced by dietary 3-aminotriazole. Vitamin E also prevented the decrease in vitamin C levels in the aqueous and vitreous humor and partially prevented the increase in lens malondialdehyde. Varma, Change, Sharma, Kuck, and Richards[3] were able to slow the progress of a hereditary cataract in the Emory mouse using *dl*-α-tocopherol acetate (30 mg/kg food). Also *in vivo,* daily subcutaneous injections of 961 IU vitamin E in soybean oil decreased the level of cataractogenesis resulting from streptozotocin-induced diabetes in rats.[4] The lenses of rats treated with vitamin E were found to have higher levels of sorbitol than those of untreated diabetic rats. This indicated that vitamin E was acting at a step in cataract formation subsequent to the well-known osmotic stress[5] previously believed to be the sole cause of sugar cataracts.

358

There is also some evidence from epidemiological studies relating cataract incidence to level of vitamin E in the diet, that vitamin E may be of benefit in the prevention of cataract formation. Bunce and Hess[6] found a cataract incidence in young rats of 6% (compared to 0% in the control group), resulting from a maternal diet low in vitamin E. Preliminary results of a case control study by Robertson,[7] of patients taking at least 400 IU of vitamin E a day for the previous 10 years, showed that patients with cataracts were four times less likely to be regular consumers of supplementary vitamin E than were their matched controls.

In support of the findings of the previous study, Evans[8] has included, in his list of recommended supplements for those with cataracts, 450 IU vitamin E a day for 2 weeks followed by a maintenance level of 300 IU vitamin E a day. Evans has reported some success, over the last 35 years, in slowing and reversing the progression of cataracts, but his patients receive more than one dietary supplement. Therefore it is not possible to attribute this success only to the use of vitamin E.

Because formation of a cataract has been linked to leakage of protein from the lens,[9-11] it was decided to monitor vitamin E treatment by measuring the leakage of γ-crystallin into the aqueous and vitreous humors using a radioimmunoassay (RIA).

METHODS

The following procedures were as previously described[12] with the following differences: the rats had initial body weights of 190-260 g, the duration of the experiment was 6 weeks, and either vitamin E (Covitol F-1000) or its acetate (Covitol 1360 or Covitol 400 C) or succinate (Covitol 1210) derivative (all a generous gift from Henkel Corp, Minneapolis, MN, USA) was added to ground rat chow at 2,850 IU/kg food.

Analysis of serum samples was accomplished by HPLC using the extraction method of Nierenberg and Lester[13] with the following differences: the HPLC was a Gilson gradient HPLC system interfaced with a Tatung TCS-7000 (40 megabyte hard disk) running 714 HPLC System Controller Software, and the column was a Waters 10 μm RP-18 irregular (300 $\times$ 3.9 mm) Bondpack column. The volumes used in the extraction procedure were 250 μL serum, 35 μL acetonitrile, 125 μL of butanol/ethyl acetate (1/1), and 75 μL of 120% K_2HPO_4. Samples of each group were doped with known amounts of α-tocopherol to monitor recovery, and α-tocopheryl-acetate was used as an internal standard.

RESULTS

The mean γ-crystallin levels in the vitreous humors are shown in TABLE 1. The two diabetic control groups had mean γ-crystallin vitreous humor levels (8.43 ng/ μL and 7.46 ng/μL) that did not differ from each other but were significantly ($p < 0.001$) higher than the mean level in the vitreous humor of the normal control group (1.23 ng/μL). Both diabetic groups treated with dietary vitamin E acetate showed no change in vitreous humor γ-crystallin levels at 9.14 ng/μL and 7.02 ng/ μL from their respective control groups at 8.43 ng/μL and 7.46 ng/μL. Dietary

TABLE 1. γ-Crystallin (ng/μL)[a]

	Normal	Diabetic (gum acacia)	
No Treatment	1.23 ± 0.11	8.43 ± 0.69	7.46 ± 0.45
	n = 27	n = 10	n = 38
Vitamin E Acetate (gum acacia)		9.14 ± 0.34 n = 11	
Vitamin E Acetate			7.02 ± 0.74 n = 10
Vitamin E			5.57 ± 0.27 n = 9
Vitamin E Succinate			5.69 ± 0.40 n = 9

[a] Concentration of γ-crystallin in vitreous humor of rats at sacrifice, after 6 weeks of diabetes and/or dietary vitamin E (2,850 IU/kg food), performed as described in the text. Shown are the mean ± SEM for each group and the number of rats in each group.

treatment of diabetic rats with vitamin E resulted in a significantly ($p < 0.001$) lower mean level (27%) of vitreous humor γ-crystallin of 5.57 ng/μL. Vitamin E succinate in the diet of diabetic rats also resulted in a significant ($p < 0.01$) reduction (26%) in the mean level of vitreous humor γ-crystallin (5.69 ng/μL) when compared to the mean level found in the diabetic control group (7.46 ng/μL).

The mean serum glucose level of the normal control group (125 mg/dL) was within the expected range (TABLE 2). Both diabetic control groups had mean serum glucose levels (508 mg/dL and 540 mg/dL) that were significantly ($p < 0.001$) elevated above that of the normal control group, but did not differ from each other. The diabetic groups receiving vitamin E acetate and vitamin E had mean serum glucose levels of 593 mg/dL and 558 mg/dL, respectively, which were not different from the level of the diabetic control group (540 mg/dL). The diabetic group receiving vitamin E acetate on gum acacia had a mean serum glucose level (577 mg/dL) that

TABLE 2. Serum Glucose (mg/dL)[a]

	Normal	Diabetic (gum acacia)	
No Treatment	125 ± 2	508 ± 28	540 ± 14
	n = 35	n = 10	n = 44
Vitamin E Acetate (gum acacia)		577 ± 24 n = 12	
Vitamin E Acetate			593 ± 42 n = 12
Vitamin E			558 ± 27 n = 11
Vitamin E Succinate			439 ± 20 n = 12

[a] Serum concentration of glucose at sacrifice, after 6 weeks of diabetes and/or dietary vitamin E (2,850 IU/kg food), as described in the text. Shown are the mean ± SEM for each group and the number of rats in each group.

was very slightly (p < 0.10) higher than that of its respective control group (508 mg/dL). The diabetic group receiving vitamin E succinate had a mean serum glucose level (439 mg/dL) that was very significantly (p < 0.001) lower than that of its respective control group (540 mg/dL).

The normal control group gained a mean of 11.53% of its initial body weight over the 6 week period of the experiment (TABLE 3). The diabetic control rats receiving gum acacia gained on the average only 1.58% of their initial weight, whereas the other diabetic control rats lost an average of 6.81% of their initial weight. These two diabetic control groups differed (p < 0.005) from each other in their weight changes, but both weight changes differed significantly (p < 0.001) from the mean weight gain of the normal control group. The small mean weight gain of the diabetic group receiving vitamin E acetate on gum acacia (0.44%) did not differ from the weight gain of its control group (1.58%). The other diabetic group receiving vitamin E acetate, however, had a mean weight gain of 2.77%, which was significantly (p < 0.02) different from the mean weight loss (6.81%) of its control group. The diabetic rats receiving vitamin

TABLE 3. Percent Change in Body Weight[a]

	Normal	Diabetic (gum acacia)	
No Treatment	11.53 ± 0.68 n = 26	1.58 ± 2.33 n = 10	−6.81 ± 1.41 n = 44
Vitamin E Acetate (gum acacia)		0.44 ± 2.96 n = 12	
Vitamin E Acetate			2.77 ± 3.67 n = 12
Vitamin E			−2.72 ± 2.07 n = 11
Vitamin E Succinate			7.21 ± 3.70 n = 12

[a] Percent change in the weight of each rat, over the 6 weeks of diabetes and/or dietary vitamin E (2,850 IU/kg food). Shown are the mean ± SEM for each group and the number of rats in each group.

E succinate showed an average weight gain of 7.21%, which differed very significantly (p < 0.001) from the weight loss of its control group, but did not differ from the mean weight gain of the normal control group. The mean weight loss (2.72%) experienced by the diabetic group receiving vitamin E did not differ from that of its control group (6.81%).

The γ-crystallin levels found in the aqueous humor are shown in TABLE 4. The mean γ-crystallin level of 0.24 ng/μL found in the aqueous humor of the normal control rats was very significantly (p < 0.001) less than the levels found in the aqueous humor of either of the control diabetic groups (1.59 ng/μL and 1.15 ng/μL). The levels in these two diabetic control groups also differed (p < 0.001) from each other. None of the four treated diabetic groups had levels of aqueous humor γ-crystallin that differed from their respective control groups.

None of the normal control rats were observed to have cataracts (TABLE 5). The two diabetic control groups had mean cataract scores of 1.05 and 1.25, which did not differ from each other, but which were very significantly (p < 0.001) greater than that

TABLE 4. γ-Crystallin (ng/μL)^a

	Normal	Diabetic (gum acacia)	
No Treatment	0.24 ± 0.05 n = 27	1.59 ± 0.05 n = 9	1.15 ± 0.06 n = 40
Vitamin E Acetate (gum acacia)		1.30 ± 0.04 n = 11	
Vitamin E Acetate			0.99 ± 0.11 n = 11
Vitamin E			1.13 ± 0.16 n = 10
Vitamin E Succinate			1.04 ± 0.13 n = 12

^{a} Concentration of γ-crystallin in aqueous humor of rats at sacrifice, after 6 weeks of diabetes and/or dietary vitamin E (2,850 IU/kg food), performed as described in the text. Shown are the mean ± SEM for each group and the number of rats in each group.

of the normal control group. Neither of the vitamin E acetate-treated groups or the vitamin E succinate-treated group, with cataract scores of 1.46, 1.04, and 1.25, respectively, differed from their respective control groups. The vitamin E-treated group had a mean cataract score (1.73) that was higher ($p < 0.005$) than that of its control group (1.25).

The two diabetic control groups had mean general body conditions (4.20 and 3.93) that did not differ from each other, but that were significantly ($p < 0.005$) less than that (4.97) of the control group (TABLE 6). None of the four treated diabetic groups showed any significant change in general body condition as a result of treatment.

The mean lens ATP levels (TABLE 7) of the two diabetic control groups (0.49 μg/mg and 0.50 μg/mg) did not differ from each other: both were 50% lower ($p < 0.001$) than the mean level of 0.98 μg/mg found in the normal control group. None of the treated diabetic groups showed any change in lens ATP level as a result of the treatment.

The normal control group had a mean lens weight of 98.69 mg (TABLE 8). The

TABLE 5. Cataract Grade per Lens^a

	Normal	Diabetic (gum acacia)	
No Treatment	0.00 ± 0.00 n = 70	1.05 ± 0.13 n = 20	1.25 ± 0.08 n = 88
Vitamin E Acetate (gum acacia)		1.46 ± 0.16 n = 24	
Vitamin E Acetate			1.04 ± 0.15 n = 24
Vitamin E			1.73 ± 0.13 n = 22
Vitamin E Succinate			1.25 ± 0.14 n = 24

^{a} Graded severity of cataracts, determined as described in the text, 1–3 days prior to sacrifice after 6 weeks of diabetes and/or dietary vitamin E (2,850 IU/kg food). Shown are the mean ± SEM of each group and the number of lenses in each group.

TABLE 6. General Body Condition[a]

	Normal	Diabetic (gum acacia)	
No Treatment	4.97 ± 0.02	4.20 ± 0.24	3.93 ± 0.01
	n = 35	n = 10	n = 44
Vitamin E Acetate (gum acacia)		3.67 ± 0.18	
		n = 12	
Vitamin E Acetate			3.67 ± 0.30
			n = 12
Vitamin E			3.64 ± 0.15
			n = 11
Vitamin E Succinate			3.92 ± 0.28
			n = 12

[a] General body condition, evaluated as described in the text, 1–3 days prior to sacrifice, after 6 weeks of diabetes and/or dietary vitamin E (2,850 IU/kg food). Shown are the mean ± SEM of each group and the number of rats in each group.

two diabetic control groups had mean lens weights (81.22 mg and 89.33 mg) that differed significantly ($p < 0.001$) from each other and from that of the normal control group ($p < 0.001$). The lenses of the diabetic group receiving vitamin E acetate on gum acacia had an average weight (81.35 mg) that did not differ from that of its control group. The diabetic rats receiving vitamin E acetate and vitamin E succinate showed mean lens weights of 80.46 mg and 78.27 mg, respectively, which were both very significantly ($p < 0.001$) less than that of their control group. The mean lens weight of the diabetic group receiving vitamin E at 85.08 mg was also less ($p < 0.02$) than that of the diabetic control group.

The lens weights expressed as a percent of initial body weight are shown in TABLE 9. The mean value for the normal control group (0.038) was not different than that of the diabetic control group receiving gum acacia (0.039). The other diabetic control group had a mean value of 0.044, which did differ ($p < 0.001$) from that of the normal control group. The diabetic group receiving vitamin E acetate on gum acacia had a mean value (0.042) that was greater ($p < 0.001$) than that of its control group. The other diabetic group receiving vitamin E acetate and the group receiving vitamin E

TABLE 7. ATP (μg/mg) Lens Wet Weight[a]

	Normal	Diabetic (gum acacia)	
No Treatment	0.98 ± 0.02	0.49 ± 0.03	0.50 ± 0.03
	n = 13	n = 10	n = 24
Vitamin E Acetate (gum acacia)		0.38 ± 0.02	
		n = 12	
Vitamin E Acetate			0.05 ± 0.02
Vitamin E			0.42 ± 0.02
			n = 11
Vitamin E Succinate			0.45 ± 0.03
			n = 11

[a] Concentration of ATP in lenses of rats at sacrifice, after 6 weeks of diabetes and/or dietary vitamin E (2,850 IU/kg food), performed as described in the text. Shown are the mean ± SEM for each group and the number of rats in each group.

TABLE 8. Weight of Both Lenses (mg)[a]

	Normal	Diabetic (gum acacia)	
No Treatment	98.69 ± 0.86 n = 35	81.22 ± 0.96 n = 10	89.33 ± 1.01 n = 44
Vitamin E Acetate (gum acacia)		81.35 ± 0.90 n = 12	
Vitamin E Acetate			80.46 ± 1.47 n = 12
Vitamin E			85.08 ± 1.29 n = 11
Vitamin E Succinate			78.27 ± 1.62 n = 12

[a] Combined weight of both lenses, determined after removal of lenses as described in the text, after 6 weeks of diabetes and/or dietary vitamin E (2,850 IU/kg food). Shown are the mean ± SEM for each group and the number of rats in each group.

TABLE 9. Lens Weight as Percent of Initial Body Weight[a]

	Normal	Diabetic (gum acacia)	
No Treatment	0.038 ± 0.001 n = 26	0.039 ± 0.001 n = 10	0.044 ± 0.001 n = 44
Vitamin E Acetate (gum acacia)		0.042 ± 0.001 n = 12	
Vitamin E Acetate			0.039 ± 0.001 n = 12
Vitamin E			0.041 ± 0.001 n = 11
Vitamin E Succinate			0.037 ± 0.001 n = 12

[a] Weight of the combined lenses from each rat, expressed as a percentage of the rat's initial body weight. Shown are the mean ± SEM of each group and the number of rats in each group. The groups treated with all forms of vitamin E received 2,850 IU/kg food.

TABLE 10. Serum Vitamin E (VE) Concentration

Treatment Diet	Number of rats	Concentration μg/mL ± SE	Relative Concentration ± SE
Normal Normal	8	3.7 ± 0.6	1.00 ± 0.16
Normal + VE	5	7.8 ± 1.7	2.12 ± 0.46
Normal + VES[a]	8	10.4 ± 0.8	2.82 ± 1.07
Diabetic Normal	5	5.8 ± 2.8	1.49 ± 0.72
Diabetic + VE	5	16.2 ± 5.5	4.40 ± 1.49
Diabetic + VES	5	34.8 ± 8.5	9.45 ± 2.31

[a] Vitamin E succinate

succinate had mean values (0.039 and 0.037, respectively) that were both lower ($p < 0.001$) than that of the control group. The diabetic group receiving vitamin E also had a mean value (0.041) that was lower ($p < 0.005$) than that of its control group.

Although it was not possible to analyze serum samples from rats receiving vitamin E acetate for tocopherol, because these were unfortunately lost, some serum samples from rats receiving free tocopherol and tocopherol succinate in a later experiment were analyzed (TABLE 10). Treatment groups showed elevations in serum tocopherol when compared to the appropriate controls (TABLE 10). Diabetic rats showed a slight but not statistically significant increase in serum tocopherol levels (1.49) as compared to normal rats. Rats treated with free tocopherol showed a significant elevation of 2.12 above untreated rats, whereas diabetic rat levels were elevated significantly: 2.95 for treatment with tocopherol, and 6.34 times for treatment with tocopherol succinate.

DISCUSSION

A mean decrease in γ-crystallin leakage in the vitreous humor occurred in the diabetic groups receiving vitamin E as d-α-tocopherol and as d-α-tocopheryl succinate. The mean serum glucose level of the diabetic group receiving dietary vitamin E (tocopherol) did not differ from that of the control group, but the mean level in the diabetic group receiving vitamin E succinate was very significantly lower than that of the control group. There is a direct, incomplete relationship between serum glucose level and γ-crystallin level in the vitreous humor. Therefore, some of the vitreous humor leakage reduction in the group receiving vitamin E succinate may have been directly a result of less stress on the animals as reflected in the lower mean serum glucose level, although the larger percent elevation in serum tocopherol in this group argues against this.

The diabetic group receiving vitamin E succinate experienced a weight gain, over the 6 weeks of the experiment, that was the same as that of the normal control group. The diabetic group receiving vitamin E succinate, however, had a lower initial body weight than did the normal control group, which means the group receiving vitamin E succinate did not experience a weight gain equivalent to the weight gain of the normal control group. The mean weight gain was, however, highly significant in the diabetic group receiving vitamin E succinate compared to the weight loss experienced by the respective control diabetic group. This may be accounted for by the elevation in serum tocopherol levels.

Streptozotocin-induced diabetes resulted in an increase in γ-crystallin leakage into the aqueous humor, but no change in leakage was found as a result of dietary vitamin E treatment. The level of γ-crystallin in the aqueous humor is one-fifth to one-eighth that in the vitreous humor: therefore, any difference between treatment groups will be similarly reduced in the aqueous humor as compared to the vitreous humors. The levels of γ-crystallin in the aqueous humors were close to the detection limit for the RIA, due to the small volumes of humor available from each animal. Therefore, measurement of γ-crystallin leakage into the vitreous seems to be a more reliable index of treatment efficacy than does leakage into the aqueous humor.

No difference in mean visual cataract score between the treated and untreated diabetic groups was seen, even though a difference was detected in mean γ-crystallin vitreous humor levels. The reduction in γ-crystallin was, however, only 25%, which is enough to be significant, but apparently the difference in damage was not large enough to be seen as a change from one visual cataract score to another. Visual scoring of a cataract is more subjective than measurement of protein leakage, and there are more increments available to express leakage than there are to express visual cataract scoring. Another dietary treatment (BHT) that resulted in a large reduction in mean vitreous humor leakage, in the range 40-60%, showed a reduction also in mean cataract score.[12] This is consistent with the idea that protein leakage into the vitreous is a more sensitive indicator of cataract-inducing lens damage than is the visual cataract score.

Vitamin E, regardless of the form in which it is administered, is absorbed from the intestine as the free tocopherol.[13] Hydrolases for removing the ester from vitamin E are supplied by the pancreas, which also supplies the bile necessary for the absorption of the tocopherol. Therefore, inadequate pancreatic hydrolases would interfere with the absorption of vitamin E when it is administered as the acetate form. This could be accentuated in streptozotocin-induced diabetes as a result of pancreatic damage from streptozotocin.

The need for pancreatic enzymes to hydrolyze vitamin E esters preparatory to absorption is reflected in the differing serum or plasma vitamin E levels attained with administration of different forms of vitamin E. In humans, no differences were found in relative absorption of free vitamin or ester by Burton et al.,[14] but in another study, administration of unesterified vitamin E resulted in tocopherols being retained in the serum for a longer period than when the acetate form was given.[15] Horwitt, Elliott, Kanjananggulpan, and Fitch[16] measured serum tocopherol levels in humans after dietary administration of various forms of vitamin E. The relative increase in serum tocopherols was 71.2, 60.9, and 41.2% for d-α-tocopherol, d-α-tocopheryl acetate, and d-α-tocopheryl succinate, respectively. Although these studies have been performed on humans and although all species do not respond to vitamin E administration with the same levels of serum tocopherol,[17,18] it is clear that there are differences in all animals in the ability of the various forms of vitamin E to produce tocopherol in the body. Therefore, the differing ability to reduce vitreous humor γ-crystallin leakage of the acetate versus the succinate and alcohol forms of vitamin E administered in these experiments may reflect the rats' abilities to absorb each of these forms.

Vitamin E treatment was begun for each of the treated groups within hours of streptozotocin injection, even though pretreatment of rats with vitamin E has been shown to have a protective effect against streptozotocin.[19] This protective effect may have contributed to the lower mean serum glucose level in the diabetic group receiving vitamin E succinate.

The best known function of vitamin E is probably its ability to react with free radical intermediates of lipid peroxidation and with the peroxides.[20] Vitamin E has been shown to react with hydroxyl (OH·), perhydroxyl (HO_2·), and superoxide (O_2·) radicals.[21] Although the hydroxyl radical is potentially the most efficient oxidant,[21] the perhydroxy radicals can react directly with unsaturated lipids.[22] The superoxide radical cannot oxidize lipids but may assist the degradative process by reacting with vitamin E.[21]

Malondialdehyde is one of the products of lipid peroxidation, and levels of malondialdehyde have been shown to reflect the amount of lipid peroxidation occurring in a tissue.[23] Vitamin E administration has been shown to reduce the age-related increase in malondialdehyde levels in liver and serum of rats,[24] whereas vitamin E deficiency in rats has been shown to lead to increased malondialdehyde excretion.[25] Bhuyan and Bhuyan[26] have shown increased malondialdehyde in lenses as a result of many types of cataract, with vitamin E administration leading to a decrease in the malondialdehyde level. Therefore, one of the functions of vitamin E in the lens most probably is protection of lipids from oxidation.

Vitamin E has been shown to be capable of penetrating into monolayers of various phospholipids,[27] liposomes,[28] and sarcoplasmic reticulum of skeletal muscle.[29] In 1982, Burlakova, Kukhtina, Sarycheva, Khrapova, and Aristarkhova,[30] showed that, even though the chroman structure of vitamin E had the antiradical properties, the side chain was necessary to anchor the vitamin E in the membranes. The presence of vitamin E in membranes has been correlated with the fluidity of the membrane,[30] its permeability[28] and conductivity.[31] The studies of Baig and Laidman[32] indicated a polar interaction between the phenolic head groups of α-tocopherol and the phosphate group of the phospholipid, possibly involving hydrogen bonding. Similarly, Erin, Skrypin, and Kagan[32] suggested hydrogen bonding between the OH group of the dihydroben-zopyran nucleus of tocopherol and the carbonyl group of the fatty acid. They also reported possible hydrophobic interactions between the fatty acyl chains and the methyl group of the tocopherol nucleus. A proposed interaction between vitamin E and membrane phospholipids has been shown.[33]

It appears, therefore that vitamin E may have two functions in the membrane: it can prevent lipid peroxidation and physically stabilize the membrane. Mino and Sugita[33] demonstrated the incorporation of tocopheryl acetate into membranes. They found that the vitamin E acetate so incorporated was not converted into the tocopherol form; therefore, vitamin E acetate used *in vitro* may offer some protection through stabilization of the membrane but is not able to prevent oxidative damage to the membrane.

Vitamin E has also been shown capable of repairing free radicals derived from the 1-electron oxidation of the amino acids tryptophan and tyrosine,[34] and methionine and histidine.[35] This oxidation of amino acids may explain the oligomerization of membrane proteins that has been shown to occur in retinal and skeletal muscle in conjunction with lipid peroxidation.[36] Kagan, Archipenko, and Kozlov[37] demonstrated membrane protein-linking involving the Ca^{2+}-ATPase along with lipid peroxidation. The presence of vitamin E in membranes has been shown to protect the Ca^{2+}-ATPase from this damage.[38,39]

It is critical to the lens to maintain low internal Ca^{2+} levels, which is accomplished by an active Ca^{2+}-ATPase.[40] Inhibition of this calcium pump was shown to lead to calcium accumulation and lens opacification.[41] Protection from oxidation of the pro-teins of the calcium pump may be, therefore, another way in which vitamin E can reduce cataract formation.

Peroxidation of lipids has been shown to lead also to formation of DNA free radicals.[42] Popov and Konev[43] established in Ehrlich ascites carcinoma cells that, as processes of lipid peroxidation were intensified, the rate of DNA synthesis decreased. The existence of a high-affinity tocopherol binding receptor protein in rat liver nuclei has been demonstrated.[44] The presence of such a vitamin E-binding protein may help to explain how vitamin E was able to prevent free radical damage to DNA[42] and $K_2Cr_2O_7$-induced DNA degradation.[45]

Vitamin E has also been shown capable of inducing RNA synthesis.[46,47] In the lens, the epithelial cells, but not the fiber cells, are actively involved in DNA and RNA synthesis; therefore, any protection against oxidation of nucleic acids, which vitamin E might offer, would be of paramount importance for the integrity of the epithelial layer and the differentiation of these cells into fiber cells.

Lipid peroxides have been shown to modulate the biosynthesis of prostaglandins.[48,49] The major arachidonic acid pathway in rabbit lens has been shown to be through the lipoxygenase enzyme.[50] Bovine epithelial lens cells *in vitro* have been shown to form leukotriene B_4, which is a product of the lipoxygenase pathway.[51] Although the lipoxygenase pathway may be the major arachidonate pathway in the lens, the lens has been shown capable of synthesizing prostaglandins by way of the cyclooxygenase pathway.[52] Ono, Obara, and Hatano,[53] found that administration of prostaglandin E_1 (PGE_1) to rats for 3 days encouraged phospholipid turnover, especially of phosphatidylcholine in the lens. The presence of PGE_1 ($10^{-3}M$) in the incubation medium of rabbit lens was shown to cause increased sodium and decreased potassium content of the lens with resultant lens opacification.[54] Both streptozotocin-induced diabetes[55] and vitamin E deficiency have been shown to result in an unbalanced production ratio of thromboxane A^2 (TXA_2) and prostaglandin I_2 (PGI_2) in platelets and serum. Gilbert, Zebrowski, and Chan[56] and Karpen, Pritchard, Arnold, Cornwell, and Panganamala[57] have reported the restoration of normal PGI_2/TXA_2 balance in platelets and serum by vitamin E. The addition of vitamin E to the diet may assist in preventing pathological changes in the lens as well.

Another way in which vitamin E may be able to protect against the hyperglycemia of streptozotocin diabetes is through control of the enzymes involved in glucose utilization. Ulasevich, Grozina, and Vorobyora[55] reported that vitamin E (50 mg daily) increased the ability of rat erythrocytes to use glucose 2.4-fold. There was simultaneous activation of aldolase and phosphohexosisomerase by 34% and 48%, respectively. A decreased level of glucose in all tissues, including the lens, resulting from the presence of high levels of vitamin E, may result in less stress on the lens with a resultant decrease in cataract formation.

Vitamin E may also have an indirect affect on the integrity of the lens through its interaction with other protective compounds. Vitamin E has been shown to modulate tissue retinol levels *in vitro* and *in vivo* by influencing retinal palmitate hydrolysis.[56] The incorporation together into liposomes of vitamin A and E was shown to lead to an increase of the antioxidant effects over vitamin E alone.[57] The ability of vitamin E to act as an antioxidant is greatly affected by the levels of vitamin C.[58-60] Vitamin E also has been shown to have an effect on the enzymes involved in the synthesis and metabolism of glutathione.[61-63]

There appear to be many ways, therefore, in which vitamin E may protect the lens from damage that might lead to cataract formation. That oxidative damage seems to be a major factor in cataract is indicated by the variety of *in vitro* cataract models in which we have found vitamin E to be effective in preventing lens damage: hygromycin B cataract (*in vitro*),[64] x-ray-induced cataract (*in vitro*),[65] galactose-induced (*in vitro*),[66] steroid (solumedrol)-induced (*in vitro*),[67] diabetic cataract (*in vitro*[68] and *in vivo*[4]), and cataract induced by elevated temperature (*in vitro*).[69] The actual mechanisms operating in the prevention of cataract remain to be worked out.

SUMMARY

Normal and streptozotocin diabetic female Wistar rats were given vitamin E in the diet as the tocopherol, acetate, or succinate form (2,850 IU/kg food). At the end of 6 weeks, the rats were examined for weight gain or loss, general body condition, and cataracts. At sacrifice, blood was collected for measurement of serum glucose, and γ-crystallin levels were measured in aqueous and vitreous humors using a radioimmunoassay. One lens was homogenized in 8 M guanidinium chloride for ATP analysis.

In normal rats, γ-crystallin was detected in both aqueous and vitreous humors, with the higher concentration in the vitreous humor. Diabetes caused a sixfold increase in γ-crystallin in both the aqueous and vitreous humors. Diabetes also led to a significant worsening in general body condition, loss of body weight, formation of cataracts, and decrease in lens ATP levels. Addition of vitamin E and vitamin E succinate, but not vitamin E acetate, to the diet resulted in reduction of γ-crystallin leakage into the vitreous humors and an increase in body weight. There was no improvement noted for the lens ATP levels, the general body condition, or visual cataract score. Neither streptozotocin-induced diabetes nor vitamin E in the diet appeared to affect the weight of the lenses.

REFERENCES

1. VARMA, S. D., N. A. BEACHY & R. D. RICHARDS. 1982. Photochem. Photobiol. **36:** 623-626.
2. BHUYAN, K. C., D. K. BHUYAN & S. M. PODOS. 1982. Ann. N.Y. Acad. Sci. **393:** 169-171.
3. VARMA, S. D., D. CHAND, Y. R. SHARMA, J. F. KUCK & R. D. RICHARDS. 1984. Curr. Eye Res. **3:** 35-57.
4. ROSS, W. M., M. O. CREIGHTON, P. J. STEWART-DEHAAN, M. SANWAL, M. HIRST & J. R. TREVITHICK. 1982. Can. J. Ophthalmol. **17:** 61-66.
5. KINOSHITA, J. H., L. O. MEROLA & E. DIKMAK. 1962. Exp. Eye Res. **1:** 405-410.
6. BUNCE, G. E. & J. L. HESS. 1976. J. Nutr. **106:** 222-229.
7. ROBERTSON, J. M. 1985. Does supplementary vitamin E prevent cataracts? Progress Report, April 1, 1984-March 31, 1985, National Health Research and Development Program, Health and Welfare, Canada. #6606-2445-43.
8. EVANS, S. C. 1978. Nutrition in eye health and disease. Roberts Publications. 28-34.
9. CHARLTON, J. M. & R. VAN HEYNINGEN. 1968. Exp. Eye Res. **7:** 47-55.
10. PIATIGORSKY, J., H. N. FUKUI & J. H. KINOSHITA. 1978. Nature **274:** 558-562.
11. BRINKMAN, C. J. J. & R. M. BROEKHUYSE. 1980. Ophthalmol. Res. **12:** 230-234.
12. LINKLATER, H. A., T. DZIALOSZYNSKI, H. L. MCLEOD, S. E. SANFORD & J. R. TREVITHICK. 1986. Exp. Eye Res. **43:** 305-313.
13. NIERENGERG, D. W. & D. C. LESTER. 1985. J. Chromatography **345:** 275-284.
14. BURTON, G. W., K. U. INGOLD, D. O. FOSTER, S. C. CHENG, A. WEBB, L. HUGHES & E. LUSZTYK. 1988. Lipids. **23:** 834-840.
15. BAKER, H., O. FRANK, B. DE ANGELIS & S. FEINGOLD. 1980. Nutr. Rep. Int. **21:** 531-536.
16. HORWITT, M. K., W. H. ELLIOTT, P. KANJANANGGULPAN & C. D. FITCH. 1984. Fed. Proc. **43:** 394.
17. WEBER, F., U. GLOOR, J. WURSCH & O. WISS. 1964. Biochem. Biophys. Res. Commun. **14:** 189-192.
18. DAM, H. & E. SONDERGAARD. 1964. Z. Ernahrungswiss **5:** 73.
19. SLONIM, A. E., M. L. SURBER, D. L. PAGE, R. A. SHARP & I. M. BURR. 1983. J. Clin. Invest. **71:** 1282-1288.
20. TAPPEL, A. L. 1962. Vitam. Horm. **20:** 493-510.
21. FUKUZAWA, K. & J. M. GEBICKI. 1983. Arch. Biochem. Biophys. **266:** 242-251.
22. GEBICKI, J. M. & B. H. H. BIELSKI. 1981. J. Am. Chem. Soc. **103:** 7020-7022.
23. WILLSON, R. L. 1978. Free radicals and tissue damage: Mechanistic evidence from radiation studies. *In* Biochemical Mechanisms of Liver Injury. C. deDuve & O. Hayaishi, Eds.: 233-245. Elsevier. Amsterdam.
24. TAKEUCHI, N., N. IRITANI, E. FUKUDA & F. TANAKA. 1978. Effects of long-term administration and deficiency of alpha-tocopherol on lipid metabolism of rats. *In* Tocopherol, Oxygen, and Biomembranes. C. deDuve & O. Hayaishi, Eds.: 257-272. Elsevier. Amsterdam.
25. DRAPER, H. H., L. POLENSEK, M. HADLEY & L. G. MCGIRR. 1984. Lipids **19:** 836-843.

26. BHUYAN, K. C. & D. K. BHUYAN. 1983. Molecular mechanism of cataractogenesis. II. Evidence of lipid peroxidation and membrane damage. *In* Oxy Radicals and Their Scavenger Systems. Vol. II. Cellular and Medical Aspects. R. A. Greenwald & G. Cohen, Eds.: 349-356. Elsevier. Amsterdam.
27. MAGGIO, B., A. T. DIPLOCK & J. A. LUCY. 1977. Biochem. J. **161:** 111-121.
28. DIPLOCK, A. T., J. A. LUCY, M. VERRINDER & A. ZIELENIEWSKI. FEBS LETT. **82:** 341-344.
29. ERIN, A. N., M. M. SPIRIN, L. V. TABIDZE & V. E. KAGAN. 1983. Biokhimiya **48:** 1855-1861.
30. BURLAKOVA, E. B., E. N. KUKHTINA, I. K. SARYCHEVA, N. G. KHRAPOVA & S. A. ARISTARKHOVA. 1982. Biokhimiya **47:** 987-992.
31. AGADZHANOV, M. I., S. A. BADZHINYAN, K. G. KARAGEZYAN & V. G. MKHITARYAN. 1979. Dokl. Akad. Nauk. SSSR. **244:** 1496-1499.
32. BAIG, M. M. A. & D. L. LAIDMAN. 1983. Biochem. Soc. Trans. **11:** 601-602.
33. DIPLOK, A. T. & J. A. LUCY. 1973. FEBS Lett. **29:** 205-210.
34. HOEY, B. M. & J. BUTLER. 1984. Biochim. Biophys. Acta **791:** 212-218.
35. BISBY, R. H., S. AHMED & R. B. CUNDALL. 1984. Biochem. Biophys. Res. Commun. **119:** 245-251.
36. KORCHAGIN, V. P., L. B. BRATKOVSKAYA, A. A. SHVEDOVA, V. YU. ARCHIPENKO, V. E. KAGAN & S. A. SHUKOLYUKOV. Biokhimiya **45:** 1767-1772.
37. KAGAN, V. E., V. YU. ARCHIPENKO & YU. P. KOZLOV. 1983. Biokhimiya **48:** 158-166.
38. ANANIEVA, L. K., I. I. IVANOV, L. V. TABIDZE & V. E. KAGAN. 1984. Biokhimiya **49:** 60-66.
39. TABIDZE, L. V., V. B. RITOV, V. E. KAGAN & YU. P. KOSLOV. 1983. Bull. Exp. Biol. Med. **96:** 1548-1550.
40. HIGHTOWER, K. R., V. LEVERENZY & V. N. REDDY. 1980. Invest. Ophthalmol. **19:** 1059-1066.
41. HIGHTOWER, K. R. & V. N. REDDY. 1981. Curr. Eye Res. **1:** 197-207.
42. NAKAYAMA, T., M. KODAMA & C. NAGATA. 1984. Agric. Biol. Chem. **48:** 571-572.
43. POPOV, G. A. & V. V. KONEV. 1984. Biokhimiya **49:** 1199-1202.
44. NAIR, P. P., R. M. PATNAIK & J. W. HANSWIRTH. 1978. Cellular transport and binding of d-α-tocopherol. *In* Tocopherol, Oxygen and Biomembranes. C. deDuve & O. Hayaishi, Eds.: 121-130. Elsevier. Amsterdam.
45. KALININA, L. M. & S. R. MINSEITOVA. 1983. Genetika **19:** 1941-1947.
46. RAJARAM, O. V., P. FATTERPAKER & A. SREENIVASAN. 1973. Biochem. Biophys. Res. Commun. **52:** 459-465.
47. HAUSWIRTH, J. W. & P. P. NAIR. 1972. Ann. N.Y. Acad. Sci. **203:** 111-122.
48. SAMUELSSON, B., E. GRANSTROM & M. HAMBERG. 1966. On the mechanism of the biosynthesis of prostaglandins. *In* Prostaglandins. S. Bergstrom & B. Samuelsson, Eds.: 31-44.
49. DAKHIL, T. & W. VOGT. 1962. J. Physiol. **160:** 21p-22p.
50. GUIVERNAU, M., A. TERRAGNO, M. W. DUNN & N. A. TERRAGNO. 1982. Invest. Ophthalmol. **32:** 214-217.
51. LONCHAMPT, M.-O., C. BONNE, F. REGNAULT, J. P. MASSE, C. COQUELET & D. SINCHOLLE. 1983. Prostaglandins Leukotrienes Med. **10:** 381-387.
52. FLEISHER, L. N. & M. C. MCGAHAN. 1985. Exp. Eye Res. **40:** 711-719.
53. ONO, S., Y. OBARA & M. HATANO. 1973. Ophthalmol. Res. **4:** 281-283.
54. PATERSON, C. A. & B. A. ECK. 1971. Ophthalmol. Res. **2:** 246-249.
55. FALANGA, A., M. G. DONI, F. DELAINI, DE B. VITTI, L. IMBERTI, M. G. DONATI & G. DEGAETANO. 1983. Am. J. Physiol. **245:** H867-H870.
56. GILBERT, V. A., E. J. ZEBROWSKI & A. C. CHAN. 1983. Horm. Metab. Res. **15:** 320-325.
57. KARPEN, C. W., K. A. PRITCHARD, JR., J. H. ARNOLD, D. G. CORNWELL & R. V. PANGANAMALA. 1982. Diabetes **31:** 947-951.
58. BASCETTA, E., F. D. GUNSTONE & J. C. WALTON. 1983. Chem. Phys. Lipids **33:** 207-210.
59. HARRISON, W. H., J. R. GANDER, E. R. BLAKLEY & P. D. BOYER. 1956. Biochim. Biophys. Acta **21:** 150-158.

60. ROUSSEAU, C., C. RICHARD & R. MARTIN. 1984. J. Chim. Phys. Phys. Chim. Biol. **81:** 137-138.
61. YANG, N. Y. J. & T. D. DESARI. 1978. Glutathione peroxidase and vitamin E interrelationship. *In* Tocopherol, Oxygen and Biomembranes. C. deDuve & O. Hayaishi, Eds.: 233-245. Elsevier. Amsterdam.
62. KRUGLIKOVA, A. A., G. V. DONCHENKO, O. P. SHVACHKO & A. V. KARPOV. 1983. Biokhimiya **48:** 639-644.
63. LANKIN, V. Z., A. K. TIKHAZE, D. R. RAKITA, POMOINETSKII & A. M. VIKHERT. 1983. Biokhimiya **48:** 1555-1559.
64. CREIGHTON, M. O., J. R. TREVITHICK, S. E. SANFORD & T. W. DUKES. 1982. Exp. Eye Res. **34:** 467-476.
65. ROSS, W. M., M. O. CREIGHTON, W. R. INCH & J. R. TREVITHICK. 1983. Exp. Eye Res. **36:** 645-653.
66. CREIGHTON, M. O., W. M. ROSS, P. J. STEWART-DEHAAN, M. SANWAL & J. R. TREVITHICK. 1985. Exp. Eye Res. **40:** 213-222.
67. CREIGHTON, M. O., M. SANWAL, P. J. STEWART-DEHAAN & J. R. TREVITHICK. 1983. Exp. Eye Res. **37:** 65-75.
68. TREVITHICK, J. R., M. O. CREIGHTON, W. M. ROSS, P. J. STEWART-DEHAAN & M. SANWAL. 1981. Can. J. Ophthalmol. **16:** 32-38.
69. STEWART-DEHAAN, P. J., M. O. CREIGHTON, M. SANWAL, W. M. ROSS & J. R. TREVITHICK. 1981. Exp. Eye Res. **32:** 51-60.

Vitamin E Intake and Risk of
Cataracts in Humans[a]

JAMES MCD. ROBERTSON, ALLAN P. DONNER,
AND JOHN R. TREVITHICK

*Departments of Epidemiology and
Biostatistics and Biochemistry
Faculty of Medicine
The University of Western Ontario
London, Ontario, N6A 5C1, Canada*

INTRODUCTION

According to the World Health Organization, cataracts are the leading cause of blindness worldwide.[1] The vast majority of cataracts are of the senile variety and, although surgical treatment is usually successful, the more desirable goal of primary prevention depends on the discovery of the causes of the condition.

Prevalence and Incidence of Cataracts

A comprehensive survey, conducted in the population of Framingham, Massachusetts,[2] revealed a prevalence of cataracts of 15% in people 55 years of age and over. In those over 75 years, 45% of men and 48% of women suffered from the disease. Applying the age-specific rates from the Framingham study to the population of the United States[3] gives an estimated prevalence of cataracts of almost 10.5 million cases in 1988 (TABLE 1), with over one and one-half times as many women as men affected. The preponderance in women rises from a ratio of 1.2 in 55- to 64-year-olds to 2.2 in people 75 years of age and over.

Other investigators[4] used the Framingham data to estimate the five-year incidence rates of senile cataracts. The rates rose from 1.2% in those 50 to 55 years of age to over 10% in people 75 years of age and over. Based on these figures, the accrual of new cases of senile cataracts in the United States from 1988 through 1992 would be some 3.6 million (TABLE 2). Adding these to the preexisting patients gives a total of 14 million cases by 1993, assuming none are treated.

[a] This work was supported by the National Health Research and Development Program, Health and Welfare Canada, Grant No. 6606-2445.

TABLE 1. Estimated Prevalence of Senile Cataracts, United States, 1988[a]

Age (years)	Numbers of cases in thousands		
	Men	Women	Total
55–64	433	539	972
65–74	1,663	1,889	3,552
≥ 75	1,852	4,110	5,962
Total	3,948	6,538	10,486

[a] Calculated by applying the prevalence figures from reference 2 to the estimated population figures from reference 3.

Costs of Treatment

The average cost of surgery and hospitalization of a cataract patient in the United States is $5,410.00.[5] Thus a conservative estimate of the cost of treatment in the five-year period, 1988 to 1992, is $49.4 billion (TABLE 3). Despite the treatment of about 9 million patients, over 4 million would still exist at the beginning of 1993, treatment for which would cost an additional $22.6 billion. These figures indicate that measures to prevent cataracts could have a major impact on the costs of health care.

Possible Causes

Current theories suggest that osmotic stress operating by way of the aldose reductase pathway[6–14] and/or oxidative stress due to the accumulation of free radicals[15–19] are involved in the pathogenesis of cataracts. A number of chemicals, including several antioxidants,[20–29] have demonstrated preventive or ameliorative actions in experimentally induced cataracts both in vivo and in vitro. Extrapolation of these findings to the aging human being[30–32] implies that adequate or supplementary doses of the antioxidant vitamins C and E may have preventive potential in senile cataracts. This evidence alone seems insufficient, however, to justify a preventive trial of these agents.

TABLE 2. Estimated Five-Year Incidence of Senile Cataracts, United States, 1988–1992[a]

Age	Numbers of cases in thousands		
	Men	Women	Total
55–64	178	203	381
65–74	505	663	1,168
≥ 75	729	1,357	2,086
Total	1,412	2,223	3,635

[a] Calculated by applying the estimated incidence figures from reference 4 to the estimated population figures from reference 3.

TABLE 3. Estimated Costs of Cataract Treatment, United States, 1988–1992

Assume: 25% of prevalent cases and 12.5% of incident cases are treated per year.
    Cost of surgery and hospitalization = $5,410/case.
Number of cases treated: 9,127,700.
Cost of treatment: $49.4 billion or $9.9 billion/year.
Prevalence at 1 Jan. 1993: 4,177,000 ($22.6 billion).
These estimates exclude the costs of corrective lenses and legal blindness in untreated people.

The authors have located only two epidemiologic studies of factors that may influence the occurrence of cataracts. The Framingham Study[33] found several variables, including age, sex, height, education, hypertension, vital capacity, and hand grip strength to be associated with the disease. As these investigators rightly pointed out, however, the results of the univariate analyses should be interpreted with caution because several of these variables are interrelated. The results of the second study[34] indicated that cataract patients tended to have lower serum levels of at least two of the vitamins, C, E, or carotenoids, than did cataract-free subjects. The findings were statistically significant only when the vitamins were entered into the analysis as a combined index rather than separately.

The foregoing evidence of the potential role of antioxidants in the pathogenesis of cataracts suggests that further investigation of the problem in humans is justified.

THE PRESENT STUDY

The aim of the study reported here was to determine if subjects who were free of cataracts consumed more supplementary vitamin E than did similar people affected with the condition.

Methods

In this case-control study, 175 cataract patients, 55 years of age and over, and a like number of cataract-free, control subjects, all of whom were patients of five ophthalmologists in London, Ontario, Canada, were interviewed in their residences by two trained interviewers. The interview, which contained no open-ended questions, covered basic demographic and personal data, self-reported health, the use of analgesics and steroids, and details of vitamin supplementation, with and without minerals, including dosage and duration of use. No attempt was made to assess dietary vitamin intake inasmuch as retrospective investigations of diet are often inaccurate and because the source of research subjects was the relatively homogeneous, predominantly white, population of the city of London and the surrounding southwestern Ontario counties.

Cataract cases were patients with lenticular opacities that impaired vision. In fact, all of these patients had either just undergone, or were awaiting, cataract surgery. Controls were cataract-free subjects who were individually matched with cases on age (± 5 years) and sex. These matching factors were chosen because of their strong associations with senile cataracts.[33] Because it is difficult to find older people whose lenses are totally clear, subjects with small opacities that did not affect their vision were included as controls. This contamination of the control group with mildly affected subjects likely reduced the chances of detecting case-control differences and tended to minimize the size of those that were detectable.

The data were first submitted to univariate analysis to assess the comparability of cases and controls and to identify potential confounding variables. Case-control pairs that were discordant with respect to vitamin supplementation were then entered into a paired, multiple logistic regression analysis[35] that controlled the effects of the confounding variables. To evaluate the possibility of a dose-response relationship, only case-control pairs in which both members reported taking supplementary vitamins were included. The total doses of vitamins were calculated by combining the daily doses with the duration of supplementation in years. Doses of vitamins in single and multiple vitamin supplements were included and, if supplementation took place only during the winter, it was counted as 0.5 years. The mean case-control differences were tested for significance by the paired *t* test.

Results

Inasmuch as the possible effects of vitamins C and E in senile cataracts were the focus of this study, we excluded the 23 case-control pairs with diabetes: 16 pairs in which the case was affected, six in which the control was diabetic, and one in which the status of the control was unknown. The final analysis thus included 152 case-control pairs, 59 of which were male and 93 female (TABLE 4).

The univariate analyses, presented in TABLE 5, revealed that the cases were significantly more likely to be rural residents (odds ratio (OR) = 5.50, p = 0.001), less likely to consume five or more cups of tea per day (OR = 0.39, p = 0.02), and to be regular consumers of supplementary vitamins C and E (OR = 0.54, p = 0.08 and OR = 0.52, p = 0.01, respectively).

The high proportion of cases from rural areas was not surprising, because London is the major medical center for the southwestern Ontario region. Nonetheless, inasmuch as place of residence and tea consumption were associated with case-control status and could also be associated with a tendency to vitamin supplementation, making them potential confounding variables, it was necessary to eliminate their influence in

TABLE 4. Age and Sex Distributions of Subjects Included in the Analysis

Age	Men		Women	
	Cases	Controls	Cases	Controls
55–59	4	4	11	11
60–64	12	12	17	17
65–69	15	15	28	28
70–74	9	9	23	23
75–79	12	12	11	11
80–84	5	5	1	1
≥ 85	2	2	2	2
Total	59	59	93	93

TABLE 5. Univariate Comparison of the 152 Cataract Cases with the Matched Control Group

Variable	Cases	Controls
1. Height (cm) mean ± SD	167.6 ± 9.6	167.6 ± 8.5
2. Weight (kg) mean ± SD	69.7 ± 13.9	69.2 ± 12.5
3. Sociodemographic characteristics		
Ethnic origin[a]: % Canadian	67	61
Place of birth: % Canada	80	84
Place of residence: % rural	42	14
Education (%)		
≤ Grade 7	6	5
Grade 8–11	54	46
High school graduate	25	27
Community college	5	7
University	10	15
Usual occupation (%)		
Scientific/technical	5	6
Management/administration	9	9
Social science/artistic	1	2
Teaching	2	4
Clerical/sales/service	30	39
Production	14	8
Transportation/handling	2	3
Construction	2	3
Farming/outdoor	12	5
Housekeeper	22	20
Other	1	1
Employment status (%)		
Employed full-time	16	12
Employed part-time	6	6
Retired, normal	48	55
Retired, disability	3	3
Unemployed	0	1
Housekeeper	27	23
Marital status (%)		
Never married	5	9
Married	70	72
Widowed	20	15
Divorced/separated	5	4
4. Personal habits		
Cigarette smoking (%)		
Never smoked	51	52
Current smoker	20	16
Exsmoker	29	32
Coffee		
Percent drinking 5 or more cups per day	15	13
Tea		
Percent drinking 5 or more cups per day	7	18
Alcohol consumption (%)		
Beer, ≥ 5 bottles per week	5	5
Wine, ≥ 5 glasses per week	3	3
Spirits, ≥ 5 drinks per week	11	7

TABLE 5. Univariate Comparison of the 152 Cataract Cases with the Matched Control Group—*Continued*

Variable	Cases	Controls
5. Self-reported health in previous 5 years		
General health (%)		
Excellent	31	37
Good	48	41
Fair	16	17
Poor	5	5
Hypertension (%)	36	43
Arthritis (%)	53	61
Heart disease (%)	18	20
6. Drug consumption (%)		
Acetylsalicylic acid		
Regular	13	14
Occasional/never	87	86
Acetaminophen		
Regular	5	3
Occasional/never	95	97
Ibuprofen		
Regular	5	3
Occasional/never	95	97
Corticosteriods		
Regular	2	1
Occasional/never	98	99
7. Supplementary vitamin use (%)		
Multiple vitamins		
Daily	17	14
Occasional/never	83	86
Vitamin A		
Daily	5	4
Occasional/never	95	96
Vitamin B (all types plus B complex)		
Daily	9	13
Occasional/never	91	87
Vitamin C[b]		
Daily	12	20
Occasional/never	88	80
Vitamin D		
Daily	3	3
Occasional/never	97	97
Vitamin E[c]		
Daily	22	38
Occasional/never	88	62

[a] Defined as father's place of birth.
[b] Takes separate vitamin C supplement or a B complex plus C supplement. Excludes those taking multiple vitamin supplements containing vitamin C.
[c] Excludes those taking multiple vitamin supplements containing vitamin E.

the further examination of the effects of the vitamins. Accordingly, the effects of residence and tea consumption were controlled by submitting the informative case-control pairs, that is, those that were discordant with respect to vitamin supplementation, to paired multiple logistic regression analysis. This amounted to 40 pairs in the case of vitamin C alone, 76 pairs for vitamin E alone, and 25 pairs for combined vitamin C and E supplements. These analyses (TABLE 6) indicated that, in contrast to the controls, cataract patients were only 30% as likely to have taken supplementary vitamin C and only 44% as likely to have consumed supplementary vitamin E; for combined vitamin consumption, the figure was 32 percent. Despite the wide confidence, limits in the case of vitamin C and vitamins C and E combined, the adjusted odds ratios retained their statistically significant deviations from 1.0.

Similar results were obtained when cigarette smoking and arthritis, in addition to place of residence and tea drinking, were entered into the analysis (vitamin C: OR = 0.25, 95% confidence limits (C.L.) = 0.06-0.97; vitamin E: OR = 0.40, 95% C.L. = 0.22-0.73). Re-analysis of the data including the 23 case-control pairs with diabetes did not alter the results substantially. In the case of vitamin C, the adjusted odds ratio was 0.32 (95% C.L. = 0.14-0.74); for vitamin E, the ratio was 0.41 (95% C.L. = 0.24-0.71).

The daily doses of vitamins C and E taken by most of the subjects were 300 to 600 mg and 400 IU, respectively. In attempting to detect a dose-response relationship, only case-control pairs in which both members reported taking supplementary vitamins were used, 12 pairs for vitamin C and 11 pairs for vitamin E. The total doses were calculated as described above. The results are shown in TABLE 7. Both differences were in the expected direction, but that for vitamin E was statistically nonsignificant. Sample sizes in these secondary analyses, however, were small, and the standard deviation was large in the case of vitamin E.

CONCLUSION

Assuming that dietary vitamin intake in these subjects was unrelated to vitamin supplementation, the results of this study suggest that the consumption of supplementary vitamins C and E may reduce the risk of senile cataracts by at least 50 percent. That these results complement those of a previous study[34] lends importance to confirming and extending these findings.

TABLE 6. Matched Pairs; Multiple Logistic Regression Analysis of the Effects of Vitamins C and E with the Effects of Residence and Tea Drinking Controlled

Variable	Case-control pairs	Coefficient ± SE	Adjusted odds ratio	95% confidence limits	Significance level (p)
Vitamin C	40	−1.19 ± 0.46	0.30	0.12-0.75	0.01
Vitamin E	76	−0.82 ± 0.29	0.44	0.24-0.77	0.004
Vitamin C and E	25	−1.12 ± 0.58	0.32	0.11-0.99	0.05

TABLE 7. Mean Case-Control Differences in Total Dosage of Vitamins C and E

	Vitamin C (n = 12)	Vitamin E (n = 11)
Mean difference	67.12×10^3 mg $\times$ year	32.97×10^3 IU $\times$ year
SD	19.51	70.81
t-value	3.44	0.47
Probability	0.006	> 0.05

SIGNIFICANCE

Association or Causation?

This study demonstrated a statistical association between supplementary vitamin consumption and freedom from senile cataracts. In the absence of experimental studies in human beings, however, the only direct method of determining causation, the probability of the relationship being causal, rests on the strength of the epidemiologic evidence. Six aspects must be evaluated (TABLE 8). The strength of the association refers to the ratio of disease rates in those with and without the exposure of interest. In this study, the odds ratios of 0.44 for vitamin E and 0.30 for vitamin C, representing two and one-half to threefold decreases in risk, suggest a strong relationship. Although the evidence for a dose-response relationship is less certain, the authors believe it provides fair support for causality. The results of this study are consistent with those of the only other investigation[34] of this association in humans. Inasmuch as the question posed to respondents concerned supplementary vitamin consumption over the previous five years, the requirement that exposure precede outcome appears to be fairly well fulfilled. The specificity of the association is difficult to judge because most disease is multifactorial and the vitamins involved potentially affect all tissues of the body. On the other hand, considerable data from animal experimentation support the causal nature of the observed association. In summary, the authors believe that these results provide fair to good evidence for a causal association between supplementary vitamin C and E consumption and freedom from senile cataracts.

Implications for Prevention

The authors estimate that almost 10.5 million prevalent cases of senile cataracts existed in the United States in 1988 (TABLE 1), with a further 3.6 million new cases expected by the end of 1992 (TABLE 2). This will occasion considerable personal suffering and reduced function as well as a heavy economic burden. Although most cataracts respond well to surgical treatment, this approach to even 50% of the combined prevalent and incident cases would cost the United States health care system a minimum of $38 billion. Because the disease results in progressive blindness, failure to provide adequate treatment adds a further burden to both the health and welfare systems.

TABLE 8. Strength of the Epidemiologic Evidence for the Vitamin/Cataract Association

	Good	Fair	Poor
1. Strength of association	×		
2. Dose-response relationship		×	
3. Consistency of association		×	
4. Time sequence		×	
5. Specificity of association		×	
6. Biological plausibility	×		

TABLE 9 illustrates the cost involved in providing supplementary vitamins C and E for the entire population group in which the risk of senile cataracts starts to rise and the savings that might be expected from the potential preventive effect suggested by the results of this study. Inasmuch as it is not yet possible to identify people at high risk of developing cataracts, the entire group would require supplementation. Nonetheless, net savings of $2.7 billion would result. This method of preventing or postponing a large proportion of senile cataracts is simple and inexpensive with no known side effects, and the potential humane and economic impacts are large. Consequently, a randomized, controlled trial of vitamin supplementation in cataract prevention appears to be justified.

SUMMARY

Experimental evidence suggests that oxidative stress due to the accumulation of free radicals plays a role in the pathogenesis of cataracts and that the process can be prevented or ameliorated by antioxidants. In addition, a recent study found that cataract patients tended to have lower serum levels of vitamins C, E, or carotenoids than did control subjects. This investigation, which compared the self-reported consumption of supplementary vitamins by 175 cataract patients with that of 175 individually matched, cataract-free subjects, revealed that the latter group used significantly more supplementary vitamins C and E ($p = 0.01$ and 0.004, respectively).

TABLE 9. Estimated Cost Savings in Cataract Treatment and Costs of Supplementary Vitamins C and E, Assuming a 60% (odds ratio = 0.40) Reduction in Risk, United States, 1988–1992.

Population ≥ 55 years, 1988: 52,070,000
Expected cases of senile cataracts: 3,635,000
Cases prevented by supplementation: 2,181,000
Cost of supplementation: $9.1 billion[a]
Savings on treatment: $11,8 billion
Net savings: $2.7 billion

[a] Based on a retail price for supplementary vitamins C and E of $35.00 per person per year.

Inasmuch as the observed reduction in risk of cataracts was at least 50%, a randomized, controlled trial of vitamin supplementation in cataract prevention seems justified.

ACKNOWLEDGMENTS

We acknowledge the cooperation of Dr. C. Dyson, Dr. D. C. McFarlane, Dr. D. W. Mills, Dr. A. C. Tokarewicz, and Dr. N. R. Willis, Department of Ophthalmology, Victoria Hospital-Westminster Campus, London, Ontario, Canada and the technical assistance of Linda Turner and Helen Martin.

REFERENCES

1. World Health Organization. 1982. Weekly Epidemiol. Record **57:** 145-146.
2. KAHN, H. A., H. M. LEIBOWITZ, J. P. GANLEY *et al.* 1977. The Framingham Eye Study. I. Outline and major prevalence findings. Am. J. Epidemiol. **196:** 17-32.
3. United States Bureau of the Census. 1984. Projections of the population of the United States by age, sex, and race: 1983 to 2080. *In* Current Population Reports, Series P-25, No. 952. U.S. Government Printing Office. Washington, D.C.
4. PODGOR, M. J., M. C. LESKE & F. EDERER. 1983. Incidence estimates for lens changes, macular changes, open-angle glaucoma and diabetic retinopathy. Am. J. Epidemiol. **118:** 206-212.
5. Metropolitan Life Insurance Company. 1987. Regional variations in costs of cataract surgeries. *In* Statistical Bulletin **68**(4): 24-30.
6. HU, T. S., M. DATILES & J. H. KINOSHITA. 1983. Reversal of galactose cataract with sorbinol in rats. Invest. Ophthalmol. Vis. Sci. **24:** 640-644.
7. UNAKAR, N. J. & J. V. TSUI. 1983. Inhibition of galactose-induced alterations in ocular lens with sorbinol. Exp. Eye Res. **36:** 685-694.
8. BEYERS-MEARS, A. & E. CRUZ. 1985. Reversal of diabetic cataract by sorbinol, an aldose reductase inhibitor. Diabetes **34:** 15-21.
9. BEYERS-MEARS, A., E. CRUZ & E. VARAGIANNIS. 1985. Reversal of stage-I sugar cataract by sorbinol, an aldose reductase inhibitor. Pharmacology **31:** 188-196.
10. SIMARD-DUQUESNE, N., E. GRESELIN, R. GONZALEZ & D. DVORNIK. 1985. Prevention of cataract development in severely galactosemic rats by the aldose reductase inhibitor, tolrestat. Proc. Soc. Exp. Biol. Med. **178:** 599-605.
11. BEYER, T. A. & N. J. HUTSON. 1986. Introduction: Evidence for the role of the polyol pathway in the pathophysiology of diabetic complications. Metabolism **35** (4 Suppl. 1): 1-3.
12. KADOR, P. F., Y. AKAGI & J. H. KINOSHITA. 1986. The effect of aldose reductase and its inhibition on sugar cataract formation. Metabolism **35** (4 Suppl. 1): 15-19.
13. YEH, L. A., C. E. RAFFORD, T. A. BEYER & N. J. HUTSON. 1986. Effects of the aldose reductase inhibitor sorbinol on the isolated cultured rat lens. Metabolism **35** (4 Suppl. 1): 4-9.
14. VARMA, S. D. 1986. Inhibition of aldose reductase by flavonoids; possible attenuation of diabetic complications. Prog. Clin. Biol. Res. **213:** 343-358.
15. JERNIGAN, H. M., H. N. FUKUI, J. D. GOOSEY & J. H. KINOSHITA. 1981. Photodynamic effects of rose bengal or riboflavin on carrier-mediated transport systems in rat lens. Exp. Eye Res. **32:** 461-466.
16. BHUYAN, K. C. & D. K. BHUYAN. 1984. Molecular mechanism of cataractogenesis: III. Toxic metabolites of oxygen as initiators of lipid peroxidation and cataract. Curr. Eye Res. **3:** 67-81.

17. VARMA, S. D., D. CHAND, Y. R. SHARMA, J. F. KUCK, JR. & R. D. RICHARDS. 1984. Oxidative stress on lens and cataract formation: Role of light and oxygen. Curr. Eye Res. 35-57.
18. LOHMANN, W., W. SCHMEHL & J. STROBEL. 1986. Nuclear cataract: Oxidative damage to the lens. Exp. Eye Res. **43:** 859-862.
19. ONO, S., S. SHIMIZU, H. TAKAHASHI & H. HIRANO. 1986. Effects of dexamethasone phosphate on the formation of ester forms of riboflavin in the lens. Ophthalmic Res. **18:** 279-281.
20. CREIGHTON, M. O. & J. R. TREVITHICK. 1979. Cortical cataract formation prevented by vitamin E and glutathione. Exp. Eye Res. **29:** 689-693.
21. CREIGHTON, M. O., J. R. TREVITHICK, S. E. SANFORD & T. DUKES. 1982. Modelling cortical cataractogenesis. IV. Induction by hygromycin B *in vivo* (swine) and *in vitro* (rat lens). Exp. Eye Res. **34:** 467-476.
22. CREIGHTON, M. O., M. SANWAL, P. J. STEWART-DEHAAN & J. R. TREVITHICK. 1983. Modelling cortical cataractogenesis. V. Steroid cataracts induced by solumedrol partially prevented by vitamin E *in vitro.* Exp. Eye Res. **37:** 65-76.
23. CREIGHTON, M. O., W. M. ROSS, P. J. STEWART-DEHAAN, M. SANWAL & J. R. TREVITHICK. 1985. Modelling cortical cataractogenesis. VII. Effects of vitamin E treatment on galactose-induced cataracts. Exp. Eye Res. **40:** 213-222.
24. ROSS, W. M., M. O. CREIGHTON, W. R. INCH & J. R. TREVITHICK. 1983. Radiation cataract formation diminished by vitamin E in rat lenses *in vitro.* Exp. Eye Res. **36:** 645-653.
25. ROSS, W. M., M. O. CREIGHTON, J. R. TREVITHICK, P. J. STEWART-DEHAAN & M. SANWAL. 1983. Modelling cortical cataractogenesis. VI. Induction by glucose *in vitro* or in diabetic rats: Prevention and reversal by glutathione. Exp. Eye Res. **37:** 559-573.
26. STEWART-DEHAAN, P. J., M. O. CREIGHTON, M. SANWAL, W. M. ROSS & J. R. TREVITHICK. 1981. Effects of vitamin E on cortical cataractogenesis induced by elevated temperature in intact rat lenses in medium 199. Exp. Eye Res. **32:** 51-60.
27. GUPTA, P. P., D. J. PANDEY, A. L. SHARMA, R. K. SRIVASTAVA & S. S. MISHRA. 1984. Prevention of experimental cataract by alpha-tocopherol. Indian J. Exp. Biol. **22:** 620-622.
28. LIBONDI, T., M. MENZIONE, M. IULIANO, M. DELLA CORTE, F. LATTE & G. AURICCHIO. 1985. Changes of some biochemical parameters of the lens in galactose-treated weaned rats with and without vitamin E therapy. Ophthalmic Res. **17:** 42-48.
29. LINKLATER, H. A., T. DZIALOSZYNSKI, H. L. MCLEOD, S. E. SANFORD & J. R. TREVITHICK. 1986. Modelling cortical cataractogenesis. VIII. Effects of butylated hydroxytoluene (BHT) in reducing protein leakage from lenses of diabetic rats. Exp. Eye Res. **43:** 305-314.
30. BENSCH, K. G., J. E. FLEMING & W. LOHMANN. 1985. The role of ascorbic acid in senile cataract. Proc. Natl. Acad. Sci. USA **82:** 7193-7196.
31. RINGVOLD, A., H. JOHNSEN & S. BLIKA. 1985. Senile cataract and ascorbic acid loading. Acta Ophthalmol. (Copenh.) **63:** 277-280.
32. CHANDRA, D. B., R. VARMA, S. AHMAD & S. D. VARMA. 1986. Vitamin C in the human aqueous humor and cataracts. Int. J. Vit. Nutr. Res. **56:** 165-168.
33. KAHN, H. A., H. M. LEIBOWITZ, J. P. GANLEY *et al.* 1977. The Framingham Eye Study. II. Association of opthalmic pathology with single variables previously measured in the Framingham Heart Study. Am. J. Epidemiol. **196:** 33-41.
34. JACQUES, P. F., L. T. CHYLACK, JR., R. B. MCGANDY & S. C. HARTZ. 1988. Antioxidant status in persons with and without senile cataract. Arch. Ophthalmol. **106:** 337-340.
35. POSNER, B. & C. H. HENNEKENS. 1978. Analytical methods in matched pair epidemiological studies. Int. J. Epidemiol. **7:** 367-372.

Vitamin E and Cancer Prevention in an Animal Model[a]

YEU-MING WANG[b], MADHU PUREWAL,
BEVERLY NIXON, DONG-HUI LI, AND
DOROTA SOLTYSIAK-PAWLUCZUK

Department of Experimental Pediatrics
The University of Texas M. D. Anderson Cancer Center
Houston, Texas 77030

Evidence for the preventive effect of vitamin E on specific forms of cancer includes epidemiological surveys, experiments using animal models, and to a lesser degree case-control studies in humans. The adequate levels of α-tocopherol in human diets in Western countries and other more advanced nations has provided a poor environment for the epidemiological study of an association between vitamin E and cancer. An inverse relationship between circulating α-tocopherol and cancer, however, has been found in a few recent prospective studies of lung cancer in this country,[1] breast cancer in England,[2] and a combined group of cancers unrelated to smoking among Finnish men.[3] Vitamin E is being tested clinically as a potential preventive agent for colon cancer; unfortunately, ascorbic acid is being tested along with it.[4] This combination precludes definitive conclusions on the utility of either vitamin singly. The investigations of vitamin E and cancer were stimulated by the irreproducible finding of Rowntree *et al.*,[5] that crude wheat germ oil induced sarcomas in rats. Wheat germ oil is naturally enriched with vitamin E. This study has never been reproduced. To date, more than 20 reports have demonstrated that animals fed vitamin E, mostly in ester form, have fewer or later-appearing tumors after administration of a carcinogen or UV radiation than animals that do not receive the vitamin. There are also a few reports of the inefficacy of vitamin E as a cancer preventive agent in animals.[6]

We used our model of the daunorubicin-induced mammary tumors in Sprague Dawley (SD) rats and prevention of these tumors by prior injection or ingestion of α-tocopherol acetate to examine the interaction between the two agents and establish a more detailed mechanistic explanation of how vitamin E works in this particular model.[7] Our results with this system suggested that in 8-9-week-old female SD rats, *dl*-α-tocopheryl acetate given at 1.8 g/m^2/day intraperitoneally for four days prior to a single injection of daunorubicin (10 mg/kg or 60 mg/m^2) through a tail vein produced a significantly lower incidence ($p < 0.05$) of tumors than appeared in rats treated with daunorubicin alone. In one of the experiments, 24/54 animals injected with only daunorubicin had histologically proven mammary tumors, whereas 9/38

[a]Our research results presented in this manuscript were supported in part by Grant CA-35363 from the National Cancer Institute, Bethesda, Maryland, and by a Grant from the American Institute for Cancer Research, Washington, D.C.

[b]Y.-M. Wang died on April 28, 1989.

animals treated with both α-tocopheryl acetate and daunorubicin had mammary cancer.[6] (The 60 mg/m^2 daunorubicin dose is a usual single dose out of nine consecutive doses given to humans.)

The increase in α-tocopherol concentration, however, was less than 100% in mammary gland and fat areas 24 hours after four injections of high doses of α-tocopheryl acetate. Therefore, to investigate whether the effect of α-tocopherol occurs in the early stage of tumor development, weanling female SD rats were fed α-tocopheryl acetate-free or α-tocopheryl acetate-supplemented diets (containing 0, 100, 1000, and 10,000 mg α-tocopheryl acetate per kg diet) for 6 weeks.

Single mammary epithelial cells were isolated from these rats,[8] and biochemical studies were performed. Using a high-performance liquid chromatographic method,[9] we found that mammary epithelial cells had increased cellular α-tocopherol concentrations in those rats fed diets higher in α-tocopheryl acetate. The increment of α-tocopherol content was from less than 13 μg/10^9 cells in animals fed the deficient diet to 332 μg/10^9 cells in animals fed the 10,000 mg/kg diet.

Since the increment of intracellular α-tocopherol was indeed significant, we started to look at the effect of α-tocopherol on daunorubicin in three areas: Does α-tocopherol alter the distribution of daunorubicin and in particular the daunorubicin concentration in the target cell mammary epithelial cells? Does α-tocopherol alter the metabolic profile of daunorubicin in mammary epithelial cells by changing the cellular metabolic machinery? Does α-tocopherol protect the integrity of cellular DNA, the presumed target of carcinogenesis?

The effect of α-tocopherol on [^{3}H]daunorubicin distribution was tested in animals fed at zero or 10,000 mg α-tocopheryl acetate/kg diet, given for 6 weeks. The distribution and clearance of the drug and the carcinogen differed in various tissues. For instance, the bell-shaped curve of daunorubicin clearance in the ovary in vitamin E-deficient rats and mammary epithelial cells was distinctly different from those for the liver and kidney. In addition, our previously unpublished results indicated that these ^{3}H counts fully represented daunorubicin and its metabolites in tissue. The distribution, as calculated by the area under the curve (AUC) of [^{3}H]daunorubicin counts showed that the AUC of daunorubicin in the mammary epithelial cells was twice the AUC in the liver.

Daunorubicin clearance was affected by vitamin E status only in the rat ovary. There was no significant difference in tritium counts in mammary epithelial cells between animals fed a vitamin E-deficient diet and high vitamin E diets. One point that needs to be reemphasized here is that the drug concentration under the curve was approximately two times higher in mammary epithelial cells than in the liver. We and others have already established that the drug itself is more mutagenic and carcinogenic[10] and induces more DNA strand breaks than some of its metabolites.[8] We have also established that mammary epithelial cells metabolize daunorubicin minimally as compared with tissues such as the liver. Therefore, the increased area under the curve of mammary epithelial cells becomes very significant.

Our results indicated that α-tocopherol has no effect on drug clearance in mammary epithelial cells. It does, however, significantly affect the AUC of daunorubicin in the ovary. Also, although the initial tissue drug concentration is not as high as in other tissues, the mammary epithelial cells appear incapable of pumping out the carcinogen and cannot detoxify it by metabolizing it. The increased AUC suggests that the cell may recycle the carcinogen, thus producing free radicals and oxygen anions intracellularly.

The ingestion of α-tocopheryl acetate had little effect on the distribution of [^{3}H]daunorubicin in mammary epithelial cells or the glutathione (GSH) concentration

(344 nmol per 10^9 cells for animals given the deficient diet and 384 ± 144 nmol per 10^9 cells for those fed 10,000 mg α-tocopheryl acetate per kg of diet for 6 weeks *in vivo*). Therefore, the influence of α-tocopheryl acetate ingestion on intracellular GSH and the enzymes relevant to free radical production, free radical neutralization, and daunorubicin detoxification were investigated. Our preliminary investigation showed that challenge by the addition of daunorubicin (9 μM) to these isolated cells of up to 1 hour of incubation did not significantly alter the intracellular GSH level. Whether there were any significant free SH group modifications in the microcellular environment, such as the nucleus, is yet unknown. A drug concentration of 167 μM, however, would result in a 50% oxidation of GSH in 45 minutes.

The effect of α-tocopheryl acetate on cellular enzymes is not dramatic but is interesting. Thus far we have quantitated xanthine oxidase, oxidized glutathione (GSSG) reductase, Se-GSH peroxidase, quinone reductase, and daunorubicin reductase. Se-GSH peroxidase and glutathione S-transferase activity were 10 to 20 times higher in livers than in mammary epithelial cells. The quinone reductase activity was

TABLE 1. Influx of [^{3}H]Daunorubicin into Isolated Mammary Epithelial Cells[a]

Experiment	Fraction	3 Minutes	30 Minutes	60 Minutes	120 Minutes
1	Postnuclei	17		25	
	Nuclei	83		75	
2	Postnuclei	30		34	
	Nuclei	70		66	
3	Postnuclei	11	16		10
	Nuclei	89	83		90
4	Postnuclei	43	41		25
	Nuclei	57	58		75

[a] Each experiment was performed in cells isolated from one animal, and 3 to 6×10^6 cells/mL were used in each experiment. Due to the scarcity of the cells isolated, experiments at many time points could not be performed. [^{3}H]Daunorubicin obtained from New England Nuclear was further purified by HPLC for use in these experiments.

10 times lower in mammary cells. Daunorubicin reductase was higher in the liver but was negligible in mammary epithelial cells. The activity of xanthine oxidase was also quantitated. Our observation for mammary epithelial cells is similar to that of George Catignani and his collaborators[11] for mammalian liver. The activity and protein copies were regulated by the status of vitamin E adequacy. Xanthine oxidase is known to metabolize doxorubicin, an analogue of daunorubicin, and to generate doxorubicin-related free radicals and oxygen anions.[12] These molecules in turn result in cellular damage.

At this moment, we cannot assign the significance of the enzymes in the postnuclear fraction of the mammary epithelial cells for several reasons. First, the *in vitro* experimentation on the transport of anthracycline antibiotics indicated that 50% to 70% or more of intracellular [^{3}H]daunorubicin was found in the nuclear fraction in less than 5 minutes (TABLE 1). The presence of α-tocopherol did not alter the movement of the radioactivity into the cell. Second, we still lack the fine print of the metabolic pattern of [^{3}H]daunorubicin in the mammary nuclear fraction. This is also related to the question of whether cellular nuclei are capable of metabolizing the drug substantially or whether nuclei-free sulfhydryl groups and their potential generation or regeneration system affect the outcome of the drug action in the nuclear fraction.

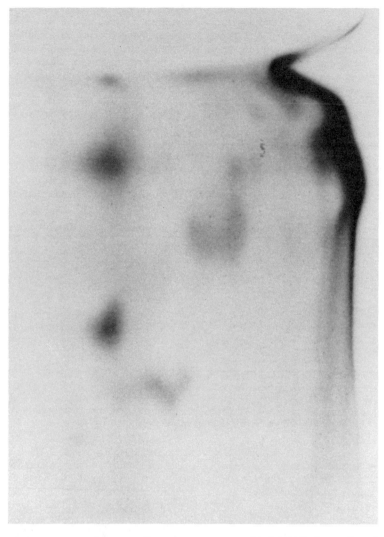

FIGURE 1. An autoradiogram of ^{32}P-labeled mammary epithelial DNA I spots from 9-week-old female Sprague-Dawley rats fed diets containing 0 (left panel) and 10,000 (right panel) mg/kg *dl*-α-tocopheryl acetate for 6 weeks. For detailed experimental procedure, please see Li.[16] Kodak XAR-5 film and DuPont Lighting Plus Intensifying Screen and films were used and processed at −80°C for 17 hours.

Furthermore, in recent years, laboratory observations have suggested that anthracycline antibiotics exert their cytotoxicity by interaction at the cell membrane level without entering the cell.[13,14] If this indeed is the case, the thought that the cellular membrane is the target of the cytotoxicity, and on the other hand, nuclear DNA is

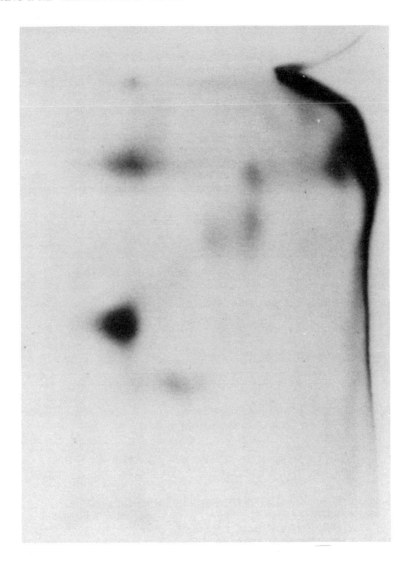

the target of carcinogenesis would indicate that those drugs would not effect carcinogenesis, although there is yet no direct experimental approach to resolve this issue.

These arguments lead us to the investigation of the effect of α-tocopherol on the stability of mammary epithelial DNA. Two experiments have been performed. The first involves a ^{32}P-postlabeling assay of mammary fat pad DNA from animals fed different amounts of α-tocopheryl acetate to show whether a cellular DNA modification results from the feeding of α-tocopheryl acetate. This modification could be induced by the direct interaction of α-tocopherol or its metabolites with DNA or indirectly by altered cellular metabolism resulting from the vitamin feeding. The second experiment analyzes DNA single strand breaks induced by daunorubicin in mammary epithelial cells.

An enhanced ^{32}P-postlabeling assay was used to detect an adduct-like nonpolar covalent DNA modification. This technique was first developed by Randerath and his collaborators,[15] and we used it to illustrate that both qualitative and quantitative vitamin E-associated differences were found in liver and kidney DNA.[16]

The ^{32}P two-dimensional profile DNA on mammary fat pad from rats fed with different amounts of α-tocopheryl acetate is shown in FIGURE 1. Obvious differences were seen in the two groups of animals: the vitamin E-deficient animals and those animals fed with 10,000 mg α-tocopherol acetate per kg diet. Although the significance of this observation needs to be further explored, an increased intensity of one spot is evident. We have also undertaken another experiment to explore the effect of α-tocopheryl acetate on the stability of the mammary cellular DNA.

TABLE 2. Median Survival after a Single Injection of Daunorubicin (10 mg/kg) through Tail Vein of Female SD Rats Fed Diets Containing Various Amounts of dl-α-Tocopheryl Acetate[a]

Dietary α-Tocopheryl Acetate Content (mg/kg)	Median Survival Time (Days)			
	AIN - 76A		Draper	Purina Chow
	Expt. 1	Expt. 2		
0	32	43	94	ND[b]
100	92	102	155	> 255[c]
1,000	104	126	186	ND
10,000	97[d]	126	184	ND

[a] Weanling female SD rats were fed a vitamin E–containing diet for 6 weeks before a single injection of daunorubicin. After the daunorubicin injection, animals were maintained on the same diet (AIN-76A and Draper diets, Bethlehem, PA). Twenty-five animals were used in each feeding experiment.

[b] Not done.

[c] The content of dl-α-tocopheryl acetate in the diet equaled 89 mg/kg by HPLC.[9]

[d] The deaths of some of the animals were due to viral infection.

Alkaline elution techniques were used to compare the frequencies and type of DNA lesions in mammary cells. Mammary cells, at 10^6 cells per mL, were incubated with 1.5, 4.0, and 10.0 μg drug for 1 hour. After incubation, the cells were pelleted at 200 × g for 4 minutes, washed once with Hanks' balanced salt solution, and resuspended in phosphate-buffered saline. DNA single-strand breaks (SSB) were assessed in the absence of proteinase K.[8]

The results indicated that α-tocopherol can significantly modify the effect of daunorubicin-induced DNA SSB. DNA SSB were substantially reduced by the increase in the level of α-tocopheryl acetate in the diet. Ten micrograms daunorubicin per 10^6 cells resulted in 0.518 ± 0.379 DNA SSB per 10^6 nucleotides in vitamin E-deficient cells, as compared with a significantly lower 0.151 ± 0.029 DNA SSB per 10^6 nucleotides at the highest level of α-tocopheryl acetate supplementation (TABLE 2). It is apparent that vitamin E-supplemented cells can resist the oxidation induced by daunorubicin.

These results, in our judgment, warranted animal experimentation. Therefore, weanling female SD rats were fed with 0, 100, 1,000, and 10,000 mg/kg diet for 6 weeks, and then a single dose of daunorubicin at a dose of 10 mg/kg (60 mg/m^2) was injected through a tail vein. Two basal dietary formulas were used: first, the AIN-76A diet and then the Draper's diet. The results are shown in TABLE 2 and were indeed disappointing. Neither diet sustained the drug-induced toxicities. The animals died prematurely with kidney failure. These results suggested a nutritional inadequacy in both diets. Because our earlier results in the animals fed with normal Purina Chow showed that 50% of the animals had one or more mammary tumors in 8½ months, the shortened life span with both AIN-76A and Draper diets made these two diets unsuitable for our carcinogenesis studies. Experiments with both diets, however, inevitably pinpointed that α-tocopherol supplementation can prolong the life span of these animals despite daunorubicin toxicity. We are currently planning to supplement Purina Chow with α-tocopheryl acetate to perform a carcinogenesis experiment with two or three groups of animals.

Our animal trials revealed that in this animal model, vitamin E can effectively prevent or delay the onset of daunorubicin-induced carcinogenesis. The significant biochemical interaction between α-tocopherol and daunorubicin might happen early after daunorubicin injection. The results indicated, however, that α-tocopherol did not alter the distribution of daunorubicin *in vivo* or affect influx or efflux of the parent drug, the carcinogen. The effect of daunorubicin on postnuclear fraction sulfhydryl group concentration appeared unimportant in relation to carcinogenesis, and α-tocopherol did not have any influence on the regulation of some GSH-related enzymic activities and their biosynthesis. The relevant enzymes have intrinsically different activities in mammary epithelial cells, however, either favoring the genesis of drug-induced free radicals or reducing cellular ability to neutralize the free radical.

The inability of mammary epithelial cells to metabolize the drug *in vitro* and the long retention time of the drug in these cells *in vivo* further suggest that the parent drug may thus recycle itself to generate free radicals in the presence of abundant amounts of free radical-producing enzymes, such as xanthine oxidase. Xanthine oxidase activity and the protein copy have an inverse relationship with the intracellular content of α-tocopherol. In addition, our results clearly demonstrated that an increased cellular concentration of α-tocopherol can significantly reduce the drug-induced DNA SSB in mammary epithelial cells. This finding and that of the vitamin control of xanthine oxidase might be important to the contribution of the vitamin to the prevention of the carcinogenesis. The significance of the finding of the modification of the DNA by α-tocopherol, however, has yet to be explored.

ACKNOWLEDGMENTS

The authors wish to express their gratitude to Ms. Rosalyn Zenon for typing and editing this manuscript and to Dr. Steven Culbert for his critical review and comments. The ^{32}P-postlabeling experiment was performed at Dr. Kurt Randeraths's laboratory.

REFERENCES

1. MENKES, M. S., G. W. COMSTOCK, J. P. VUILLEUMIER, K. J. HELSING, A. A. RIDER & R. BROOKMEYER. 1986. Serum β-carotene, vitamins A and E, selenium and risk of lung cancer. N. Engl. J. Med. **315:** 1250-1254.

2. WALD, N. J., J. BOREHAM, H. HAYWARD & R. D. BULBROOK. 1986. Plasma retinol-beta-carotene and vitamin E levels in relation to the future risk of breast cancer. B. J. Cancer 49: 321-324.
3. KNEKT, P., A. ARAMOA, J. MAATELA et al. 1988. Serum vitamin E and risk of cancer among Finnish men during a 10-year follow-up. Am. J. Epidemiol. 127: 28-41.
4. MCKEOWN-EYSSEN, G., C. HOLLOWAY, V. JAZMAJI, E. BRIGHT-SEE, P. DION & W. R. BRUCE. 1988. A randomized trial of vitamins C and E in the prevention of recurrence of colorectal polyps. Cancer Res. 48: 4701-4705.
5. ROWNTREE, L. G., A. STEINBERT, G. M. DORRANCE & E. F. CRICCONE. 1937. Sarcoma in rats from the ingestion of a crude wheat germ oil made by ether extraction. Am. J. Cancer 31: 359-372.
6. WANG, Y. M. 1985. Mechanisms and prevention of chemotherapy-induced cancers: Interaction of anthracycline antibiotics and α-tocopherol. In Vitamins and Cancer — Human Cancer Prevention by Vitamins and Micronutrients. F. L. Meyskens, Jr. & K. Prasad, Eds.: 213-228. Humana Press.
7. SOTYSIAK-PAWLUCZUK, D. & Y-M. WANG. 1988. α-Tocopherol as a potential modifier of anthracycline antibiotics toxicities. In Handbook of Free Radicals and Antioxidants in Biomedicine. C. Weber, Ed. Vol. II. CRC Press. Boca Raton, FL.
8. HOWELL, S. K., C. S. HAIDLE & Y. M. WANG. 1986. Daunorubicin-induced DNA lesions in isolated rat hepatocytes and mammary epithelial cells. Biochim. Biophys. Acta 868: 254-261.
9. HOWELL, S. K. & Y. M. WANG. 1982. Quantitation of physiological alpha-tocopherol, metabolites, and related compounds by reversed-phase high performance liquid chromatography. J. Chromatog. 227: 174-180.
10. MARQUARDT, H. 1979. DNA-The critical cellular target in chemical carcinogenesis? In Chemical carcinogenesis and DNA. Vol. 2: 159-179. CRC Press. Boca Raton, FL.
11. CATAGNANI, G. L., F. CHYTIL & W. J. DARBY. 1974. Vitamin E deficiency: Immunological evidence for increased accumulation of liver xanthine oxidase. Proc. Natl. Acad. Sci. USA 71: 1966-1968.
12. PAN, S. S. & N. R. BACHUR. 1980. Xanthine oxidase catalyzed reductive cleavage of anthracycline antibiotics and free radical formation. Mol. Pharmacol. 17: 95-99.
13. TOKES, Z. A., K. E. ROGERS & A. ROMBAUM. 1982. Synthesis of adriamycin-coupled polyglutaraldehyde microspheres and evaluation of their cytostatic activity. Proc. Natl. Acad. Sci. USA 79: 2026-2030.
14. TRITON, T. R. & G. YEE. 1982. The anticancer agent adriamycin can be actively cytotoxic without entering cells. Science 217: 248-250.
15. REDDY, M. V. & K. RANDERATH. 1986. Nuclease P1-mediated enhancement of sensitivity of ^{32}P-postlabeling test for structurally diverse DNA adducts. Carcinogenesis 7: 1543-1551.
16. LI, D., Y. M. WANG, R. NATH, S. PARETH & K. RANDERATH. 1988. Vitamin E effect on age-dependent DNA modification (I-compounds) in rat liver and kidney. Proc. Am. Assoc. Cancer Res. 29: 146.

Cancer Mortality and Vitamin E Status

H. B. STÄHELIN,[a] K. F. GEY, M. EICHHOLZER,
E. LÜDIN, AND G. BRUBACHER

Geriatric Clinic
Kantonsspital, University of Basel
4031 Basel, Switzerland
and
Department of Vitamin Research
F. Hoffmann-La Roche Ltd.
CH-4002 Basel, Switzerland

INTRODUCTION

Migration studies and secular trends suggest that human cancer may be dependent to a large extent on exogenous influences.[1] Dietary factors may act on initiation or promotion of tumors or exert a protective effect at various levels of carcinogenesis.[2] This may involve a ubiquitous mechanism like scavenging free radicals or the interference with specific processes such as nitrosamine formation or cellular proliferation and differentiation.[3]

Aggressive oxygen species such as the superoxide anion, the hydroxyl radical, and singlet oxygen have been implicated in cancerogenesis. Essential antioxidants, for example, beta-carotene and the vitamins A, C, and E are part of the body's multilevel defence system against oxygen radicals. These compounds may be considered as natural inhibitors[4] affecting cancer initiation or promotion.

Vitamin E protects fatty acids of cell membranes against peroxidation and may thus inhibit the formation of tumor-promoting compounds.[5] The action of vitamin E probably depends on the presence of ascorbic acid. Thus vitamins may act synergistically.

Different cancer incidences in populations imply possibilities of cancer prevention. Hence, hypotheses derived from metabolic and molecular studies have to be verified in epidemiological studies and finally proven by successful intervention.

VITAMIN E AND CANCER

Evidence is mounting that the uptake and plasma concentration of beta-carotene is inversely associated with cancer, particularly cancer of the lung.[6,7] The findings are

---

[a] Send correspondence to Prof. Dr. Med. H. B. Stähelin, Medizinisch-geriatrische Klinik, Kantonsspital Basel, CH-4031 Basel, Switzerland.

less clear for vitamin A[8-11] and even more controversial for vitamin C.[2,12,13] Despite the important membrane protective action of vitamin E, the relation of alpha-tocopherol to cancer in humans is far from clear. Animal studies are rare, but indicate that alpha-tocopherol may protect against cellular damage produced by active oxygen.[14,15] Vitamin E is effective as an antioxidant at high oxygen concentrations.[16] Vitamin E also inhibits endogenous nitrosation reactions leading to the formation of cancerigenic nitrosamines.[2] Its reaction may even be more complicated, for in a study by Sumijoshi,[17] vitamin E deficiency promoted the initiation of colon tumors induced by 1,2 dimethylhydrazine (DMHC), but inhibited the growth. By contrast, Temple and El-Khabib[18] found in vitamin E-supplemented mice a higher colon tumor incidence. Vitamin E was shown to affect experimentally induced skin, cheek pouch, and fore-stomach carcinogenesis and, to enhance, to have no effect on, or to inhibit colon carcinogenesis. The results depended on selenium status and dietary fat.[19] In human volunteers, the addition of vitamin E and C to the diet decreased fecal mutagenicity significantly.[20]

TABLE 1. Vitamin E and Cancer: Prospective Studies

Study	All	Lung	Cancer Stomach	Colon	Breast
Willett	(+)[a]	0[c]	0	0	0
Wald					+
Salonen	+[b]	(+)			
Nomura		0	0	0	
Risch			0		
Menkes		+			
Knekt	+	(+)	0	0	0
Kok	+	(+)			

[a] (+) = trend
[b] + = significant association
[c] 0 = no association

In the last years several, case control studies based on serum vitamin E have been reported, analyzing vitamin E and subsequent cancer development. From these data no firm conclusions may be drawn. The present state is summarized in TABLE 1.

An association between low vitamin E was observed for all cancer, by Salonen et al.,[21] in nonsmoking men. The risk was particularly high in subjects with coexisting low vitamin E and selenium status (relative risk 11.4). Knekt in 1988 observed a similar trend but only in nonsmoking young subjects and thus in cancer not related to smoking.[22] For females, Knekt[23] reported a statistically significant relative risk for low alpha-tocopherol for all sites and epithelial cancers but no association for cancers in tissue under estrogen control. Willett[10] in 1984 could not find any correlation between cancer and alpha-tocopherol levels.

Lung cancer was significantly inversely associated in the study by Menkes et al.[24] Other studies noted lower values without reaching statistical significance.[11,21,22] Others found no association.[10,25] In stomach cancer as well as colorectal cancer no relationship at all could be demonstrated.[22,25-27] In breast cancer, no association was observed by

Willett[10] and Knekt,[23] a finding that is in contrast to Wald,[8] who found in cases significant lower mean values and a significant increased risk in the lowest quintile.

THE PROSPECTIVE BASEL STUDY

The Basel Study was started originally in 1960 as a survey on cardiovascular diseases. To it was added, at the follow-up in 1971-1973 (Basel Study (BS) III)—as a unique feature of an epidemiological study of this size—the analysis of plasma vitamins, as well as other laboratory parameters and life-style variables.[28] At this time, 2974 men and 688 women were evaluated. Recently a mortality follow-up was completed,[29] and cancer deaths were analyzed with regard to antioxidant vitamins, cholesterol, and smoking.[13] In the period from 1973 until 1985 (12 years), 204 men died from cancer. The cancer cases were grouped as follows: all cancer (International Classification of Diseases (ICD) 8th revision 140-239; n = 204), lung cancer (ICD 162; n = 68), stomach cancer (ICD 151; n = 20), and gastrointestinal cancer (ICD 151, 153; n = 37).

In contrast to most other studies that used the case control approach, we are able to compare the investigated variables in cancer cases to the total number of noncancer cases. Here the results of the plasma vitamin E are given.

The statistical analysis was divided into two parts: (1) a description of the data (to illustrate differences, appropriate significance tests were done (analysis of covariants adjusted for smoking habits and age)); and (2) a risk analysis, where the analysis of explanatory variables was based on Cox's proportional hazard regression model for survival data.[30,31] Subjects below quartile (Q) 1 were considered at risk and compared to higher quartiles.

Inasmuch as alpha-tocopherol is transported in lipoproteins,[32] lipid adjustment is mandatory.[33] TABLE 2 gives correlation coefficients for fat soluble vitamins and plasma lipids in the Basel Study obtained in BS III. The best fit for alpha-tocopherol was observed for betalipoproteins. Because this measurement is not available in other epidemiological studies, however, we used the slightly inferior fit by taking the sum of total cholesterol and triglycerides in order to assure comparability. Hence all alpha-tocopherol values were adjusted to a cholesterol and triglyceride of 330 mg/dL. Inasmuch as most studies do not have fasting blood samples, triglycerides were not routinely determined. Hence, most studies adjusted, if at all, for cholesterol, which is a good estimate of LDL.

Again BS III offers the possibility to evaluate the contribution of triglycerides. In BS III, fasting plasma samples were obtained each Tuesday between 7 and 9 A.M. and immediately analyzed. These results allowed us to estimate the various intercorrelations and to correct accordingly. The values in TABLE 2 are Pearson's correlation coefficients of log values. It becomes evident that only adjustment to the sum of cholesterol and triglycerides (in mg/dL) allows a lipid-independent estimation of vitamin E as well as of vitamin A status. In the case of beta-carotene, adjustment to cholesterol alone is sufficient.

There is, incidentally, no correlation between retinol and beta-carotene plasma levels (r = 0.06), which confirms the observation by Olsen that in affluent Western societies, plasma levels of beta-carotene and retinol behave independently.[34] It can also be noted that after adjustment, a significant, albeit small, correlation exists between vitamin E and both vitamin A and beta-carotene (TABLE 2).

TABLE 2. Correlation of Plasma Vitamins with Plasma Lipids
Pearsons Correlation Coefficients
BS III (1971–1973), n = 2974

	Vitamin A	Beta-carotene	Vitamin C	Cholesterol	Triglyceride	β-lipoprotein	Cholesterol and Triglycerides
Vitamin E	0.34	0.21	0.02	0.56	0.50	0.72	0.64
adjusted	0.11	0.23	0.09	0.16	-0.10	0.24	0.00
Vitamin A		-0.03	-0.02	0.25	0.39	0.39	0.41
adjusted		-0.06	0.01	0.02	0.02	0.05	0.00
Beta-carotene			0.16	0.23	-0.06	0.06	0.05
Vitamin C				-0.05	-0.06	-0.06	-0.08
Cholesterol					-0.07	0.62	0.67
Triglycerides					0.34	0.74	0.90
β-lipoprotein							0.84

RESULTS

Of the 2974 men investigated in 1971-1973 (BS III), 204 died from cancer (6.9%). The total mortality was 553 (18.6%) and will not be considered further. As mentioned above, females, due to the low number of deaths in the observation period, were excluded from the analysis. Bronchial cancer was, with 68 cases, by far the most common cancer, followed by stomach cancer (n = 20) and colon cancer (n = 17). Gastrointestinal cancer, thus, made up 37 cases (rectum excluded). The mean age of the survivors, in BS III, was 50 ± 9.3 years. Mean age of cancer cases was, as expected, significantly higher: 60.47 ± 7.6 years (p <0.01). In BS III, one-third of the survivors were cigarette smokers, that is, 72% of the subjects who died from lung cancer (p <0.01) and 47.6% of all cancer cases (p <0.01). Smoking was not more prevalent than in survivors among stomach and gastrointestinal cancer cases.

A comparison of the mean vitamin E values among the different groups considered revealed no differences. By contrast, vitamin A, beta-carotene, and vitamin C were found to be associated with cancer mortality either at distinct sites or with overall cancer mortality (TABLE 3).

RISK ANALYSIS FOR VITAMIN E AND CANCER

Subjects with lipid-adjusted alpha-tocopherol values below Q 1 (12.9 mg/L) were considered at risk and compared with subjects with higher values. For this analysis, age, smoking, vitamin A, beta-carotene, vitamin C, cholesterol, and the computed oxidative potential (the molar product of the lipid-adjusted vitamins A, E, beta-carotene, and vitamin C (CIA-VIT)) were simultaneously considered. Only for bronchial cancer was there a tendency toward increased risk for low alpha-tocopherol levels, albeit statistically not significant (p = 0.16). In all cancer, stomach and gastrointestinal cancer, no effect was noted. Smoking proved to be, as expected, associated with cancer and caused a greatly increased risk. Unexpectedly, subjects with cholesterol values below Q 1 (5.16 mmol/L) were found to be at a significantly elevated risk for cancer death.

DISCUSSION

In the 12-year cancer mortality follow-up, we could no longer observe the statistically significant lower vitamin E concentration in gastrointestinal cancer and in all cancer observed in the 7-year follow-up.[35] In accordance with Menkes,[24] Knekt,[22] and Kok,[11] we could on the other hand observe a tendency to a higher risk for lung cancer associated with low vitamin E.

The discrepancy in our previous findings may be explained by the use of Cox's proportional hazard regression model[30] in the 12-year follow-up and the adjustment to cholesterol and triglycerides. In the 7-year follow-up, the model by Peto was used.[35]

TABLE 3. Mean Plasma Vitamin Concentrations in Survivors and in Cancer Victims in the Basel Study, 1973–1985

| N | Survivors 2421 | All 204 | Cancer | | |
			Bronchial 68	Stomach 20	Gastrointestinal 37
Vit. E (adjusted) mg/L	14.9(2.9)[a]	14.9(2.9)	14.5(3.4)	14.7(3.4)	14.8(2.9)
Vit. A (adjusted) μmol/L	2.81(0.57)	2.81(0.67)	2.77(0.70)	2.60(0.48)[c]	2.79(0.66)
Carotene μmol/L	0.43(0.27)	0.34(0.24)[b]	0.30(0.20)[b]	0.28(0.18)[b]	0.37(0.28)[c]
Vit. C μmol/L	52.8(21.7)	47.6(25.4)[b]	52.4(30.3)	42.8(21.8)[c]	45.9(21.6)

[a] Standard deviation.
[b] $p < 0.01$.
[c] $p < 0.05$.

As can be noted from TABLE 2, the method chosen for adjustment may influence substantially the individual risk assignment.

Nevertheless, the inconclusive epidemiological findings contrast to the large biological importance of vitamin E in protecting membranes against oxidative damage.[36] Again some of the discrepancies can be explained by different study designs. Case-control studies are less powerful than the comparison of cases to almost 3000 noncases, as in our study. Another fact that makes direct comparison difficult is the loss of vitamin E under various storage conditions. Indeed, the reported vitamin E concentrations are in other studies clearly below alpha-tocopherol concentrations observed in BS III. Knekt[22] reported, for his over 800 cases, a mean value of 8.03 mg/L, and for controls, 10.03 mg/L (TABLE 4). In another study by Knekt, Q 1 was < 7.9 mg/L, and a higher risk was observed, particularly in the presence of low cholesterol.[37] Similarly, Kok et al. reported lower mean vitamin E levels (7.2 in cases vs 8.5 mg/ L in controls). Salonen[21] had even lower values, that is, between 4.6 in smoking cases and 5.6 in nonsmoking controls, values that are comparable to Wald's[8] (4.7 mg/L in cases vs 6.0 mg/L in controls). Menkes et al.[24] reported values closer to the ones in the BS: 10.5 versus 11.9, a difference statistically significant as well a significantly higher risk for subjects below Q 1. Finally, Willett[26] with unadjusted alpha-tocopherol levels between 11.6 and 12.6 mg/L could not detect an increased risk attributable to low vitamin E. In our study, alpha-tocopherol was determined immediately after venipuncture; hence, no storage loss occurred. The lower values in cancer cases and controls in other studies in comparison to our results (TABLE 4) may reflect storage loss, but also probably a better vitamin E intake in our population, inasmuch as vitamin E intake significantly predicts plasma alpha-tocopherol levels.[38]

Because significant association of low vitamin E with cancer was found in cohorts with low values,[8,11,21,22] the question of a threshold effect arises. The significant association of lung cancer, by Menkes et al.,[24] with higher values, however, argues against such an interpretation. The BS has no data on selenium. Animal experiments as well as epidemiological findings suggest that the coexistence of low selenium in conjunction with low vitamin E increases cancer risk substantially.[19] Whether this is of importance in the BS cohort remains open.

Finally, low CIA-Vit (computed antioxidative potential of plasma vitamins (adjusted for lipids)) was a risk for stomach cancer in subjects older than 60 years. Neither beta-carotene nor vitamin E alone reach statistical significance. CIA-Vit is probably mostly affected by beta-carotene, which may vary several fold (see TABLE 3), whereas the variations of other antioxidants contributing to CIA-Vit are much

TABLE 4. Plasma Vitamin E Concentration in Different Studies

Study	Vitamin E Concentration		
	Cases	Controls	
Wald 1984	4.7	6.0	mg/L
Salonen 1985	4.6	5.6	mg/L
Kok 1987	7.2(2.0)[a]	8.5(3.0)	mg/L
Knekt 1988	8.0(2.6)	10.3(3.3)	mg/L
Menkes 1986	10.5(3.2)	11.9(4.9)	mg/L
Willett 1984	11.6	12.6	mg/L
Basel Study 1973/1985	14.9(2.9)	14.9(2.9)	mg/L

[a] Standard deviation.

smaller. Hence, variations of beta-carotene, not alpha-tocopherol, may to a large extent determine the CIA-Vit value. Thus, the observed association of an increased risk in stomach cancer and subjects above 60 years of age reflect more beta-carotene than the other components.

In addition, the significant correlation of beta-carotene with vitamin E ($r = 0.23$) may obscure in our logistic model an independent effect. It may also reflect the fact that subjects with good vitamin E intake also tend to have high beta-carotene concentrations.

In conclusion, we have found more evidence to show that low vitamin E is associated with an overall increased risk for cancer, albeit the association seems not very strong in the affluent Western societies that we studied. In addition, the interpretation of the available epidemiological data is made more difficult by major methodological problems. Thus, albeit definite proof of an association of low vitamin E and cancer is still lacking, the result of the Basel Study indirectly supports a correlation of low vitamin E with high cancer incidence.

REFERENCES

1. DOLL, R. & R. PETO. 1981. The causes of cancer: quantitative estimates of avoidable risks of cancer in the United States today. J. Natl. Cancer Inst. **66:** 1192-1308.
2. BERTRAM, J. S., L. N. KOLONEL & F. L. MEYSKENS. 1987. Rationale and strategies for chemoprevention of cancer in humans. Cancer Res. **47:** 3012-3031.
3. OLSON, J. A. 1972. The biological role of vitamin A in maintaining epithelial tissues. Isr. J. Med. Sci. **8:** 1170-1178.
4. METTLIN, C. 1984. Diet and the epidemiology of human breast cancer. Cancer **53:** 605-611.
5. LEVIJ, I. S. & A. POLLIACK. 1968. Potentiating effect of vitamin A on 9-10 dimethyl 1-2 benzanthracene-carcinogenesis in the hamster cheek pouch. Cancer **22:** 300-306.
6. STÄHELIN, H. B., F. RÖSEL, E. BUESS & G. BRUBACHER. 1984. Cancer, vitamins and plasma lipids: Prospective Basel Study. J. Natl. Cancer Inst. **73:** 1463-1468.
7. STÄHELIN, H. B., M. EICHHOLZER, E. LÜDIN, F. BERNASCONI, J. THURNEYSEN, F. GEY & G. BRUBACHER. 1989. Antioxidant vitamins, and the risk of death from cancer of specific sites in the Basel Prospective Study. Submitted.
8. WALD, N., M. IDLE & J. BORCHAM. 1984. Low serum vitamin A and subsequent risk of cancer. Lancet **2:** 813-819.
9. PELEG, I., S. HEYDEN, M. KNOWLES & C. G. HANNES. 1984. Serum retinol and risk of subsequent cancer; extension of the Evans County Georgia Study. J. Natl. Cancer Inst. **73:** 1455-1458.
10. WILLETT, W. C., B. F. POLK, B. A. UNDERWOOD *et al.* 1984. Relation of serum vitamins A and E and carotenoids to the risk of cancer. N. Engl. J. Med. **310:** 430-434.
11. KOK, F. J., C. M. DUIJN, A. HOFMAN *et al.* 1987. Micronutrients and the risk of lung cancer. N. Engl. J. Med. **316:** 1416.
12. KROMHOUT, D. 1987. Essential micronutrients in relation to carcinogenesis. Am. J. Clin. Nutr. **45:** 1361-1367.
13. STÄHELIN, H. B., K. F. GEY & G. BRUBACHER. 1987. Plasma vitamin C and cancer death: the prospective Basel Study. Ann. N.Y. Acad. Sci. **498:** 124-131.
14. CERUTTI, P. A. 1985. Prooxidant states and tumor promotion. Science **227:** 375-81.
15. SUMMERFIELD, F. W. & A. L. TAPPEL. 1984. Vitamin E protects against methyl-ethyl peroxide-induced peroxidative damage to rat brain DNA. Mutat. Res. **122:** 113-120.
16. BURTON, G. W. & K. U. INGOLD. 1984. Beta-carotene: an unusual type of lipid antioxidant. Science **224:** 569-573.
17. SUMIYOSHI, H. 1985. Effects of vitamin E deficiency on 1,2 dimethylhydrazine-induced intestinal carcinogenesis in rats. Hiroshima J. Med. Sci. **34:** 363-369.

18. TEMPLE, N. J. & S. M. EL-KHABIB. 1987. Cabbage and vitamin E: their effect on colon tumor formation in mice. Cancer Lett. **35:** 71-77.
19. BIRT, D. F. 1986. Updates on the effect of vitamins A, C and E and selenium on carcinogenesis. Proc. Soc. Exp. Biol. Med. **183:** 311-320.
20. DION, P. W., E. B. BRIGHT-SEE, C. C. SMITH & W. R. BRUCE. 1982. The effect of dietary ascorbic acid and alpha-tocopherol on fecal mutagenicity. Mutat. Res. **102:** 27-37.
21. SALONEN, J. T., R. SALONEN, R. LAPPETETAINEN et al. 1985. Risk of cancer in relation to serum concentrations of selenium and vitamins A nd E: matched case control analysis of prospective data. Br. Med. J. **290:** 417-420.
22. KNEKT, P., A. AROMAA, J. MAATELA et al. 1988. Serum vitamin E and risk of cancer among Finnish men during a 10-year follow-up. Am. J. Epidemiol. **127:** 28-41.
23. KNEKT, P. 1988. Serum vitamin E level and risk of female cancers. Int. J. Epidemiol. **17:** 281-288.
24. MENKES, M. S., G. W. COMSTOCK, J. P. VUILLEUMIER, K. J. HELSING, A. A. RIDER & R. BROOKMEYER. 1986. Serum beta-carotene, vitamins A and E, selenium and the risk of lung cancer. N. Engl. J. Med. **315:** 1250-1254.
25. NOMURA, A. M. J., G. N. STEMMERMANN, L. K. HEILBRUNN et al. 1985. Serum vitamin levels and the risk of cancer of specific sites in men of Japanese ancestry in Hawaii. Cancer Res. **45:** 2369-2372.
26. ATUKORALA, S., T. K. BARN, J. W. T. DICKERSON, D. DONALDSON & A. SAKULA. 1979. Vitamin A, zinc and lung cancer. Br. J. Cancer **40:** 927-931.
27. RISCH, H. A., M. JAIN, N. W. CHOI et al. 1985. Dietary factors and the incidence of cancer of the stomach. Am. J. Epidemiol. **122:** 947-955.
28. WIDMER, L. K., H. B. STÄHELIN, C. NISSEN & A. DA SILVA. 1981. Basler Studie: Venen-, Arterienkrankheiten, koronare Herzkrankheit bei Berufstätigen. Bern, Huber.
29. STÄHELIN, H. B., J. THURNEYSEN, E. BUESS, F. RÖSEL et al. 1988. Todesfälle und Todesursachen im 20-Jahres Follow-up der Basler Studie. Schweiz. Med. Wochenschr. **118:** 1039-1047.
30. COX, D. R. 1972. Regression models and life tables. J. Roy. Stat. Soc. Series B **34:** 187-220.
31. BMDP STATISTICAL SOFTWARE, UNIVERSITY OF CALIFORNIA. 1983. Berkeley.
32. JÜRGENS, G., H. F. HOFT, G. M. CHISOLM III & H. ESTERBAUER. 1987. Modification of human serum low density lipoprotein by oxidation—Characterization and pathophysiological implications. Chem. Phys. Lipids **45:** 315-336.
33. BRUBACHER, G., H. B. STÄHELIN & J. P. VUILLEUMIER. 1974. Beziehung zwischen Beta-Lipoproteingehalt des Serums und Plasma Vitamin E-Gehalt. Ein Beitrag zur Frage der Beurteilung des Vitamin E-Status beim Menschen. Int. Z. Vitamin. Ernaehrungsforsch. **44:** 521-526.
34. OLSEN, J. A. 1984. Serum levels of vitamin A and carotenoids as reflector of nutritional status. J. Natl. Cancer Inst. **73:** 1439-1444.
35. GEY, K. F., G. B. BRUBACHER & H. B. STÄHELIN. 1987. Plasma levels of antioxidant vitamins in relation to ischemic heart disease and cancer. Am. J. Clin. Nutr. **45:** 1368-1377.
36. NIKI, E. 1987. Interaction of ascorbate and α-tocopherol. Ann. N. Y. Acad. Sci. **498:** 186-199.
37. KNEKT, P., A. REUNANEN, A. AROMAA et al. 1988. Serum cholesterol and risk of cancer in a cohort of 39,000 men and women. J. Clin. Epidemiol. **41:** 519-530.
38. STRYKER, W. S., L. KAPLAN, E. A. STEIN, M. J. STAMPFER, A. SOBER & W. C. WILLETT. 1988. The relation of diet, cigarette smoking, and alcohol consumption to plasma beta-carotene and alpha-tocopherol levels. Am. J. Epidemiol. **127(2):** 283-296.

Vitamin E: The Status of Current Research and Suggestions for Future Studies

WILLIAM A. PRYOR

Biodynamics Institute
Louisiana State University
Baton Rouge, Louisiana 70803

The Society for Free Radical Research organized an informal discussion group on vitamin E research at a meeting in 1986 in Düsseldorf. Despite the fact that this meeting ran in competition with one of the regularly scheduled sessions, the attendance at the vitamin E meeting was large and enthusiastic, and a great deal of exciting science was reported. After this stimulating session, several of us realized that an international conference on vitamin E would be very timely and useful, and so this New York Academy of Sciences meeting was born.

The timing was perfect. All of the persons that attended both the New York Academy of Sciences meeting on vitamin E held in November 1982 and this meeting agreed that a watershed had been reached in the scientific study of vitamin E. It is unfortunate, but true, that our scientific understanding of vitamin E has developed more or less in parallel with a nonscientific literature that sometimes is scandalously inaccurate. This is partly because the original rat fetus resorption assay caused an unfortunate association in the lay press of vitamin E and sexual potency.[1-3] Some of the controversy arises because vitamin E is an antioxidant that protects biological systems against damage by free radicals, and the free radical literature itself has been amazingly controversial for more than 100 years, with leading chemists at the turn of the century arguing whether radicals could or could not exist.[4,5]

The papers presented at this meeting make abundantly clear that we have entered an era of well-planned and carefully performed scientific studies on vitamin E. The new biochemical studies that were described, the new animal data, the human clinical trials, and the human epidemiological data that were presented all reflect a substantial new body of literature pointing out new roles for vitamin E.

A NEW ERA IN PREVENTIVE MEDICINE

The new attitude toward vitamin E arises partly because of a sweeping new view of nutrition that has gained dominance in the last few years.[6-9] In the USA in 1900, the primary causes of death were pneumonia, influenza, tuberculosis, and similar contagious diseases; heart disease was responsible for only 8% of the deaths, and cancer for just 4 percent. In 1983, however, the contagious diseases were under control;

none was responsible for more than 1% of deaths, whereas heart and cardiovascular diseases were responsible for nearly half of the deaths and cancer for nearly a quarter.[10] These new killer diseases are more easily prevented than cured. For example, D. H. Hegsted remarked in his 1985 Atwater Award address[11] that we are now in an era for industrial nations in which chronic diseases are the "... primary health concern. ... Most of us will die from one or more of those diseases—coronary heart disease, cancer, stroke, hypertension, or diabetes. Major improvements in the health of Americans depend on bringing these diseases under control. The major opportunities in nutrition lie in this area. ..." A similar point of view was expressed recently with regard to cancer by Boutwell,[12] who stated that, "In experimental animals, protection against both genetically-determined and intentionally-induced cancer is provided by diet. Therefore, optimism is justified that reduction in human cancer morbidity and mortality through nutrition can be accomplished."

It is becoming increasingly clear that the important chronic killer diseases, such as cancer, heart and blood vessel diseases, osteoarthritis, emphysema, and (perhaps) diabetes and cirrhosis involve radical reactions in some stage in their development.[6,13,14] Vitamin E is the principal, lipid-soluble, chain-breaking antioxidant and radical scavenger in human tissue.[15] Therefore, there is reason to hope that vitamin E may provide important protection against and/or delay the onset of these life-limiting processes.

It also has become clear in recent years that oxidative stress is an inescapable result of aerobic metabolism. When life became dependent upon oxygen and when respiration became the principal energy-producing process, a continuing level of oxidative damage to tissue had to be endured. The level of damage is quite striking. For example, humans excrete in the urine over 1,000 molecules of oxidatively damaged thymine per cell per day.[16] Similarly, deoxyguanosine is oxidized to 8-hydroxydeoxyguanosine in animals subjected to oxidative stresses of a variety of types.[17] Compounds that react with thiobarbituric acid (TBA) are found in human plasma in greater amounts for humans with a variety of disease conditions (such as atherosclerosis) than in normal patients.[18] Both animals and humans continually exhale ethane and pentane from the conversion of n-3 and n-6 polyunsaturated fatty acids (PUFA) to hydroperoxides and the subsequent decomposition of these hydroperoxides.[19,20] It was recently reported, in fact, that the amounts of pentane exhaled in breath correlate significantly with the vitamin E status of human patients.[20]

Although the current literature gives good hope for a beneficial effect for vitamin E on a variety of pathologies, the data are not yet complete.[6-9,21] There currently are 28 human trials in progress, sponsored by the National Cancer Institute, that are examining the role of various micronutrients in the development of cancer, using a prospective, double-blind protocol.[22] As the results of these studies begin to appear, the possible role of vitamin E (as well as, *e.g.,* ascorbate and beta-carotene) in preventing cancer will become clearer. Nevertheless, the evidence that is now available both from animal and human studies is very encouraging.[23,24]

FUTURE RESEARCH DIRECTIONS

Where do we go from here? The advances and new science presented at this meeting are impressive, especially in view of the fact that only eight years have elapsed since the previous New York Academy of Sciences vitamin E meeting. New scientists with new perspectives are entering the field. For example, I was impressed with the number of reports on proteins: the purification of tocopherol-binding and transport proteins, the binding of tocopherol to enzymes, and the enzyme-catalyzed reduction of the tocopheroxyl radical by ascorbate.

BIOCHEMICAL RESEARCH

From a biochemical perspective, three areas seem to me to need development. First, we have now entered the era of the measurement of absolute rate constants for a variety of oxidative processes involving tocopherol. The rate constants for the propagation and termination steps for the autoxidation of several PUFA and PUFA-containing lipids have been measured in micelles, but values are needed for systems that more closely model biological bilayers. A discussion held several years[25] ago asked whether the rate constants obtained with styrene as the oxidizable substrate in chlorobenzene solution might also apply to aqueous systems; we now know that the rate constants are substantially different for PUFA autoxidation in micelles relative to styrene oxidation in chlorobenzene.[26] The reactions of peroxyl radicals with lipids and with tocopherol in a bilayer, however, are only just beginning to be studied, and further data of this type are needed.[26,27]

Second, evidence is accumulating for the reduction of the α-tocopheroxyl radical by various reducing agents such as glutathione (GSH) and ascorbate, and rate constants for these processes need to be determined in a bilayer system. An extremely important line of investigation asks: Is the re-reduction of the α-tocopheroxyl radical by a biological reducing agent such as GSH or ascorbate enzymatically catalyzed? Present evidence indicates that it is. If a cofactor role were identified for vitamin E as part of an enzyme-controlled cascade of reducing equivalents, the implications would be vast. For example, it might be possible to design an enzyme-based test for vitamin E status that would provide fresh insights over the tests now used.

The third biochemical area that appears to be important to me, as I remarked above, concerns the interaction of vitamin E with proteins. How is tocopherol carried through plasma and cellular fluids to membranes or to other storage depots? Do changes in the levels of plasma lipoproteins have implications about vitamin E status for humans?

MEASURES OF OXIDATIVE STRESS

It would be very useful to have an established battery of (preferably noninvasive) methods for determining the instantaneous status of an organism with regard to the oxidative stress caused by toxins, exercise, mental stress, diseases, or by aging itself. Tests presently developed include the detection of oxidized thymine derivatives in urine, 8-hydroxydeoxyguanosine in tissue or urine, TBA-reactive substances in plasma, PUFA and antioxidant concentration changes in fat depots, ethane/pentane exhalation, and the detection of products (such as hydroperoxides, malonaldehyde and its precursors, alkenals, etc.) from oxidized PUFA. Do these tests agree? Can they validate each other? Are some more useful in some circumstances than others? If reliable tests were established, the protective and moderating effects of vitamin E against stress could be more easily established.

One group of papers in the literature suggests how interesting this field could be. Cigarette smoke puts a chronic oxidative burden on the lung.[28] Vitamin E is depleted in the alveolar fluid of smokers.[29] In addition, pentane exhalation is elevated in smokers, but interestingly, plasma malonaldehyde is not elevated.[30] Thus, radical production is elevated by smoking, but the effects can be seen only by techniques sensitive to changes within the lung.

VITAMIN E AND THE INFLAMMATORY PROCESS

The possible role of tocopherol in changing the balance of the products from the arachidonic acid cascade should be studied further. The current literature indicates that α-tocopherol is a mild antiinflammatory compound. What are the mechanisms involved? Possibilities include control of lipases and the release of arachidonic acid, control of the radical flux (and feedback control of prostaglandin (PG) and thromboxane (TX) production), and direct interaction of α-tocopherol itself with one or more of the PG synthetase complex of enzymes.

PHARMACOKINETICS

What are the rates and controlling factors for the uptake of the tocopherols by various tissues? What are the products of tocopherol metabolism? For example, does the ratio of alpha-tocopherol to its quinone provide a measure of the oxidative stress on a tissue? Some of these problems must be studied in animals using radio-labeled tocopherol isomers. Some can be studied directly in humans, however, using the deuterium-labeled tocopherol methods pioneered by the National Research Council group and reported on at this meeting.

VITAMIN E AND LIFE EXPECTANCY

Some antioxidants extend the mean (but not the maximum) lifespan of laboratory mammals, but alpha-tocopherol does not have this effect. If the free radical theory is correct, and if oxidative stress is an important lifespan-limiting factor, then why does tocopherol not have an effect similar to certain of the synthetic antioxidants and radiation-protectant drugs, such as 2-mercaptoethanol? Is the reason, as some have suggested, that a homeostasis in total antioxidant status of tissue is maintained?[13,31,32] This is an important question worth further study.

Another area worthy of research concerns the implications of other life-extension methods on free radical biology. The technique of reducing caloric intake is the most powerful method known for extending lifespan, producing extensions of 30 to 50 percent.[33,34] For this reason it is important to ask: What is the effect of caloric restriction on measures of oxidative stress or on tocopherol pharmacokinetics? I believe these questions are critical probes of the free radical theory of aging.

VITAMIN E AND HUMAN DISEASES

An area of critical importance, and one in which I believe great progress has been made since the 1982 vitamin E meeting,[2] is the role of vitamin E in delaying or preventing the critical, chronic lifespan-limiting diseases. In these areas we need to know biochemical mechanisms, and animal models must be developed.

In studies on humans, a number of papers dealing with retrospective serum bank studies of cardiovascular diseases and cancer were reported at this meeting. Prospective intervention trials involving micronutrients such as the tocopherols, ascorbate, beta-carotene, and selenium are currently ongoing. As the results of these trials become known, our knowledge of free radical biology and the ability of antioxidants to improve human health will be greatly strengthened.

Impressive new evidence was presented at this meeting that senile cataracts and the age-related decrease in the immune response are influenced by vitamin E status. Vitamin E also could influence age-related maculopathy, arthritis, and the decline in the neurological function with age. Exciting results on the involvement of oxidative processes in marking HDL for uptake by macrophages and on the involvement of radicals in tumor initiation and promotion have been presented. In view of our aging population and the tremendous health implications of these issues, further research in these areas offers great prospects for the future.

REFERENCES

1. LUBIN, B. & L. J. MACHLIN, EDS. 1982. Vitamin E: Biochemical, Hematological, and Clinical Aspects. Ann. N.Y. Acad. Sci. Vol. 393. New York Academy of Sciences. New York.
2. PRYOR, W. 1982. Free radical biology: xenobiotics, cancer, and aging. In Vitamin E: Biochemical, Hematological, and Clinical Aspects. B. Lubin & L. J. Machlin, Eds. Vol. 393: 1-22. New York Academy of Sciences. New York.
3. MACHLIN, L. J. 1980. Vitamin E. Dekker. New York, NY.
4. PRYOR, W. 1988. A festschrift volume celebrating the 20th anniversary of the discovery of superoxide dismutase. Free Rad. Biol. Med. 5: 271-273.
5. PRYOR, W. 1968. Organic free radicals. Chem. Eng. News 46: 70-89.
6. PRYOR, W. 1987. Views on the wisdom of using antioxidant vitamin supplements. Free Rad. Biol. Med. 3(3): 189-191.
7. DIPLOCK, A. T. 1987. Dietary supplementation with antioxidants. Is there a case for exceeding the recommended dietary allowance? Free Rad. Biol. Med. 3(3): 199-201.
8. JACOBSON, H. N. 1987. Dietary standards and future developments. Free Rad. Biol. Med. 3(3): 209-213.
9. BIERI, J. G. 1987. Are the recommended allowances for dietary antioxidants adequate? Free Rad. Biol. Med. 3(3): 193-197.

10. LEAF, A. 1988. The aging process: Lessons from observations in man. Nutr. Rev. **46**: 40-44.
11. HEGSTED, D. M. 1985. Nutrition: The changing scene. Nutr. Rev. **43**(12): 357-367.
12. BOUTWELL, R. K. 1988. An overview of the role of diet and nutrition in carcinogenesis. *In* Nutrition, Growth and Cancer. 81-104. Alan R. Liss. New York, NY.
13. PRYOR, W. A. 1987. The free-radical theory of aging revisited: A critique and a suggested disease-specific theory. *In* Modern Biological Theories of Aging. H. R. Warner, R. N. Butler & R. L. Sprott, Eds: 89-112. Raven Press. New York, NY.
14. PRYOR, W. A. 1984. *In* Free Radicals in Molecular Biology, Aging, and Disease. D. Armstrong, R. S. Sohal, R. G. Cutler & T. F. Slater, Eds.: 13-54. Raven Press. New York, NY.
15. BURTON, G. W. & K. U. INGOLD. 1981. Autoxidation of biological molecules. 1. The antioxidant activity of vitamin E and related chain-breaking phenolic antioxidants *in vitro.* J. Am. Chem. Soc. **103**: 6472-6477.
16. AMES, B. N. 1989. Endogenous DNA damage as related to cancer and aging. Mutat. Res. Special Ed. 2-6.
17. KASAI, H., P. F. CRAIN, Y. KUCHINO, S. NISHIMURA, A. OOTSUYAMA & H. TANOOKA. 1986. Formation of 8-hydroxyguanine moiety in cellular DNA by agents producing oxygen radicals and evidence for its repair. Carcinogenesis **7**: 1849-1851.
18. YAGI, K. 1984. Increased serum lipid peroxides initiate atherogenesis. BioEssays **1**: 58-60.
19. DILLARD, C. J., V. C. GAVINO & A. L. TAPPEL. 1983. Relative antioxidant effectiveness of α-tocopherol and γ-tocopherol in iron-loaded rats. J. Nutr. **113**: 2266-2273.
20. VAN GOSSUM, A., R. KURIAN, J. WHITWELL & K. N. JEEJEEBHOY. 1988. Decrease in lipid peroxidation measured by breath pentane output in normals after oral supplementation with vitamin E. Clin. Nutr. **7**: 53-57.
21. DRAPER, H. H. & R. P. BIRD. 1987. Micronutrients and cancer prevention: Are the RDAs adequate? Free Rad. Biol. Med. **3**(3): 203-207.
22. Anonymous. 1984. Backgrounder. p. 3. National Cancer Institute. Bethesda, MD.
23. MIRVISH, S. S. 1986. Effects of vitamins C and E on N-nitroso compound formation, carcinogenesis, and cancer. Cancer **58**: 1842-1850.
24. WALD, N. J., S. G. THOMPSON, J. W. DENSEM & J. BOREHAM. 1987. Serum vitamin E and human cancer. *In* Clinical and Nutritional Aspects of Vitamin E. O. Hayaishi & M. Mino, Eds.: 73-82. Elsevier. Amsterdam.
25. Ciba Foundation Symposium 101. 1983. Biology of vitamin E. Pitman. London.
26. PRYOR, W. A., T. STRICKLAND & D. F. CHURCH. 1988. Comparison of the efficiencies of several natural and synthetic antioxidants in aqueous sodium dodecyl sulfate micelle solutions. J. Am. Chem. Soc. **110**: 2224.
27. BARCLAY, L., K. A. BASKIN, S. J. LOCKE & M. R. VINQUIST. 1989. Absolute rate constants for lipid peroxidation and inhibition in model biomembranes. Can. J. Chem. **67**: 1366-1369.
28. PRYOR, W. A., D. G. PRIER & D. F. CHURCH. 1983. Electron-spin resonance study of mainstream and sidestream cigarette smoke: Nature of the free radicals in gas-phase smoke and in cigarette tar. Environ. Health Perspect. **47**: 345-355.
29. PACHT, E. R., H. KASEKI, J. R. MOHAMMED, D. G. CORNWELL & W. B. DAVIS. Deficiency of vitamin E in the alveolar fluid of cigarette smokers. J. Clin. Invest. **77**: 789-796.
30. SHARIFF, R., E. HOSHINO, J. ALLARD, C. PICHARD, R. KURIAN & K. N. JEEJEEBHOY. Vitamin E supplementation in smokers. Am. J. Clin. Nutr. **47**(4): 758.
31. BALIN, A. K. 1982. Testing the free radical theory of aging. *In* Testing the Theories of Aging. R. C. Adelman & G. S. Roth, Eds.: 138-185. CRC Press. Boca Raton, FL.
32. SOHAL, R. S. & R. G. ALLEN. 1985. Relationship between metabolic rate, free radicals, differentiation and aging; a unified theory. *In* Molecular Biology of Aging. A. D. Woodhead, A. D. Blackett & A. Hollaender, Eds.: 75-104. Plenum. New York, NY.
33. LAGANIERE, S. & B. P. YU. 1987. Anti-lipoperoxidation action of food restriction. Biochem. Biophys. Res. Commun. **145**(3): 1185-1191.
34. WALFORD, R. L., S. B. HARRIS & R. WEINDRUCH. 1987. Dietary restriction and aging: Historical phases, mechanisms and current directions. J. Nutr. **117**: 1650-1654.

Pharmacokinetic Modeling and Bioavailability of *RRR* and *All-Racemic* Alpha-Tocopheryl Acetate in Human Blood Components[a]

R. V. ACUFF,[b] K. E. FERSLEW, E. A. DAIGNEAULT,
R. H. ORCUTT, S. S. THEDFORD, AND
P. E. STANTON

Departments of Pharmacology and Surgery
East Tennessee State University
Johnson City, Tennessee 37614

Bioavailability is both the rate and extent of absorption of a substance from a dosage form to reach circulation. Different forms of vitamin E, though apparently chemically equivalent, may not be bioequivalent; therefore, differences in the forms may produce significant differences in their degree of pharmacological effect and/or clinical response.[1] It has been suggested that the relative biological activity of the different forms of vitamin E could be related to the vitamin's bioavailability.

This investigation was undertaken to determine if there are differences between absorption, distribution, elimination, or overall bioavailability of *RRR* and *all rac* in plasma or red blood cells (RBC) following a single, oral administration of a pharmacological dose. Plasma alpha-tocopherol concentrations per mg plasma lipid (cholesterol, triglycerides, phospholipids) were also modeled to determine if alpha-tocopherol bioavailability is related to plasma lipid kinetics.

MATERIAL AND METHODS

Twenty-seven healthy, male volunteers (18-40 yr) participated in the study. Twenty-four subjects were given three 400 mg doses of either *RRR* or *all rac*-alpha-tocopheryl acetate in soft gelatin capsules with breakfast. Three subjects (placebo controls) were administered similar capsules containing corn oil stripped of toco-

[a]This work was supported by Eastman Chemical Products, Inc., Kingsport, TN.

[b]To whom all correspondence should be addressed at the Division of Clinical Nutrition, Department of Surgery.

pherols. Doses were administered as a double-blind randomized crossover design. A fasted venous blood sample (15 mL) was obtained five days, three days, and one day prior to dosing. Additional samples were obtained at 0, 1, 2, 4, 6, 8, 12, and 14 hours postadministration. Fasted samples were obtained before breakfast at 24, 48, 72, 96, and 120 hours postadministration.

Plasma and RBC were separated by centrifugation. Tocopherol contents were determined by HPLC.[2] Plasma cholesterol and triglyceride levels were determined enzymatically (Sigma Chemical Co., St. Louis, MO) and evaluated spectrophotometrically. Phospholipids were extracted from plasma with chloroform:methanol (2:1) and phosphorus content determined by the method of Fiske and Subbarow.[3]

Plasma and RBC alpha-tocopherol concentrations as well as plasma alpha-tocopherol levels per mg of plasma cholesterol, triglyceride, or phospholipids were pharmacokinetically modeled[4] on individual concentration-time data. Statistical evaluation included analysis of variance (ANOVA), Tukey's honestly significant difference (HSD), and *t* tests (Systat, Inc., Evanston, IL).

RESULTS AND DISCUSSION

Plasma pharmacokinetic data indicate that the *RRR* formulation has a greater bioavailability than does *all rac* as shown by area under the curve (AUC_{0-t}). This increased bioavailability cannot be attributed to a single pharmacokinetic component but is the result of several factors contributing to the overall effect. The data indicate that the bioavailability of alpha-tocopherol given orally as the acetate ester is to a degree stereoselective and discriminative in favor of the *RRR* enantiomer and agree with previously published data for *RRR* and *all rac*-alpha-tocopherol.[5,6]

Mean RBC concentration-time profiles indicate no significant difference in RBC alpha-tocopherol concentrations among treatment groups during the baseline period. Significant differences ($p < 0.05$) in RBC alpha-tocopherol concentrations occurred at 4, 6, and 14 hours, suggesting a preferential *in vivo* binding of the *RRR* enantiomer to the erythrocyte membrane.

Modeling of plasma alpha-tocopherol per mg of lipid concentration showed no significant differences in any pharmacokinetic parameters between *RRR* and *all rac*. Our data show that a dietary influx of lipid occurs between zero and 24 hours. This effect is not evident for the concentration-time points at 24 hours and beyond because these samples were obtained following a twelve-hour fast. The lack of agreement in the various pharmacokinetic parameters for plasma alpha-tocopherol per mg lipid reflects the lack of correlation to lipid kinetics.

REFERENCES

1. WAGNER, J. G. 1979. Bioavailability. *In* Fundamentals of Clinical Pharmacology. 337-358. Drug Intelligence Publications, Inc. Hamilton, IL.
2. BIERI, J. G., T. J. TOLLIVER & G. L. CATIGNANI. 1979. Simultaneous determination of alpha-tocopherol and retinol in plasma or red cells by high pressure liquid chromatography. Am. J. Clin. Nutr. **32:** 2143-2149.

3. FISKE, C. H., C. C. HARVEY, C. H. DAHM, JR. & M. T. SEARCY. 1972. Relationship between tocopherol and serum lipid levels for determination of nutritional adequacy. Ann. N. Y. Acad. Sci. **203:** 223-235.
4. BROWN, R. D. & J. E. MANNO. 1978. Estrip, a BASIC computer program for obtaining initial polyexponential parameter estimates. J. Pharmacol. Sci. **67:** 1687-1691.
5. FERSLEW, K. E., E. A. DAIGNEAULT, R. V. ACUFF, T. W. WOOLLEY & P. E. STANTON. 1987. Pharmacokinetics and bioavailability of *RRR* and *all-rac* steroisomers of alpha-tocopherol in humans after single oral administration. J. Clin. Pharmacol. **27:** 217.
6. DAIGNEAULT, E. A., K. E. FERSLEW, R. V. ACUFF & P. E. STANTON. 1987. Double blind randomized crossover study of bioavailability of d and dl alpha tocopherol in humans. P.2 P604. 10th International Congress of Pharmacology (International Union for Pharmacology). Sidney, Australia.

Dynamic Properties of the Phospholipid Bilayer of the Erythrocyte Membrane in the Presence of α-Tocopherol

T. ARAISO AND T. KOYAMA

Section of Physiology
Research Institute of Applied Electricity
Hokkaido University
060 Sapporo, Japan

The one-month oral administration of α-tocopherol-nicotinate to healthy human subjects caused a decrease in the membrane viscosity in erythrocyte.[1] The measurement was made with a time-resolved fluorescence depolarization technique. With this technique the two factors, which relate to the molecular dynamics of phospholipid bilayer, that is, the membrane viscosity and wobbling angle of phospholipids, can be measured separately.[2] Both factors seem to be closely related with the permeation of small molecules such as lactate, phosphate, and glucose through membranes.[3] But these factors have never been studied in human erythrocytes that were enriched with α-tocopherol (TOC) *in vitro*. In the present study, these factors were measured in membrane ghosts prepared from TOC-incubated blood with a subnanosecond time-resolved fluorescence depolarization technique using a fluorophore, diphenyl-hexatriene (DPH).

Four milliliters of blood was drawn into a heparinized 10 mL injection syringe from the antecubital vein; 0.1 mL of 1 M glucose solution was added to the blood sample, and 6 mL of a gas mixture (95% O_2 and 5% CO_2) was sucked into the syringe. This syringe was gently rotated at the rate of 60 rpm in a 37°C thermostated bath for one hour. Then the sample was divided into two portions, each 2 mL, in a 5 mL syringe. To one portion was added the TOC solution (Supplied from Eisai Pharmaceutical Co., Tokyo) at the final concentration of 0.5 mg/mL. To another portion was added 0.01 mL solvent, (HOC-60, polyoxyethylene-hydrogenated castor oil derivatives, 60 mole ether, Nikko Chemical, Tokyo). Both syringes were filled with the gas mixture. They were rotated at the rate of 60 rpm for 4 hours at 37°C. Then membrane ghosts were prepared from these blood samples by a routine method and incubated with dispersed DPH. Anisotropy decay curves were measured with the time-resolved fluorometer that consists of a Nd-YAG Q-switch pulsed laser as a light source of pulsed excitation and a streak camera system as a detector of the DPH fluorescence. The overall time resolution of this system was 200 picoseconds.

Examples of the anisotropy decay curve, r(t), are shown in FIGURES 1 and 2. The r(t) curve for TOC-incubated membrane ghosts (FIG. 1) reached a higher steady value ($r_\infty = 0.175$, and wobbling diffusion rate = 4.4×10^7 sec^{-1}) than the curve

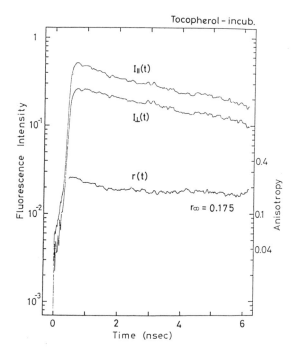

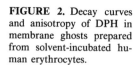

FIGURE 1. Decay curves of polarized fluorescence, $I_{\parallel}(t)$ and $I_{\perp}(t)$, and emission anisotropy, $r(t)$, of DPH in membrane ghosts prepared from α-tocopherol-incubated human erythrocytes.

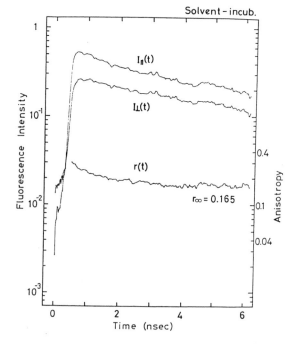

FIGURE 2. Decay curves and anisotropy of DPH in membrane ghosts prepared from solvent-incubated human erythrocytes.

for the solvent-incubated ones (r_∞ = 0.165, and wobbling diffusion rate = 4.9 × $10^7 \sec^{-1}$) (FIG. 2).

The membrane viscosity calculated from these curves increased from 0.90 of the solvent-incubated membrane ghosts to 1.05 poise of the TOC-incubated ones. This viscosity change can be interpreted on the basis of the molecular motion of phospholipid from the fact that the wobbling angle decreased from 32° to 28°. There is evidence that transient low-density spaces are formed in the lipid bilayer as the result of the movement of the hydrocarbon chains of phospholipid molecules and that the wobbling angle obtained from DPH fluorescence represents the size of the transient low-density space (submitted for publication). The incorporation of TOC acts to reduce the range of movements of phospholipid molecules and the frequency of development of transient low-density spaces. These effects are reflected in a decrease in the wobbling angle.

Thus, the *in vitro* application of TOC produces an increase in the membrane viscosity and a decrease in the wobbling angle, both acting to rigidify the erythrocyte membranes. This agreement is consistent with the reported nature of TOC that the TOC molecules incorporated into membranes causes an increase in the density of the hydrocarbon chains in the lipid bilayer. The previous result, obtained in an *in vivo* study where the enrichment with TOC was induced by the oral administration of TOC-nicotinate, was probably due to the small increase in the TOC concentration in erythrocyte membranes and to a small change in phospholipid constituents in erythrocyte membranes.

REFERENCES

1. KOYAMA, T. & T. ARAISO. 1988. J. Nutr. Sci. & Vitaminol. **34:** 449-457.
2. ARAISO, T., Y. SHINDO, T. ARAI, J. NITTA, Y. KIKUCHI & T. KOYAMA. 1986. Biorheology **23:** 467-483.
3. ARAISO, T. & T. KOYAMA. 1987. J. Physiol. Soc. Jpn. **49:** 1-11. (in Japanese).

The Effect of Vitamin E on the Immunosuppressive Effects of n-6 Polyunsaturated Fatty Acids

ADRIANNE BENDICH

Clinical Nutrition
Hoffmann-La Roche, Inc.
Nutley, New Jersey 07110

Vitamin E, at concentrations above that found in standard laboratory animal diets, significantly enhances many aspects of immune function.[1,2] Immunodepression has been associated with high levels of n-6 dietary polyunsaturated fats (n-6 PUFA).[3,4] The objective of this study was to determine whether dietary vitamin E can protect T- and B-cell proliferative responses from the immunosuppressive effects of dietary n-6 PUFA.

METHODS

Male weanling rats were fed vitamin E-deficient, purified diets supplemented with 0, 15, 50, 200, or 1000 mg/kg *all-rac* alpha-tocopheryl acetate with either vitamin E-free 10% lard (SF) or 10% corn oil (n-6 PUFA) as the fat source. Animals were fed the diets for seven to eight weeks and lightly anesthetized with Metofane. Blood was collected by cardiac puncture using 5% EDTA as an anticoagulant. Plasma vitamin E levels were determined by HPLC. Total plasma lipids were determined spectrophotometrically.[5] The spleens were removed aseptically, and T- and B-cell proliferative responses to the T-cell mitogens, concanavalin A (Con A), phytohemagglutinin (PHA), and the B-cell mitogen, lipopolysaccharide (LPS), were determined as previously described.[1] Lymphocyte populations were analyzed using a fluorescence-activated cell sorter.

RESULTS AND CONCLUSIONS

T- and B-cell responses were depressed when the fat source was PUFA, compared with SF at all levels of vitamin E used. As the level of vitamin E in the diets increased, the degree of immunosuppression by PUFA was reduced. PUFA-fed rats given 200 mg/kg vitamin E had B-cell mitogen responses that were not significantly different

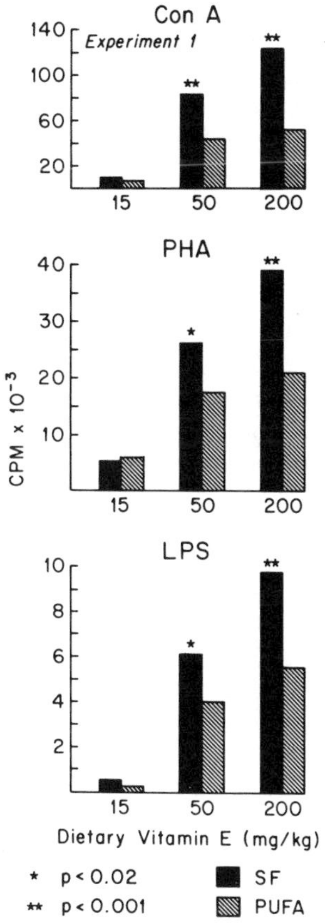

Con A

PHA

LPS

FIGURE 1. Effect of dietary vitamin E and fat type on lymphocyte mitogen responses.

* p < 0.02   ■ SF
** p < 0.001   ▨ PUFA

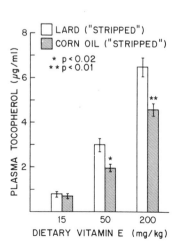

FIGURE 2. Effect of fat source on plasma tocopherol in rats.

than those of SF-fed rats given 50 mg/kg vitamin E. By contrast, PUFA-fed rats given 200 or 1000 mg/kg vitamin E had consistently depressed T-cell mitogen responses that did not reach the level of stimulation found in the SF-fed rats given 50 mg/kg vitamin E (FIG. 1). Thus, B-cell responses were more significantly enhanced by high levels of dietary vitamin E than T-cell responses.

Plasma vitamin E levels were significantly lower in the PUFA group compared with the SF group fed 50-1000 mg/kg of dietary vitamin E (FIG. 2). There were no changes in subcellular populations of lymphocytes. Therefore, the type of dietary fat and the level of vitamin E significantly affects lymphocyte functions.

REFERENCES

1. BENDICH, A., E. GABRIEL & L. J. MACHLIN. 1986. J. Nutr. **116:** 675-681.
2. MEYDANI, S. N., M. MEYDANI, C. P. VERDON, A. A. SHAPIRO, J. B. BLUMBERG & K. C. HAYES. 1986. Mech. Ageing Dev. **34:** 191-201.
3. ERICKSON, K. L. 1986. Mechanisms of dietary fat modulation of tumorigenesis: Changes in immune responses. *In* Dietary Fat and Cancer. C. Ip, D. F. Birt, A. E. Rogers & C. Mettlin, Eds.: 555-586. Alan R. Liss. New York, NY.
4. VITALE, J. J. & S. A. BROITMAN. 1981. Cancer Res. **41:** 3706-3710.
5. ZOELLNER, N. & K. KIRSCH. 1962. Z. Gesamte Exp. Med. **135:** 545-547.

Vitamin E Deficiency as a Causative Factor in Equine Degenerative Myeloencephalopathy

L. L. BLYTHE, A. M. CRAIG, E. D. LASSEN, AND
B. D. HULTGREN

College of Veterinary Medicine
Oregon State University
Corvallis, Oregon 97331
and
College of Veterinary Medicine
University of Minnesota
St. Paul, Minnesota 55108

Equine degenerative myeloencephalopathy (EDM) is a degenerative neurological disease of young horses.[1] The predominant clinical features of the disease are an insidious-to-acute onset of ataxia, paresis, hyporeflexia, and dysmetria in horses usually less than three years of age. The clinical signs can progress to quadriplegia, but may stabilize in some animals and remain static. There is no premortem diagnostic test, and the definitive diagnosis is made on the classic histopathological findings of neuroaxonal dystrophy in the nucleus cuneatus and nucleus gracilis of the medulla oblongata and in Clark's nucleus throughout the spinal cord. Swollen axons (spheroids) are present in varying amounts at all levels of the spinal cord and are believed to be evidence of large neuronal dieback. Premature accumulation of lipofuscin-like pigment in neurons, macrophages, and extracellular spaces in the affected area is also a prominent feature of the disease. Familial predisposition has been reported in multiple breeds, but sporadic cases are common.[2-4]

Vitamin E deficiency has been proposed as part of the pathogenesis in EDM, based on the following four factors. (1) Low serum vitamin E has been documented in a number of affected horses during the first year of life. This is not diagnostic for the disease, inasmuch as many young horses can have similar low values. In addition, serum vitamin E values have been shown to be poor indicators of vitamin E status. (2) The clinical progression and pathological features of EDM are similar to those seen in both experimental rats and monkeys and in clinical human cases of vitamin E deficiency. (3) A decrease in incidence of EDM from 40% to less than 10% in a susceptible herd has been reported with prophylactic vitamin E supplementation.[3] Finally, a clinical response of diseased horses to long-term massive vitamin E therapy (6000 IU/day) has been evidenced by authors.

A family of Appaloosa horses with a high incidence of EDM is being used as a model to study the pathophysiology of the disease.[2] The incidence of clinical signs and confirmed disease in these foals ranges from 70 to 85%, whereas nonrelated foals raised with them remain normal. Research is focused currently on defining if EDM is 1) a simple antioxidant deficiency from either malabsorption, lack of blood carrier lipoproteins, deficits in lipoprotein receptor sites, storage deficits, or increased excretion, or 2) an inherent defect in their lipid metabolism that renders them more susceptible to oxidative stress when antioxidant capacities, especially vitamin E, are low.

An oral vitamin E absorption test has been developed for horses using a dosage elevation of 198 mg/kg body weight of vitamin E (dl-alpha tocopherol, Hoffmann-La Roche Inc., Nutley, NJ, USA). Preliminary results in 18 horses show no differences in the serum vitamin E values between normal and EDM-affected horses. These data support normal vitamin E absorption in EDM-diseased horses. Current research is focused on evaluating blood carrier lipoproteins and the pharmacodynamics of vitamin E in normal and EDM-diseased horses.

REFERENCES

1. MAYHEW, I. G., A. DELAHUNTA, R. H. WHITLOCK et al. 1977. J. Am. Vet. Med. Assoc. 170: 195-201.
2. BLYTHE, L. L. 1986. Proceedings of the Eastern States Veterinary Conference. Orlando, FL. Abstr. 160.
3. MAYHEW, I. G., C. M. BROWN, H. D. STOWE et al. 1987. J. Vet. Int. Med. 1: 45-50.
4. BEECH, J. & M. HASKINS. 1987. Am. J. Vet. Res. 48: 109-113.

Vitamin E as an Anticarcinogen[a]

CARMIA BOREK

Radiological Research Laboratory
Department of Radiation Oncology
and
Department of Pathology / Cancer Center
Columbia University
New York, New York 10032

INTRODUCTION

Epidemiologists estimated that over 80% of human cancer is due to environmental factors, and that "most human cancers would, in principle, be preventible if the main risk and anti-risk factors could be identified."[1,2] The role of diet in the etiology of cancer has been known for some time, and a number of studies have suggested that the absence of certain dietary components, notably antioxidants, contributes to a substantial portion of human malignancies.[1,2]

Vitamin E is a hydrophobic, peroxyl radical-trapping, chain-breaking antioxidant found in the lipid fraction of living organisms. Its main function is to protect the lipid material of an organism from oxidation.[3]

The potential of vitamin E as a cancer preventive agent has been of interest for some time.[4–6] Several epidemiological studies have demonstrated an inverse relationship between levels of serum vitamin E and cancer rates.[4,5]

Individuals whose intake of vitamin E was above average showed a lower risk of lung cancer,[4] whereas those with prediagnostic low serum levels of vitamin E were found to have an increased incidence of the disease.[5,6] Studies in animals have demonstrated that vitamin E can prevent the growth of tumors induced in animals by chemical carcinogens[7–9] and inhibit the effects of tumor promoters in enhancing carcinogenesis.[10]

VITAMIN E AS AN ANTICARCINOGEN *IN VITRO*

Cell cultures offer a powerful tool in carcinogenesis research. In these *in vitro* systems, cells are grown under defined conditions free from complex homeostatic mechanisms that prevail *in vivo*. These systems afford us the opportunity to assess at a cellular level the carcinogenic potential of physical and/or chemical agents,[11] and

[a]This work was supported by Grant No. CA-12536 from the National Cancer Institute, and by a contract from the National Foundation for Cancer Research.

to identify factors that inhibit transformation and act as cancer preventive agents. Work in our laboratory has focused on the potential of vitamin E as an anticarcinogen in radiation and chemically induced transformation in cell cultures. Our studies to evaluate the inhibitory effects of vitamin E in radiation and chemically induced transformation were conducted with the mouse cell line C3H/10T-1/2.[12]

When cells were pretreated with vitamin E (alpha-tocopherol succinate) at 7 μM for 1-2 days and then exposed to either benzo(a)pyrene, a widespread carcinogen, tryptophane pyrolsate, a carcinogen in broiled food, vitamin E dramatically inhibited transformation as compared to controls that were not pretreated with the vitamin[12] (FIG. 1). We studied the effect of vitamin E on lipid peroxidation initiated in cells following exposure to radiation, using the TBA assay.[13] We found a reduction in lipid peroxidation in cells pretreated with vitamin E as compared to the untreated, indicating that the action of vitamin E in protecting the cells was mediated, in part, by inhibiting lipid peroxidation and its damaging free radical-mediated consequences.[13]

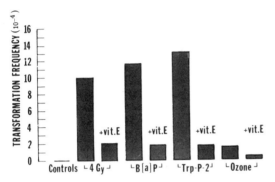

FIGURE 1. The inhibition of radiation and chemically induced transformation by vitamin E in mouse C3H/10T-1/2 cells. Data in part from references 12, 14, and 16.

VITAMIN E INHIBITS OZONE CARCINOGENESIS

Ozone (O_3), a reactive species of oxygen, is an important natural constituent of the atmosphere, and a key component in oxidant smog. Recently we reported that ozone acts as a carcinogen and as a synergistic cocarcinogen with x-irradiations.[14] We now find that cells pretreated with vitamin E at 7 μM and then exposed to ozone became refractory to transformation by ozone (FIG. 1). The enhanced levels of lipid peroxidation products and free radical intermediates found in ozone-exposed cells,[14] which may be associated with its oncogenic properties, are reduced when vitamin E treatment precedes ozone exposure.[13]

INTERACTION OF VITAMIN E AND VITAMIN C

The synergistic interaction between vitamins E and C as antioxidants are known.[15] Vitamin C spares vitamin E by reducing the vitamin E radical to regenerate vitamin

E. Vitamin E scavenges lipid peroxyl radical (LOO·) to interfere with chain propagation. The resulting vitamin E radical is reduced by ascorbate to regenerate vitamin E.[15]
We conducted studies to test if vitamin E and vitamin C were synergistic in their capacity to prevent transformation. We pretreated cells with vitamin E, 7 μM, and vitamin C (0.1 mg/mL), alone or in combination. Our work indicates that vitamin E and vitamin C act in concert to inhibit transformation in a manner that appears to be synergistic in nature.[13]
The role of vitamin E in protecting the organism from oxidative stress is a critical one. As observed from experiments *in vivo* and *in vitro* and from human studies, vitamin E in its capacity as an antioxidant can protect against neoplastic development. Because vitamin E is consumed in linear fashion during oxidative processes, and exposure to a variety of environmental carcinogens (radiation, chemicals, ozone) increases oxidant stress, it is critical for us to maintain a high level of vitamin E in our tissues. This would be of great value for enhancing our defense against the malignant process induced by the plethora of cancer-causing oxidants around us.[16]

REFERENCES

1. DOLL, R. & R. PETO. 1981. The causes of cancer: Quantitative estimates of avoidable risks of cancer in the United States today. J. Natl. Cancer Inst. **66:** (6) 1193-1194.
2. AMES, B. N., R. MAGAW & L. S. GOLD. 1987. Ranking possible carcinogenic hazards. Science **230:** 271-279.
3. MENZEL, D. B., N. J. ROEHM & S. D. LEE. 1972. Vitamin E: The biological and environmental antioxidant. J. Agric. Food Chem. **20:** 481-486.
4. MENKES, M. S., G. W. COMSTOCK, J. P. VUILLEUMIER, K. J. HELSING, A. A. RIDER & R. BROOKMEYER. 1986. Serum beta-carotene vitamins A and E, selenium, and the risk of lung cancer. N. Engl. J. Med. **315:** 1250-1254.
5. SALONEN, J. T., R. SALONEN, R. LAPPETELAINEN, P. H. MAENAPAA, G. ALFTHAN & P. PUSKA. 1985. Risk of cancer in relation to serum concentrations of selenium and vitamins A and E: Matched case-control analysis of prospective data. Br. Med. J. **290:** 917-920.
6. HAENSZEL, W., P. CORREA, A. LOPEZ, C. CUELLO, G. ZARAMA, D. ZAVALA & E. FONTHAM. 1985. Serum micronutrient levels in relation to gastric pathology. Int. J. Cancer **36:** 43-48.
7. SHKLAR, G. 1982. Oral mucosal carcinogenesis inhibition by vitamin E. J. Natl. Cancer Inst. **68:** 791-797.
8. ODUKOYA, O., F. HAWACH & G. SHKLAR. 1984. Retardation of experimental oral cancer by topical vitamin E. Nutr. Cancer **6:** 98-104.
9. SADEK, I. 1984. Vitamin E and its effect on skin papilloma. *In* Vitamins, Nutrition, and Cancer. K. N. Prasad, Ed.: 118-122. Karger. Basel.
10. CHAN, J. T. & H. S. BLACK. 1978. The mitigating effect of dietary antioxidants on chemically-induced carcinogenesis. Experientia **34:** 110-111.
11. BOREK, C. 1987. The induction and regulation of radiogenic transformation *in vitro:* Cellular and molecular mechanisms. *In* Mechanisms of Cellular Transformation by Carcinogenic Agents. D. Grunberger & S. Goff, Eds.: 151-195. Pergamon. New York, NY.
12. BOREK, C., A. ONG, H. MASON, L. DONAHUE & J. E. BIAGLOW. 1986. Selenium and vitamin E inhibit radiogenic and chemically induced transformation *in vitro* via different mechanisms of action. Proc. Natl. Acad. Sci. USA **83:** 1490-1494.
13. BOREK, C. 1989. The role of free radicals and antioxidants in cellular and molecular carcinogenesis *in vitro*. *In* Medical, Biochemical and Chemical Aspects of Free Radicals. O. Hayaishi, E. Niki, M. Kondo & T. Yoshikawa, Eds: 1461-1469. Elsevier. Amsterdam.

14. BOREK, C., M. ZAIDER, A. ONG, H. MASON & G. WITZ. 1986. Ozone acts alone and synergistically with ionizing radiation to induce *in vitro* neoplastic transformation. Carcinogenesis **7:** 1611-1613.
15. NIKI, E., T. SAITO, A. KAWAKAMI & Y. KAMIYA. 1984. Inhibition of oxidation of methyl linoleate in solution by vitamin E and vitamin C. J. Biol. Chem. **259:** 4177.
16. BOREK, C. 1987. Radiation and chemically induced transformation: Free radicals, antioxidants and cancer. Br. J. Cancer **55:** 74-86.

Relationship between Dose of Vitamin E Administered and Blood Level[a]

M. F. BRIN, S. FAHN, S. LOFTUS, D. McMAHON, AND E. FLASTER

Neurological Institute
College of Physicians and Surgeons
Columbia University
New York, New York 10032

Supplemental vitamin E (VE) may have a role in ameliorating symptoms or retarding progression of neurologic and medical disease. For the neurologist, there are potential applications in slowing the progression of Parkinson's disease, reducing cerebral edema after brain or spinal cord injury, reducing the incidence of intraventricular hemorrhage in the newborn, and relieving symptoms of tardive dyskinesia. In designing a clinical trial, it would be helpful to know what dose of administered vitamin produced the optimum level of serum vitamin E. We sought to answer this question.

Our study was approved by the Human Investigation Committee. Eighteen healthy volunteers were randomly assigned to 3 groups taking dl-alpha-tocopherol on a twice-a-day schedule (BID) at a total dose of 1000 IU/day (group I), 2000 IU/day (group II), or 3000 IU/day (group III). Vitamin E was taken for 4 weeks with a 4-week washout period. Blood was monitored for 8 weeks for vitamin E, thyroid function, and cholesterol in addition to other chemistries. Serum vitamin E was determined using a high pressure liquid chromatography technique.

Abdominal bloating was the only dose-related side effect noted, present in 3 subjects in group III: one subject stopped the supplement when he developed frank diarrhea during week 3, and another had sufficient discomfort that he discontinued the supplement at the end of week two.

Serum levels were corrected for baseline levels in the analysis (TABLE 1A). Inspection of the uptake curves revealed that the vitamin level plateaued by week 2. Therefore, the levels analyzed were the average of blood sample results from weeks 2-4. Adjusted peak average ("wk 4") serum vitamin E was 27.1, 42.6, and 34.0 µg/mL in the three respective groups; ($p < 0.05$ group I vs II only; TABLE 1B, FIGURE 1). There was no consistent effect on cholesterol. T3 was slightly higher in group I (1.08) versus group II (1.02) $p = 0.02$ (TABLE 1B, FIGURE 1); there were no differences among the groups for T4 or thyroid-stimulating hormone (TSH). Within group III, TSH was slightly, but significantly ($p < 0.01$) higher for week 4 versus week 0, using an analysis of covariance.

These data suggest that supplemental VE at a dose of 2000 IU/day is reasonable for clinical trials. Higher doses are unlikely to result in higher blood levels and may

[a] This work was supported by Hoffmann-La Roche and the Parkinson's Disease Foundation.

TABLE 1A. Average Results

Assay	Group	Week 0	Week 4	Week 8	Week 4 minus Week 0
Vitamin E	I	9.2	23.9	10.3	14.7
(peak, μg/mL)	II	13.0	45.4	13.4	32.4
	III	11.5	34.4	12.1	22.9
Cholesterol	I	173.0	170.5	182.8	−2.5
(mg/dL)	II	212.5	208.3	218.2	−4.2
	III	196.6	199.5	197.0	2.9
T3	I	1.04	1.09	1.06	0.04
(Percent)	II	1.00	0.99	1.02	−0.01
	III	1.08	1.09	1.10	0.01
T4	I	6.08	6.24	6.05	0.16
(μg/dL)	II	6.47	6.58	6.75	0.11
	III	5.95	5.97	5.47	0.02
TSH	I	2.07	2.50	2.17	0.42
(IU/mL)	II	1.85	2.32	2.03	0.47
	III	1.78	2.28	1.98	0.50[a]

[a] $p < 0.01$ for week 4 significantly higher than baseline (analysis of covariance).

TABLE 1B. Least Squares Adjusted Means for Week 4

Assay	Group	Week 4	SE
Vitamin E	I	27.1[a]	3.12
(peak, μg/mL)	II	42.6	3.08
	III	34.0	2.94
Cholesterol	I	193.1	6.9
(mg/dL)	II	197.9	6.8
	III	189.6	6.5
T3	I	1.08[b]	0.016
(Percent)	II	1.02	0.015
	III	1.06	0.015
T4	I	6.23	0.24
(μg/dL)	II	6.38	0.23
	III	6.18	0.23
TSH	I	2.27	0.21
(IU/mL)	II	2.37	0.19
	III	2.42	0.19

[a] $p < 0.05$ for group I significantly less than group II.
[b] $p = 0.02$ for group I significantly greater than group II.

VITAMIN E--ADJUSTED MEANS

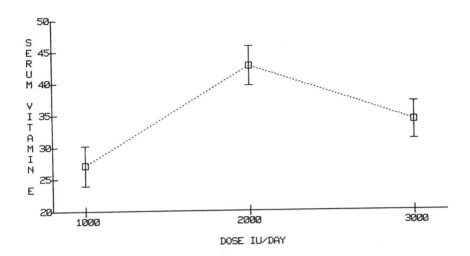

SERUM T3--ADJUSTED MEANS

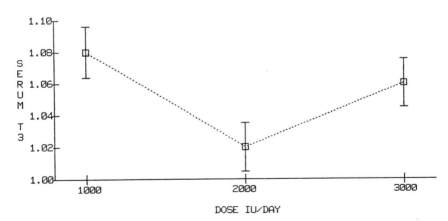

FIGURE 1. Graphs showing adjusted means for serum vitamin E (top) and T3 (bottom). The results for group I and group II are significantly different (see TABLE IB).

cause diarrhea on a BID schedule. Changes in thyroid function were not clinically meaningful. Additional studies will be required to explore the relationship between blood level and resultant tissue concentrations.

ACKNOWLEDGMENTS

We are grateful to the attending and support staff of the Columbia Presbyterian Medical Center for their participation as subjects in this study.

Increased Vitamin E Content in the Lungs of Chronic Cigarette-Smoked Rats

CHING K. CHOW, GERRY R. AIRRIESS, AND
CHARUS CHANGCHIT

Department of Nutrition and Food Science
University of Kentucky
Lexington, Kentucky 40506

Oxidative damage to the lung may be caused directly by the action of oxidants and free radicals in cigarette smoke, or indirectly by reactive oxygen species generated by alveolar macrophage and polymorphonuclear leukocytes following cigarette smoking. The status of vitamin E, a major biological antioxidant, may determine the cellular susceptibility to the effects of cigarette smoking.[1] We have recently found that the levels of vitamin E in the lungs of guinea pigs were significantly increased following exposure to cigarette smoke.[2] In the present research the effect of chronic cigarette smoking on the status of vitamin E was studied in rats.

MATERIAL AND METHODS

Ninety-six 7-week-old male Sprague-Dawley rats were randomly divided into four groups and exposed to either mainstream smoke (MS), sidestream smoke (SS), or sham smoke (SH), or served as room controls (RC) for 8, 16, 24, or 32 weeks. Smoke was generated by a peristaltic pump machine,[3] using the high nicotine Kentucky reference cigarette, 2R1, and was delivered to exposure chambers following an initial dilution to 35% strength with air (MS). SS was delivered to animals constantly at 25% of the original concentration through a collecting device placed around the cigarette. The animals were exposed to smoke through the nose while being restrained once daily, one cigarette/session at 10 puffs/cigarette. The animals in the sham group (SH) were "sham-smoked" on the same type of smoking machine, set for exposure conditions, except for the absence of smoke. RC animals were not subjected to smoking or handling as in the other three groups. After the 8, 16, 24, or 32 week-smoking period, four to eight rats from each group were killed following blood withdrawal. Vitamin E levels in the plasma and homogenates of lungs, kidneys, and livers were measured using a high-performance liquid chromatographic procedure with fluorescence detection.[4] Data were analyzed using analysis of variance followed by Newman's multiple comparison test.

425

TABLE 1. Vitamin E Levels in the Lungs and Plasma of Cigarette-Smoked Rats

Tissue	Exposure Time	MS	SS	SH	RC
Lung	8 weeks	$10.1 \pm 1.6^{a,b}$	7.5 ± 2.1^c	8.2 ± 2.1^c	7.4 ± 2.3^c
		(8)	(8)	(8)	(8)
	16 weeks	11.6 ± 1.6^b	8.1 ± 1.9^c	7.6 ± 1.5^c	8.3 ± 1.6^c
		(8)	(8)	(8)	(8)
	24 weeks	12.9 ± 1.1^b	7.1 ± 1.2^c	7.5 ± 1.3^c	7.7 ± 2.0^c
		(4)	(4)	(4)	(4)
	32 weeks	15.8 ± 2.6^b	7.3 ± 1.6^c	8.0 ± 1.4^c	7.5 ± 1.8^c
		(4)	(4)	(4)	(4)
Plasma	8 weeks	2.5 ± 0.5^b	2.5 ± 0.4^b	2.4 ± 0.4^b	3.5 ± 0.4^c
		(8)	(8)	(8)	(8)
	16 weeks	2.3 ± 0.3^b	2.6 ± 0.4^b	2.5 ± 0.3^b	3.3 ± 0.2^c
		(8)	(8)	(8)	(8)
	24 weeks	2.9 ± 0.2^b	3.0 ± 0.5^b	3.0 ± 0.7^b	3.9 ± 0.4^c
		(4)	(4)	(4)	(4)
	32 weeks	2.7 ± 0.4^b	2.5 ± 0.1^b	2.9 ± 0.5^b	4.0 ± 0.4^c
		(4)	(4)	(4)	(4)

[a] Mean $\pm$ standard deviation. The data are expressed as $\mu g/mL$ plasma or $\mu g/g$ tissue. The means that do not share the same superscript are statistically significant. The number of animals in each group is shown in the parenthesis.

TABLE 2. Vitamin E Levels in the Kidneys and Livers of Cigarette-Smoked Rats

Tissue	Exposure Time	MS	SS	SH	RC
Kidney	8 weeks	$9.9 \pm 1.7^{a,b}$	10.2 ± 1.5^b	9.4 ± 1.3^b	10.9 ± 1.5^b
		(8)	(8)	(8)	(8)
	16 weeks	9.4 ± 1.2^b	11.0 ± 1.3^b	9.6 ± 0.8^b	13.8 ± 1.4^c
		(8)	(8)	(8)	(8)
	24 weeks	10.3 ± 0.5^b	$10.3 \pm 1.3^{b,c}$	$10.2 \pm 1.6^{b,c}$	11.7 ± 0.8^c
		(4)	(4)	(4)	(4)
	32 weeks	9.6 ± 0.5^b	9.7 ± 0.7^b	$10.3 \pm 1.1^{b,c}$	11.4 ± 1.4^c
		(4)	(4)	(4)	(4)
Liver	8 weeks	10.2 ± 1.1^b	$11.3 \pm 1.7^{b,c}$	9.9 ± 1.2^b	12.6 ± 2.1^c
		(8)	(8)	(8)	(8)
	16 weeks	10.1 ± 1.6^b	11.5 ± 1.6^b	$12.1 \pm 1.8^{b,c}$	13.3 ± 1.6^c
		(8)	(8)	(4)	(4)
	24 weeks	10.3 ± 1.1^b	9.9 ± 1.6^b	9.9 ± 1.7^b	11.6 ± 1.7^b
		(4)	(4)	(4)	(4)
	32 weeks	9.5 ± 1.6^b	9.1 ± 0.5^b	9.2 ± 1.3^b	10.1 ± 0.7^b
		(4)	(4)	(4)	(4)

[a] Mean $\pm$ standard deviation. The data are expressed as $\mu g/g$ tissue. The means that do not share the same superscript are different statistically ($p < 0.05$). The number of animals in each group is shown in the parenthesis.

RESULTS AND DISCUSSION

The effect of cigarette smoking on the tissue levels of vitamin E are summarized in TABLES 1 and 2. Relative to the SH group, the levels of vitamin E (alpha-tocopherol) increased significantly in the lungs of rats exposed to MS, but not to SS, for either 8, 16, 24, or 32 weeks. Relative to the SH group, cigarette smoking did not have a significant effect on the levels of vitamin E in the plasma, liver, or kidney of MS or SS groups. The vitamin E levels in the plasma of the RC group, however, were significantly ($p < 0.05$) higher than those of MS, SS, or SH. Similarly, the levels of vitamin E in the kidneys of the RC group were found to be higher than the MS group after 16, 24, and 32 weeks of exposure, and in the liver after 8 and 16 weeks.

The increased levels of vitamin E in the lungs of MS rats observed in this research are compatible with the previous studies using guinea pigs as experimental animals.[2] Because the experimental animals were fed a diet that contained an adequate amount of vitamin E, it is unclear whether higher levels of vitamin E in the lungs of smoked animals resulted from the mobilization of their body stores. Nevertheless, the results obtained from the smoking studies suggest that this adaptive response may protect the pulmonary tissue of chronically exposed animals against oxidative damage.

REFERENCES

1. CHOW, C. K., L. H. THACKER, R. CHEN & R. B. GRIFFITH. 1984. Environ. Res. **34:** 8-17.
2. AIRRIESS, G. R., C. CHANGCHIT, L. C. CHEN & C. K. CHOW. 1988. Nutr. Res. **8:** 653-661.
3. GRIFFITH, R. B. & S. STANDAFER. 1985. Toxicology **35:** 13-24.
4. HATAM, L. J. & H.J. KAYDEN. 1979. J. Lipid Res. **20:** 639-645.

Activated Neutrophil-Induced Membrane Damage in Vitamin E-Deficient Erythrocytes

S. CLASTER, A. QUINTANILHA, B. DE LUMEN,
D. CHIU, AND B. LUBIN

Children's Hospital Medical Center of Northern California
Oakland, California 94609
and
University of California
Berkeley, California 94720

Red blood cells (RBC) deficient in vitamin E ($-E$) have increased susceptibility to oxidant stress. Activated neutrophils (AN) are one potential source of oxidants *in vivo*. We have previously demonstrated that AN induce formation of malondialdehyde (MDA) and K^+ leak when incubated with human RBC,[1,2] and that sickle RBC, which are $-E$, are more susceptible to such damage. AN-induced K^+ leak was found to be due primarily to a mechanism involving proteases and cationic proteins released following neutrophil activation. To further explore how products of AN affect $-E$ RBC, we incubated $-E$ rat RBC with human AN and measured MDA generation and passive potassium leak. We found that $-E$ RBC exposed to AN for two hours generated significantly higher levels of MDA (49.81 ± 7.65 nmol MDA/g Hb) than did normal RBC (29.25 ± 1.59 nmol MDA/g Hb). At 30 minutes of exposure, a marked increase in K^+ leak (4.23 nmol $K^+/10^{13}$ RBC) was measured in $-E$ RBC compared to normal RBC (1.52 nmol $K^+/10^{13}$ RBC) (FIG. 1). After one hour of exposure to AN, $-E$ RBC displayed significant hemolysis. We then studied red cell membrane properties that might contribute to the increased susceptibility to AN in $-E$ RBC. We analyzed the phospholipid composition of membranes from both supplemented and deficient rats by treating RBC with sphingomyelinase and phospholipase A_2. No change in phospholipid composition or organization was detected in the deficient group as compared to the supplemented controls. Specifically, we did not detect phosphatidylserine (PS) on the outer membrane leaflet, nor did we find a decrease in phosphatidylethanolamine (PE). Using SDS polyacrylamide gel electrophoresis, we were unable to detect any high molecular weight cross-linked material in membranes from deficient rats, nor did we note any difference in membrane proteins between the two groups. Analysis of sulfhydryl (SH) groups in deficient and supplemented RBC membranes using dithiolnitrobenzene showed similar numbers of SH groups in both types of membranes (48.8 nM SH/mg/mL protein, supplemented vs 48.0 nM SH/mg/mL protein, deficient). We did find that even in the absence of exposure to AN, $-E$ RBC had increased MDA levels. Presence of MDA was paralleled by an increased binding of phospholipid liposomes (TABLE 1). Similar increases in liposome binding were also observed in normal RBC previously treated with oxidants. It is possible that alterations in the cell surface of $-E$ RBC, as reflected by increased

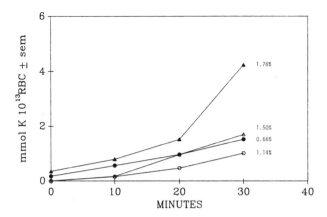

FIGURE 1. RBC were incubated at 37°C in buffer alone (phosphate-buffered saline with 0.1 mM ouabain and 10 mM glucose, pH 7.4) or with AN and passive K$^+$ leak measured in 10 minute intervals. Symbols: buffer (open); AN (closed); vitamin E-deficient (triangles); vitamin E-supplemented (circles). Percent hemolysis is shown for the final time point (30 minutes only). At 45 minutes, the percent hemolysis for vitamin E-deficient RBC was 11.8%, an amount that invalidated K$^+$ leak measurements. The values shown represent the mean of two determinations.

TABLE 1. Liposome Binding[a]

	nmol Liposomes Incorporated/10^8 RBC ± SEM	
Supplemented animals	5.42 ± .46	
N=6		
Deficient animals	12.5 ± 1.45	p < .001
N=10		
Human RBC, control	1.41 ± .06	
N=5		
Human RBC, H$_2$O$_2$ + azide	2.77 ± .13*	*p < .001
N=7		
Human RBC, X/XO	4.89 ± .16*	
N=8		

[a] The binding of PS-phosphatidylcholine (PC) liposomes to vitamin E-deficient and vitamin E-supplemented RBC as well as to human RBC was performed according to the method of Schwartz *et al.*[3] Oxidation of RBC was induced by treatment of RBC with 1-5 mM H$_2$O$_2$ plus azide (0.4 mM) or by addition of xanthine plus xanthine oxidase (50 mM). RBC counts were performed on a Coulter-S-Plus. The difference between deficient and supplemented RBC was significant at p < .001, as was the difference between control human RBC and those treated with oxidants.

liposome binding, could promote binding by cationic proteins and proteases released from AN to these cells and result in the marked K^+ leak and hemolysis we observed. These results suggest that $-E$ RBC are particularly sensitive to damage by AN. Both oxidant and nonoxidant insults by AN contribute to this susceptibility and may play a role in the infection-mediated hemolysis observed in congenital hemolytic anemias associated with low RBC vitamin E levels.

REFERENCES

1. CLASTER, S., D. T.-Y. CHIU, A. QUINTANILHA & B. LUBIN. 1984. Blood **64:** 1079.
2. CLASTER, S., A. QUINTANILHA, M. A. SCHOTT, D. T. Y. CHIU & B. LUBIN. 1986. J. Lab. Clin. Med. **109:** 201.
3. SCHWARTZ, R. S., N. DUZGUNES, D. T.-Y. CHIU & B. LUBIN. 1983. J. Clin. Invest. **71:** 1570.

Decrease of Alpha-Tocopherol and Beta-Carotene by High-Dose Radiochemotherapy Preceding Bone Marrow Transplantation

MICHAEL R. CLEMENS,[a] CLAUDIA LADNER,
HELMUT SCHMIDT, GERHARD EHNINGER,
HERMANN EINSELE, K. FRED GEY,[b] AND
HANS DIERCK WALLER

Eberhard-Karls-Universität Tübingen
Medizinische Klinik
Federal Republic of Germany
and
[b] *Hoffmann-La Roche & Co. Ltd.*
CH-4002 Basel, Switzerland

INTRODUCTION

Conditioning regimens preceding bone marrow transplantation (BMT) consist of high-dose chemotherapy, generally in combination with total body irradiation (TBI). These regimens approach the limit of tolerance for several tissues. Lipid peroxidation has been suggested as one of the main causes of radiation damage. Cyclophosphamide (CP), frequently used in conditioning chemotherapy, depletes hepatic glutathione, thus potentially initiating peroxidative processes and enhancing radiation-induced tissue damage. Therefore, we measured lipid hydroperoxides (LOOH) in blood and investigated whether an abnormal breakdown of antioxidants, such as alpha-tocopherol (TOC) and beta-carotene (CAR), follows the conditioning therapy, which may be involved in the pathogenesis of severe and early posttransplant complications.

METHODS

Nineteen consecutive patients with acute leukemias, chronic granulocytic leukemia, severe aplastic anemia (SAA), myelodysplastic syndrome, and neuroblastoma were

[a] Address for correspondence: Dr. M. R. Clemens, Medizinische Klinik, Otfried-Müller-Strasse 10, D 7400 Tübingen 1, Federal Republic of Germany.

431

studied. Additionally, one patient suffering from SAA was examined again 4 months later during the course of a second BMT consecutive to a graft failure. Patients were treated with different conditioning regimens: CP, 4 BMT; CP and TBI, 7 BMT; CP, TBI, and etoposide (ETOP), 6 BMT; CP and ETOP, 1 BMT; CP and melphalan (MELPH), 1 BMT; TBI and MELPH, 1 BMT. The day of BMT was numbered as day 0. CP was given on 2 consecutive days beginning day -4 (2 × 60 mg/kg body weight). ETOP was given on day -4 (1 × 30 mg/kg body weight). TBI (12 Gy; lung shielding at 10 Gy) was fractionated (3 days twice daily 2 Gy), beginning on day -7. MELPH was given on day -3 (180 mg/m^2). The supportive nutritional therapy consisted of 500 mL lipid emulsion, 10% daily (Intralipid^R), which contains about 4 mg TOC. Additionally, 5 mg TOC acetate was given i.v. with a multivitamin preparation. Infusion of lipid emulsion and vitamins started on day -7 iv and did not contain CAR. Measurements of cholesterol (CHOL), TOC, and CAR were carried out as previously described.[1] LOOH were determined in serum by using the CHOD-Iodide method (Merck No. 14106).

RESULTS

LOOH in serum were expressed as μmol/mg CHOL, inasmuch as the CHOL-rich fraction of lipoproteins is carrying the major part of LOOH. Patients who did not receive TBI (RT$^-$) showed no significant changes of LOOH concentrations following conditioning therapy and BMT (FIG. 1). By contrast, patients treated with TBI (RT$^+$) exhibited a significant increase of serum LOOH of about 100% ($p =$ 0.036) following conditioning therapy (FIG. 1). Analysis of variance supported the difference between both groups (RT$^+$ and RT$^-$) ($p = 0.047$).

The ratio alpha-tocopherol/cholesterol (T/C) in serum dropped in both groups of patients (RT$^+$: day -8: 5.06 ± 1.22 nmol/μmol; day +12: 3.91 ± 1.11; $p <$ 0.01; RT$^-$: day -8: 6.58 ± 1.85; day +12: 3.7 ± 1.17; $p < 0.05$). Analysis of variance supported the significant decrease of the T/C ratio in serum from day -8

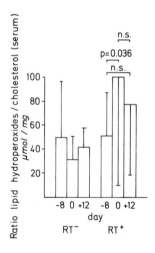

FIGURE 1. Lipid hydroperoxides/cholesterol ratio in serum. RT$^-$ patients treated without (n = 6); RT$^+$ treated with total body irradiation (12 Gy) (n = 14). Calculation of significance indicated in the figure by paired t test; no significant changes in group RT$^-$. Analysis of variance shows a significant difference between both groups ($p = 0.047$). Day 0 is the day of bone marrow transplantation. Mean values ± SD.

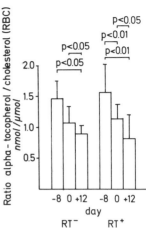

FIGURE 2. Alpha-tocopherol/cholesterol molar ratio in plasma. For further explanation, see FIGURE 1. Analysis of variance shows no difference between the two groups.

to day $+12$ ($p < 0.001$). There was no significant difference, however, between the 2 groups (RT^+ vs RT^-; main effect $p = 0.6$; 2-way interaction $p = 0.056$). Congruent data for the T/C ratio in red cell membranes are shown in FIGURE 2. Again, there is no difference between the 2 groups (RT^+ vs RT^-), but changes in the time course as calculated by the t test (FIG. 2) and by analysis of variance ($p < 0.001$).

The CAR/CHOL ratio in serum from patients of group RT^+ dropped from 0.11 $\pm$ 0.78 μmol/mmol (day -8) to 0.04 $\pm$ 0.03 (day $+12$) ($p < 0.01$). Patients in the RT^- group did not exhibit significant changes of the CAR/CHOL ratio during the follow-up. Analysis of variance shows significant differences between the two groups and during the follow-up (both $p < 0.005$). Patients treated with TBI had about 50% less CAR prior to conditioning therapy than patients not treated with TBI. This finding could be due to previously applicated chemotherapy in the RT^+ group.

DISCUSSION

Our results clearly demonstrate that TOC and CAR have not been maintained on the initial basis of concentrations as determined prior to the conditioning therapy. The intravenously applicated amount of TOC (about 9 mg daily) covers the recommended dietary allowance (RDA: women 8 mg, men 10 mg TOC equivalents). Diplock[2] suggested that the present RDA will prove to be too low and that there are cogent reasons for the recognition of CAR as a vitamin in its own right. Our results support this suggestion in respect of special situations appearing with an enhanced requirement for antioxidants. A particular recommendation for the supplementation of antioxidants in patients undergoing highly toxic cancer treatment is required, because the deleterious effects of chemotherapy, radiotherapy, and total parenteral nutrition with a high content of PUFA accumulate.

There may be multifarious causes for the loss of antioxidants in patients undergoing conditioning therapy before BMT. Interestingly, two very different biological antioxidants are consumed. Surprisingly, different conditioning regimens (RT^+ vs RT^-), independently of the drugs used for chemotherapy, lead to comparable losses of antioxidants. The expected cumulative effect of TBI in combination with chemotherapy was not found in respect to the breakdown of antioxidants; however, it appears by measuring the LOOH in blood. Loss of TOC in combination with markedly reduced CAR levels might actually render organs much more susceptible to free radical-induced tissue damage. Activated granulocytes appearing during hematopoietic reconstitution and graft-versus-host reaction may serve as a source of oxygen radicals. On the basis of our results, we propose intervention studies investigating the effect of high-dose CAR and TOC administration on the toxicity of intensive cancer chemotherapy protocols.

REFERENCES

1. GEY, K. F., G. B. BRUBACHER & H. B. STAHELIN. 1987. Plasma levels of antioxidant vitamins in relation to ischemic heart disease and cancer. Am. J. Clin. Nutr. **45:** 1368-1377.
2. DIPLOCK, A. T. 1987. Dietary supplementation with antioxidants. Is there a case for exceeding the recommended dietary allowance? Free Rad. Biol. Med. **3:** 199-201.

Antioxidant Status of Smokers and Nonsmokers

Effects of Vitamin E Supplementation

GARRY G. DUTHIE, JOHN R. ARTHUR,
W. PHILIP T. JAMES, AND
HAZEL M. VINT

Rowett Research Institute
Greenburn Road
Aberdeen, Scotland, U.K. AB1 6UX

INTRODUCTION

Inasmuch as free radicals are implicated in the pathogenesis of many diseases, including heart disease and cancer, some authors suggest that the RDA for certain antioxidants should be increased,[1] whereas others disagree.[2] Smokers, a group at high risk from heart disease and cancer, inhale large amounts of potentially injurious free radicals derived from tobacco.[3] The aim of this study was to assess whether such a sustained free radical load affected indices of lipid peroxidation and antioxidants in blood of smokers and whether oral vitamin E supplementation influenced these parameters.

MATERIAL AND METHODS

Twenty male smokers (mean age $\pm$ SE; 48 $\pm$ 0.5 years) and 20 male nonsmokers (46 $\pm$ 0.4 years) were age-matched and allocated to one of four treatment groups that formed a 2 $\times$ 2 factorial: smokers versus nonsmokers and placebo versus vitamin E supplementation. Smokers used 15-25 cigarettes/day. Each subject took one capsule/day of either a supplement of 1000 mg α-tocopheryl acetate or a placebo containing only 20 μg total vitamin E. The selenium content of the capsules was negligible (0.005-0.044 μg).

After 14 days, a blood sample was withdrawn from each subject. The susceptibility of washed erythrocytes to 6% hydrogen peroxide was assessed as malonaldehyde production after 90 min incubation.[4] Previously described methods were used to assess the indices of lipid peroxidation, antioxidants, and antioxidant-related enzymes shown in TABLE 1. Data were analyzed using analysis of variance[5] and where appropriate age was included as a covariate.

435

TABLE 1. Indices of Lipid Peroxidation, Antioxidants, and Antioxidant Enzymes in Blood of Smokers and Nonsmokers

Parameter	Smokers	Smokers +E[a]	Nonsmokers	Nonsmokers +E	Smoking effect	Vitamin E effect	SED[e]
Plasma							
Conjugated dienes (U/mL)	219	197	179	165	c	NS	15.4
Malonaldehyde (nMoles/mL)	2.3	1.7	1.7	1.7	NS	NS	0.3
Vitamin E (µg/mL)	8.3	21.2	9.3	16.6	NS	d	2.2
Vitamin C (µMoles/mL)	26.2	29.1	46.4	52.4	b	NS	9.2
Uric acid (µMoles/mL)	4.7	4.7	4.7	4.6	NS	NS	0.3
Ceruloplasmin (EU/L)	105	94	89	97	NS	NS	6.5
Erythrocyte							
Vitamin E (µg/mL)	0.6	1.2	0.7	1.0	NS	d	0.2
Glutathione peroxidase (U/mL)	2.8	2.6	2.8	2.9	NS	NS	0.35
Glucose-6-phosphate dehydrogenase (U/g Hb)	4.2	3.6	5.0	5.3	d	NS	0.49
Superoxide dismutase (µg/mL)	108	99	97	79	NS	NS	11.7
Catalase (K/g Hb)	1673	1605	1525	1557	NS	NS	21.2
Reduced glutathione (µg/mL)	159	167	138	132	c	NS	13.4
Oxidized glutathione (µg/mL)	7.8	6.1	7.3	8.2	NS	NS	1.7

[a] + E denotes supplementation with 1000 IU vitamin E/day for 14 days.
[b] $p < 0.05$.
[c] $p < 0.01$.
[d] $p < 0.001$.
[e] Standard error of the difference.

RESULTS

Despite no significant difference in erythrocyte vitamin E between unsupplemented smokers and nonsmokers, erythrocytes of smokers had a greater tendency to peroxidize when incubated with hydrogen peroxide; this effect was abolished in the vitamin E-supplemented smokers (TABLE 1, FIG. 1). Plasma-conjugated dienes were increased in smokers. A similar trend for plasma malonaldehyde did not attain statistical significance. Erythrocytes of smokers had an increase in reduced glutathione content and lower glucose-6-phosphate dehydrogenase activity; plasma vitamin C of smokers was 45% less than in nonsmokers. These parameters were unaffected by vitamin E supplements. Neither smoking or vitamin E supplementation affected plasma uric acid concentration, and ceruloplasmin activity, erythrocyte catalase, superoxide dismutase and glutathione peroxidase activities were also unaffected. Conjugated dienes and ceruloplasmin significantly increased with age ($p < 0.001$ and $p < 0.05$, respectively).

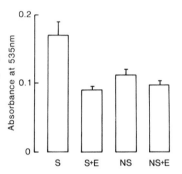

FIGURE 1. Hydrogen peroxide-induced peroxidation of erythrocytes of smokers (S) and nonsmokers (NS). +E denotes supplementation with 1000 IU vitamin E/day. Effect of smoking, $p < 0.05$; effect of vitamin E, $p < 0.001$.

DISCUSSION

These results suggest that smoking causes changes to antioxidant status. Increased erythrocyte peroxidation is associated clinically with a reduced glucose-6-phosphate dehydrogenase activity,[6] and the decreased activity of this enzyme in the erythrocytes of smokers may contribute to their increased susceptibility to hydrogen peroxide. Decreased activity of glucose-6-phosphate dehydrogenase may reflect inhibition by extracellar or intracellular lipid hydroperoxides,[7] which can arise through exposure of endogenous fatty acids to a free radical load. Increased erythrocyte glutathione may indicate an adaptive response to the increased oxidant stress[8] incurred by smokers, and the lower plasma vitamin C concentration is likely to be due to an increased turnover in response to increased oxidant stress.[9]

The elevation in conjugated dienes in plasma indicates that smokers incur abnormal oxidative stress. As vitamin E supplementation abolishes enhanced erythrocyte peroxidation of smokers, it is possible that smokers have an increased requirement for antioxidants. The clinical significance of such results is unclear, but it is possible that a prolonged increase in antioxidant intake could ameliorate free radical-mediated damage in smokers and thereby decrease the risk of developing diseases such as coronary heart disease and cancer.

REFERENCES

1. DIPLOCK, A. T. 1987. Free Rad. Biol. Med. **3:** 199-201.
2. BIERI, J. G. 1987. Free Rad. Biol. Med. **3:** 193-197.
3. CHURCH, D. F. & W. A. PRYOR. 1985. Environ. Health Perspect. **64:** 111-126.
4. CYNAMON, H. A., J. N. ISENBERG & C. H. NGUYEN. 1985. Clin. Chim. Acta **151:** 169-176.
5. WELCH, B. L. 1938. Biometrika **29:** 350-362.
6. CLEMENS, M. R. & H. D. WALLER. 1987. Chem. Phys. Lipids **45:** 251-268.
7. KHANDWALA, A. & J. B. L. GEE. 1973. Science **182:** 1364-1365.
8. GOHIL, K., C. VIGUIE, W. C. STANLEY, G. A. BROOKS & L. PACKER. 1988. J. Appl. Physiol. **64:** 115-119.
9. DRAPER, H. H. & R. P. BIRD. 1987. Free Rad. Biol. Med. **3:** 203-207.

Mobilization of Vitamin E to the Lung under Oxidative Stress[a]

NABIL M. ELSAYED

Division of Toxicology
Letterman Army Institute of Research
Presidio of San Francisco
San Francisco, California 94129

Vitamin E is a fat-soluble vitamin with many proven and attributed functions. After almost 60 years of research, its mechanism of action and its requirement in humans remain controversial. One function that is generally accepted is its ability to act as a biological antioxidant[1] and free radical quencher capable of breaking chain reactions, thus protecting from oxidative damage. There is now increasing evidence that vitamin E plays an important role in the cellular antioxidant defenses against environmental stresses, such as air pollution and carcinogens.

For a number of years, we have studied the antioxidant properties of vitamin E in the lung and its ability to protect against oxidant air pollutants, namely, nitrogen dioxide (NO_2) and ozone (O_3).[2-4] We have reported previously that lung vitamin E content increased significantly after NO_2 or O_3 exposures,[2,4] and we have postulated that vitamin E may have been mobilized to the lung under oxidative stress possibly by a mechanism similar to that suggested by Kitada *et al.*[5,6] This increase in lung vitamin E content after oxidative stress was also reported by other investigators using NO_2 and tobacco smoke.[7,8]

To test this postulate, pregnant rats, 10 days from term, were fed a vitamin E-deficient diet. The offspring were fed the same deficient diet. After 8 weeks, half of the rats were supplemented with vitamin E (1000 IU/kg) for 2 additional weeks, and the other half continued to receive the deficient diet. One hour before exposure to O_3, both vitamin E-supplemented and -deficient rats were injected ip with ^{14}C-labeled *dl*-α-tocopheryl acetate (10 μCi/rat) and exposed to 0.5 ppm O_3 for 5 days. After exposure, vitamin E content and uptake were evaluated in seven rat organs. In general, vitamin E content reflected the dietary level, but the uptake was greater in deficient rats independent of the oxidative stress, possibly reflecting relative saturation of the supplemented rats with the vitamin. The relative (ozone/air) values of vitamin E content were not markedly altered after exposure, except in the lungs (TABLE 1), where it decreased in deficient rats, but increased in supplemented rats. The relative uptake increased in all organs, except for adipose tissue of both dietary groups and brain of supplemented rats, where it decreased. In the lungs, the relative uptake increased in both groups, but the increase was greater in supplemented rats (TABLE 1). The marked increase in lung vitamin E content and uptake after oxidative stress supports the concept of mobilization to the lung when the vitamin is sufficiently available in the body.

[a]This work was done in part at the University of California, Los Angeles.

439

TABLE 1. Effect of Exposure to 0.50 ± 0.05 ppm of Ozone Continuously for Five Days on Lung Vitamin E Content and [^{14}C]Vitamin E Uptake of Deficient and Supplemented Rats[a]

	Content (μg/g)		Uptake (dpm × 1000/g)	
	Deficient	Supplemented	Deficient	Supplemented
Air	0.34 ± 0.23	25.80 ± 3.33	17.81 ± 3.91	3.84 ± 0.33
Ozone	0.21 ± 0.04	34.81 ± 1.35	22.77 ± 3.41	9.49 ± 0.73
Change	−38%	+35%[b]	+28%	+147%[b]

[a] Dietary regimens are explained in the text. Results are expressed as mean ± SD, n=4.
[b] Significantly different from air; Student's t test, $p < 0.05$.

ACKNOWLEDGMENT

^{14}C-labeled dl-α-tocopheryl acetate was a gift from Dr. Lawrence J. Machlin, Hoffmann-La Roche Inc. Nutley, New Jersey.

REFERENCES

1. TAPPEL, A. L. 1962. Vitamin E as the biological antioxidant. Vitam. Horm. 20: 493-510.
2. ELSAYED, N. M. & M. G. MUSTAFA. 1982. Dietary antioxidants and the biochemical response to oxidant inhalation. I. Influence of dietary vitamin E on the biochemical effects of nitrogen dioxide exposure in rat lung. Toxicol. Appl. Pharmacol. 66: 319-328.
3. ELSAYED, N. M., R. KASS, M. G. MUSTAFA, A. D. HACKER, J. J. OSPITAL, C. K. CHOW & C. E. CROSS. 1988. Effect of dietary vitamin E level on the biochemical response of rat lung to ozone inhalation. Drug Nutr. Interact. 5: 373-386.
4. ELSAYED, N. M. 1982. Influence of vitamin E on polyamine metabolism in ozone-exposed rat lungs. Arch. Biochem. Biophys. 255: 392-399.
5. KITADA, S., E. F. HAYS & J. F. MEAD. 1980. A lipid mobilizing factor in serum of tumor-bearing mice. Lipids 15: 168-174.
6. KITADA, S., E. F. HAYS & J. F. MEAD. 1981. Characterization of a lipid mobilizing factor from tumors. Prog. Lipid Res. 20: 823-826.
7. SAGAI, M., T. ICHINOSE, H. ODA & K. KUBOTA. 1982. Studies on biochemical effects of nitrogen dioxide. II. Changes of the protective systems in rat lungs and of lipid peroxidation by acute exposure. J. Toxicol. Environ. Health. 9: 153-164.
8. AIRRIESS, G. R., C. CHAGCHITT, L-C. CHEN & C. K. CHOW. 1988. Increased vitamin E levels in the lungs of guinea pigs exposed to mainstream smoke. Nutr. Res. 8: 653-661.

Retrospective Evaluation of Vitamin E Therapy in Parkinson's Disease

STEWART A. FACTOR[a] AND WILLIAM J. WEINER[b]

[a] Department of Neurology
Albany Medical College
Albany, New York 12208

[b] Department of Neurology
University of Miami
Miami, Florida 33101

Parkinson's disease (PD) is a progressive neurologic disorder of unknown etiology, which is the result of degeneration of dopaminergic neurons in the substantia nigra (SN). It has been postulated that free radical-mediated lipid peroxidation of cell membranes may be implicated in the pathogenesis of PD.[1] Evidence indicating that lipid peroxidation is increased in PD[2] and that natural protective mechanisms may be deficient[3,4] has been reported. Vitamin E is an antioxidant that concentrates in the hydrophobic interior of cell membranes. It acts to interfere with the chain reaction initiated by free radicals that leads to membrane lipid peroxidation, and thus may protect against the progressive degeneration of SN neurons and later the progression of PD.

We retrospectively evaluated 14 PD patients who have been self-administering vitamin E for reasons other than PD for 1 to 20 years (mean 6.9) at doses of 400-3200 IU per day (mean 1067). The mean age of these patients was 68.6 and mean duration of disease 6.9 years. Severity of disease was compared to that of 14 age- (mean 70.1) and duration- (6.8 yr) matched PD controls not taking vitamin E (chosen from our patient population by a blinded observer). The comparison was performed using three accepted scales for measuring severity of disease and level of disability in patients with PD: the Unified Parkinson's Disease scale,[5] Hoehn and Yahr staging scale,[6] and the Schwab and England activities of daily living scale. The Unified PD scale has four parts: mentation, activities of daily living, motor examination, and complications of therapy. Comparison was performed for the overall score as well as the individual parts.

The vitamin E group had a significantly lower unified PD score than controls (mean 26.3 vs 37.1; $p < 0.05$), suggesting less severe disease. Hoehn and Yahr, and Schwab and England scores also reflected a trend toward less severe disease in the vitamin E group. We also examined eight of these PD patients who could be matched with their respective controls for daily levodopa dose (463 mg vs 488 mg), as well as age and duration of PD. The vitamin E group had significantly lower mean unified PD scores than controls (21.1 vs 38.3; $p < 0.05$). This was reflected most prominently in mean scores of the activities of daily living portion (6.9 vs 12.8; $p = 0.05$) and the complications of therapy portion (0.88 vs 3.50; $p < 0.05$). In addition, the mean Schwab and England score was significantly higher in the vitamin E group than controls (90.6 vs 78.7; $p < 0.05$). These findings indicate that the vitamin E group had significantly less severe disease than controls. Three of our patients were taking vitamin E at doses of 400, 1600, and 3200 IU per day for 2, 17, and 13 years, respectively, prior to the onset of PD. Our results suggest that vitamin E does not prevent the onset of PD; however, it may slow the natural progression of the disorder.

REFERENCES

1. HALLIWELL, B. & J. M. C. GUTTERIDGE. 1985. Trends Neurosci. **8:** 22-26.
2. DEXTER, D., C. CARTER, F. AGID *et al.* 1986. Lancet **2:** 639-640.
3. KISH, S. J., C. MORITO & O. HORNYKIEWICZ. 1985. Neurosci. Lett. **58:** 343-346.
4. PERRY, T. L., D. V. GODIN & S. HANSEN. 1982. Neurosci. Lett. **33:** 305-310.
5. Parkinson Study Group. 1987. Neurology 37(Suppl. 1): 278.
6. HOEHN, M. M. & M. D. YAHR. 1967. Neurology **17:** 427-442.

Vitamin E in Preterm Infants during the First Year of Life

MARIA LUCIA SILVEIRA FERLIN,
FRANCISCO EULÓGIO MARTINEZ,
SALIM MOYSÉS JORGE,
ARTHUR LOPES GONÇALVES, AND
INDRAJID D. DESAI

Medical School
University of São Paulo
14049, Ribeirão Preto, SP
São Paulo, Brazil

INTRODUCTION

Preterm newborns are considered a high-risk group with respect to vitamin E deficiency, which can lead to hemolytic anemia.[1] Maternal nutrition, birthweight, gestational age, dietary vitamin E content, iron, polyunsaturated fatty acids, and absorption ability[2,3] are factors that predispose to the onset of vitamin E deficiency. The objectives of this study were to determine vitamin E levels in preterm infants during the first year of life, the influence of these levels on early and late prematurity anemia, and the effect of iron prophylaxis on these levels.

MATERIAL AND METHODS

Twenty-five preterm infants were followed longitudinally during the first year of life. Subjects were born at the University Hospital, Faculty of Medicine of Ribeirão Preto, USP with birthweight < 1800 g and gestational age of 30 to 36 weeks. Eleven children (group I) received 2 mg/kg/day of iron by the oral route in the form of ferrous sulfate from the 15th day of life, and 14 children (group II) received the same amount of iron from the second month of life. Iron supplementation at this dose was continued for both groups until the end of the first year of life. Plasma concentrations of vitamin E[4] and total lipids,[5] globular resistance to hydrogen peroxide,[6] and hematocrit were determined at birth and at 2, 4, 6, 9-10, and 12 months.

RESULTS AND DISCUSSION

The vitamin E/total lipid ratio did not differ between groups at birth. At 2 months, 6 (55%) of the infants in group I showed an inadequate vitamin E/total lipid ratio as opposed to only 1 (7%) in group II ($p < 0.05$), considering 0.6 mg/g to be the lower normal limit[7] (FIG. 1). Hemoglobin and hematocrit reached minimum values at this age (TABLE 1). Data analysis suggests that early iron treatment (15 days)

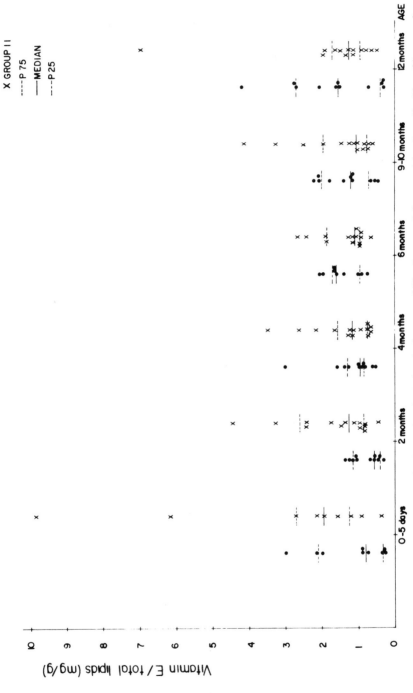

FIGURE 1. Values of the vitamin E/total lipids (mg/g) ratio during the first year of life of preterm infants receiving 2 mg/kg/day of iron p.o. from 15 days (group I) and from 2 months of age (group II).

TABLE 1. Hemoglobin Levels, Hematocrit, Vitamin E, Vitamin E/Total Lipid Ratio, and Red Cell Resistance to Hydrogen Peroxide in Preterm Infants Receiving Iron from the 15th Day (Group I) and from Two Months (Group II) of Age

Age		0–5 days GI[a]	0–5 days GII[b]	2 months GI	2 months GII	4 months GI	4 months GII	6 months GI	6 months GII	9–10 months GI	9–10 months GII	12 months GI	12 months GII
Hemoglobin (g/dL)	Median	18.2	19.3	10.2	9.9	10.3	11.0	10.0	11.5	11.4	11.6	12.4	11.8
	P25[c]	17.9	16.1	9.4	9.1	9.8	9.8	9.7	9.8	10.2	11.1	10.4	10.6
	P75[d]	19.6	20.8	10.8	10.6	11.1	11.4	10.7	12.3	12.4	12.8	13.1	12.3
Hematocrit (percent)	Median	57	57	31	29	32	32	34	34	37	35	38	37
	P25	53	50	29	27	31	30	33	33	36	34	35	35
	P75	58	61	32	31	35	34	36	37	39	38	39	40
Vitamin E (mg/dL)	Median	0.21[e]	0.41[e]	0.40	0.42	0.41	0.45	0.63	0.53	0.56	0.52	0.57	0.46
	P25	0.16	0.37	0.26	0.40	0.38	0.35	0.45	0.45	0.36	0.43	0.28	0.43
	P75	0.47	0.63	0.57	0.53	0.52	0.51	0.73	0.77	0.67	0.61	0.73	0.61
Ratio Vitamin E/Total Lipids (mg/g)	Median	0.8	2.0	0.6[e]	1.2[e]	1.0	1.1	1.6	1.1	1.2	1.1	1.5	1.3
	P25	0.3	1.2	0.4	0.9	0.8	0.7	1.0	1.0	0.7	0.8	0.4	0.9
	P75	2.1	2.7	1.1	2.3	1.3	1.6	1.7	1.8	2.0	2.0	2.7	1.7
RBC[f] Resistance to H_2O_2	Median	50	56	51	53	39	32	16	19	16	41	14	32
	P25	19	51	34	33	14	18	13	16	5	21	12	23
	P75	76	64	83	83	88	48	28	38	24	74	26	58

[a] GI = Group I.
[b] GII = Group II.
[c] P25 = percentile 25.
[d] P75 = percentile 75.
[e] $p < 0.05$.
[f] RBC = red blood cells.

may have interfered with the levels and nutritional adequacy of vitamin E, though without worsening early prematurity anemia.

From 4 months to the end of the first year of life, only 8% of all children in the two groups showed inadequate vitamin E/total lipid ratios at 4 and 9 months, and only 17% showed the same at 12 months (FIG. 1). There was no relationship between the late anemia detected in the infants and vitamin E levels (TABLE 1).

The elevated erythrocyte hemolysis index observed in the presence of hydrogen peroxide (> 20%)[7] at all ages suggests that this test is inappropriate for the detection of vitamin E deficiency and that other factors may be involved that cause greater red cell fragility. The present findings do not support the appropriateness of offering prophylactic vitamin E to preterm infants, even when they are supplemented early with iron, at the dose of 2 mg/kg/day.

REFERENCES

1. OSKI, F. A. & L. A. BARNESS. 1967. Vitamin E deficiency: A previously unrecognized cause of hemolytic anemia in the premature infant. J. Pediatr. **70**(2): 211-220.
2. GROSS, S. & D. K. MELHORN. 1974. Vitamin E-dependent anemia in the premature infant. J. Pediatr. **85**(6): 753-759.
3. EHRENKRANZ, R. A. 1980. Vitamin E and the neonate. Am. J. Dis. Child. **134**(12): 1157-1166.
4. HANSEN, L. G. & W. J. WARWICK. 1966. A fluorometric micro method for serum tocopherol. Am. J. Clin. Pathol. **36**(6): 133-138.
5. AMENTA, J. S. 1970. A rapid extraction and quantification of total lipids and lipid fractions in blood and feces. Clin. Chem. **16**(4): 339-346.
6. ROSE, C. S. & P. GYORGY. 1952. Specificity of hemolytic reaction in vitamin E deficient erythrocytes. Am. J. Physiol. **168**(2): 414-420.
7. FARRELL, P. M., S. L. LEVINE, M. D. MURPHY & A. J. ADAMS. 1978. Plasma tocopherol levels and tocopherol-lipid relationship in a normal population of children as compared to healthy adults. Am. J. Clin. Nutr. **31**(4): 1720-1726.

Antioxidant Therapy and Uptake of Human Oxidized LDL by Macrophages

J. C. FRUCHART, J. SAUZIERES,[a] V. CLAVEY, AND
M. O. PLANCKE

Service de Recherche sur les Lipoproteines et l'Athérosclérose
Institut Pasteur de Lille
1 rue du Pr. Calmette
59019 Lille, France
[a] Laboratoire Negma
584 rue Fourny
78530 Buc, France

There is now substantial evidence that blood monocytes are precursors of certain foam cells in the early stage of atherogenesis[1] and that the major portion of cholesterol in atheroma is derived from plasma low density lipoproteins (LDL). Macrophages can take up and degrade native LDL but at a rather low rate and generally without marked accumulation of cholesterol.[2] By contrast, a biologically modified form of LDL, generated by incubation of native LDL with cultured endothelial cells or arterial smooth cells or macrophages,[3] is degraded much faster than native LDL by a high-affinity binding site, the "scavenger receptor," resulting in stimulation of the cholesterol ester deposit in the macrophage. This modification is accompanied by a number of striking changes, including an increase in electrophoretic mobility, an increase in density, a change in phospholipid composition, a degradation of the apoprotein B, and the generation of peroxides.[3,4] Most of the same changes can be induced by oxidizing LDL in the presence of cupric ïons in the absence of cells.[5] Because the scavenger receptor is not down-regulated, it is necessary to prevent LDL modification. D. Steinberg *et al.* have shown that *in vitro*, vitamin E, a free radical scavenger, suppresses LDL modification induced by endothelial cells or cupric solution.[4] They also demonstrated that long-term antioxidant treatment reduces, in WHHL rabbits, LDL uptake in atherosclerotic areas.[6]

The present study was designed to test the sensibility to copper-catalyzed oxidation of LDL from hypercholesterolemic patients under different treatments including an antioxidant therapy. Twenty hypercholesterolemic men (Fredrikson's type IIA) were randomized in four treatment groups : placebo, fenofibrate (300 mg/d), vitamin E (1 g/d), and fenofibrate plus vitamin E. Two months later, LDL (d = 1.019-1.063 g/mL) were isolated from fasting blood plasma by ultracentrifugation and studied as described by Steinberg.[7] Briefly, each LDL sample was individually labeled with carrier-free ^{125}I; then 200 μg [^{125}I]LDL was incubated at 37°C for 24 h in 2 mL of F-10 medium with 5 μM Cu^{2+}. At the end of the modifying incubation, medium was transferred to a mouse peritoneal macrophage culture at a final concentration of 10

447

μg/mL [^{125}I]LDL. Susceptibility of LDL to oxidation was evaluated by the rate of LDL uptake by macrophages during a 5-hour incubation. As compared to the placebo group, LDL uptake was identical in the fibrate group, meaning that fibrate has no effect on LDL oxidation; by contrast, in vitamin E, and fenofibrate plus vitamin E groups, LDL uptake was decreased by 19.9 and 22.4%, respectively ($p < 0.01$) (FIG. 1). The LDL isolated from patients treated with vitamin E were resistant to oxidative modification. In plasma, vitamin E is transported in lipoproteins, mainly in LDL, so that it offers maximum protection of the lipoproteins against the *in vivo* peroxidation process.

Because recent reports suggest that oxidation of LDL is relevant to atherogenesis,[6–10] LDL must be considered not only in terms of its plasma concentration but also in terms of its tendency to be modified. With this information in mind, the combination of a cholesterol-lowering agent with an inhibitor of LDL modification, such as vitamin E, might be a particularly effective regimen.

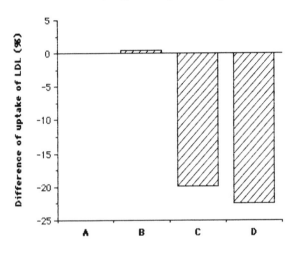

FIGURE 1. Uptake of copper-oxidized LDL from treated patients by cultured mouse peritoneal macrophages. A = placebo; B = fenofibrate; C = vitamin E; D = fenofibrate + vitamin E.

REFERENCES

1. SCHAFFNER, T., K. TAYLOR, E. J. BARTUCCI, K. FISCHER-DZOGA, J. M. BEESON, S. GLAGOV & R. W. WISSLER. 1980. Am. J. Pathol. **100:** 57-80.
2. GOLDSTEIN, J. L., Y. K. BASU & M. S. BROWN. 1979. Proc. Natl. Acad. Sci. USA **76:** 333-337.
3. JURGENS, G., H. F. HOFF, G. M. CHILSOM III & H. ESTEBAUER. 1987. Chem. Phys. Lipids **45:** 315-356.
4. STEINBRECHER, U. P., S. PARTHASARATHY, D. S. LEAKE, J. L. WITZTZUM & D. STEINBERG. 1984. Proc. Natl. Acad. Sci. USA **81:** 3883-3887.
5. MOREL, D. W., J. R. HESSLER & G. M. CHILSOM III. 1983. J. Lipid Res. **24:** 1070-1076.
6. CAREW, T. E., D. C. SCHWENKE & D. STEINBERG. 1987. Proc. Natl. Acad. Sci. USA **84:** 7725-7729.
7. PARTHASARATHY, S., S. G. YOUNG, J. L. WITZTZUM, R. C. PITTMAN & D. STEINBERG. 1986. J. Clin. Invest. **77:** 641-644.
8. CLEVIDENCE, B. A., R. E. MORTON, G. WEST, D. M. DUSEK & H. F. HOFF. 1984. Arteriosclerosis **4:** 196-207.
9. HABERLAND, M. E., D. FONG & L. CHENG. 1988. Science **241:** 216-218.
10. SCHAIKH, M., S. MARTINI, J. R. QUINEY, P. BASKERVILLE, A. E. LAVILLE, N. L. BROWSE, R. DUFFIELD, P. R. TURNER & B. LEWIS. 1988. Atherosclerosis **69:** 165-172.

Increased Platelet-Activating Factor (PAF) Synthesis in Polymorphonuclear Leukocytes of Vitamin E-Deficient Rats[a]

KENJI FUKUZAWA, YASUHIRO KUROTORI,
AKIRA TOKUMURA, AND
HIROAKI TSUKATANI

Faculty of Pharmaceutical Sciences
Tokushima University
1-78 Shomachi
Tokushima 770, Japan

Platelet-activating factor (1-O-alkyl-2-acetyl-sn-glycero-3-phosphocholine (PAF)) is a potent phospholipid mediator that causes the aggregation of platelets, the stimulation of leukocytes, and their release of factors with various inflammatory and vasoactive actions.[1] This bioactive phospholipid is synthesized in a variety of blood cells, including polymorphonuclear leukocytes (PMN).

Platelet aggregability is reported to be elevated in vitamin E-deficient animals,[2] and vitamin E has been shown to inhibit platelet aggregation due to its actions in inhibiting lipid peroxidation and regulating the turnover of arachidonic acid, the major precursor of biologically active eicosanoids.[2-4] Phospholipid metabolism is also observed to be modulated by the vitamin E status of the animal.[5-7] No evidence of a biological relation between vitamin E and PAF, however, has been reported. In the present investigation, we examined the influence of dietary vitamin E and *in vitro* addition of vitamin E on the biosynthesis and catabolism of PAF in rat PMN.

MATERIAL AND METHODS

Chemicals

[^{3}H]PAF(1-O-[^{3}H]octadecyl-2-acetyl-sn-glycero-3-phosphocholine, 80 Ci/mmol) was purchased from Amersham Corporation. Unlabeled PAF and lyso-PAF (1-O-

[a] This study was supported in part by a Research Grant (62560087) from the Japanese Ministry of Education, Science, and Culture.

octadecyl-*sn*-glycero-3-phosphocholine) were obtained from Feinchemikalien. [³H]Acetyl-CoA (1.6 Ci/mmol) was from New England Nuclear. Unlabeled acetyl-CoA, FMLP (*N*-formyl-L-methionyl-L-leucyl-L-phenylalanine) and cytochalasin B came from Sigma Chemical Company. PMSF (phenylmethylsulfonyl fluoride) were obtained from Nakarai Chemicals. Percoll came from the Pharmacia Company. Silica gel-60 plates were purchased from Merck. α-Tocopherol was kindly supplied from the Eisai Co. Ltd.

Animals

Male Wistar strain rats, initially weighing 30-50 g, were divided into a vitamin E-deficient group and vitamin E-sufficient group and given rat chow containing α-tocopherol acetate at less than 0.1 IU/100 g and 50 IU/100 g, respectively, for 16-20 weeks. Rats weighing about 230-280 g were used for experiments. At this time, the mean α-tocopherol contents of the serum of the vitamin E-sufficient and -deficient groups were 13.1 ± 0.9 μg/mL (n = 20) and less than 0.2 μg/mL (n = 20), respectively, as determined by the method of Abe and Katsui.[8]

Preparation of PMN Cells

Rat peritoneal PMN were obtained from male Wistar strain rats 15-16 hr after intraperitoneal injection of sodium caseinate.[9] The cells were separated by centrifugation at 300 g for 5 min, and a highly purified preparation of neutrophils (> 95%) was obtained by Percoll gradient centrifugation.

Biosynthesis of PAF

Reaction mixtures containing 1×10^7 PMN cells/mL Krebs Ringer phosphate buffer (KRP) and 2 mM PMSF, a serine hydrolase inhibitor, were incubated at 37°C for 15 minutes. The mixture was then centrifuged at 120 g for 2 min at 4°C to remove PMSF, and the PMN were resuspended in the same volume of fresh KRP. Then 3 mL portions (3×10^7 cells) were stirred with 10^{-6} M FMLP, 0.5 μg/mL cytochalasin B and 1 mM CaCl$_2$ for 12 minutes. Reactions were terminated by the addition of 10 mL of chloroform/methanol (1:2, v/v), and lipids were extracted by the method of Blight and Dyer.[10] After evaporation of solvent, the residues were dissolved in 100 μL of chloroform/methanol (2:1) and subjected to TLC on silicagel-60 plates with chloroform/methanol/water (65:35:7) as solvent. Bands of PAF were scraped off and extracted by the method of Blight and Dyer. The solvent was evaporated, and the concentration of PAF was determined by assay of its ability to aggregate washed rabbit platelets.[11] Student's t test was used to calculate the significance of differences.

Acetyltransferase Assay

The activity of lyso-PAF:acetyl-CoA acetyltransferase (EC 2.3.1.67) was assayed by a modification of the method of Albert and Snyder.[12] The acetylation reaction was carried out at 37°C in basic medium containing 60 mM Tris-HCl (pH 7.5), 0.2% fatty acid-free bovine serum albumin, 10 μM $CaCl_2$, 2 mM PMSF (an inhibitor of acetylhydrolase), 12 μM lyso-PAF, 2 μCi of [^{3}H]acetyl-CoA, 130 μM acetyl-CoA, and about 0.2 mg protein of cell lysate in a final volume of 2 milliliters. The reaction was started by the addition of [^{3}H]acetyl-CoA. After incubation, radioactive PAF was extracted and purified, and its radioactivity was assayed in a liquid scintillation counter.

Acetylhydrolase Assay

The activity of PAF acetylhydrolase (EC 3.1.1.48) was determined by the method of Blank *et al.*[13] with minor modifications. The reaction mixture consisted of 60 mM

TABLE 1. Effect of Dietary Vitamin E on PAF Production in FMLP-Activated Rat PMN Cells[a]

| Group | PAF (pmoles/10^6 cells/12 min) | | |
	Exp. 1	Exp. 2	Exp. 3
E-Deficient	354	248	345
E-Sufficient	153	131	227

[a] n = 3-4

Tris-HCl (pH 7.5), 80 μCi of [^{3}H]PAF, 50 μM PAF, 0.8% fatty acid-free bovine serum albumin, 0.1 mM EDTA (to inhibit acetyltransferase), and about 0.2 mg protein of cell lysate in a final volume of 2 milliliters. The reaction was carried out at 37°C, and then radioactive PAF and lyso-PAF were extracted, purified, and measured in a liquid scintillation counter.

RESULTS AND DISCUSSION

TABLE 1 shows the effect of dietary vitamin E on FMLP-induced biosynthesis of PAF by PMN from rat peritoneum. In each experiment, PMN obtained from three or four rats were incubated with FMLP for 12 min at 37°C. Vitamin E deficiency increased PAF production. This increase could be attributed to increased synthesis and/or decreased catabolism of PAF in vitamin E-deficient animals. Acetylation of lyso-PAF by acetyltransferase [1] is the main pathway for the biosynthesis of PAF, and deacetylation of PAF by acetylhydrolase [2] is the first step in its conversion to biologically inactive lyso-PAF in PMN.

$$\text{lyso-PAF + acetyl-CoA} \xrightarrow{\text{acetyltransferase}} \text{PAF} \qquad [1]$$

$$\text{PAF} \xrightarrow{\text{acetylhydrolase}} \text{lyso-PAF + CH}_3\text{COOH} \qquad [2]$$

As shown in TABLE 2, when lyso-PAF and [³H]acetyl-CoA were incubated with PMN homogenates at 37°C, [³H]PAF production by PMN of vitamin E-deficient rats was about twice that of PMN of vitamin E-sufficient rats. There was no difference, however, between the activities of acetylhydrolase in the two groups, measured as degradation of PAF (TABLE 2) and formation of lyso-PAF (data not shown) on incubation of [³H]PAF with PMN homogenates. In the case of phosphatidylcholine, the major phospholipid in mammalian tissue, vitamin E deficiency is reported to increase both its biosynthesis and catabolism through acylation and deacylation at its sn-2 position.[5-7]

Next, we examined whether the lower activity of acetyltransferase in vitamin E-sufficient rats was attributable to direct inhibition of the enzyme by α-tocopherol. A physiological concentration of α-tocopherol (40 ng/mL of incubation medium) and a 10-fold higher concentration (400 ng/mL) were added to samples of homogenate of PMN from vitamin E-deficient rats and incubated with lyso-PAF and [³H]acetyl-CoA. No difference was found in [³H]PAF production with and without added α-tocopherol (data not shown), indicating that the acetyltransferase was not directly inhibited by α-tocopherol.

Kinetic data on the acetyltransferases from the two groups are shown in FIGURE 1. The K_m and V_{max} values of the enzymes for acetyl-CoA were determined from double reciprocal plots. The K_m values of the vitamin E-deficient and -sufficient groups were similar (225 and 216 μM, respectively), but their V_{max} values were different (6.4 and 3.6 nmoles/min/mg protein). These results suggest that in vitamin E deficiency the acetyltransferase was not activated but increased in amount.

PAF was first characterized by its platelet-aggregating activity,[14] but later it was shown to have a wide spectrum of biological activities on physiological and pathological processes.[1] Our findings should be helpful in further studies on other effects of PAF besides elevated platelet aggregation in vitamin E-deficient animals.

TABLE 2. Effect of Dietary Vitamin E on the Activities of Lyso-PAF: Acetyl-CoA Acetyltransferase and PAF Acetylhydrolase in Rat PMN Homogenates[a]

Group	Acetyltransferase	Acetylhydrolase
	(nmoles/min/mg protein)	
E-Deficient	2.28 ± 0.07	4.26 ± 0.71
E-Sufficient	1.06 ± 0.10	4.26 ± 0.06
	$p < 0.001$	NS

[a] n = 6

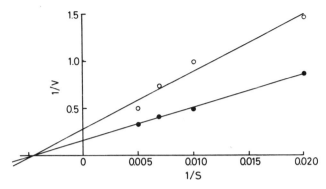

FIGURE 1. Double reciprocal plot of lyso-PAF:acetyl-CoA acetyltransferase activity of vitamin E-deficient ● and -sufficient ○ rats. V, PAF (nmoles/min/mg protein); S, acetyl-CoA (μM).

ACKNOWLEDGMENT

The authors are grateful to Eisai Co. Ltd., Tokyo for generous gifts of vitamin E-deficient and -sufficient rat chow.

REFERENCES

1. BRAQUET, P., L. TOUQUI, T. Y. SHEN & B. B. VARGAFTIG. 1987. Perspectives in platelet-activating factor research. Am. Soc. Pharmacol. Exp. Ther. **39:** 97-145.
2. KARPEN, C. W., A. J. MEROLA, R. V. TREWYN, D. G. CORNWELL & R. V. PANGANAMALA. 1981. Modulation of platelet thromboxane A_2 and arterial prostacyclin by dietary vitamin E. Prostaglandins **22:** 651-661.
3. OKUMA, T., H. TAKAHASHI & H. UCHINO. 1980. Generation of prostacyclin-like substance and lipid peroxidation in vitamin E-deficient rats. Prostaglandins **19:** 527-536.
4. STEINER, M. & J. ANASTASI. 1976. Vitamin E. An inhibition of the platelet release reaction. J. Clin. Invest. **57:** 723-737.
5. CHAN, A. C., B. FRAGISKOS, C. E. DOUGLAS & P. C. CHOY. 1985. Increased arachidonate incorporation in perfused heart phospholipids from vitamin E-deficient rats. Lipids **20:** 328-330.
6. DOUGLAS, C. E., A. C. CHAN & P. C. CHOY. 1986. Vitamin E inhibits platelet phospholipase A_2. Biochim. Biophys. Acta **876:** 639-645.
7. CAO, Y.-Z., K. O., P. C. CHOY & A. C. CHAN. 1987. Regulation by vitamin E of phosphatidylcholine metabolism in rat heart. Biochem. J. **247:** 135-140.
8. ABE, K. & G. KATSUI. 1975. Fluorometric determination of tocopherol in serum. Jpn. J. Food Nutr. **28:** 277-280.
9. CUNNINGHAM, F. M., M. J. H. SMITH, A. W. FORD-HUTCHINSON & J. R. WALKER. 1979. Migration of peritoneal polymorphonuclear leucocytes in the rat. J. Pathol. **128:** 15-20.
10. BLIGHT, E. & W. J. DYER. 1959. A rapid method of total lipid extraction and purification. Can. J. Biochem. Physiol. **37:** 911-917.
11. TOKUMURA, A., J. YOSHIDA, T. MARUYAMA, K. FUKUZAWA & H. TSUKATANI. 1987. Platelet aggregation induced by ether-linked phospholipids. Inhibitor actions of bovine serum albumin and structural analogues of platelet activating factor. Thromb. Res. **46:** 51-63.

12. ALBERT, D. H. & F. SNYDER. 1983. Biosynthesis of 1-alkyl-2-acetyl-sn-glycero-3-phosphocoline (platelet-activating factor) from 1-alkyl-2-acyl-sn-glycero-3-phosphocoline by rat alveolar macrophages. J. Biol. Chem. **258:** 97-102.
13. BLANK, M. L., A. A. SPECTOR, T. L. KADUCE, T. LEE & F. SNYDER. 1986. Metabolism of platelet activating factor (1-alkyl-2-acetyl-sn-glycero-3-phosphocoline) and 1-alkyl-2-acetyl-sn-glycerol by human endothelial cells. Biochim. Biophys. Acta **876:** 373-378.
14. BENVENISTE, J., P. M. HENSON & C. G. COCHRANE. 1972. Leukocyte-dependent histamine release from rabbit platelets: The role of IgE, basophils and a platelet activating factor. J. Exp. Med. **136:** 1356-1377.

Effects of Dietary Restriction on Weight and Alpha-Tocopherol Concentration of Tissues in Rats

FUMIKO HIRAHARA

Division of Food Science
National Institute of Nutrition
Tokyo, 162 Japan

Fundamental to the general theories of the physiological action of vitamin E is an understanding of the dynamics of vitamins in the body, and adipose tissue is considered an important depot for it.[1,2] Bieri concluded, however, that the tissues other than adipose tissue contained a labile pool of alpha-tocopherol (TOC), which mobilized rapidly.[3] Machlin also reported that even during fasting, adipose tissue TOC was not mobilized readily.[4] The present study was designed to study the effects, under food restriction, of TOC distribution in adult male rats, as a part of the role of TOC in various organs and tissues.

Sprague-Dawley male rats, weighing 290 to 340 g (320.0 ± 13.1 g) were divided into four groups of six each. They were fed one of four diets for four weeks: (1) a basal diet, *ad libitum* feeding (control); (2) a food-restriction diet (FR), 70% of the control; (3) an FR diet with supplemental TOC; and (4) a vitamin E-deficient diet. TOC (by HPLC[5]) and thiobarbituric acid-reactive substance (TBA-RS) values (by colorimetry[6]) were determined in the principal organs and tissues.

The results demonstrated that TOC supplementation induced the reduction of TBA-RS values in the liver but not in adipose tissue. Although adipose tissue weight of rats fed the FR diets was apparently smaller than those of the rats fed the *ad libitum* diets (TABLE 1), there was no significant difference between the control and

TABLE 1. Tissue and Organ Weight (grams)

Tissue	Control	70% FR	70% FR + TOC	Vitamin E-deficient
Liver	$12.4 \pm 1.19^{a,b}$	10.4 ± 0.53^c	9.7 ± 0.51^c	13.0 ± 1.06^b
Heart	1.1 ± 0.06^b	0.9 ± 0.02	0.9 ± 0.04	1.1 ± 0.05^b
Kidney	3.0 ± 0.31^b	2.6 ± 0.15	2.3 ± 0.13	3.0 ± 0.18^b
Spleen	0.9 ± 0.19^b	0.6 ± 0.01^c	0.6 ± 0.08^c	0.8 ± 0.11^b
Lung	2.5 ± 0.98^b	2.2 ± 0.49^b	2.1 ± 0.51^b	2.7 ± 0.81^b
Testis	3.4 ± 0.23^b	3.3 ± 0.29^b	3.4 ± 0.13^b	3.5 ± 0.38^b
Retroperitoneum Fat Pad	6.8 ± 1.87^b	2.7 ± 0.58^c	3.2 ± 0.43^c	8.0 ± 1.63^b
Epididymal Fat Pad	5.0 ± 0.75^b	3.4 ± 0.20	3.8 ± 0.18	5.9 ± 0.85^b

[a] Mean $\pm$ SD. Means in the same line not sharing a common supperscript are significantly different ($p < 0.05$).

the FR groups in tissue TOC concentration (μg TOC/g tissue) except in adipose tissue. Therefore, total TOC content (μg TOC/whole tissue) of the tissues decreased significantly in the FR groups in liver, heart, spleen, kidney, and lung. On the other hand, TOC concentration of adipose tissue increased almost twice as much as that of the control, but per tissue there were not significant differences between the control and FR groups (FIG. 1). The fatty acid composition was not different among the groups. These results suggest that there are separate mechanisms for the efflux of triglyceride and TOC from adipose tissue.

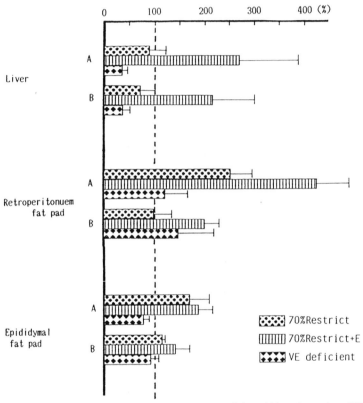

FIGURE 1. The percentage of TOC content per gram of tissue(A) and per tissue(B) in the principal tissues of rats fed the control diet, the food-restricted diet (70%), the food-restricted diet with added TOC, and the vitamin E-deficient diet.

REFERENCES

1. McMasters, V., T. Howard, L. W. Kinsell, J. Van der Veen & H. S. Olcott. 1967. Am. J. Clin. Nutr. **20:** 622-626.
2. Engelhart, F. R., J. R. Geraci & B. L. Walker. 1975. Comp. Biochem. Physiol. **52B:** 561-562.

3. BIERI, J. G. 1972. Ann. N. Y. Acad. Sci. **203:** 181-191.
4. MACHLIN, L. J., J. KEATING, J. NELSON, M. BRIN, P. PILIPSKI & O. N. MILLER. 1979.
    J. Nutr. **109:** 105-109.
5. HIRAHARA, F. & M. YAMAGUCHI. 1984. Jpn. J. Nutr. (in Japanese) **42:** 21-30.
6. OHKAWA, H., N. OSHISHI & K. YAGI. 1979. Anal. Biochem. **95:** 351-358.

Photooxidative Inactivation of Membrane-Bound Enzymes

Pathological Significance of Heme-Related Metabolites

MASAYASU INOUE AND YUKIO ANDO

Department of Biochemistry
Kumamoto University Medical School
Kumamoto 860, Japan

Reactive oxygens have been postulated to play critical roles in the pathogenesis of various diseases. Despite extensive studies on peroxidative damage of membranous lipids as a cause of oxygen-induced tissue injury, only limited information is available for the inactivation of membranous proteins. To understand better the pathological significance of reactive oxygen in membrane deterioration in various diseases, we tested the effect of $o_2 \cdot^{-}$ on γ-glutamyltransferase (GGT) and alkaline phosphatase (AP), enzymes that anchor the external surface of plasma membranes in the presence or absence of various scavengers.

RESULTS AND DISCUSSION

To test the effect of photooxidation on renal brush border membrane-bound AP and GGT, membrane samples were irradiated at 10°C in the presence of porphyrin-related metabolites (FIG. 1). Photolysis induced a rapid inactivation of AP and GGT; among various metabolites tested, protoporphyrin showed the most potent activity to inactivate the enzyme. Inactivation of AP was prevented by the presence of albumin or serum; the protective effect of serum was more potent than that of the same concentration of albumin. FIGURE 2 shows the effect of various antioxidants on bilirubin-induced AP inactivation. The rate of inactivation was markedly reduced by the presence of various antioxidants; tryptophan was most effective in protecting AP, suggesting that singlet oxygens were responsible for the inactivation. Bilirubin-catalyzed inactivation of the enzyme was also inhibited by normal serum. Analbuminemic rat serum also protected AP; however, its protective effect was lower than that of normal serum. This suggests that both albumin and nonalbumin components of serum are responsible for preventing photooxidation inactivation. Thus, membranous enzymes and other functional molecules in some tissues exposed to light, such as skin

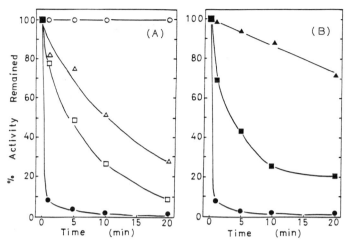

FIGURE 1. Photooxidative inactivation of membrane-bound AP by porphyrin-related metabolites. (A) Incubation medium contained in a final volume of 1 mL, 60 μg of renal brush border membranes, 20 mM phosphate buffer, pH 7.4, either 10 μM of coproporphyrin □, protoporphyrin ●, or 0.2 mM bilirubin △. Photooxidation was started at 10°C by irradiation, as described previously.[1] The membrane samples were also incubated with 0.2 mM bilirubin without photolysis ○. (B) Protoporphyrin-catalyzed photooxidation was also performed in the presence of 0.3 mM rat albumin ■ or 50% serum ▲.

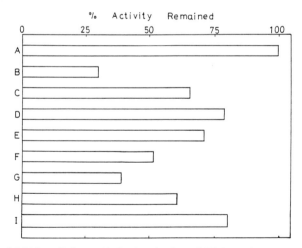

FIGURE 2. Inhibition of photooxidative inactivation of AP by various scavengers. Photooxidation of membranous AP was carried out for 15 min at 10°C in the presence of 0.2 mM bilirubin and various scavengers. A, incubated without photolysis; B, photooxidized without scavengers; C, photooxidized in the presence of 0.2 mM tryptophan; D, 2 mM tryptophan; E, 1 mM vitamin C; F, 1 mM α-tocopherol; G, 2 mM reduced glutathione; H, 50% normal rat serum; I, 50% analbuminemic rat serum. Other conditions were the same as in FIG. 1.

and eye, would undergo oxidative inactivation when levels of photosensitizable metabolites increased in patients with hyperbilirubinemia and porphyria. Inasmuch as hazardous metabolites with a long half-life can be generated under oxidative stress, tissues other than skin and eye may also be perturbed by such diseases.

REFERENCE

1. ITOH, K., M. INOUE & Y. MORINO. 1984. Enzyme **31:** 143-153.

Vitamin E and Membrane Abnormalities in Red Cells of Sickle Cell Disease Patients and Newborn Infants

SUSHIL K. JAIN

Department of Pediatrics
Louisiana State University School of Medicine
Shreveport, Louisiana 71130

Vitamin E is known to protect the red blood cell (RBC) membrane by scavenging peroxidation processes and stabilizing the membrane bilayer. Studies of sickle cell patients have shown that their RBC have a greater amount of peroxidative lipid damage and accumulation of malondialdehyde (MDA) in the membranes than do the RBC of normal patients.[1-4] We have recently found that the plasma of sickle cell patients also contains increased levels of MDA. In the present study, we found that oral supplementation of vitamin E (400 IU/day) to these patients significantly reduced the amount of membrane lipid peroxidation products in both RBC and plasma. Previous studies have shown that MDA accumulation in the RBC can decrease its deformability[5,6] and can induce irreversible sickling of discoid sickle cells.[2] Our results suggest that vitamin E supplementation to sickle cell patients decreases lipid peroxidation and lowers MDA levels in RBC (FIG. 1), which may increase RBC deformability and reduce irreversible sickling of sickle cells as observed by Natta *et al.*[7]

It has been known for many years that RBC from newborns are more susceptible to peroxide-induced lipid peroxidation and hemolysis. Newborns also have low levels of plasma vitamin E, presumably due to its limited transport across the placenta. We have found that fresh, untreated RBC of newborns have nearly two-fold amounts of MDA as measured by thiobarbituric acid reactivity.[8] Further, we observed that in RBC of some newborns, phosphatidylserine (PS) is present in the outer membrane bilayer, in contrast to the presence of PS only in the inner membrane bilayer of adult RBC (TABLE 1). There was a significant correlation between the PS externalization and increased *in vitro* coagulability of neonatal RBC as measured by Russel's viper venom clotting time.[9] Further, newborn infants with lower plasma vitamin E levels had greater *in vitro* coagulability of RBC, which suggests that supplementation of vitamin E to newborns or to expecting mothers may prevent some of the coagulation abnormalities frequently encountered in the neonatal period.

[a] This study was supported in part by a Grant from the NIH, #RO1 HL30247, and Grants-in-aid from Hoffmann-La Roche Inc. and the National Diabetes Association.

461

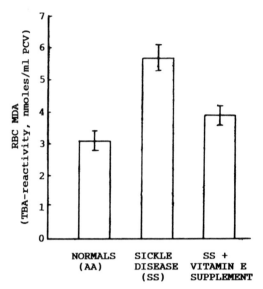

FIGURE 1. The effect of vitamin E supplementation on the level of malondialdehyde (MDA), an end product of lipid peroxidation in RBC of sickle cell disease patients. Values are mean ± SE of 19 normals, 15 sickle cell disease (SS), and 15 vitamin E-supplemented SS patients. Sickle cell disease patients were given orally 400 IU vitamin E capsules daily for 2-3 months. Note a decrease in the level of lipid peroxidative damage in RBC of patients after vitamin E supplementation.

TABLE 1. Plasma Vitamin E and Phosphatidylserine (PS) Externalization across the Membrane Bilayer and Coagulability of Red Blood Cells (RBC) in Newborns and Adults[a]

	Vitamin E in Plasma (μg/mL)	PS Externalization in RBC (percent of total)	*In vitro* Clotting Time of RBC (seconds)
Newborns (10)	1.7 ± 0.2	4 ± 1	8.3 ± 0.4
Adults (9)	5.4 ± 0.7	0	9.8 ± 0.4

[a] Values are mean ± SE. Number of subjects is given in parenthesis. Differences in values between newborns and adults are statistically significant ($p < 0.01$). Newborn values are from blood of fresh placental cord obtained immediately after delivery. Adult values are from blood of any healthy volunteer. PS externalization was assessed by treating RBC with bee venom phospholipase-A_2. *In vitro* clotting time of RBC was measured in a fibrometer using Russell's viper venom.[9]

ACKNOWLEDGMENT

The author thanks Ms. Barbara McRoberts for editing this manuscript.

REFERENCES

1. DAS, S. K. & R. C. NAIR. 1980. Superoxide dismutase, glutathione peroxidase, catalase and lipid peroxidation of normal and sickled erythrocytes. Br. J. Haematol. **41:** 223-234.
2. JAIN, S. K. & S. B. SHOHET. 1984. A novel phospholipid in irreversibly sickled cells: Evidence for *in vivo* peroxidative membrane damage in sickle cell disease. Blood **63:** 362-367.
3. HEBBEL, R. P. & W. J. MILLER. 1984. Phagocytosis of sickle erythrocytes: Immunological and oxidative determinants of hemolytic anemia. Blood **64:** 733-741.
4. CHIU, D. & B. LUBIN. 1980. Abnormal vitamin E and glutathione peroxidase levels in sickle cell anemia: Evidence for increased susceptibility to lipid peroxidation *in vivo*. J. Lab. Clin. Med. **94:** 542-548.
5. PFAFFEROTT, C., H. J. MEISELMAN & P. HOCHSTEIN. 1982. The effect of malondialdehyde on erythrocyte deformability. Blood **59:** 12-15.
6. JAIN, S. K., N. MOHANDAS, M. R. CLARK & S. B. SHOHET. 1983. The effect of malondialdehyde, a product of lipid peroxidation, on the deformability, dehydration and ^{51}Cr-survival of erythrocytes. Br. J. Haematol. **53:** 247-255.
7. NATTA, C. L., L. J. MACHLIN & M. BRIN. 1980. A decrease in irreversibly sickled erythrocytes in sickle cell anemia patients given vitamin E. Am. J. Clin. Nutr. **33:** 968-971.
8. JAIN, S. K. 1986. Membrane lipid peroxidation in erythrocytes of the newborn. Clin. Chim. Acta **161:** 301-306.
9. JAIN, S. K. 1986. Presence of phosphatidylserine in the outer membrane bilayer of newborn human erythrocyte. Biochem. Biophys. Res. Commun. **136:** 914-920.

Bilateral Stage 3-Plus Retinopathy of Prematurity (ROP)

Effect of Treatment (Rx) with High-Dose Vitamin E

L. H. JOHNSON,[a] G. E. QUINN,[b] S. ABBASI,[a]
M. DELIVORIA-PAPADOPOULOS,[d] G. PECKHAM,[c]
AND F. W. BOWEN JR.[a]

[a] Section on Newborn Pediatrics
Pennsylvania Hospital
Philadelphia, Pennsylvania 19107

[b] Department of Ophthalmology
[c] Division of Neonatology
Children's Hospital of Philadelphia
Philadelphia, Pennsylvania 19104

[d] Neonatal/Perinatal Medicine
Hospital of the University of Pennsylvania
Philadelphia, Pennsylvania 19104

ROP is an oxidant disease of the incompletely vascularized retina. Increasing evidence suggests that its initiation, progression, and long-term outcome are modulated by the balance between oxidant stress and antioxidant defenses.[1,2]

ROP of stage 3-plus severity with $\geq$ 5 contiguous or 8 cumulative clock hours of extraretinal neovascularization (ERNV) in zones 1 or 2 (International Classification of ROP) carries a poor visual prognosis.[3,4] It was designated as severe ROP and threshold for treatment (Rx) in the Multicenter Trial of Cryotherapy for ROP (Cryo Trial). Untreated bilateral ROP of this severity[4,5] results in a 50% incidence of zone 1 retinal detachment, retinal fold involving the macula or retrolental tissue mass ($\geq$ grade 3 cicatricial (CIC) ROP).

We report here the results, by worse eye grade, of high-dose vitamin E Rx of bilateral severe ROP in 33 $\leq$ 1250 gram birth weight (BW) infants ($\bar{x}$ BW 789 g $\pm$ SD 186) cared for in the University of Pennsylvania Perinatal Complex between 1981 and 1986 when enrollment in the Cryo Trial began. At diagnosis (Dx) of threshold ROP in at least one eye ($\bar{x}$ age Dx 10.5 weeks $\pm$ SD 1.7) and after informed consent had been obtained, vitamin E was administered by the intravenous, intramuscular, and/or oral route to maintain serum E levels of 3 to 5 mg/dL until ROP was clearly regressing or CIC ROP had developed. The Hoffmann-La Roche parenteral preparation of dl-alpha-tocopherol free alcohol was used on an investigator's IND permit.

TABLE 1. Long-term Outcome following Treatment of Bilateral Severe ROP with High-dose Vitamin E (Worse Eye Grade)[a]

Grade ROP	≤ Grade-1 CIC	Grade-2 CIC	≥ Grade-3 CIC
No. of Infants	16	9	8
Percent of Infants	48.5%	27.5%	24.2%

[a] Reese classification for CIC ROP.[7]

Serum E levels were monitored twice weekly during active disease and weekly or biweekly thereafter. There were no complications of Rx and no apparent decrease in resistance to infection as reported in a clinical trial of prophylactic vitamin E using 5 mg/dL serum levels from birth until completion of retinal vascularization.[6] This may relate to the much shorter duration of Rx (usually 2 to 4 weeks) and the delayed onset of severe ROP (usually 2 months after birth), by which time host defenses are significantly more adequate and broadly based than in the newborn.

As seen in TABLE 1, only 24% of infants developed ≥ grade 3 CIC ROP or worse; 48.5% had a normal posterior pole and little or no peripheral scarring (≤ Gr 1 CIC). This is a high incidence of very favorable outcome. By way of comparison, the Cryo Trial (1986-1987) reported[5] an unfavorable outcome (≥ grade 3 CIC ROP) in 23% of eyes randomized to cryotherapy versus one of 48% for eyes assigned to no treatment ($\bar{x}$ BW = 801 g $\pm$ SD 171; $\bar{x}$ age Dx 11.4 weeks $\pm$ SD 2.6). TABLE 2 presents representative data for a single infant from our series.

TABLE 2. Details of Response to Vitamin E Therapy in One Infant with Severe ROP (Birthweight = 980 g; Gestational Age = 27 weeks)[a]

Grade	The International Classification of ROP (ICROP) (ou = both eyes, od = right, os = left)	Serum E (mg/dL)	Age days
1+ ou	Marked posterior pole dilatation and tortuosity, poor pupillary dilatation; 360° demarcation line in zone 2. Increase oral E supplement	0.5	69
2+ os	Rapid progression, "Rush" ROP	1.9	71
3+ od	Poor pupillary dilatation Begin IV vitamin E		
3+ ou	Progressive retinopathy, ERNV in all quadrants. Continue IV vitamin E	4.0	76
3+ ou	Stable od. Early resolution os. Continue IV vitamin E	4.1	83
	Stable od (decreased ERNV); resolving ROP os. Resume oral E.	3.3	93
	Resolving ROP ou. Good pupillary dilatation. Continue oral E.	3.0	101
Resolved 3+ ROP	Normal posterior pole. No peripheral scar (exam under anesthesia). Severe myopia od, mild myopia os.		2½ yr

[a] Baby WS. Clinical diagnoses included respiratory distress, acidosis, hypotension, repeated pneumothoraces, episodes of apnea, bradycardia, and suspected sepsis. Rx with artificial ventilation, 43 days; oxygen therapy, 139 days.

These results, though tentative because of the small numbers involved and the nonrandomized nature of the study, suggest that Rx of severe ROP with above physiologic serum E levels has a favorable risk/benefit ratio and deserves study in a multicenter clinical trial. Ideally, the protocol for such a trial should involve a two-tiered, sixway randomization: the first at 2-plus ROP to E Rx or no Rx, and the second at threshold ROP to E Rx or Cryo Rx.

REFERENCES

1. HITTNER, H. M., M. E. SPEER, A. J. RUDOLPH et al. 1984. Pediatrics **73:** 238-249.
2. JOHNSON, L., G. E. QUINN, S. ABBASI et al. 1989. J. Pediatr. **114:** 827-838.
3. An International Classification of Retinopathy of Prematurity. 1984. Pediatrics **74:** 127-130.
4. PALMER, E. A. & D. PHELPS. 1986. Commentary. Pediatrics **77:** 428-429.
5. Multicenter Trial of Cryotherapy for Retinopathy of Prematurity. 1988. Pediatrics **81:** 697-706.
6. JOHNSON, L., F. W. BOWEN, S. ABBASI et al. 1985. Pediatrics **75:** 619-638.
7. REESE, A. B., M. J. KING & W. C. OWENS. 1953. Am. J. Ophthalmol. **36:** 1333.

Selective Damage to the Cardiac Conduction System in Vitamin E– and Selenium-Deficient Calves

SEAMUS KENNEDY AND DESMOND A. RICE

Veterinary Research Laboratories
Stormont, Belfast BT4 3SD, Northern Ireland

Most reports of cardiac alterations in vitamin E and selenium (E-Se)-deficient animals document necrosis of the contractile myocardium but indicate that cells of the cardiac conduction system are unaffected. Nutritional myopathy commonly develops in E-Se-deficient cattle following access to pasture in the spring.[1] We have developed an experimental model for this disease.[2] It is based on feeding a low E-Se diet (1.0 mg kg^{-1} alpha-tocopherol; 0.03 mg kg^{-1} Se) to calves for several months, followed by dietary supplementation with polyunsaturated fatty acids (PUFA) to mimic ingestion of large quantities of linolenic acid from grass. Selective damage to the cardiac conduction system is a feature of our model.[3]

Autofluorescent, acid-fast, periodic-acid-Schiff-positive lipopigment granules develop in Purkinje cardiocytes after a few weeks of feeding the low E-Se diet (FIG. 1). Ultrastructurally, these granules appear as cytolysosomes containing altered mitochondria and other cell debris. More severe damage is characterized by necrosis of Purkinje cells. Such cells contain many cytolysosomes and highly electron-dense granules with electron-lucent foci that resemble classic lipofuscin (FIG. 2). Mitochondrial calcification and plasmalemmal lysis are seen in necrotic cells, but the external lamina remains intact. Necrotic cells are invaded by macrophages that phagocytose cell debris and lipopigment granules. Postnecrotic resolution of the lesions is by fibrosis.

Calves killed after 127-137 days of E-Se-depletion have relatively mild alterations of the contractile myocardium. Dietary supplementation with PUFA intensifies Purkinje cell damage and also induces severe necrosis of the contractile myocardium.

We do not know whether Purkinje lesions in our calves are the result of vitamin E deficiency, Se deficiency, or combined E-Se deficiency. Accumulation of lipopigment supports a role for lipoperoxidation in development of the lesions. Dietary supplementation with PUFA increases the severity of the lesions, further supporting such a mechanism. We do not know whether Purkinje cells are more susceptible to injury than contractile cardiocytes, because they have (1) a higher rate of production of lipoperoxidation protagonists; (2) lower concentrations of lipoperoxidation antagonists, such as vitamin E, glutathione peroxidase, superoxide dismutase, catalase, vitamin C, and vitamin A; or (3) another mechanism.

Lesions of the contractile myocardium in our calves are similar to those of Keshan disease of humans in China. Alterations of the conduction system are not similar, however, (Bo qi Gu, personal communication). Our model is an attractive method of studying damage and repair to the cardiac conduction system and has potential value for evaluating the role of Purkinje cell damage in cardiac arrhythmias.

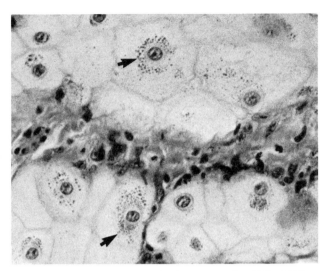

FIGURE 1. Purkinje cells of the cardiac conduction system of an E-Se-deficient calf contain many lipopigment granules (arrows); (Periodic acid-Schiff stain).

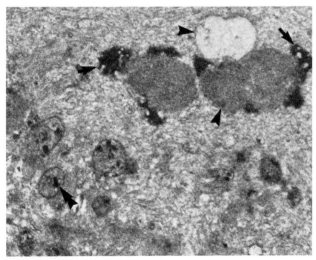

FIGURE 2. Cytolysosomes (arrowheads), lipofuscin granules (arrows), and damaged mitochondria with matrical densities (double arrowhead) are in necrotic Purkinje cardiocyte of E-Se-deficient calf; (electromicrograph × 11,400).

REFERENCES

1. MCMURRAY, C. H. & P. K. MCELDOWNEY. 1977. A possible prophylaxis and model for nutritional myopathy in young cattle. Br. Vet. J. **133:** 535-542.
2. KENNEDY, S., D. A. RICE & W. B. DAVIDSON. 1987. Experimental myopathy in vitamin E- and selenium-depleted calves with and without dietary polyunsaturated fatty acids as a model for nutritional degenerative myopathy in ruminant cattle. Res. Vet. Sci. **43:** 384-394.
3. KENNEDY, S. & D. A. RICE. 1988. Selective morphologic alterations of the cardiac conduction system in calves deficient in vitamin E and selenium. Am. J. Pathol. **130:** 315-325.

Vitamin E Modulation of Retrovirus-Induced Immune Dysfunctions and Tumor-Cell Proliferation[a]

KIMBERLY KLINE, GWENDOLEN S. COCHRAN,
ELIZABETH R. HUGGINS, THOMAS J. MORGAN,
ARUNDHATI RAO, AND BOB G. SANDERS

Division of Nutrition
University of Texas
Austin, Texas 78712

Vitamin E has been demonstrated to be a potent biomodulator of immune functions and tumorigenesis in studies of uninfected and retrovirus-infected chickens as well as in *in vitro* studies of retrovirus-transformed tumor cells. The avian retroviruses studied were reticuloendotheliosis and avian erythroblastosis viruses. These viruses induce a general suppression of the host immune response system monitored *in vitro* as reduced mitogen-induced T-lymphocyte proliferative responses and transiently expressed T suppressor cell activity, as well as thymus atrophy and disruption and fatal lymphoid leukosis or erythroleukemia.

Vitamin E (*d*-alpha tocopherol dissolved in an ethanol/polyethylene glycol vehicle) administered by i.p. injection at two-day intervals at a dose of 0.1 mg/g body weight enhanced mitogen-mediated T lymphocyte proliferation by spleen cells of uninfected chickens, reduced retrovirus-induced suppression of host T lymphocytes, reduced retrovirus-induced T suppressor cell activity (TABLE 1), and enhanced tumorigenesis. Supplementation of spleen cells from infected chickens with *d*-alpha-tocopherol acid succinate *in vitro* reduced retrovirus-suppressed mitogen-mediated responses, and reduced T suppressor cell activity. Supplementation of retrovirus-transformed tumor cell line C4#1 with *d*-alpha-tocopherol acid succinate arrested cell proliferation without affecting cell viability. Analyses of several markers suggested that the arrested proliferation was not due to vitamin E induction of differentiation/maturation.

It was important to determine if the biomodulating effects of vitamin E succinate were due to an antioxidant effect. Accordingly, other antioxidants (BHT, $CuSO_4$, and mannitol) were shown not to exhibit the biomodulating properties found with vitamin E. Although inconclusive, the biomodulating properties of vitamin E may involve mechanisms other than an antioxidant effect.

Immune functions are mediated by immune cell interactions and a host of immunoregulatory molecules. Retroviruses suppress immune responses by several mech-

[a] This research was supported by the American Institute for Cancer Research (AICR) Grant 87A69 and PHS Grant number CA45422, awarded by the National Cancer Institute, DHHS.

TABLE 1. Modulation of Reticuloendotheliosis Virus–Induced T Suppressor Cell Activity by *in Vivo* Vitamin E Supplementation

		Effect of Spleen Cells from Infected Chickens on the Mitogen-Induced Proliferative Response of Spleen Cells from Uninfected Chickens in Co-culture[a]					
Treatment[b]	Tumor Challenge[c]	+Con A (cpm)[d]	Percent Suppression[e]	+PHA (cpm)	Percent Suppression	+PWM (cpm)	Percent Suppression
Vitamin E	+	50,160 ± 1,334	0[f]	30,772 ± 1,020	13	10,560 ± 363	3
Vehicle	+	18,248 ± 664	50	15,056 ± 334	57	4,406 ± 223	59
Vehicle	–	36,444 ± 875		35,240 ± 509		10,856 ± 579	

[a] T suppressor cell activity was examined 5 days following tumor challenge. Co-culture analyses were performed at a 1:1 ratio.

[b] Vitamin E, at 0.1 mg/g body weight was administered at 2-day intervals by intraperitoneal injection starting 3 days posthatch. Vehicle contained 5% ethanol in 10% polyethylene glycol 8000 (v/v)/g body weight. Vitamin E and vehicle solutions were prepared fresh immediately prior to injection.

[c] Tumor challenge was with 1×10^4 BB5 reticuloendotheliosis virus–transformed tumor cells.

[d] Mean [³H]TdR uptake in cpm of triplicate cultures at 66 hours after 18-hour pulse of isotope.

[e] Percent suppression in comparison to age-matched, unchallenged, vehicle treated control: $100\% - \dfrac{\text{Mean cpm of experimental group co-culture}}{\text{Mean cpm of control response}} \times 100$.

[f] Analysis of Con A–induced proliferation in co-culture revealed 38% enhancement rather than suppression.

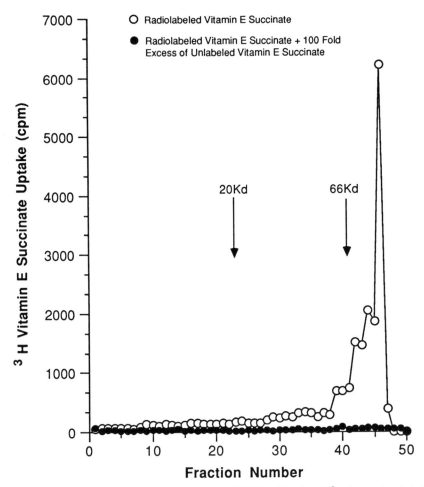

FIGURE 1. Reticuloendotheliosis virus-transformed C4#1 cells at 1×10^7/mL were incubated with 5 μL radiolabeled vitamin E succinate (d-alpha [^{3}H]tocopherol succinate; Amersham 17.4 Ci/mmol) for 30 minutes (O). Binding inhibition studies involved incubating the C4#1 cells with 5 μL radiolabeled vitamin E succinate plus a 100-fold excess of unlabeled vitamin E succinate (d-alpha-tocopherol acid succinate; Sigma; ●). Following labeling, cells were washed and fractionated; nuclei were collected by centrifugation, and soluble nuclei fractions were separated by centrifugation on a 5-20% sucrose gradient. Bovine serum albumin (66 kDa) and carbonic anhydrase (29 kDa) served as molecular mass markers.

anisms; here, only two are mentioned: elimination or alteration of specific immune cell subpopulations, and induction of host immunosuppressive cells and/or immunosuppressive molecules. A possible mechanism for vitamin E effects on retrovirus-induced immune suppression may involve (1) vitamin E interactions with arachidonic acid,[1] which result in interference with retrovirus-induced immune suppressive prostaglandin E_2 production, thereby eliminating prostaglandin E_2-dependent T suppressor cell activity;[2] and (2) up-regulation of T_{helper} cell-dependent immunoregulatory molecules such as interleukin-2.

Assuming that the biomodulating properties of vitamin E are through a mechanism not associated with the antioxidant effect, one would expect vitamin E to enter the cell and perhaps be transported to the nucleus by way of a ligand receptor-mediated process. Studies in progress, using [^{3}H]vitamin E succinate, show that the tritiated vitamin E is taken in by tumor cells, and that the tritiated vitamin E is associated with the cell nucleus. Furthermore, sucrose gradient centrifugation studies revealed a 66-70 kDa vitamin E binding molecule in soluble nuclei fractions (FIG. 1). Specificity of binding was shown by the ability of 100-fold excess of unlabeled vitamin E succinate to inhibit the binding of the tritiated vitamin E succinate.

In summary, these studies suggest that vitamin E is a potent biomodulator and that a vitamin E receptor mechanism of action may be involved.

REFERENCES

1. CARPENTER, M. J. 1986. *In* Vitamins and Cancer. F. L. Meyskens & K. N. Prasad, Eds.: 199-211. Humana Press. Clifton, NJ.
2. CHOUAIB, S., L. CHATENOUD, D. KLATZMANN & D. FRADELIZI. 1984. J. Immunol. **132**(4): 1851-1857.

Synergistic Inhibition of Oxidation in RBC Ghosts by Vitamins C and E

MASAYUKI MIKI,[a] TADASHI MOTOYAMA, AND
MAKOTO MINO

Department of Pediatrics
Osaka Medical College
Takatsuki, Osaka 569, Japan

INTRODUCTION

Recently the possible interaction of vitamins C and E has received much attention, and a number of investigations have been performed to explore the synergistic inhibition of oxidation by their combination.[1] Nevertheless, a question still remains whether such an interaction between vitamin C and the vitamin E radical can take place in biological systems, where lipophilic vitamin E resides within the membrane, and hydrophilic vitamin C resides in the aqueous region. In this study, we use azo compounds as radical initiators. This enables us to control the site of initial radical generation and could supply evidence for their interaction in biomembranes.

MATERIAL AND METHODS

Ghost membranes were prepared by Burton's method[2] from RBC of adult male Wistar rats, which were maintained on a vitamin E-deficient or control diet.[3] The ghosts obtained were suspended in buffered saline with EDTA. Initiating radicals were generated by the thermal decomposition of azo compounds[3] 2,2'-azobis(2-amidinopropane)dihydrochloride (AAPH) and 2,2'-azobis (2,4-dimethyl-valeronitrile) (AMVN). The oxidations in ghost suspension were initiated either by the addition of water-soluble AAPH or by the incubation with unoxidizable liposomes containing lipid-soluble AMVN and carried out in air at 37° or 56°C, respectively. The rate of oxygen uptake was followed with oxygen electrode, which gives a good measure of the rate of membrane oxidation. When water-soluble antioxidants, vitamin C, urate, and glutathione were added individually to the reaction medium, their effects on membrane oxidation and on vitamin E consumption were examined.

[a] Address correspondence to Masayuki Miki, M.D., c/o Prof. W. A. Pryor, 711 Choppin, Biodynamics Institute, Louisiana State University, Baton Rouge, LA 70803.

RESULTS AND DISCUSSION

When ghost suspensions were incubated with liposomes containing AMVN, the oxidation of ghosts was initiated mainly within the membrane lipid bilayer.[1] The oxygen uptake of ghosts was observed at a rapid and constant rate. Vitamin E in the membranes could interrupt the chain propagation efficiently and suppress the oxidation to form an induction period, during which it could be consumed linearly. When the radicals were generated from AAPH initially in the aqueous region, water-soluble

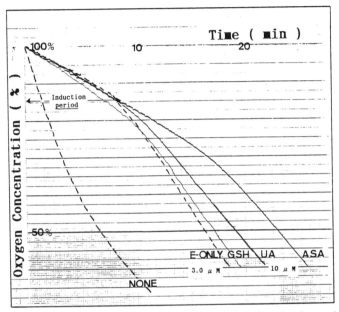

FIGURE 1. Inhibition of oxidation of ghosts in aqueous dispersions by the combination of vitamin E and water-soluble antioxidants. The oxidation was initiated by the incubation with liposomes (1.54 mM free cholesterol, 1.54 mM dimyristoyl-phosphatidylcholine) containing 1.0 mM AMVN in air at 56°C. The dashed lines show the oxygen consumption in vitamin E-deficient or -sufficient (3.0 μM) ghosts. The solid lines show the oxygen consumption in vitamin E-sufficient ghosts when ascorbate (ASA), urate (UA), and glutathione (GSH) were added individually to the reaction medium at 10 μM.

antioxidants, in the order of urate > vitamin C > glutathione suppressed the oxidation of ghosts by scavenging the radicals before they attacked the membranes. These antioxidants, however, could not trap lipid peroxyl radicals induced by AMVN. In the presence of vitamin E, only the addition of vitamin C in the reaction medium could greatly lengthen the induction period (FIG. 1). These results strongly suggest that vitamin C in the aqueous phase was more accessible to the vitamin E radical than to the lipid peroxyl radical in biomembranes and could show the synergistic antioxidant effect. During the AMVN-induced oxidation in the presence of vitamins C and E, vitamin C in the aqueous phase decreased first to maintain membrane vitamin E, which was consumed after vitamin C disappeared (FIG. 2A). This reaction indicates

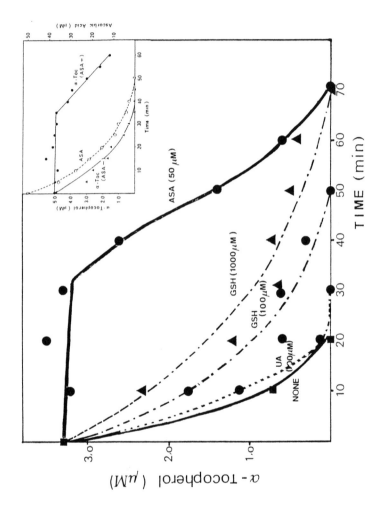

FIGURE 2. The sparing actions of water-soluble antioxidants for membrane vitamin E. (Inset) Consumption of vitamin E (solid lines) and vitamin C (dotted line) during the oxidation of ghosts induced by AMVN, as described in FIG. 1. Solid line (▲) shows the rate of decay of vitamin E in the absence of vitamin C. (Large figure) Consumption of vitamin E was shown when ascorbate (ASA; ●-solid line), glutathione (GSH; ●-broken line, ▲-broken line), and urate (UA; ●-dotted line) were added individually to the reaction medium at the indicated concentration. ■-Solid line shows the rate of decay of vitamin E in the absence of water-soluble antioxidants.

that vitamin E in membranes scavenges the lipid peroxyl radical induced by AMVN, and the resulting vitamin E radical is reduced to regenerate vitamin E by vitamin C in the aqueous phase. Any sparing action for vitamin E was hardly observed with glutathione or urate (FIG. 2B).

REFERENCES

1. NIKI, E. 1987. Interaction of ascorbate and α-tocopherol. Ann. N.Y. Acad. Sci. **498**: 186-199.
2. BURTON, G. W., K. U. INGOLD & K. E. THOMPSON. 1981. An improved procedure for the isolation of ghost membranes from human red blood cells. Lipids **16**: 946.
3. MIKI, M., H. TAMAI, M. MINO, Y. YAMAMOTO & E. NIKI. 1987. Free-radical chain oxidation of rat red blood cells by molecular oxygen and its inhibition by α-tocopherol. Arch. Biochem. Biophys. **258**(2): 373-380.

Tissue α-Tocopherol, Thiobarbituric Acid-Reactive Substances (TBA-RS), and Glutathione Levels in Rats Fed Algal Proteins[a]

G. V. MITCHELL, M. Y. JENKINS, AND E. GRUNDEL

Division of Nutrition
Food and Drug Administration
Washington, DC 20204

In recent years, the algal proteins have been promoted as alternative protein sources, adjuvants in diets for weight reduction and dietary supplements of beta carotene. Studies in our laboratory have indicated that diets containing the algal protein, Spirulina, may interfere with the utilization of the fat-soluble vitamins A and E.[1] The importance of vitamin E as a biological antioxidant is well-documented.[2] The purpose of the present study was to extend knowledge about the effect of algal proteins on plasma and liver alpha-tocopherol levels and to determine the susceptibility of selected tissues from algal-fed rats to lipid peroxidation.

Male weanling Sprague-Dawley rats were fed for six weeks a casein-control diet or the same diet containing either Spirulina or Chlorella as the protein source instead of casein. Diets were adequate in all nutrients and specifically contained 18% protein and 50 IU/kg of added *all rac*-alpha tocopherol. Plasma and liver were extracted with hexane, and alpha-tocopherol was determined by reversed phase high-performance liquid chromatography (HPLC). Lipid peroxidation was measured by determining tissue thiobarbituric acid-reactive substances (TBA-RS),[3] and liver-reduced glutathione was measured by HPLC.[4]

No significant reduction in the weight gain was noted when the algal-fed rats were compared to the casein controls (TABLE 1). There was a slight reduction in the food efficiency for rats fed the Spirulina diet, however, when compared to the other two groups. Both algal diets caused a significant reduction in plasma and liver levels of alpha-tocopherol when compared to the casein control diet. The liver TBA-RS levels were inversely related to the liver tocopherol levels. Both algal proteins caused more than a fourfold increase in liver and heart TBA-RS when compared to casein. Beta carotene, a naturally occurring component present in algal proteins, functions as an antioxidant.[2] The increased intake in dietary beta carotene, however, by the algal-fed

[a] The studies reported herein were conducted according to the principles set forth in the *Guide for the Care and Use of Laboratory Animals,* Institute of Laboratory Animals Resources, National Research Council, NIH Pub. No. 85-23.

478

TABLE 1. Effect of Dietary Treatments on Rat Growth and TBA-RS, Vitamin E, and Glutathione Levels in Selected Tissues[a]

	Casein Control	Spirulina	Chlorella
Weight gain, g	224 ± 6.4[d]	223 ± 4.6[d]	237 ± 5.5[d]
Food efficiency[b]	32 ± 0.1[e]	29 ± 0.3[d]	31 ± 0.4[e]
Plasma α-tocopherol (mg/dL)	1.1 ± 0.07[e]	0.2 ± 0.02[d]	0.2 ± 0.03[d]
Liver α-tocopherol (μg/g)	14.1 ± 0.50[e]	2.7 ± 0.27[d]	2.9 ± 0.16[d]
Liver TBA-RS[c] (nmoles/g)	23 ± 0.9[d]	123 ± 15.0[e]	105 ± 13.3[e]
Heart TBA-RS (nmoles/ heart)	6 ± 0.3[d]	24 ± 4.7[e]	31 ± 3.3[e]
Liver glutathione (μmoles/g)	3.5 ± 0.31[e]	1.5 ± 0.19[d]	1.9 ± 0.18[d]

[a] Values are means plus SEM for n = 10. Values in the same horizontal row not sharing a common superscript letter are significantly different from each other at $p < 0.05$.
[b] Food efficiency = weight gain/food intake × 100.
[c] TBA-RS = thiobarbituric acid–reactive substances measured as malondialdehyde.

rats did not prevent the production of high levels of TBA-RS. In addition, glutathione, a component of the secondary oxidative defense system, was significantly lower in the livers of algal-fed rats than in those of the casein-fed group. These results suggest that the bioavailability of vitamin E is reduced in diets of rats fed the algal proteins. This may explain some of the alterations in the oxidative defense system of the algal-fed rats.

REFERENCES

1. JENKINS, M. Y. & G. V. MITCHELL. 1986. Nutr. Res. 6(9): 1083-1094.
2. MACHLIN, L. J. & A. BENDICH. 1987. Fed. Am. Soc. Exp. Biol. 1: 441-445.
3. BUCKINGHAM, K. W. 1985. J. Nutr. 115: 1425-1435.
4. COTGREAVE, I. A. & P. MOLDEUS. 1986. J. Biochem. Biophys. Methods 13: 231-249.

Alpha-Tocopherol in Microsomal Lipid Peroxidation[a]

MICHAEL E. MURPHY, HEINER SCHOLICH,
HERIBERT WEFERS, AND HELMUT SIES [b]

Institut für Physiologische Chemie I
Universität Düsseldorf
D-4000 Düsseldorf, F.R.G.

INTRODUCTION

The reactivity of vitamin E with free radicals is considered its major biochemical function. Studies by Ingold and associates have provided information about the rate constants with which vitamin E reacts with peroxyl radicals. The latter are generated from polyunsaturated fatty acids after hydrogen abstraction by the addition of an oxygen molecule (FIG. 1). The formation of the chromanoxyl radical from the tocopherols (reaction 3b in FIG. 1) occurs with rate constants of about $10^{-6} M^{-1} s^{-1}$.[1] This reaction is the basis for the proposal by Tappel[2] that vitamin E functions as an *in vivo* antioxidant that protects tissue lipids from free radical attack (see also ref. 3). Vitamin E has been described as the only lipid-soluble chain-breaking antioxidant in human blood plasma and erythrocyte membranes,[4] and it seems that alpha-tocopherol is the optimized structure for biological antioxidant effectiveness. The phytyl side chain is required for optimum antioxidant activity in biological membranes.[5] Most likely it is involved in the proper positioning of the vitamin, given its lipophilic properties.[6] The antioxidant properties of vitamin E *in vitro* and *in vivo* have been analyzed,[7] and the current state of knowledge on the biochemical function of vitamin E together with the relevant literature have been compiled by Machlin.[8]

It is possible that the biological activity of vitamin E is fully accounted for by its antioxidant properties. The effect of the reaction shown in FIGURE 1 would be that the radical chain of lipid peroxidation is interrupted, if the vitamin E radical can be repaired and by itself does not lead to further propagation reactions. The hydroperoxide generated from the peroxyl radical may undergo further nonradical repair reactions, for example, the reduction to the corresponding alcohol by peroxidase reactions and the excision of the peroxidized fatty acid from the phospholipids in the membrane.

[a]The work was supported by the Deutsche Forschungsgemeinschaft, by the National Foundation for Cancer Research, and by the Krebsforschung International e.V., Frankfurt. M.E.Murphy was supported by a Grant from the Deutscher Akademischer Austauschdienst (DAAD).

[b]Address for correspondence: Prof. Dr. Helmut Sies, Institut für Physiologische Chemie I, Universität Düsseldorf, Moorenstr. 5, D-4000 Düsseldorf, F.R.G.

At present, one should be open to further potential effects of vitamin E because of the high degree of specificity. For example, there could be special biochemical reactions that can be effectively modulated. This refers to some of the enzymatic transformations of arachidonic acid. In addition, vitamin E can react with singlet molecular oxygen.[9–11]

REGENERATION OF ALPHA-TOCOPHEROL FROM THE CHROMANOXYL RADICAL

One of the active fields of interest in vitamin E research currently focuses on the processes related to the regeneration of vitamin E. Several possibilities exist: the radical

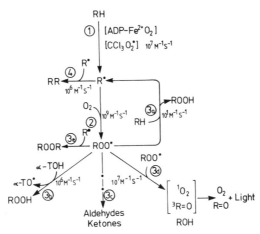

FIGURE 1. Relationships in the lipid peroxidation process initiated by free radicals. Reaction 1 is the initiation step, generating the carbon-centered lipid radical R•, which, in the presence of oxygen, is rapidly converted to the corresponding lipid peroxyl radical, ROO• (reaction 2). Several further reactions are depicted. The reaction of vitamin E is shown as reaction 3b, and further fragmentation reactions are indicated as well as dimerization and propagation reactions. Literature is referred to in ref. 22. (T. Noll *et al.*[22] With permission from Academic Press.)

might react with a peroxyl radical to form a nonradical product; the radical may interact with another one, forming a vitamin E dimer; and the radical may be reduced to regenerate vitamin E itself. Also, other products could potentially be generated. The repair of the vitamin E radical to generate the bona fide vitamin E is, of course, the major biological reaction of interest. Various reductants have been considered. Several groups[12–16] reported on the free radical interaction between vitamin E and vitamin C, extending earlier work on fat autoxidation by Golumbic and Mattill.[17] The ascorbyl radical that would be generated can be repaired in the aqueous phase. Another compound of interest has been glutathione, which also has been shown to be able to regenerate vitamin E. This area of research has recently been reviewed by McCay[18] and Niki.[19]

As shown in FIGURE 2, the action of the antioxidant capacity can be identified as a lag phase before the onset of lipid peroxidation. In this case, a microsomal system of membrane lipid peroxidation is employed (see also ref. 20), and at zero time, the reaction is started by providing NADP$^+$ for the NADPH regenerating system, which drives the lipid peroxidation. It is shown in FIGURE 2 that the addition of 1 mM ascorbate or, instead, 1 mM GSH is capable of prolonging the lag phase in this system, as in other types of systems employed in the literature cited above. It should be mentioned that GSH has another influence on lipid peroxidation, because it slows down the rate of lipid peroxidation when the process has started and the antioxidants have been depleted. Current research is directed to protein factors that might be involved in these effects, not discussed here in detail.

It should be noted that the interaction of ascorbate and glutathione with vitamin E explain their effect on the lag phase regarding the protection of microsomal membranes against lipid peroxidation. This is underlined by the complete absence of a protective effect on the lag phase by either ascorbate or glutathione in microsomes that are depleted of tocopherol.[21] This means that in experiments, as in FIGURE 2 carried out with microsomes from alpha-tocopherol-depleted animals, the lag phase

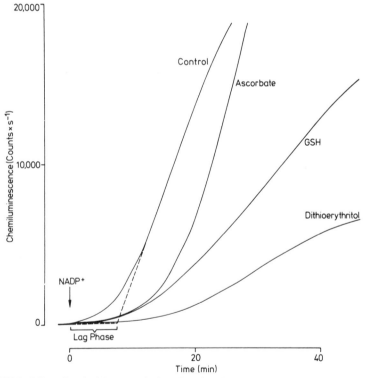

FIGURE 2. Effect of antioxidants on the lag phase in microsomal lipid peroxidation. Rat liver microsomes were examined in a lipid peroxidation system, monitoring low-level chemoluminescence. The addition of ascorbate (1 mM) or GSH (1 mM) or dithioerythritol (1 mM) are shown to increase the lag phase. In similar experiments (not shown) from microsomes from tocopherol-deficient animals the lag phase was diminished to about 1 min.[21]

TABLE 1. The Protection by Ascorbate and Glutathione against Microsomal Lipid Peroxidation Is Dependent on Vitamin E[21]

Addition	Concentration mM	Control Microsomes Lag Phase (min)	Tocopherol-Deficient Microsomes Lag Phase (min)
None		9.3 ± 0.6	1.6 ± 1.2
Ascorbate	1	28.5 ± 7.5	2.0 ± 0.1
	3	87.0 ± 13	2.7 ± 0.3
Glutathione, GSH	1	16.2 ± 1.2	1.2 ± 0.8
	3	16.3 ± 1.1	0.1 ± 0.1

was decreased to about 2 min (TABLE 1), and the addition of the further antioxidants did not have any protective effect.[21] Other biological thiols, such as dihydrolipoate are also capable of exhibiting antioxidant activity dependent on alpha-tocopherol.[23,24]

LOSS OF ALPHA-TOCOPHEROL

Based on previous work in model systems, notably by Niki and associates,[19] it would be anticipated that the time course of microsomal lipid peroxidation would first exhibit a depletion of vitamin E to levels approaching zero before the onset of the peroxidation of lipids. As shown in FIGURE 3, however, and as also observed by Ursini (personal communication, 1988), it is noteworthy that parameters of lipid peroxidation can be observed when much of the total alpha-tocopherol is still measurable. In a detailed study of the time course of depletion, a two-phase loss of alpha-tocopherol during NADPH-initiated lipid peroxidation was detected, involving a slow phase followed by a more accelerated phase.[24] The lag phase before the start of the rapid loss was similar to the lag phase before the onset of chemoluminescence (TABLE 2). Low-level chemoluminescence and thiobarbituric-reactive material started to rise at an alpha-tocopherol content of about 0.38 nmol/mg protein, that is, about 86% of the initial content. During subsequent lipid peroxidation, the alpha-tocopherol content decreased to about 0.03 nmol/mg protein at the time of maximal chemoluminescence. These observations indicate that in hepatic microsomal lipid peroxidation there are inhomogeneities, based, for example, on uneven distribution of the antioxidant. The asymmetry between the inner and outer leaflet of the bilayer or lateral clustering, therefore, has considerable interest.

CONCLUDING REMARKS

It has become evident from this brief survey that the interactions between hydrophobic domains in the membrane and indeed also in other locations, such as LDL particles on the one hand, and the water-soluble antioxidants on the other, are of potentially crucial importance in the maintenance of a biological steady state of antioxidant defense. Some of these aspects were reviewed recently.[25,26]

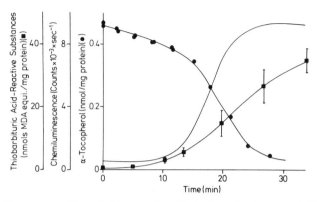

FIGURE 3. Time course of loss of alpha-tocopherol (●), chemoluminescence (solid line), and accumulation of thiobarbituric acid-reactive substances (■) in microsomal lipid peroxidation.[24] Rat liver microsomes (0.5 mg protein/mL) were added to 0.1 M potassium phosphate buffer, pH 7.4, containing $ADP/FeCl_3$ and a NADPH-regenerating system. The reaction was started by the addition of $NADP^+$ at zero time. For evaluation of this experiment, typical of 4 different incubations, see TABLE 2.

ACKNOWLEDGMENT

Excellent technical assistance was provided by Ursula Rabe.

TABLE 2. Relationship between Low-level Chemoluminescence, Loss of Alpha-Tocopherol, and the Accumulation of Thiobarbituric Acid-Reactive Substances[24,a]

Parameter	Control Microsomes	Tocopherol-Deficient Microsomes
Low-level chemoluminescence		
Lag phase (min)	12.3 ± 1.1	< 1.0
Maximal slope (%max.rate/min)	7.8 ± 0.6	7.1 ± 0.8
Loss of alpha-tocopherol		
Lag phase (min)	13.5 ± 1.6	—
Rate of loss (pmol/min × mg protein)		
Initial (slow phase)	5.8 ± 0.3	—
Second (fast phase)	27.3 ± 2.1	—
Initial content (nmol/mg protein)	0.44 ± 0.01	0.04 ± 0.005
Accumulation of thiobarbituric acid-reactive substances		
Lag phase (min)	12.3 ± 1.5	2.6 ± 0.2
Maximum rate (%max. rate/min)	3.9 ± 0.4	3.2 ± 0.2
Maximum accumulation (nmol MDA equiv/mg protein)	47.1 ± 1.0	35.1 ± 2.5

[a] Compare FIGURE 3.

REFERENCES

1. BURTON, G. W. & K. U. INGOLD. 1981. Autoxidation of Biological Molecules. 1. The antioxidant activity of vitamin E and related chain-breaking phenolic antioxidants *in vitro.* J. Am. Chem. Soc. **103**: 6472-6477.
2. TAPPEL, A. L. 1962. Vitamin E as the biological lipid antioxidant. Vitam. Horm. **20**: 493-510.
3. DIPLOCK, A. T. & J. A. LUCY. 1973. The biochemical modes of action of vitamin and selenium: a hypothesis FEBS Lett. **29**: 205-210.
4. BURTON, G. W., A. JOYCE & K. U. INGOLD. 1983a. Is vitamin E the only lipid-soluble, chain-breaking antioxidant in human blood plasma and erythrocyte membranes? Arch. Biochem. Biophys. **221**: 281-290.
5. NIKI, E., A. KAWAKAMI, M. SAITO, Y. YAMAMOTO, J. TSUCHIYA & Y. KAMIYA. 1985. Effect of phytyl side chain of vitamin E on its antioxidant activity. J. Biol. Chem. **260**: 2191-2196.
6. SIMIC, M. G.1981. Vitamin E radicals. *In* Oxygen and Oxyradicals in Chemistry and Biology. M. A. J. Rodgers & E. L. Powers, Eds.: 109-115. Academic Press. New York.
7. BURTON, G. W., K. H. CHEESEMAN, T. DOBA, K. U. INGOLD & T. F. SLATER. 1983b. Vitamin E as an antioxidant *in vitro* and *in vivo. In* Biology of vitamin E. 4-14. Pitman. London.
8. MACHLIN, L. J. 1984. Vitamin E. *In* Handbook of vitamins. Nutritional, Biochemical, and clinical aspects. L. J. Machlin, Ed.: 99-145. Marcel Dekker. New York and Basel.
9. FAHRENHOLTZ, S. R., F. H. DOLEIDEN, A. M. TROZZOLLO & A. A. LAMOLA. 1974. On the quenching of singlet oxygen of alpha-tocopherol. Photochem. Photobiol. **20**: 505-508.
10. FOOTE, C. S., T. Y. CHING & G. G. GELLER. 1974. Chemistry of singlet oxygen-XVII. Rates of reaction and quenching of alpha-tocopherol and singlet oxygen. Photochem. Photobiol. **20**: 511-513.
11. NEELY, W. C., J. M. MARTIN & S. A. BARKER. 1988. Products and relative reaction rates of the oxidation of tocopherols with singlet molecular oxygen. Photochem. Photobiol. **48**: 423-428.
12. PACKER, J. E., T. F. SLATER & R. L. WILLSON. 1979. Direct observation of a free radical interaction between vitamin E and vitamin C. Nature **278**: 737-738.
13. LEUNG, H. W., M. J. VANG & R. D. MAVIS. 1981. The cooperative interaction between vitamin E and vitamin C in suppression of peroxidation of membrane phospholipids. Biochim. Biophys. Acta **664**: 266-272.
14. NIKI, E., J. TSUCHIYA, R. TANIMURA & Y. KAMIYA. 1982. Regeneration of vitamin E from alpha-chromanoxyl radical by glutathione and vitamin C. Chem. Lett. 789-792.
15. NIKI, E., T. SAITO, A. KAWAKAMI & Y. KAMIYA. 1984. Inhibition of oxidation of methyl linoleate in solution by vitamin E and vitamin C. J. Biol. Chem. **259**: 4177-4182.
16. LAMBELET, P., F. SAUCY & J. LÖLIGER. 1985. Chemical evidence for interactions between vitamins E and C. Experientia **41**: 1384-1388.
17. GOLUMBIC, C. & H. A. MATTILL. 1941. Antioxidants and the autoxidation of fats. XIII. The antioxygenic action of ascorbic acid in association with tocopherols, hydroquinones and related compounds. J. Am. Chem. Soc. **63**: 1279-1280.
18. MCCAY, P. B. 1985. Vitamin E: Interactions with free radicals and ascorbate. Annu. Rev. Nutr. **5**: 323-340.
19. NIKI, E. 1987. Interaction of ascorbate and α-tocopherol. Ann. N.Y. Acad. Sci. **498**: 186-198.
20. CADENAS, E., M. GINSBERG, U. RABE & H. SIES. 1984. Evaluation of alpha-tocopherol antioxidant activity in microsomal lipid peroxidation as detected by low-level chemiluminescence. Biochem. J. **223**: 755-759.
21. WEFERS, H. & H. SIES. 1988. The protection by ascorbate and glutathione against microsomal lipid peroxidation is dependent on vitamin E. Eur. J. Biochem. **174**: 353-357.
22. NOLL, T., H. DE GROOT & H. SIES. 1987. Distinct temporal relation among oxygen uptake, malondialdehyde formation, and low-level chemiluminescence during microsomal lipid peroxidation. Arch Biochem. Biophys. **252**: 284-291.

23. BAST, A. & G. R. M. M. HAENEN. 1988. Interplay between lipoic acid and glutathione in the protection against microsomal lipid peroxidation. Biochim. Biophys. Acta. **963:** 558-561.
24. SCHOLICH, H., M. E. MURPHY & H. SIES. 1989. Antioxidant activity of dihydrolipoate against microsomal lipid peroxidation and its dependence on alpha-tocopherol. Biochim. Biophys. Acta. **1001:** 256-261.
25. SIES, H. 1989. Relationship between free radicals and vitamins: an overview. *In* Elevated dosages of vitamins. P. Walter, H. Stähelin & G. Brubacher, Eds.: 215-223. Hans Huber Publ. Stuttgart.
26. SIES, H. 1986. Biochemistry of oxidative stress. Angew. Chem. Int. Ed. Engl. **25:** 1058-1071.

Tocopherol Concentrations of Leukocytes in Neonates

TOHRU OGIHARA, MUNENORI MIYAKE,
NAOHISA KAWAMURA, HIROSHI TAMAI,
MAKOTO KITAGAWA, AND MAKOTO MINO

Department of Pediatrics
Osaka Medical College
Takatsuki, 569, Japan

We have reported that newborn infants have erythrocyte (RBC)-tocopherol concentrations corresponding to a level found in normal adults, despite the low plasma tocopherol levels.[1] Recently some investigators demonstrated that the LDL receptor mechanism mediates the delivery of tocopherol to cells.[2] RBC do not have LDL receptors, and it has been demonstrated that HDL plays a greater role in the delivery of tocopherol to RBC than the other lipoproteins.[3] Moreover, neonates generally show low LDL levels. In the present work, we have examined tocopherol concentrations of neonatal leukocytes before and after oral administration of tocopherol compared with data from adults, and we attempt to reveal whether tocopherol levels of cells possessing LDL receptors are well-regulated or not in neonates.

Blood samples of neonates at birth were obtained through the umbilical vein from term AFD (appropriate for dates) babies. Oral administration of dl-α-tocopheryl nicotinate (provided by Eisai Co., Ltd.) for 7 days was performed as follows: during the initial 2 days, 80 mg/kg/day of tocopherol was given to neonates (term AFD babies at the 7th day after birth) and 1200 mg/day to male adults; then during the following 5 days, 40 mg/kg/day was given to neonates and 600 mg/day to adults, respectively. Mononuclear cells (MN) and polymorphonuclear cells (PMN) were prepared simultaneously by Ficoll-Hypaque centrifugation. Lipoproteins were separated by ultracentrifugation according to Hatch and Lees' method. Tocopherol was measured by HPLC with electrochemical detection (IRICA Amperometric E-520 detector).

In newborn infants, we found that tocopherol levels in both MN and PMN were only about half the levels of male adults. Plasma tocopherol levels were extremely low, and LDL total lipids decreased to a quarter of the adult levels at birth. During the first week of life, tocopherol levels of leukocytes gradually increased and reached about three-quarters of adult values. Plasma tocopherol levels and LDL total lipid levels were almost double, but still only half the adult values. Percent distribution of tocopherol in individual lipoproteins coincided with those of total lipids in neonates and adults, as previously reported[1] (TABLE 1).

When tocopherol was given orally, plasma tocopherol was elevated to higher levels in adults compared with neonates, but no significant difference was observed on the 7th day after administration. On the contrary, RBC tocopherol levels in neonates readily reached statistically significant higher levels than in adult cases. These findings

TABLE 1. Alpha-Tocopherol Concentrations in Plasma, RBC, and Leukocytes, and the Distribution of Tocopherol and Three Major Lipids in Lipoprotein Fractions[a]

	Neonates		Male Adults (n = 20)
	At Birth (n = 11)	At the 7th Day (n = 11)	
Alpha-Tocopherol			
MN	4.8 ± 2.0	6.3 ± 2.2	8.3 ± 2.6
PMN	2.7 ± 0.6	3.5 ± 1.1	5.5 ± 1.5
RBC	179 ± 33	199 ± 45	207 ± 19
Plasma	237 ± 62	481 ± 81	899 ± 201
VLDL	14 ± 8(6%)	60 ± 25(13%)	158 ± 85(19%)
LDL	68 ± 20(30%)	162 ± 47(35%)	352 ± 129(42%)
HDL	143 ± 43(64%)	233 ± 39(52%)	328 ± 63(39%)
Total Cholesterol			
Plasma	70 ± 20	145 ± 28	199 ± 25
VLDL	3 ± 2(5%)	8 ± 5(6%)	13 ± 8(7%)
LDL	23 ± 8(37%)	60 ± 29(48%)	106 ± 29(61%)
HDL	36 ± 11(58%)	56 ± 7(45%)	55 ± 9(32%)
Phospholipid			
Plasma	99 ± 24	146 ± 26	200 ± 30
VLDL	5 ± 2(5%)	8 ± 5(6%)	19 ± 11(10%)
LDL	18 ± 5(20%)	33 ± 13(26%)	69 ± 19(37%)
HDL	69 ± 19(75%)	86 ± 18(68%)	101 ± 15(53%)
Triglyceride			
Plasma	24 ± 8	70 ± 29	103 ± 59
VLDL	6 ± 2(26%)	27 ± 16(45%)	52 ± 9(60%)
LDL	8 ± 3(35%)	17 ± 4(28%)	22 ± 7(25%)
HDL	9 ± 6(39%)	16 ± 5(27%)	13 ± 5(15%)
Total Lipids			
Plasma	193 ± 52	334 ± 127	469 ± 94
VLDL	14 ± 6(8%)	45 ± 22(14%)	83 ± 43(19%)
LDL	49 ± 16(28%)	110 ± 38(35%)	197 ± 43(52%)
HDL	114 ± 36(64%)	158 ± 45(51%)	168 ± 26(38%)

[a] Values are the mean ± SD (μg/10 cells for MN and PMN, μg/dL packed cells for RBC, μg/dL for plasma, mg/dL for lipids). Total lipids were estimated by the addition of total cholesterol, phospholipids, and triglycerides. The percent distributions relevant to the sum of the values in the three fractions are expressed in parentheses.

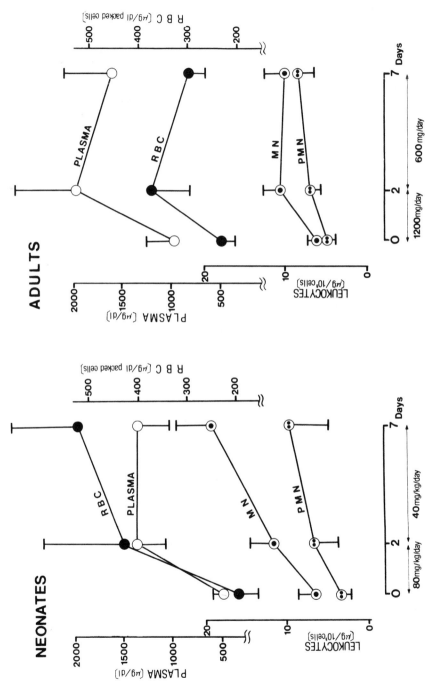

FIGURE 1. Changes of tocopherol concentrations in plasma, RBC, and leukocytes after oral administration of *dl*-alpha-tocopheryl nicotinate. Values are the mean ± SD. Eleven full-term AFD neonates at the 7th day after birth and 7 male adults (aged 26 to 34 years) were given tocopherol orally.

may be explained by relatively large amounts of HDL in neonates from which tocopherol may be easily transferred to RBC. Leukocyte tocopherol levels were also elevated to a higher extent in neonates than in adults, reaching significantly higher levels of MN at the 7th day after administration (FIG. 1). These data would lead us to predict that the LDL receptor mechanism in neonates may act more efficiently than in adults. Some investigators reported that HDL enriched in apoprotein E may take the part of LDL in neonates,[4] and this may also account for our findings. Further study is required in neonates to clarify tocopherol distribution in parenchymal cells other than peripheral circulating leukocytes.

REFERENCES

1. OGIHARA, T., M. MIKI, M. KITAGAWA & M. MINO. 1988. Distribution of tocopherol among human plasma lipoproteins. Clin. Chim. Acta 174: 299-306.
2. TRABER, M. G. & H. J. KAYDEN. 1984. Vitamin E is delivered to cells via the high affinity receptor for low-density lipoprotein. Am. J. Clin. Nutr. 40: 747-751.
3. KAYDEN, H. J. & L. BJORNSON. 1972. The dynamics of vitamin E transport in the human erythrocytes. Ann. N. Y. Acad. Sci. 203: 127-140.
4. INNERARITY, T. L., T. P. BERSOT, K. S. ARNOLD, K. H. WEISGRABER, P. A. DAVIS, T. M. FORTE & R. W. MAHLEY. 1984. Receptor binding activity of high-density lipoproteins containing apoprotein E from abetalipoproteinemic and normal neonate plasma. Metabolism 33: 186-195.

In Vitro Model to Assess Alpha-Tocopherol Efficacy

Protection against UV-Induced Lipid Peroxidation

E. PELLE, D. MAES, G. A. PADULO, E-K. KIM, AND
W. P. SMITH

Estée Lauder Research and Development
Melville, New York 11747

Alpha-tocopherol is a well-characterized antioxidant that inhibits lipid peroxidation. Because lipid peroxidation has been detected in human skin,[1] the topical application of alpha-tocopherol and other antioxidants to protect skin from peroxide-causative factors, such as ultraviolet (UV) radiation, is an important area of research. As a first step towards developing effective strategies to counteract the damage caused by UV radiation on the skin, we wanted to assess the relative efficacy of alpha-tocopherol and other antioxidants by examining their ability to prevent UV-induced lipid peroxidation with a simple and reliable *in vitro* technique.

Liposomes were chosen as the target for peroxidation because of their resemblance to cellular bilayer structures that are conducive to membrane intercalation by alpha-tocopherol. In addition, the use of liposomes allows interaction with an aqueous environment that plays a significant role in free radical/antioxidant reactions. As shown in FIGURE 1A, liposomes were prepared by injecting 36 μmol of soybean phosphatidylcholine (PC) in ethanol into phosphate-buffered saline, pH 7.4, and then dispersed by mixing for one minute. In our model system, both lipophilic and hydrophilic antioxidants were tested. Lipophilic antioxidants, such as alpha-tocopherol, were premixed with PC and then injected into buffer together. Hydrophilic antioxidants, such as ascorbic acid, were premixed with the aqueous buffer before injection of PC. The concentration of the lipophilic antioxidants ranged from 1 to 10 molepercent of the liposome and from 1 to 10 mM in buffer for hydrophilic antioxidants. Lipophilic antioxidants were incorporated into the lipid bilayer region, whereas hydrophilic antioxidants were either outside or encapsulated within the liposome.

After preparation, liposomes either treated or untreated with antioxidants were exposed to UV radiation (FIG. 1B). An unexposed sample was also prepared and used as a control. Both UVB and UVC were used. UVB was used at doses comparable to causing an erythemic response in type 2/3 human skin. UVC, though not biological, was found to produce an effect analogous to UVB but at a much accelerated rate and used routinely in our assays.

During exposure, aliquots were removed for assaying lipid peroxides (FIG. 1C). Lipid peroxidation was determined spectrophotometrically by an increase in thiob-

A

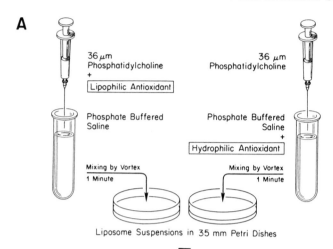

36 μm
Phosphatidylcholine
+
Lipophilic Antioxidant

36 μm
Phosphatidylcholine

Phosphate Buffered
Saline

Phosphate Buffered
Saline
+
Hydrophilic Antioxidant

Mixing by Vortex
1 Minute

Mixing by Vortex
1 Minute

Liposome Suspensions in 35 mm Petri Dishes

B

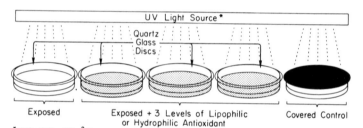

UV Light Source*

Quartz
Glass
Discs

Exposed

Exposed + 3 Levels of Lipophilic
or Hydrophilic Antioxidant

Covered Control

*UVC = 2.8 mJ/Cm²/Sec
*UVB = 0.11 mJ/Cm²/Sec
Incubation temp: ambient

C

Thiobarbituric Acid Reacting
Material Assay

0.2 ml liposome suspension
(aliquots taken
at various hours
of irradiation)

3 ml
20% trichloroacetic acid
+
1 ml
1% thiobarbituric acid

• Incubated 100 °C, 25 min
• Centrifuged 500xg, 10 min
• Absorbance measured 532 nm

Gas Liquid
Chromatography

1.2 ml liposome suspension

4.2 ml
chloroform/methanol (2:1)

• Mixed 2 min
• Centrifuged 500xg, 10 min
• CHCL₃ layer removed
  and dried with N₂
• Lipid weighed
• 0.05% BHT added
• Lipid methylated
• Injection on OV-351 capillary column

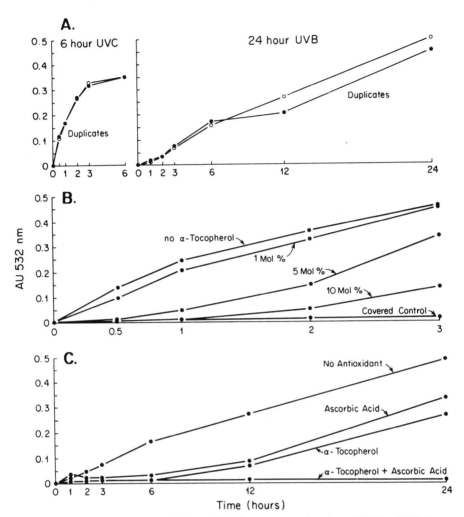

FIGURE 2. (A) Increased peroxidation of PC liposomes as a function of UVC or UVB dose over time. Peroxidation was measured by an increase in absorbance of TBARM over time. (B) Peroxidation by UVC inhibited by increasing amounts of alpha-tocopherol. (C) Peroxidation by UVB inhibited by 5 mole-percent alpha-tocopherol, 5 mM ascorbic acid, and total inhibition with both mixed together.

arbituric acid-reacting materials (TBARM) measured at 532 nanometers. To further substantiate the production of lipid peroxides by UV radiation in our system, we also measured the decrease in polyunsaturated fatty acid substrate by way of capillary gas liquid chromatography.[2] Typically, an aliquot of 2.4 μmol of PC bilayers without antioxidants yielded an average of 3 nmol/mL TBARM ($e_{532\ nm}$ = 150,000) after 2 hr of UVC irradiation or 14 hr of UVB irradiation (FIG. 2A).

FIGURE 1. (A) Liposomal preparation and incorporation of antioxidants, (B) irradiation of liposomes, and (C) assay for peroxidation products.

As illustrated in FIGURE 2B, irradiated liposomes (UVC) exhibited significantly higher amounts of lipid peroxides than irradiated liposomes containing alpha-tocopherol in a dose- and concentration-dependent manner. The effectiveness of alpha-tocopherol to inhibit peroxidation was determined by the percent decrease in absorbance. For example in FIGURE 2B, 5 mole-percent alpha-tocopherol is equivalent to 58% inhibition at the 2-hr time point. In a similar experiment, liposomes containing 5 mole-percent alpha-tocopherol were mixed in buffer containing 5 mM ascorbic acid and then exposed to UVB (FIG. 2C). In this experiment, ascorbic acid and alpha-tocopherol alone were inhibitory, but when exposed together there was a total inhibition of peroxidation. Another experiment demonstrated these two antioxidants to act synergistically, which is in agreement with other scientific reports.[3]

Using this model system, we have compared the relative antioxidant potential of alpha-tocopherol to several other lipophilic antioxidants. In order of decreasing effectiveness, we found BHA > catechin > BHT > alpha-tocopherol > chlorogenic acid. In addition, we observed alpha-tocopherol to lose its potency and become a pro-oxidant when stored at ambient temperatures over a period of one week. Lastly, our data suggest that peroxyl radicals may be selectively generated in our model system. Thus, it may provide a means to differentiate the multifunctional antioxidant nature of alpha-tocopherol.

REFERENCES

1. MEFFERT, H., W. DIEZEL & N. SONNICHSEN. 1976. Experientia 32: 1397-1398.
2. SELIGMAN, M. L., J. A. MITAMURA, N. SHERA & H. B. DEMOPOULOS. 1979. Photochem. Photobiol. 29: 549-558.
3. PACKER, J. E., T. F. SLATER & R. L. WILSON. 1979. Nature 278: 737-738.

Oxygen-Induced Retinopathy in the Rat

Role of Vitamin E in Defending against Peroxidation

JOHN S. PENN AND LISA A. THUM

Cullen Eye Institute
Houston, Texas 77030

Oxygen has been known, for more than 30 years, to play a causal role in retinopathy of prematurity (ROP).[1] In the ensuing time, although careful control of oxygen administration to premature infants has reduced the incidence of ROP, the precise mechanism of cytotoxicity of oxygen on the retina has not been discovered. Inasmuch as oxygen is a causal factor, it seems reasonable to suggest that lipid peroxidation reactions are involved in the pathophysiology of the degeneration. In fact, retinal tissue serves as an excellent substrate for these reactions, because it contains an abundance of polyunsaturated fatty acids;[2] it has a high oxygen flux across its membranes;[3] and it processes light, which can initiate radical formation.[4]

The adult retina normally has a variety of antioxidants at its disposal to combat peroxidation reactions. A premature infant, however, is deficient in one important antioxidant, vitamin E, having retinal levels only one-tenth that of adults.[5] The retinal levels of other antioxidants (ascorbic acid, glutathione peroxidase, glutathione-S-transferase, and glutathione reductase) are the same or higher in premature infants than in adults.

We are developing a rat model for ROP so that we can make a careful and systematic analysis of biochemical factors that affect retinal vascular development. The rat was chosen because its retina can be damaged by oxygen, its vasculature develops in a manner similar to that of the human, and, at birth, the retina is vitamin E-deficient compared to the adult animal.

Immediately after birth, newborn rat pups and their mothers were placed in an atmosphere of 60% oxygen for 14 days. The extent of oxygen-induced retinopathy was measured in India ink-perfused retinal whole mounts as the percent of total retinal area containing intact blood vessels. The values were 59% for oxygen-exposed rats and 94% for age-matched room air controls (FIG. 1). The occurrence of peroxidation reactions during the 14-day exposure period was tested by measuring retinal levels of malondialdehyde (MDA), a toxic product of lipid peroxidation, and measuring the loss of a likely substrate, docosahexaenoic acid (TABLE 1). Both measures were consistent with the idea that lipid peroxidation had taken place. Several retinal antioxidants were also assayed, including vitamins E and C, superoxide dismutase, and three enzymes of the glutathione system. Retinal levels of vitamins E and C were

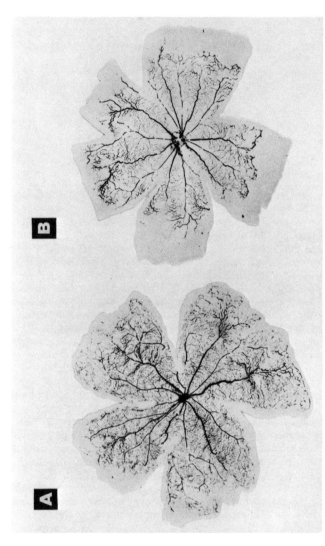

FIGURE 1. Ink-perfused retinal whole mounts from room air rats (A) and oxygen-exposed rats (B) reveal a 35% decrease in the vasculature of the latter. This decrease is manifested by a retarded progression of vessels toward the retinal periphery and a complete loss of capillaries in the central retina.

reduced in oxygen-exposed rats by 34% and 20%, respectively. Retinal levels of glutathione enzymes were not significantly different in the two groups. If lipid peroxidation is involved in the degeneration, then enhancement of antioxidants might provide some protection. In order to test this, another set of experiments was conducted in which nursing mothers were fed diets containing either 1.0 g α-tocopherol acetate/kg of food (E+) or no α-tocopherol acetate (E−). The dietary manipulation began 21-25 days prior to birth of the litters and lasted throughout the 14-day exposure. This treatment resulted in tocopherol levels in the ratling retinas that were 1.5 and 0.5 mmol/mol phospholipid, respectively, for E+ and E− room air controls and 1.5 and 0.6, respectively, for the two oxygen-exposed groups. The levels of other antioxidants were also affected. Of note was a significant increase in the retinal level of glutathione peroxidase in both the E+ and E− rats in the oxygen-exposed group. Further, the combination of dietary and atmospheric oxygen manipulations resulted in differences in the extent of retinal vasculature, with E+ exposed animals sustaining approximately 10% less vaso-obliteration than their E− counterparts.

TABLE 1. Evidence of Retinal Lipid Peroxidation

Determination	Room Air	60% Oxygen	p Value
Docosahexaenoic Acid level (mole-percent)	15.5 ± 0.8	11.0 ± 1.1	<0.02
nmol MDA/mg Retinal protein	11.1 ± 3.5	23.2 ± 1.3	<0.001

REFERENCES

1. CAMPBELL, K. 1950. Retrolental fibroplasia as a syndrome. Arch. Ophthalmol. **44:** 245.
2. FLIESLER, S. J. & R. E. ANDERSON. 1983. Chemistry and metabolism of lipids in the vertebrate retina. Prog. Lipid Res. **22:** 79-131.
3. RODIECK, R. W. 1973. In The Vertebrate Retina. D. Kennedy & R. B. Park, Eds.: 159. W. H. Freeman. San Francisco, CA.
4. DELMELLE, M. 1979. Possible implication of photooxidation reactions in retinal photodamage. Photochem. Photobiol. 29(4): 713-716.
5. NIELSEN, J. C., M. I. NAASH & R. E. ANDERSON. 1988. The regional distribution of vitamins E and C in mature and premature human retinas. Invest. Ophthalmol. Vis. Sci. 29(1): 22-26.

Evaluation of Vitamin E Deficiency in Patients with Adult Respiratory Distress Syndrome

J. PINCEMAIL,[a] Y. BERTRAND,[b] G. HANIQUE,[b]
B. DENIS,[b] L. LEENAERTS,[b] L. VANKEERBERGHEN,[b]
AND C. DEBY[a]

[a] *Institute of Chemistry*
Université de Liège
B6, Sart Tilman
4000 Liège, Belgium

[b] *Clinique St. Jean*
rue des Marais 104
1000 Bruxelles, Belgium

Vitamin E (VE) functions primarily as a biological antioxidant and prevents, in the cell, the peroxidation of polyunsaturated fatty acids by its ability to scavenge free radicals, species suspected to be produced in some pathological diseases. In adult respiratory distress syndrome (ARDS), complement activation is implicated,[1] with possible subsequent granulocyte activation, resulting in the release of active oxygen radicals that can induce a loss of lung permeability.[2] Plasmatic VE (determined by HPLC technique), plasmatic lipid levels, and a VE/lipids ratio were measured in 12 critically ill patients and compared with those of the control group. These patients who did not receive parenteral nutrition during the study were divided into two groups. Group I (●——●) consisted of six critically ill patients with ARDS, and group II (●—·—●) comprised six severely ill patients without ARDS. In group I, the first blood sample was taken at the onset of ARDS criteria, whereas in group II, blood was drawn when the patients were admitted into the intensive care unit. The following blood samples were taken every 6 hours for 2 days.

FIGURE 1 indicates that the VE level in the two groups is significantly depressed relative to the control group ($p < 0.0001$), suggesting therefore that lipoperoxidation processes occur in a general way in critically ill patients. The evolution during the time is quite different between the two groups, however, as it clearly appears at hours 36 and 48 after the onset of their acute disease : values < 5 $\mu g/mL$ in the ARDS group and > 5 $\mu g/mL$ in the non-ARDS group ($p < 0.01$). As plasma VE concentration is dependent on circulating lipid levels, the VE/lipids ratio has been proposed as the best indicator of VE status rather than the sole determination of VE in plasma.[3] A ratio of 0.8 mg/g or less is usually considered indicative of VE deficiency.[3] Inasmuch as total plasma lipid levels are not statistically different between the two groups (data not shown), the study of VE/lipid ratios (FIG. 2) indicates that the VE decrease is more critical in patients who developed ARDS than in those

498

who did not develop it. Indeed this decrease leads to a VE deficiency, as it particularly appears at hour 48 : 0.78 mg/g for ARDS patients versus 1.54 mg/g for non-ARDS patients.

In conclusion, our findings indicate that VE should be regularly monitored in critically ill patients and that replacement therapy should be initiated to avoid insufficiency and to maximize the protection against oxidative free radical injury, especially when plasmatic VE levels are less than 5 μg/mL and associated with a VE-lipid ratio lower than 0.8, as is the case for patients developing ARDS.

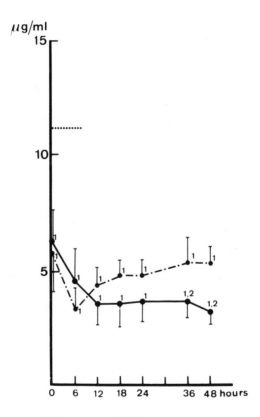

FIGURE 1. Evolution of VE level in ARDS group (●——●) and non-ARDS group (●—·—●). Values are mean ± SEM. ·······: mean normal value (n = 17). 1 : $p < 0.0001$ versus mean normal value; 2 : $p < 0.01$ versus non-ARDS group. One-way analysis of variance was used for statistics study.

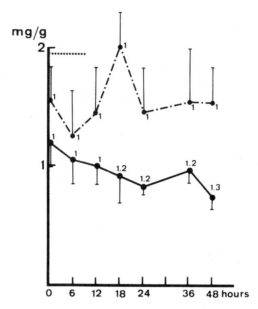

FIGURE 2. Evolution of VE/lipids ratio in ARDS group (●——●) and non-ARDS group (●—·—●). Values are mean ± SEM. ·······: mean normal value (n = 17). 1 : p < 0.0001 versus mean normal value; 2 : p < 0.05 versus non-ARDS group; 3 : p < 0.01 versus non-ARDS group. One-way analysis of variance was used for statistics study.

REFERENCES

1. DUCHATEAU, J., M. HASS, H. SCHREYEN *et al.* 1984. Complement activation in patients at risk of developing the adult respiratory distress syndrome. Am. Rev. Respir. Dis. **130:** 1058.
2. WONG, C., J. FLYEN & R. H. DEMLING. 1984. Role of oxygen radicals in endotoxin induced lung injury. Arch. Surg. **119:** 77.
3. HORWITT, M. K., C. H. HARVEY, C. H. DAHM, JR. & M. T. SEARCY. 1972. Relationship between tocopherol and serum lipid levels for determination of nutritional adequacy. Ann. N.Y. Acad. Sci. **203:** 223-236.

Neutrophil Activation Evidenced by Plasmatic Myeloperoxidase Release during Cardiopulmonary Bypass in Humans

Consequence on Vitamin E Status

J. PINCEMAIL,[a] M-L. FAYMONVILLE,[b]
G. DEBY-DUPONT,[b] A. THIRION,[a] C. DEBY,[a]
AND M. LAMY[b]

[a] Institute of Chemistry
B6, Sart Tilman

[b] Centre Hospitalier Universitaire
B33, Sart Tilman
University of Liège
4000 Liège, Belgium

Cardiopulmonary bypass (CPB) has been shown to activate alternate complement pathway and causes sequestration of neutrophils in pulmonary capillary beds.[1] It is suggested that these sequestrated neutrophils can be activated, resulting in the release of oxygen free radicals able to injure the lung by lipoperoxidation processes.[2] The aim of our study was (1) to clearly evidence neutrophil activation in CPB by the plasmatic measurement of myeloperoxidase (MPO), a specific neutrophil enzyme released by activated neutrophils in the extracellular medium, and (2) to evaluate the consequence of this neutrophil activation on plasmatic vitamin E status, which can be modified by lipoperoxidation processes.

Ten patients undergoing CPB for coronary disease treatment were investigated. Conditions of CPB were described earlier.[3] Blood samples, drawn on heparin according to the protocol described in TABLE 1, were immediately centrifuged, and plasma was frozen until assay.

Plasmatic vitamin E (VE) was determined by the HPLC technique. Human MPO was isolated from purified neutrophils of healthy volunteers with an absorbance ratio A_{430nm}/A_{280nm} equal to 0.72. Plasmatic determination of the enzyme was assessed by a radioimmunoassay technique developed in our laboratory.

Upon the beginning of CPB, the mean plasmatic MPO level progressively increases to reach maximum values at the lung reperfusion and at the end of CPB (respectively, 15.8- and 16.1-fold, the initial value of pre-CPB). During the first postoperative day, MPO returns to baseline level. The same reestablishment of pulmonary circulation

501

results in a significant increase of mean leukocyte count ($13,760$ cells/mm^3 $\pm$ $1,851$ (SEM) vs $7,200$ cells/mm^3 $\pm$ 814 (SEM) in pre-CPB). As MPO, a specific neutrophil enzyme, can go out of stimulated neutrophils,[4] our results unequivocally indicate that the sequestrated neutrophils in lung are in a highly excited state and therefore capable of inducing lipid peroxidation in lung membrane through oxygen free radical production. Lipoperoxidation processes during CPB are evidenced by the plasmatic VE level that decreases by 50% during CPB and that significantly remains lower than the initial value of pre-CPB even 24 hours post-CPB. Such an observation has been previously made by Cavarocchi et al.[5] As VE primarily acts as a potent lipidic radical scavenger, its consumption indicates that lipoperoxidation processes really occur during CPB.

In conclusion, the increase in the plasmatic MPO level, the index of the neutrophil excitation state, associated with the decrease of the plasmatic VE level, the index of lipoperoxidation processes, gives strong evidence that oxygen free radical generation is highly involved during CPB.

TABLE 1. Evolution of Myeloperoxidase (MPO) and VE Levels during CPB[a]

	Leucocyte count (cells/mm^3)	MPO (ng/mL)	VE (μg/mL)
Pre-CPB	$7,200 \pm 814$	318 ± 32	8.70 ± 1.00
Rewarming		3472 ± 171^b	4.70 ± 1.20^b
Lung reperfusion		5041 ± 1028^b	5.50 ± 1.20^b
End of CPB	$13,760 \pm 1,851^b$	5121 ± 961^b	5.00 ± 1.17^b
24 h post-CPB		446 ± 57^d	7.00 ± 1.30^c

[a] Values are mean $\pm$ SEM (n $=$ 10).
[b] $p < 0.001$ vs pre-CPB.
[c] $p < 0.05$ vs pre-CPB.
[d] Not significant. All values were corrected to baseline total proteins for hemodilution.

REFERENCES

1. HAMMERSCHMIDT, D. E. et al. 1981. Complement activation and neutropenia occurring during cardiopulmonary bypass. J. Thorac. Cardiovasc. Surg. **81:** 370-377.
2. SACHS, T. et al. 1978. Oxygen radicals mediate endothelial cell damage by complement stimulated granulocytes. J. Clin. Invest. **61:** 1161-1167.
3. FAYMONVILLE, M. E. et al. 1986. Prostaglandins E$_2$, prostacyclin and thromboxane changes during non pulsatile cardiopulmonary bypass in man. J. Thorac. Cardiovasc. Surg. **91:** 858-866.
4. BENTWOOD, B. J. & P. M. HENSON. 1980. The sequential release of granule constituents from human neutrophils. J. Immunol. **124**(2): 855-862.
5. CAVAROCCHI, N. C. et al. 1986. Superoxide generation during cardiopulmonary bypass. Is there a role for Vitamin E? J. Surg. Res. **40:** 519-527.

Vitamin E Prevents NADPH-Dependent but not NADH-Dependent Chemoluminescence by Isolated Rat Liver Nuclei

SUSANA PUNTARULO AND
ARTHUR I. CEDERBAUM[a]

Department of Biochemistry
Mount Sinai School of Medicine
New York, New York 10029

Lipid peroxidation is thought to be an important biological consequence of oxidative cellular damage. The destruction of unsaturated fatty acids, which occurs in lipid peroxidation, has been linked with altered membrane structure[1] and enzyme inactivation.[2] In addition to lipid hydroperoxides and lipid radicals,[3] lipid peroxidation may generate activated oxygen species. Vitamin E blocks lipid peroxidation in a variety of biological systems, especially liver microsomes. The role of transition state metals, particularly iron, in microsomal generation of active oxygen radicals is complex and depends on the nature of the iron chelate and the reaction under investigation.[4–6] A study was initiated to investigate the effects of various ferric complexes on oxygen radical generation by rat liver nuclei and the effect of antioxidants, including vitamin E.

In the presence of either NADH or NADPH as cofactor, nuclei catalyzed the production of hydroxyl radical (measured as ethylene production from keto-thio-methylbutyric acid), malondialdehyde (MDA) (TBA-reactive material), and chemoluminescence (CL) (TABLE 1). Iron was required to catalyze these oxidative processes; however, the effect of iron depended on the way iron was chelated. Lipid peroxidation was stimulated by the addition of either ferric-ATP or ferric-citrate but not by ferric-EDTA or ferric-Detapac. By contrast, ·OH production was stimulated by ferric-EDTA and ferric-Detapac but not by ferric-ATP or ferric-citrate. The same response of ·OH or MDA production by nuclei to the iron chelates was observed with either NADH or NADPH as the reductant (TABLE 1). The response of the light emission to ferric chelates, however, was dependent on the cofactor. NADPH-dependent CL, analogous to lipid peroxidation, was increased by ferric-ATP and citrate and decreased by ferric-EDTA or -Detapac. NADH-dependent CL, analogous to ·OH production, was increased by the latter two ferric chelates, but not by the former two (TABLE 1). These results suggest that the oxidizing species responsible for initiating the processes ultimately leading to CL were different when NADPH or NADH were the electron donors.

---

[a]To whom correspondence should be addressed.

To evaluate this possibility, the effect of radical scavenging agents was determined. NADPH-dependent CL (similar to MDA production) was not sensitive to superoxide dismutase, catalase, or the ·OH scavenger DMSO, whereas NADH-dependent light emission was sensitive to these agents. These results suggest a role for ·OH (generated by way of an iron-catalyzed Haber-Weiss type of reaction) in the NADH-catalyzed, but not the NADPH-catalyzed, CL.

Vitamin E nearly completely blocked NADPH-dependent CL in the presence of ferric citrate, consistent with its ability to inhibit lipid peroxidation (TABLE 2). Vitamin E, however, had no effect on NADH-dependent CL catalyzed by either ferric citrate or ferric-Detapac (TABLE 2), consistent with its lack of effect on ·OH production by the nuclei. Freeze-thawing the nuclei elevates the content of nuclei membrane phospholipid hydroperoxides and increases NADPH-dependent CL (data not shown). The response of the NADH-dependent CL to freeze-thawing the nuclei is dependent on the iron catalyst; light emission is increased with ferric-citrate but decreased with ferric-Detapac (TABLE 2). This suggests that freeze-thawing promotes NADH-dependent light emission by a peroxidative-type process and decreases the contribution by a ·OH-dependent process. Accordingly, vitamin E was now an effective inhibitor of CL catalyzed by ferric-citrate (a good catalyst for lipid peroxidation), but CL catalyzed by ferric Detapac (a good catalyst for ·OH generation) remained insensitive to vitamin E (TABLE 2).

Taken as a whole, these results suggest that vitamin E is effective in preventing oxygen radical generation by processes occurring in nuclei membranes, for example, lipid peroxidation, but has no effect on reactions that occur outside the membrane, for example, ·OH generation in solution. The ability of vitamin E to prevent oxidative reactions is dependent on the nature of the initiator oxidant, which in turn, is dependent on the ferric chelate used to catalyze the generation of active oxygen radicals.

TABLE 1. Effect of Ferric Chelates on Generation of Oxygen Radicals by Rat Liver Nuclei[a]

Ferric Chelate Added	Chemoluminescence		Lipid Peroxidation		·OH Production	
	NADPH[b]	NADH	NADPH	NADH	NADPH	NADH
	(area/30 min/0.5 mg)		(nmol MDA/30 min/mg)		(nmol ethylene/ min/mg)	
None	0.69	0.03	4.74	0	0.04	0.13
Ferric-Detapac	0.11	0.36	0.41	0	0.73	3.82
Ferric-EDTA	0.12	0.10	4.14	0	0.76	6.96
Ferric-citrate	1.26	0.07	8.36	11.98	0.02	0.32
Ferric-ATP	1.45	0.04	7.56	11.87	0	0.06

[a] Full details of reaction conditions are similar to those described for experiments with microsomes in ref. 6. Final concentration of iron was 50 μM, and all the ferric chelates were used in a 1:2 ratio, except ferric:ATP, which was used at a 1:20 ratio. Reactions were carried out in the presence of 3 mM NADPH or a NADPH-generating system consisting of 10 mM glucose 6-phosphate, 1.4 units of glucose-6-phosphate dehydrogenase, and 0.4 mM $NADP^+$.
[b] Samples of nuclei subjected to a cycle of freeze-thawing.

TABLE 2. Effect of Vitamin E on Chemoluminescence by Rat Liver Nuclei

Ferric chelate	Vitamin E (units/mL)	Chemoluminescence (area/30 min/0.5 mg nuclei protein)	
		NADPH	NADH
Ferric citrate	0	0.87^a	0.02	0.14^a
	0.1	0.78^a		
	0.5	0.10^a		
	1.0	0.04^a	0.02	0.04^a
Ferric Detapac	0		0.17	0.08^a
	1.0		0.17	0.09^a

^{a} Samples subjected to a cycle of freeze-thawing.

REFERENCES

1. EICHENBERGER, K., P. BOHNI, K. H. WINTERHALTER, S. KAWATO & C. RICHTER. 1982. FEBS Lett. 142: 59-62.
2. BAKER, S. P. & B. A. HEMSWORTH. 1978. Biochem. Pharmacol. 27: 805-806.
3. PORTER, N.A. 1984. In Methods in Enzymology. Vol. 105. L. Packer, Ed.: 273-282. Academic Press. Orlando, FL.
4. AUST, S. D., L. A. MOREHOUSE & C. E. THOMAS. 1985. Free Rad. Biol. Med. 1: 3-25.
5. AUST, S. D. & B. A. SVINGEN. 1982. In Free Radicals in Biology. Vol. 5. W. A. Pryor, Ed.: 1-28. Academic Press. New York, NY.
6. PUNTARULO, S. & A. I. CEDERBAUM. 1988. Arch. Biochem. Biophys. 264(2): 482-491.

Biochemical Evidence of Lipoperoxidation in Venous Stasis Ulcer

Beneficial Role of Vitamin E as Antioxidant

SAI S. RAMASASTRY, MICHAEL F. ANGEL,
KRISHNA NARAYANAN,[a] R. A. BASFORD, AND
J. WILLIAM FUTRELL

Division of Plastic Surgery
[a] Department of Biochemistry
University of Pittsburgh School of Medicine
Pittsburgh, Pennsylvania 15261

Ninety percent of patients with deep vein thrombosis will eventually develop chronic venous insufficiency leading to skin ulceration. The pathophysiology of skin ulceration associated with venous insufficiency is not totally clear. Browse[1] hypothesized that venous hypertension produced an egress of fluid and molecules into the interstitium leading to tissue ischemia and necrosis. We hypothesize that in venous insufficiency an incomplete ischemic state exists that leads to generation of free radicals, tissue necrosis, and skin breakdown. The basis for the hypothesis is as follows.

It has been previously demonstrated that experimental skin island flaps tolerate obstruction of their entire vascular pedicle (complete ischemia) better than disruption of venous outflow alone (incomplete ischemia).[2] The distal portion of such rat pedicle flaps destined to necrosis manifest greatly increased lipoperoxidation and release of free radicals.[3] The partially ischemic state is probably the basis for generation of free radicals and skin ulceration in chronic venous insufficiency.[4]

This study was undertaken to demonstrate the biochemical evidence for lipoperoxidation in venous stasis ulcer and the role of vitamin E as an antioxidant in preventing recurrence of venous stasis ulcer. Malondialdehyde (MDA), one of the byproducts of lipoperoxidation, was used as the indicator.

MATERIAL AND METHODS

Twenty patients with long-standing (more than 5 years), recurrent venous stasis ulceration were studied. The mean size of the ulcers measured 15 × 18 centimeters.

All patients underwent débridement and split-thickness skin graft coverage. The legs were kept wrapped with elastic bandages. In eight patients, biopsy of the ulcer perimeter areas (zone of partial ischemia) and biopsy of the skin graft donor site (zone of complete ischemia) from the proximal thigh for MDA analysis was carried out. Patients were divided into 2 groups: group I (n = 10) did not receive vitamin E; group II (n = 10) received vitamin E, 400 U (α-tocopheryl) orally daily.

RESULTS

Biopsy from the edge of the venous ulcers showed consistent elevation of the MDA values, suggesting increased lipoperoxidation (TABLE 1). Skin grafts are stable at 18 months, mean follow-up in 9 of 10 patients in the vitamin E group (TABLE 2). One patient had a recent small, shallow ulcer recurrence. Group I patients, though, had 100% grafts take at three weeks and had skin graft breakdown within 6 months (100%; $p < 0.001$).

CONCLUSIONS

In chronic venous insufficiency there is evidence of increased lipoperoxidation at the site of skin ulceration, and vitamin E as antioxidant prevents recurrent skin ulceration.

TABLE 1. MDA Assays of Skin Biopsies (ng/g)

Patient	(Complete Thigh Ischemia)	(Partial Ulcer Ischemia)
1	0.3	0.9
2	1.3	1.8
3	0.9	1.1
4	0.9	1.0
5	1.1	1.3
6	1.2	1.3
7	0.9	1.2
8	0.9	1.8
	0.971 ± 0.129	1.23 ± 0.10
		$p < 0.025$

TABLE 2. Result of Skin Graft at 18 Months

Group I (n = 10) Vitamin E^a	Stable in 9/10
Group II (n = 10) No Treatment	Skin graft breakdown 10/10
	$p < 0.001$

^{a} α-Tocopheryl.

REFERENCES

1. BROWSE, N. *et al.* 1982. Venous ulceration. Br. Med. J. **286:** 1920-1922.
2. HARASHINA, T., Y. SAWADA & S. WATANABE. 1977. The relationship between venous occlusion time in island flaps and flap survivals. Plast. Reconstr. Surg. **60:** 92-95.
3. ANGEL, M. F., S. S. RAMASASTRY *et al.* 1988. The critical relationship between free radicals and degree of ischemia: Evidence for tissue intolerance of marginal perfusion. Plast. Reconstr. Surg. **81:** 232.
4. ANGEL, M. F., S. S. RAMASASTRY *et al.* 1987. The causes of skin ulceration associated with venous insufficiency: A unifying hypothesis. Plast. Reconstr. Surg. **79:** 289.

Vitamin E, Glutathione Peroxidase, and Polyunsaturated Fatty Acid Concentrations of Heart and Liver in Swine with Dietetic Microangiopathy

DESMOND A. RICE AND SEAMUS KENNEDY

Veterinary Research Laboratories
Stormont, Belfast BT4 3SD, Northern Ireland

Vitamin E and selenium (E-Se) deficiency and/or polyunsaturated fatty acid (PUFA) excess in swine is associated with dietetic microangiopathy (DM),[1,2] hepatosis dietetica, myopathy, steatitis, stillbirths, and weak piglets. In spite of fourfold increases in dietary E-Se in recent years, DM still affects swine in Northern Ireland. Affected pigs die suddenly and have myocardial hemorrhage, hydropericardium, and pulmonary edema. Histologically there is fibrinoid necrosis of arterioles, hemorrhage, and necrosis of cardiocytes. This study determined the involvement of vitamin E, glutathione peroxidase (GSH-Px), and PUFA in contemporary cases of DM.

We examined 54 fattening swine that died suddenly. Of these, 27 had histological evidence of DM, and 27 pigs with no evidence of E-Se deficiency were used as controls. Feed consumed by pigs at time of death was collected where possible. Liver, kidney, and heart were analyzed for alpha-tocopherol by HPLC/fluorometry, GSH-Px by a kit (Randox Laboratories, Crumlin, Northern Ireland), and long chain fatty acids up to C22:6 (n-3) by capillary gas chromatography. Feed concentrations of vitamin E, selenium (by fluorometry), oil, and long chain fatty acids were also measured.

All pigs were in good body condition. DM pigs had fibrin clots in the pericardial sac and in the pleural and peritoneal cavities, together with pulmonary edema and hepatic congestion. Subepicardial, myocardial, and subendocardial hemorrhages were consistent findings. Thrombosis of intramural myocardial arterioles and capillaries, and multifocal myocardial necrosis were frequently seen.

Liver and heart concentrations of alpha-tocopherol were lower in DM swine than in controls (TABLE 1). This was most significant in the case of heart tissue. The relationship between heart (y) and liver (x) alpha-tocopherol concentrations was y = 0.83 $\times$ + 0.92 (R^2 = 0.28) in DM pigs compared to y = 1.04 $\times$ + 1.80 (R^2 = 0.66) in controls. Vitamin E metabolism thus appears to be severely altered in DM swine, indicating an important pathogenetic role for the vitamin in development of DM.

Selenium concentrations of heart and liver, and heart GSH-Px concentrations were similar in both groups, indicating that Se deficiency is not of primary etiological importance in DM. There were minor differences in the percentage composition of

C20:4(n-6) and C22:5(n-3) in heart. Unexpectedly, control swine had the highest concentrations of these two fatty acids. The disease was not therefore induced by excess PUFA in the DM swine. The dietary intakes of alpha-tocopherol (TABLE 1), selenium, and oil were not different between groups. DM does not therefore appear to result from dietary deficiency of alpha-tocopherol, Se, or excess of dietary PUFA.

The reason for the tissue deficiency of alpha-tocopherol has not been determined. A possible cause could be a genetic predisposition of individual pigs to maintain suboptimum concentrations of alpha-tocopherol in subcellular membranes in spite of apparently adequate dietary intakes. Such a situation could be due to an absorption problem or to inadequate absorption or transport mechanisms for alpha-tocopherol in tissues. We do not know if feeding even higher levels of vitamin E will prevent DM. Alternatively, there may be an increased rate of lipid peroxidation in subcellular membranes increasing the antioxidant requirement. This is most likely and is consistent with the lower correlation between heart and liver alpha-tocopherol in DM swine. Microthrombosis may result from prostacyclin I_2/thromboxane A_2 imbalance resulting from vitamin E deficiency,[3] or microthrombosis may result from peroxidative damage to vascular endothelium.

TABLE 1. Alpha-Tocopherol in Tissues and Feed, and GSH-Px in Tissues of DM and Control Swine

| Group | | Alpha-Tocopherol (μg/g) | | | GSH-Px (IU/mg protein) |
		Heart	Liver	Feed	Heart
DM Swine	Mean	2.63	2.02	44.1	216.10
	SD	1.34	0.84	12.7	161.96
	N	23	25	7	20
Control Swine	Mean	4.93	3.12	39.7	167.67
	SD	2.29	1.78	10.3	76.76
	N	24	26	8	24
	t test	[a]	[a]	NS[b]	NS[b]

[a] Differences were statistically significant, $p \geq 0.05$.
[b] Not significant.

These results indicate that similar studies should be carried out in other species, including humans, in order to determine whether similar alterations in vitamin E metabolism exist.

REFERENCES

1. GRANT, C. A. 1961. Morphological and aetiological studies of dietetic microangiopathy in pigs ("mulberry heart" disease). Acta Vet. Scand. 2(Suppl. 3): 1-107.
2. VAN VLEET, J. F., V. J. FERRANS & G. R. RUTH. 1977. Ultrastructural alterations in nutritional cardiomyopathy of selenium-vitamin E deficient swine. II. Vascular lesions. Lab. Invest. 37: 201-211.
3. TOIVANEN, J. L. 1987. Effects of selenium, vitamin E and vitamin C on human prostacyclin and thromboxane synthesis in vitro. Prostaglandins Leukotrienes Med. 26: 265-280.

Radiolabeling Microsomes *in Vitro* with Tritiated Alpha-Tocopherol

SUSAN M. ROBEY-BOND,[a] RICHARD D. MAVIS,[b,d]
AND JACOB N. FINKELSTEIN[c,e]

[a] *Environmental Health Sciences Center*
[b] *Department of Biophysics*
Division of Toxicology
[c] *Department of Pediatrics*
University of Rochester Medical Center
Rochester, New York 14642

Direct measurement of α-tocopherol (α-t) in peroxidizing microsomes would be useful to a variety of experimental questions. Measurement is difficult, however, because α-t is present in minute quantities in the microsomal membrane (0.16 μg/mg protein[1]). Monitoring radiolabeled α-t ([³H]α-t) in the membrane would increase sensitivity of detection of the oxidation of microsomal α-t.

Microsomes were isolated from male Long-Evans hooded rats by a modification of the method previously described.[1] We used the cytosolic α-t transfer protein (VETP) found in rat liver[2] to label microsomal membranes with [³H]α-t *in vitro*. This protein specifically transfers [d]-α-tocopherol between membranes.[2,3] To label microsomes using the cytosolic transfer protein, [³H]α-t in methanol (Amersham, 3-11 Ci/mmol, 40-50 μCi/mL, 3.7 μCi/g wet weight liver, purified by reverse phase HPLC) was added to the 16,000 × g supernatant of liver homogenate. This supernatant contains the cytosolic transfer protein and microsomes from a 40% w/v liver homogenate in 5 mM Tris maleate buffer, .15 M KCl, 1 mM EDTA, pH 7.4 at 4°C. To label microsomes in the absence of the cytosolic transfer protein, microsomes were pelleted from the 16,000 × g supernatant of liver homogenate by centrifugation (100,000 × g, 1 h, 4°C), resuspended in homogenization buffer, and [³H]α-t in methanol was added. All work with [³H]α-t was performed under an N₂ atmosphere. After incubation (shaking at 4°C or 37°C), labeled microsomes were obtained by centrifugation (100,000 × g for 1 h at 4°C). Microsomes were washed with EDTA-free buffer, repelleted, and resuspended to a concentration of approximately 10 mg microsomal protein per milliliter.

Microsomes labeled at 4°C exhibited twice the incorporation of [³H]α-t than microsomes labeled at 37°C. The protease inhibitors NEM and PMSF were added during liver homogenization to test whether the decreased labeling at 37°C was due to the activation of proteases. The presence of protease inhibitors did not affect incorporation at a given temperature. Therefore it seems unlikely that this decreased

[d] Present address: Mitre Corporation, Civil Systems Division, 7525 Colshire Dr., McLean, VA 22102-3481.
[e] To whom correspondence should be addressed.

511

labeling at 37°C is due to proteolytic decomposition of the VETP. Optimal labeling conditions were a 10 min incubation at 4°C with no protease inhibitors, which resulted in .25-.30 μCi [³H]α-t incorporated per mg protein.

These microsomes were then peroxidized, and the production of malondialdehyde (MDA) and the oxidation of [³H]α-t determined. The [³H]α-t is oxidized rapidly after initiation of lipid peroxidation (LPO) when it has been incorporated into microsomes by way of the VETP (FIG. 1). When [³H]α-t is added to microsomes in the absence of the VETP, however, the label does not oxidize during the time course of LPO (FIG. 2).

Published results of Venekei[4] demonstrate that during NADPH-Fe^{2+}-initiated LPO, α-t rapidly oxidizes and is depleted after 10 min of LPO. Thus [³H]α-t incorporated into microsomes through the VETP acts as a marker for endogenous α-t oxidation.

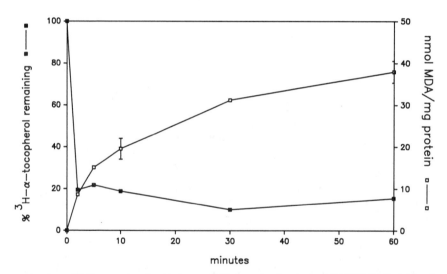

FIGURE 1. [³H]α-tocopherol oxidation and MDA production during NADPH/Fe^{2+}-initiated lipid peroxidation in microsomes. Microsomes (1.4 mg/mL) were aerobically incubated at 37°C in 50 mM Tris maleate buffer (pH 7.4), with 30 μM FeSO$_4$ and with an NADPH-generating system (1 unit glucose-6-phosphate dehydrogenase per mL, 1.5 mM glucose-6-phosphate, 250 μM NADPH) to initiate *in vitro* LPO. Lipid peroxidation was assayed by a modification of the spectrophotometric method of Buege and Aust[5] and is expressed as nmol MDA/mg microsomal protein (open squares). [³H]α-tocopherol and its nonpolar oxidation products were extracted into 2.5 mL hexane after solubilization by trichloroacetic acid (0.31 M) and triton X 100 (4% w/v). α-Tocopherol (75 μg in ethanol) was added as carrier and antioxidant. In some experiments, [³H]α-t was extracted by the method of Burton *et al.*[6] The hexane phase was removed, dried under N$_2$, resuspended in 30 μL ethanol, and spotted on preabsorbent silica gel G 250 TLC plates (Analtech). The chromatogram was developed in cyclohexane/chloroform/acetic acid (60:30:10). The α-t and α-t oxidation product, tocopherol quinone, bands were visualized with iodine, scraped, and counted by scintillation. Oxidation of [³H]α-t is expressed as percent control levels (closed squares). Rat liver microsomes were radiolabeled *in vitro* with [³H]α-t using cytosol.

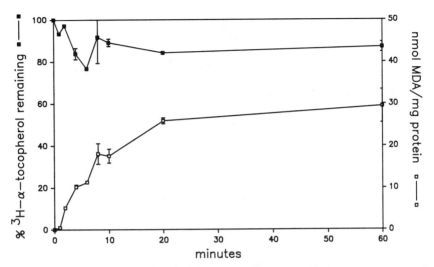

FIGURE 2. Rat liver microsomes were radiolabeled *in vitro* with [³H]α-t in the absence of cytosol. Methods are described in the FIGURE 1 legend.

REFERENCES

1. KORNBRUST, D. J. & R. D. MAVIS. 1980. Lipids **15:** 315-322.
2. MURPHY, D. J. & R. D. MAVIS. 1981. J. Biol. Chem. **256:** 10464-10468.
3. POSCH, K. C. 1988. Ph.D. thesis, University of Rochester, Rochester, NY.
4. VENEKEI, I. 1987. Biochim. Biophys. Acta **917:** 347-355.
5. BUEGE, J. A. & S. D. AUST. 1978. *In* Methods in Enzymology. S. Fleischer & L. Packer, Eds. Vol. 52: 302-310. Academic Press. New York, NY.
6. BURTON, G. W., A. WEBB & K. U. INGOLD. 1985. Lipids **20:** 29-39.

Mechanism of Interaction of Vitamin E and Glutathione in the Protection against Membrane Lipid Peroxidation

R. W. SCHOLZ, K. S. GRAHAM, E. GUMPRICHT,
AND C. C. REDDY

Department of Veterinary Science
College of Agriculture
The Pennsylvania State University
University Park, Pennsylvania 16802

Although the function of vitamin E as the major, if not only, chain-breaking, lipid-soluble antioxidant in biological membranes has been established,[1] its mode(s) of action has yet to be elucidated. One proposed mechanism of vitamin E function involves a possible glutathione-dependent system that inhibits *in vitro* lipid peroxidation. Previously, we have described a rat liver microsomal system that inhibited both enzymatic and nonenzymatic lipid peroxidation in the presence of both glutathione and microsomal vitamin E.[2] The GSH-dependent inhibition of lipid peroxidation was not observed in microsomes obtained from vitamin E-deficient rats and was independent of the selenium status of the animal. This inhibition, however, was not seen in heat-denatured microsomes, despite the continued presence of vitamin E. We therefore suggested that a microsomal heat-labile protein was likely involved in the mediation of the vitamin E-dependent, glutathione inhibition of lipid peroxidation. Other groups have also recently reported the presence of a glutathione-dependent liver microsomal factor that inhibited lipid peroxidation.[3–5] The experiments reported here were designed to investigate the nature of the GSH-dependent inhibition of lipid peroxidation in the presence or absence of vitamin E.

Weanling male Long-Evans hooded rats were fed chemically defined diets either deficient or supplemented with 150 IU *dl*-α-tocopheryl acetate/kg diet for 7 weeks.[2] *In vitro* lipid peroxidation of liver microsomes was monitored by the formation of thiobarbituric acid (TBA)-reactive products, using both NADPH-dependent enzymatic and ascorbate/ADP-dependent nonenzymatic procedures, and by the consumption of O_2 from the reaction medium.

As shown in FIGURE 1A, 5 mM GSH inhibited lipid peroxidation in this system for approximately 45 minutes. Interestingly, the addition of both GSH and oxidized glutathione (GSSG) resulted in a synergistic interaction that inhibited lipid peroxidation to a greater extent than the addition of GSH alone. GSSG alone did not inhibit lipid peroxidation of rat liver microsomes, and additional experiments (data not shown) revealed that GSH was oxidized to a limited extent to GSSG, whereas the conversion of GSSG to GSH was not observed. A possible explanation for this effect is that GSSG functions to protect a heat-labile factor(s) from inactivation, perhaps by sulfide-disulfide interchange with a sulfhydryl group on an enzyme.

A potent inhibitor of non-Se glutathione peroxidase activity, decylGSH, markedly reduced the inhibition of lipid peroxidation by GSH, suggesting that microsomal non-Se GSH-Px or another GSH-dependent enzyme may be responsible for this effect (Fig. 1B).

The addition of GSH to assays containing liver microsomes from rats supplemented with vitamin E resulted in a decreased rate of O_2 consumption during *in vitro* lipid

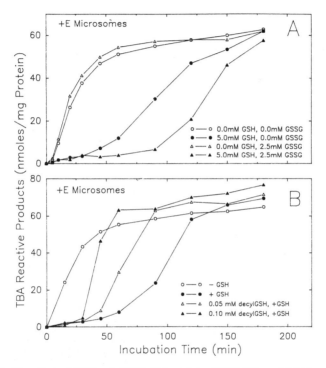

FIGURE 1. The effect of GSH and GSSG (A), and decylGSH (B), on inhibition of rat liver microsomal lipid peroxidation as monitored by the formation of TBA-reactive products. The NADPH-Fe^{++}-dependent enzymatic lipid peroxidation assay mixture contained 0.012 mM FeSO$_4$, 0.25 mM NADPH, 0.05 M Tris-HCl buffer, pH 7.4, varying concentrations of GSH, GSSG, and decylGSH (adjusted to pH 7.4 prior to addition to the mixture), and approximately 0.16 mg microsomal protein/mL.

peroxidation (Fig. 2A). GSH also decreased the magnitude and rate of TBA-reactive products formed under conditions where O_2 was limiting (Fig. 2B) and spared the consumption of α-tocopherol (Fig. 2C). GSH failed to decrease the elevated rates of O_2 consumption and TBA-reactive product formation in peroxidizing liver microsomes from vitamin E-deficient animals. The ratio of O_2 consumed to TBA-reactive products formed suggests that lipid peroxidation may be inhibited by some mechanism other than radical scavenging.

These data suggest the presence of two GSH-dependent, heat labile systems that function to inhibit microsomal lipid peroxidation. The first appears to be by way of the GSH-dependent regeneration of vitamin E from its oxidized form(s), thereby blocking radical propagation by quenching lipid peroxy radicals. The second mech-

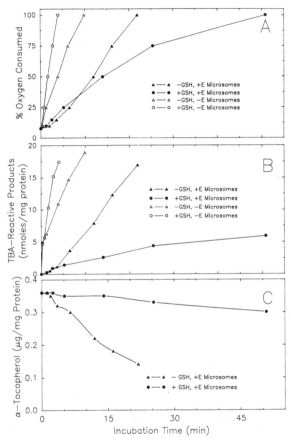

FIGURE 2. The effect of GSH on oxygen consumption (A), TBA-reactive product formation (B), and α-tocopherol disappearance (C) in an O_2-limiting, lipid peroxidation assay system. The assay system described in FIGURE 1 was used with a total volume of 3.0 mL. Approximately 1.9 mg of microsomal protein was used in these assays, and lipid peroxidation was initiated by the addition of $FeSO_4$. O_2 concentration was measured polarigraphically, and α-tocopherol was determined by HPLC.

anism may involve a microsomal Se-independent GSH-Px, which, by reducing fatty acid hydroperoxides effectively, can prevent the formation of chain-propagating radicals. If this is true, these two mechanisms should complement each other and form a GSH-dependent system that would be extremely effective in preventing lipid peroxidation.

REFERENCES

1. BURTON, G. W., A. JOYCE & K. U. INGOLD. 1983. Arch. Biochem. Biophys. **221:** 281.
2. REDDY, C. C., R. W. SCHOLZ, C. E. THOMAS & E. J. MASSARO. 1982. Life Sci. **31:** 571.
3. BURK, R. F. 1983. Biochim. Biophys. Acta **757:** 21.
4. MCCAY, P. B., E. K. LAI, S. R. POWELL & G. BREUGGMANN. 1986. Fed. Proc. **45:** 451.
5. WEFERS, H. & H. SIES. 1988. Eur. J. Biochem. **174:** 353.

Alpha-Tocopherol Ingestion from Birth and Its Effects on Serum Androgens in Rats

SHAN G. SUNDARAM, S. MANIMEKALAI, AND
P. J. GOLDSTEIN

Obstetrics and Gynecology Research Divisions
Sinai Hospital of Baltimore
Baltimore, Maryland 21215

INTRODUCTION

The probability of developing breast cancer (BC) was reported to be 2 to 8 times increased in women with fibrocystic disease of breast (FD).[1] Alpha-tocopherol (E) had been used to treat FD with some success.[2] In 1982, London *et al.*[3] showed that E therapy in FD patients was associated with a decrease in serum dehydroepian-drosterone sufate (DHEAS).[3] In 1987, Heinonen *et al.*[4] showed that a decrease in DHEAS was also associated with the incidence of BC and ovarian cancer (OC) in women. If those associations were true and not casual, it would imply that E therapy should be undertaken with caution at least in FD patients. We carried out the following study to assess the effect of E therapy from birth on the serum and tissue levels of androgens, especially DHEAS and serum-free testosterone (FT), in normal females, using a rat pup model.

MATERIAL AND METHODS

Pups were delivered from pregnant female Sprague-Dawley rats. From the time of delivery, the mothers were given 10 IU of E (liquid form from Hoffman-La Roche, Inc., Nutley, NJ) per day for 4 weeks by gavage, the pups receiving E from their mothers through maternal milk. Subsequently, the pups were given 5 IU of E per day by gavage for 4 more weeks. The adult females, pups (males and females), and an equal number of controls (without E) were sacrificed, and their sera, liver, kidney, and adipose tissue were isolated. DHEAS and FT were measured by radioimmunoassay (RIA) using appropriate RIA kits from Diagnostic Products Corporation, CA.

518

TABLE 1. Serum Dehydroepiandrosterone Sulfate and Free Testosterone Levels in Adult Female Rats[a]

	DHEAS (ng/mL)	FT (pg/mL)
Control (n = 9)	22.06 ± 2.15	0.96 ± 0.22
Vitamin E (n = 9)	25.13 ± 3.23	0.42 ± 0.12[b]

[a] The values are mean ± standard error of mean.
[b] p less than 0.05.

RESULTS AND DISCUSSION

When compared to their controls, E-treated adult females had decreased FT but similar DHEAS levels (TABLE 1). E-treated pups, female or male, did not show any change in FT levels when compared to the levels in their controls (TABLE 2). The E-treated female pups, however, had significantly elevated DHEAS levels with no change in male pups (TABLE 2). The presence of E-mediated gonadal and adrenal activities in adult females and the absence of gonadal activity in the pups may be the cause of the observed differences. It was also observed that the female pups (controls and E-treated) had significantly higher DHEAS and lower FT levels than that found in male pups, probably due to their difference in sex rather than their response to E.

In conclusion, DHEAS is found more in growing female pups than in male pups, and it is further enhanced by E therapy from birth, because low DHEAS appears to be associated with an increased risk of BC and OC, and E-induced increase in DHEAS from birth in females may be of potential use in preventing breast and ovarian tumors in later years, assuming findings in rat model can be extrapolated to humans.

TABLE 2. Serum Dehydroepiandrosterone Sulfate and Free Testosterone Levels in Female and Male Rat Pups

	DHEAS (ng/mL) Female pups (n = 15)	Male pups (n = 15)
Control	31.65 ± 2.37	17.39 ± 1.49[a]
Vitamin E	40.68 ± 4.27[a]	15.14 ± 0.90[a]
	FT (pg/mL)	
Control	0.40 ± 0.08	37.16 ± 12.38
Vitamin E	0.43 ± 0.10	26.38 ± 5.22

[a] p less than 0.05.

REFERENCES

1. DAVIS, H. H., M. SIMONS & J. B. DAVIS. 1964. Cancer **17:** 957-978.
2. ABRAMS, A. A. 1965. N. Engl. J. Med. **272:** 1080-1088.
3. LONDON, R. S., G. S. SUNDARAM, S. MANIMEKALAI, D. STRUMMER, M. M. SCHULTZ, P. P. NAIR & P. J. GOLDSTEIN. 1982. Nutr. Res. **2:** 243-247.
4. HEINONEN, P. K., T. KOIVULA & P. PYSTYMEN. 1987. Gynecol. Obstet. Invest. **23:** 271-274.

Mode of Action of Vitamin E as Antioxidant in the Membranes as Studied by Spin Labeling

MAREYUKI TAKAHASHI, JYUNICHI TSUCHIYA,
AND ETSUO NIKI

Department of Reaction Chemistry
Faculty of Engineering
The University of Tokyo
Hongo, Tokyo 113, Japan

Vitamin E (vit.E) is accepted as the most important and vital lipophilic antioxidant in biomembranes. It is known that vitamin E functions as a chain-breaking antioxidant and interrupts the chain propagation of free radical-mediated peroxidation of biological molecules and membranes by scavenging radicals. At the same time, it has been proposed that vitamin E contributes physically as a membrane stabilizer.

In this study we tried to elucidate the mode of action of vitamin E in the membranes using ESR spin label technique. ESR spin labeling has been mainly used to measure the fluidity or microviscosity of membranes. It is known that the nitroxide group of the spin probe reacts with radical species, alkyl radical or peroxy radical, and acts as an antioxidant in the autoxidation of organic substrates.[1,2] Recently it was found that this nitroxide spin probe can act as an antioxidant in the oxidation of phospholipid liposomal membranes.[3,4] 2,2'-Azobis(2,4-dimethylvaleronitrile) (AMVN) and 2,2'-azobis(2-amidinopropane) dihydrochloride (AAPH) were used as lipid-soluble and water-soluble radical initiators, respectively. They decompose thermally to give free radicals at a constant rate. When one of the spin probes, 5-, 7-, 10-, 12-, and 16-doxyl stearic acid (5-, 7-, 10-, 12-, 16-NS), was incorporated into the soybean phosphatidylcholine (PC) liposomal membranes and their oxidation was induced by AMVN, which was also incorporated into the same liposomal membranes, the spin probe was consumed at a constant rate (FIG. 1). When vitamin E was also incorporated into the PC liposomal membranes together with NS and AMVN, the rate of disappearance of the spin probe was reduced, apparently because vitamin E scavenged the peroxy radicals. We defined the parameter P as

$$P = \frac{R(\text{without vit.E}) - R(\text{with vit.E})}{R(\text{without vit.E})} \times 100(\%)$$

where, R(without vit.E) and R(with vit.E) are the rates of consumption of NS in the absence and presence of vitamin E, respectively. This parameter, P, gives a per-

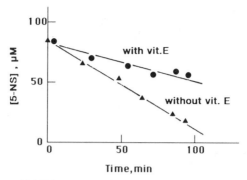

FIGURE 1. Decrease of 5-NS incorporated into 10.3 mM soybean PC liposomes in the presence and absence of vitamin E during the oxidation initiated with 4.0 mM AMVN at 50° C under air; [vit. E] = 100μM, [5-NS] = 86.7μM.

centage of peroxy radicals that are scavenged by vitamin E rather than by spin probe: if vitamin E scavenges all of the peroxy radicals, then R(with vit.e) is 0 and P = 100, whereas if all of the radicals are trapped by the spin probe and not by vitamin E, then R(without vit.E) = R(with vit.E) and P = 0. In other words, P gives the efficiency for scavenging radicals by vitamin E in the membranes. Interestingly, it was found that, as shown in FIGURE 2, the efficiency for sparing the spin probe by vitamin E decreased as the spin probe went deeper into the interior of the bilayer, suggesting that vitamin E scavenges radicals near the surface more efficiently than those residing closer to the inner region of the membranes. In order to understand the role of the phytyl side chain of vitamin E in the biological membranes,[5] we measured the effi-

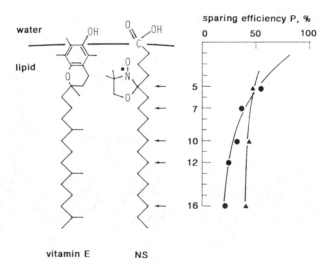

FIGURE 2. Probable location of vitamin E and NS in the PC liposomal membranes and the sparing efficiency by vitamin E(●) and PMC(▲) for the consumption of NS induced by AMVN in dimyristoylphosphatidylcholine (14:OPC) liposomal membranes at 50° C. [14:OPC] = 10.3 mM; [AMVN] = 4.0 mM; [IH] (inhibitor) = 1.0 mM; [NS] = 86.7 μM.

ciencies for sparing spin probes by 2,2,5,7,8-pentamethyl-6-chromanol (PMC), which is an analogue of vitamin E (FIG. 2). Comparing these results in FIGURE 2, it may be said that PMC scavenges radicals more easily within the membranes than vitamin E. Although the *phytyl* side chain of vitamin E is required for incorporation and retainment into the biomembranes, it appears that the phytyl side chain reduces the mobility of vitamin E within the membranes.

We also measured the sparing efficiency using AAPH, which generates radicals in the aqueous phase. The sparing efficiencies by vitamin E against the aqueous radicals were larger than those against the lipophilic radicals.

In conclusion, it was shown that vitamin E scavenges radicals at or near the surface of the membranes more easily than those that reside deep in the bilayer. Vitamin E acts as an antioxidant more effectively against the radicals coming from the outside of the membranes than against those within the bilayer.

REFERENCES

1. MASLOV, S. A. & G. E. ZAIKOV. 1987. *In* Developments in Polymer Stabilization-8. G. Scott, Ed.: 1-28. Elsevier Applied Science. London.
2. BROWNLIE, I. T. & K. U. INGOLD. 1967. Can. J. Chem. **45:** 2427-2432.
3. TAKAHASHI, M., J. TSUCHIYA & E. NIKI. 1988. J. Nutr. Sci. Vitaminol. **34:** 25-34.
4. TAKAHASHI, M., J. TSUCHIYA & E. NIKI. 1989. *In* Medical, Biochemical and Chemical Aspects of Free Radicals. O. Hayaishi, E. Niki, M. Kondo & T. YOSHIKAWA, Eds.: 833-836. Elsevier. Amsterdam.
5. NIKI, E., A. KAWAKAMI, M. SAITO, Y. YAMAMOTO, J. TSUCHIYA & Y. KAMIYA. 1985. J. Biol. Chem. **260:** 2191-2196.

Membrane-Stabilizing Effect of Vitamin E

SHIRO URANO AND MITSUYOSHI MATSUO

Tokyo Metropolitan Institute of Gerontology
35-2 Sakae-cho
Itabashiku, Tokyo 173, Japan

It has been generally believed that vitamin E acts as a biological membrane stabilizer. Diplock and Lucy proposed that methyl groups on the isoprenoid side chain of α-tocopherol may interact physicochemically with Z pockets of arachidonoyl residues of membrane phospholipids.[1] Although this theory offers a possible explanation for the membrane-stabilizing property of vitamin E, no obvious evidence has been reported to show that this interaction exists in biomembranes. For the elucidation of the membrane-stabilizing ability of vitamin E, the interaction of α-tocopherol or its model compounds with fatty acids or phospholipids has been examined in homogeneous solution and liposomes using fluorescence quenching, fluorescence polarization, and ^{13}C-NMR relaxation (T_1) techniques. The inhibitory effect of α-tocopherol and its model compounds on vitamin A-induced hemolysis has also been investigated.

In homogeneous solution, α-tocopherol as well as each of its model compounds having side chains of different length at 2-position forms a complex with an unsaturated fatty acid or a lecithin in methanol or benzene. For complex formation, the isoprenoid side chain and hydroxy group of α-tocopherol are unessential and, rather, methyl groups attached to the aromatic ring of the chromanol moiety seem to be responsible. For better interaction, more than three methylene-interrupted Z double bonds of a fatty acid are necessary.

All tocopherols decreased the fluidity of liposomes that were perturbed by the inclusion of an unsaturated fatty acid having more than one double bond, and among them, α-tocopherol was the most effective. For example, the fluidity of arachidonic acid-containing liposomes was greatly decreased by the inclusion of α-tocopherol and considerably decreased by the inclusion of its model compounds having at least one isoprene unit or a long straight chain instead of the isoprenoid side chain. Both the chromanol, however, with a methyl group instead of the side chain and phytol, had no effect. On the basis of T_1 values, it was proved that the segmental motion of the isoprenoid side chain of α-tocopherol tends to increase with an increase in the distance from the chromanol moiety, and that three methyl groups attached to the aromatic ring rather than those of the isoprenoid side chain have strong affinity to unsaturated lipids (TABLE 1).

The inhibitory effect of α-tocopherol on vitamin A-induced hemolysis was larger than those of the other naturally occurring tocopherols, and was similar to those of its model compounds having two isoprene units or a straight chain instead of the isoprenoid side chain. Phytol was inactive under the conditions used. It is of interest that the inhibitory effects of α-tocopheryl acetate and nicotinate were striking, particularly in higher concentrations, relative to that of α-tocopherol itself (FIG. 1).

TABLE 1. ^{13}C-Relaxation Times (T_1) for the Labeled Carbon Atoms of α-Tocopherol

Position (see Structure)	Temperature (°C)	T_1 (sec)			
		DPPC[a]	Egg PC	Rat Liver PC	Neat(CDCl$_3$)
5a	20	0.730	0.463	0.654	2.146
7a	20	1.100	0.715	0.748	2.208
8b	20	0.881	0.635	0.736	2.285
4'a	20	0.498	0.491	0.463	0.930
	50	0.781	0.873	0.826	
8'a	20	0.480	0.625	0.531	0.930
	50	1.140	1.163	1.031	
12'a & 13'	20	0.973	1.039	1.135	2.159
	50	2.185	1.606	1.592	
6'	20	0.127	0.161	0.177	0.477
	50	0.226	0.308	0.272[b]	

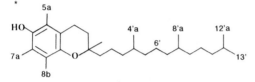

[a] Dipalmitoylphosphatidylcholine.
[b] Colored under experiment.

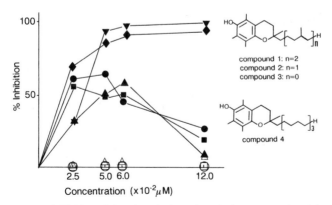

FIGURE 1. Percent inhibition of vitamin A-induced hemolysis by α-tocopherol, its derivatives, and the model compounds. The mixture of erythrocyte and $1.7 \times 10^{-3}\mu$M retinol was incubated with α-tocopherol (●), compound 1 (▲), compound 2 (○), compound 3 (□), Compound 4 (■), phytol (△), α-tocopheryl acetate (◆), or α-tocopheryl nicotinate (▼) at 37°C.

In conclusion, for the stabilization of membrane, the presence of the chromanol moiety with three methyl groups born on the aromatic ring of α-tocopherol is essential as a "space filler," similar to the effect of cholesterol, in membranes perturbed by unsaturated fatty acids, and the isoprenoid side chain acts as an "anchor" for the retention of the α-tocopherol molecule.

REFERENCE

1. DIPLOCK, A. T. & L. A. LUCY. 1973. FEBS Lett. 29: 205-210.

Cooperative Protection by Vitamins E and C of Human Erythrocyte Membranes against Peroxidation

JEROEN J. M. VAN DEN BERG, BEN ROELOFSEN,
JOS A. F. OP DEN KAMP, AND
LAURENS L. M. VAN DEENEN

Department of Biochemistry
State University of Utrecht
Padualaan 8
3584 CH Utrecht, the Netherlands

As a membrane-soluble radical scavenger, vitamin E (tocopherol) appears to be of vital importance in the protection of biological membranes against peroxidation. It was proposed by Tappel[1] that vitamin C in the water phase could regenerate membrane vitamin E from vitamin E radical, thus maintaining an active vitamin E pool. This kind of interaction between vitamins E and C and the synergistic protection of membranes resulting therefrom have been observed in solution, in model membranes, and recently in a microsomal system.[2] We have performed studies on the effect of vitamins E and C, alone as well as in combination, on lipid peroxidation in human erythrocyte white ghost membranes. Cumene hydroperoxide plus hemin-Fe^{3+} were used as oxidants, resulting in the formation of cumene (per)oxyl radicals in the membranes that initiate lipid peroxidation. The fluorescent polyunsaturated fatty acid, parinaric acid (PnA, 9,11,13,15-octadecatetraenoic acid), was used as a sensitive membrane probe for peroxidation.[3,4] Peroxidation of the conjugated double bond system of PnA is accompanied by a loss in its fluorescent properties, which can be detected in a direct, continuous, and sensitive way. Analysis of the PnA fluorescence decrease curves in peroxidation experiments yields information on the peroxidation process of PnA.

Vitamin E incorporated in the erythrocyte membranes exhibited a clearly protective effect on the peroxidation on PnA, introducing a concentration-dependent lag phase. It can be assumed that cumene (per)oxyl radicals entering the membrane primarily react with vitamin E molecules, thus preventing peroxidation of PnA.

The effect of vitamin C (ascorbate) on peroxidation is known to depend on its concentration as well as on the oxidant system. In our experiments, vitamin C appeared to have a "double dualistic" effect on PnA peroxidation (FIG. 1). The overall effect of vitamin C on peroxidation, as determined 5 or 10 min after addition of oxidants, can be pro- or antioxidant, depending on the initial vitamin C concentration (FIG. 1B, open circles). In addition, the effect apparently changes from antioxidant (lag phase, FIG. 1A) to prooxidant within the time course of an experiment at low initial vitamin C concentrations. In the presence of both vitamins (FIG. 1, closed circles), the overall effect is always protective and exceeds the sum of the individual effects.

The reaction scheme in FIGURE 2 provides an explanation for the above observations. Ascorbate can either react with radicals to slow down the peroxidation process or reduce transition metal ions. The resulting ascorbyl radical has the same principle options. As cumene (per)oxyl radical production proceeds more rapidly with Fe^{2+} than Fe^{3+}, metal ion reduction by either ascorbate or ascorbyl radical will increase the rate of radical formation, leading to enhanced peroxidation. At low vitamin C concentrations, ascorbate initially causes a lag phase by scavenging radicals. This antioxidant action, however, is continuously counteracted by the reduction of metal ions, resulting in an overall prooxidant effect. The presence of vitamin E provides ascorbate and ascorbyl radicals with an alternative for their prooxidative action. The reduction of metal ions is apparently replaced by the regeneration of vitamin E from vitamin E radical, which represents an indirect protection by ascorbate and, possibly, ascorbyl radicals.

Our findings provide further indications that high plasma vitamin C concentrations could function to maintain the low levels of erythrocyte membrane vitamin E in an active state.

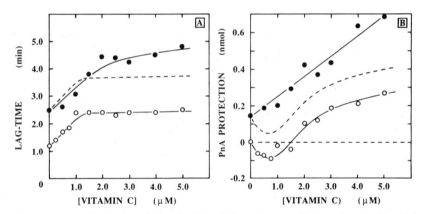

FIGURE 1. Combined effect of vitamins E and C on the peroxidation of parinaric acid in human erythrocyte white ghost membranes. Peroxidation was initiated by 500 μM cumene hydroperoxide plus 0.25 μM hemin-Fe^{3+}. General conditions: 200 μM ghost phospholipid in 2 mL buffer (10 mM Tris-HCl, 150 mM NaCl, pH 7.4), T = 25°C. Cis-parinaric acid (1.75 μM) was added by injection from a concentrated ethanolic solution. Excitation wavelength was 324 nm; emission wavelength was 413 nm. Vitamin E (*dl*-α-tocopherol) was incorporated in the membranes during a 40 min incubation at 37°C after addition from a concentrated ethanolic solution. Vitamin E concentrations are given as mole-percent relative to ghost phospholipid. Data are presented for 0 mole-percent ($\bigcirc$) and 1 mole-percent ($\bullet$) vitamin E. The dashed curves represent the theoretical effect of vitamin E plus C, calculated by adding up their individual effects. Points are means of 3 measurements. (A) Duration of the lag phase as a function of vitamin C concentration. (B) Parinaric acid protection, calculated from residual fluorescence intensities 10 min after addition of oxidants as a function of vitamin C concentration. The amount of parinaric acid protected from peroxidation after 10 min (in nmol) is defined as the amount peroxidized in the absence of added vitamins minus the amount peroxidized in the presence of added vitamins. Without addition of vitamins, 1.32 nmol of parinaric acid was peroxidized after 10 min from an initial amount of 3.0 nmol.

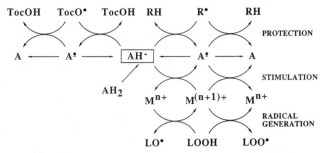

FIGURE 2. Simplified reaction scheme proposed to account for the observed effects of vitamins E and C on cumene hydroperoxide-induced parinaric acid peroxidation. The scheme can be seen to link *protection* against peroxidation (by radical scavenging) and *stimulation* of peroxidation (by metal ion reduction and subsequently enhanced *radical generation*). AH_2 : ascorbic acid; AH^- : ascorbate ; $A^{\bullet}$: ascorbyl radical ; A : dehydroascorbate ; $M^{(n+1)+}$: transition metal ion (hemin-Fe^{3+}) LOOH represents cumene hydroperoxide, but may also represent other hydroperoxide species. $R^{\bullet}$ represents a radical species (*e.g.* a cumene (per)oxyl radical). Tocopheroxyl radicals ($TocO^{\bullet}$) result from the quenching of a radical species by tocopherol ($TocOH$).

REFERENCES

1. TAPPEL, A. L. 1968. Geriatrics **23:** 97-105.
2. WEFERS, H. & H. SIES. 1988. Eur. J. Biochem. **174:** 353-357.
3. KUYPERS, F. A., J. J. M. VAN DEN BERG, C. SCHALKWIJK, B. ROELOFSEN & J. A. F. OP DEN KAMP. 1987. Biochim. Biophys. Acta **921:** 266-274.
4. VAN DEN BERG. J. J. M., F. A. KUYPERS, J. H. QJU, D. CHIU, B. LUBIN, B. ROELOFSEN & J. A. F. OP DEN KAMP. 1988. Biochim. Biophys. Acta **944:** 29-39.

Effects of α- and γ-Tocopherol (α-T, γ-T) and α-Tocotrienol (α-TT) on the Spontaneous and Induced Prostacyclin (PGI₂) Synthesis from Cultured Human Endothelial Cells (HEC) and Rat Aorta Segments *ex Vivo*

B. J. WEIMANN, H. STEFFEN, AND H. WEISER

Departments of Vitamin and Nutrition Research and
Biological Pharmaceutical Research
F. Hoffmann-La Roche Ltd.
CH-4002 Basle, Switzerland

INTRODUCTION

Treatment with vitamin E has been recommended for diseases of the cardiovasculature. Its role, however, in thrombosis and coronary diseases remains controversial.[1-6] Healthy vascular endothelium maintains a nonthrombogenic surface for circulating blood. This property may be partly related to the ability of these cells to produce inhibitors of aggregation and coagulation. PGI_2 is the most potent endogenous inhibitor of platelet aggregation. Its synthesis and release may be an important mechanism in reducing thrombosis and arteriosclerosis. Arteries of vitamin E-depleted animals produced lesser amounts of prostaglandins, although repletion restored their production.[7,8] We report on the spontaneous and thrombin-induced PGI_2 synthesis from cultured human endothelial cells treated with monolamellar liposomes carrying *all-rac*-α-T or the vehicle alone. In addition, PGI_2 was determined from aorta segments of rats used in resorption-gestation bioassays and given *RRR*-α-T, *R*-α-TT, and *all-rac*-γ-T.

METHODS

Cultures of HEC from umbilical cords and resorption-gestation assays were done as described.[9,10] Liposomes with and without *all-rac*-α-T were produced by ultrasonication using lecithin as carrier. Concentrations of PGI_2 were measured by an RIA for 6-keto-prostaglandin $F_{1\alpha}$.

RESULTS AND DISCUSSIONS

Confluent monolayers of cultured HEC maintained their typical cobblestone-like morphology, with tight and gap junctions and desmosomes. The spontaneous PGI_2 synthesis was low; thrombin, however, induced a burst-like PGI_2 formation within minutes. Cell layers treated with liposomes carrying α-T produced more PGI_2 upon stimulation with thrombin than those receiving the vehicle only. A concentration-

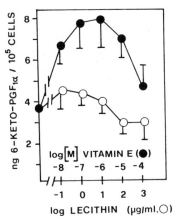

FIGURE 1. Effect of vitamin E at different concentrations on the PGI_2 synthesis from human endothelial cells induced by thrombin. Cell cultures (n = 3) were incubated for 16 hours with vitamin E-containing liposomes (●) at concentrations as indicated, whereas control cultures received liposomes only (○). In order to induce PGI_2, all cultures were then exposed to 5 U/ mL thrombin. Mean values are given ± SEM.

dependent induction was observed with an optimum around 10^{-6}M vitamin E, followed by a decrease towards higher vitamin E concentrations (FIG. 1). This decrease is most likely due to effects of high lecithin amounts on the cell membranes. Accordingly, growth of HEC was also retarded at high concentrations of the vehicle and of liposomes carrying α-T. Regarding the *ex vivo* experiments, aorta segments were obtained from rats used to test the activities of different compounds in resorption-gestation assays. The ranking order was *RRR*-α-T > *R*-α-TT > *all-rac*-γ-T. Spontaneous PGI_2 generation of aorta segments of *R*-α-TT-repleted rats was higher than that of *RRR*-α-T-repleted rats (FIG. 2). The induced synthesis will be the subject of a future study. Thrombin-induced PGI_2 formation of vitamin E-depleted as well as *all-rac*-γ-T-repleted rats was higher than the spontaneous PGI_2 release, but there were no significant differences among groups treated with different amounts of *all-rac*-γ-T, including the fully repleted group. Due to their antioxidant potential, α-T and α-TT may protect the cyclooxygenase system from the inherent destruction by oxygen radicals generated during the enzymic transformation of arachidonic acid to the prostaglandin peroxide PGH_2. In conclusion, the data suggest that some, but not all, of the vitamin E-active compounds influence the PGI_2 synthesis *in vitro* and *in vivo*.

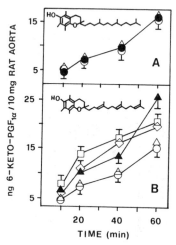

FIGURE 2. Prostacyclin synthesis from segments of rat aortas *ex vivo*. Rats were repleted with (A) 2.76 mg *RRR*-α-tocopherol (●, n = 5); and (B) 1.21 mg (◇, n = 5), 2.73 mg (□, n = 5), and 9.22 mg (▲, n = 6) *R*-α-tocotrienol per animal. Rats fed a commercial diet (△, n = 4), as well as vitamin E-depleted animals (○, n = 10), served as controls.

REFERENCES

1. HAEGER, K. 1982. Ann. N.Y. Acad. Sci. **393:** 369-375.
2. OLSON, R. E. 1973. Circulation **48:** 179-184.
3. ANDERSON, T. W. 1974. Can. Med. Assoc. J. **110:** 401-406.
4. ROBERTS, H. J. 1981. J. Am. Med. Assoc. **246:** 129-131.
5. BIERI, J. G., L. CORASH & V. S. HUBBARD. 1983. N. Engl. J. Med. **308:** 1063-1071.
6. GEY, K. F. 1986. *In* Scientific evidence for dietary targets in Europe. J. C. Somogyi, Ed.: 53-91. Karger. Basel.
7. OKUMA, M., H. TAKAYAMA & H. UCHINO. 1980. Prostaglandins **19:** 527-536.
8. CHAN, A. C. & M. K. LEITH. 1981. Am. J. Clin. Nutr. **34:** 2341-2347.
9. JAFFE, E. A., R. L. NACHMAN, C. G. BECKER & C. B. MINICK. 1973. J. Clin. Invest. **52:** 2745-2756.
10. WEISER, H. & M. VECCHI. 1981. Int. J. Vit. Nutr. Res. **51:** 100-113.

Competitive Uptake of Deuterium-Labeled α-Tocopherols in Male Rats

HAYDER A. ZAHALKA,[a] GRAHAM W. BURTON,
AND KEITH U. INGOLD

Division of Chemistry
National Research Council of Canada
Ottawa, Ontario, Canada K1A 0R6

INTRODUCTION

The major component of natural vitamin E, $2R,4'R,8'R$-α-tocopherol (*RRR*-α-T), has been shown to have a greater activity in various animal bioassays than synthetic $2RS,4'RS,8'RS$-α-tocopherol (*all-rac*-α-T; an equimolar mixture of all of the eight possible stereoisomers).[1] Vitamin E is absorbed mainly through the lymphatic pathway.[1,2] Analysis of lymph provides a direct measure of the amount of each stereoisomer that is absorbed from the gut.

We report here results of single, oral, competitive dose experiments using *RRR*-α-T and $2S,4'R,8'R$-α-tocopherol (*SRR*-α-T, an unnatural stereoisomer of vitamin E), labeled with specific numbers of deuterium atoms.[3,4] These experiments were designed to measure the relative net uptake of α-tocopherols into rat lymph from equimolar mixtures of (A) free tocopherols, (B) α-tocopheryl acetates, and (C) α-tocopherol and its acetate ester. Gas chromatography–mass spectrometry (GC-MS)[4] was employed to probe the appearance of the deuterated tocopherols in the rat lymph.

ABSORPTION OF α-TOCOPHEROLS FROM AN EQUIMOLAR MIXTURE OF (A) d_3-*SRR*-α-T AND d_6-*RRR*-α-T; (B) d_3-*SRR*-α-T-Ac AND d_6-*RRR*-α-T-Ac

FIGURES 1a and 1b present the absolute concentrations of deuterated α-tocopherols absorbed into rat lymph from mixtures A and B, respectively. The maximum absorption occurred 2.5–3.5 h (free tocopherols, FIG. 1a) and 4.5–6.0 h (acetate esters, FIG. 1b) after the administration of the single oral dose. It is clear from FIGURE 1a that the rate of absorption of the 2S and 2R epimers was similar during the first 3 h; however, after 3.5 h there was a slight discrimination in favor of natural vitamin E (*RRR*-α-T). After 8 h about 10% of the total single dose of deuterated tocopherols was recovered in the lymph.

---

[a] New address: Polysar Limited, P.O. Box 3001, Sarnia, Ontario, Canada N7T 7M2.

ABSORPTION OF DEUTERATED α-TOCOPHEROLS FROM AN EQUIMOLAR MIXTURE OF d_3-RRR-α-T-Ac AND d_6-RRR-α-T (MIXTURE C)

FIGURE 2a shows that RRR-α-T began to appear in lymph 1.0 h after feeding, and the maximum absorption occurred between 2.5-3.5 h for the free form, and 2.5-5.5 h for the acetate. From 1.0 to 3.0 h RRR-α-T was absorbed at similar rates from the two forms of vitamin E; however, after 3.5 h the amount of RRR-α-T derived from α-tocopheryl acetate exceeded that from the free tocopherol. After 8 h, about 6% of the total single dose of deuterated tocopherols was recovered in the lymph. FIGURE 2b shows that the d_6-RRR-α-T/d_3-RRR-α-T ratio was 1.35 after 1.5 h, and then decreased continuously to a value of 0.53 8 h after the administration of the tocopherols.

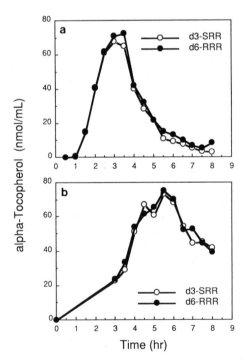

FIGURE 1. Appearance of d_3-SRR-α-T and d_6-RRR-α-T in the thoracic duct lymph of rat.[5] The rat was fed with an equimolar mixture of (**a**) d_3-SRR-α-T and d_6-RRR-α-T, and (**b**) d_3-SRR-α-T-Ac and d_6-RRR-α-T-Ac, dissolved in tocopherol-stripped corn oil. Total dose = 6 mg/kg rat body weight.

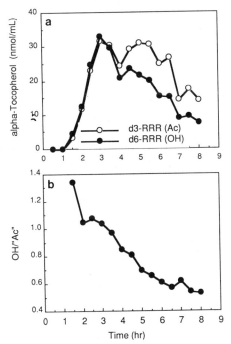

FIGURE 2. (a) Appearance of d_3-*RRR*-α-T and d_6-*RRR*-α-T in rat lymph after oral administration of an equimolar mixture of d_3-*RRR*-α-T-Ac and d_6-*RRR*-α-T, dissolved in tocopherol-stripped corn oil. (b) d_6-*RRR*-α-T/d_3-*RRR*-α-T (OH/Ac) ratio as a function of time (data derived from FIG. 2a). Total dose = 6 mg/kg rat body weight.

REFERENCES

1. MACHLIN, L. J., Ed. 1980. Vitamin E: A Comprehensive Treatise. Dekker. New York, NY.
2. BJORNEBOE, A., G. E. A. BJORNEBOE, E. BODD, B. F. HAGEN, N. KVESETH & C. A. DREVON. 1986. Biochim. Biophys. Acta **889:** 310-315.
3. INGOLD, K. U., L. HUGHES, M. SLABY & G. W. BURTON. 1987. J. Labelled Compd. Radiopharm. **24:** 817-831.
4. INGOLD, K. U., G. W. BURTON, D. O. FOSTER, L. HUGHES, D. A. LINDSAY & A. WEBB. 1987. Lipids **22:** 163-172.
5. BOLLMAN, J. L., J. C. CAIN & J. H. GRINDLAY. 1948. Am. J. Physiol. **220:** 333-336.

SUBJECT INDEX

INDEX OF CONTRIBUTORS